Pediatric Decision Making

Clinical Decision Making™ Series

Pediatric Decision Making

Third Edition

Stephen Berman, M.D., F.A.A.P.

Professor of Pediatrics
Director of Health Policy
University of Colorado Health Sciences Center
Attending Pediatrician for The Children's Hospital
Denver, Colorado

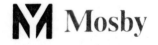 Mosby

St. Louis Baltimore Boston Carlsbad Chicago Naples New York Philadelphia Portland

London Madrid Mexico City Singapore Sydney Tokyo Toronto Wiesbaden

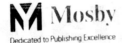

A Times Mirror
Company

Vice President and Publisher: Anne S. Patterson
Senior Managing Editor: Lynne Gery
Project Manager: Linda Clarke
Production Editor: Jennifer Harper
Production: Graphic World Publishing Services
Designer: Carolyn O'Brien
Manufacturing Manager: William A. Winneberger Jr.

THIRD EDITION
Copyright © 1996 by Mosby–Year Book, Inc.

Previous editions copyrighted 1984, 1991

Printed in the United States of America
Composition by Graphic World, Inc.
Printing/binding by Maple–Vail Book Manufacturing Group

Mosby–Year Book, Inc.
11830 Westline Industrial Drive
St. Louis, Missouri 63146

Library of Congress Cataloging in Publication Data

Berman, Stephen.
    Pediatric decision making / Stephen Berman. — 3rd ed.
        p.   cm.
    Includes bibliographical references and index.
    ISBN 0-8151-0715-3
    1. Pediatrics — Decision making.   I. Title.
    [DNLM: 1. Pediatrics. 2. Diagnosis. 3. Decision Making. WS 200
B5164p 1996]
    RJ47.B47   1996
    618.92 — dc20
    DNLM/DLC
    for Library of Congress   96-17609
                                                                     CIP

97 98 99 00 / 9 8 7 6 5 4 3 2

This book is dedicated to Elaine Gantz Berman, Shirley Berman Cole, and Sarita Gantz. Thank you for everything.

Preface

Pediatric Decision Making presents an algorithm approach to the diagnosis and management of common clinical problems. This third edition of *Pediatric Decision Making* has been expanded and extensively rewritten, and several new authors improve the book with their contributions. All the chapter authors have my deep appreciation for their dedication and effort. The format of most chapters has been modified to include a tabular form of the assessment of degree of illness. This critical section is the linchpin between diagnosis and management. It is hoped that this new form will make this text even more user friendly. Additional new chapters on problems encountered in developing countries reflect the growing realization that our world is smaller. I hope that residents and other clinicians who practice in developing areas of the world find these chapters relevant and helpful.

I would like to acknowledge a special debt of gratitude to my family; Elaine, for support and encouragement; Seth, for his competitive spirit and determination; and Ben, for his creativity and enthusiasm. A special thanks to Chris Paap for reviewing the therapy tables. Thanks to Vince Fulginiti and Doug Jones for providing me with the best job in the world; and to my wonderful colleagues in the Department, especially Roxann Headley, Don Schiff, Janet Weston, Gabriela Sebiane, Bob Roark, Mark Colloton, Bob Brayden, Allison Kempe, and Eric Simoes.

Stephen Berman, M.D.

Contributors

ROBERTA K. BEACH, M.D., M.P.H.

Associate Professor of Pediatrics, University of Colorado School of Medicine; Assistant Director of Community Health Services, Denver Department of Health and Hospitals, Denver, Colorado

STEPHEN BERMAN, M.D.

Professor of Pediatrics, University of Colorado School of Medicine; Attending Pediatrician, Child Health Clinic, The Children's Hospital; Director of Health Policy, University of Colorado Health Sciences Center, Denver, Colorado

ROBERT M. BRAYDEN, M.D.

Assistant Professor of Pediatrics, University of Colorado School of Medicine, Denver, Colorado

BONNIE W. CAMP, M.D., Ph.D.

Professor Emeritus of Pediatrics and Psychiatry, University of Colorado School of Medicine, Denver, Colorado

MICHAEL R. CLEMMENS, M.D.

Pediatrician, Annapolis Pediatrics, Annapolis, Maryland

JERROLD M. EICHNER, M.D.

Pediatric Pulmonary Fellow, University of Colorado School of Medicine, Denver, Colorado

PATRICIA H. ELLISON, M.D.

Professor of Pediatrics, University of Colorado School of Medicine, Denver, Colorado

RICHARD C. FISHER, M.D.

Associate Professor of Orthopedics, University of Colorado School of Medicine; Director of Orthopaedics, Denver General Hospital, Denver, Colorado

DOUGLAS M. FORD, M.D.

Associate Professor of Pediatrics, University of Colorado School of Medicine; Director, Home Dialysis Program, The Children's Hospital, Denver, Colorado

CARRIE A. GANONG, M.D.

Pediatric Endocrinology Fellow, The Children's Hospital, Denver, Colorado

CAROL L. GREENE, M.D.

Associate Professor of Pediatrics, University of Colorado School of Medicine; Director, Inherited Metabolic Diseases Clinic, The Children's Hospital, Denver, Colorado

ROBERT D. GROSS, M.D.

Clinical Associate Professor of Ophthalmology, University of Texas Southwestern Medical Center, Dallas, and Adjunct Associate Professor, University of North Texas Health Science Center, Fort Worth; Attending Surgeon in Ophthalmology, Cook Children's Medical Center, Fort Worth, Texas

ROXANN HEADLEY, M.D.

Assistant Professor of Pediatrics, University of Colorado School of Medicine; Medical Director, Child Health Clinic, Ambulatory Care Center and Adolescent Clinic, The Children's Hospital, Denver, Colorado

MICHAEL S. KAPPY, M.D., Ph.D.

Professor of Pediatrics, University of Colorado School of Medicine; Section Head, Endocrinology, The Children's Hospital, Denver, Colorado

PETER A. LANE, M.D.

Associate Professor of Pediatrics, University of Colorado School of Medicine; Director, Colorado Sickle Cell Treatment and Research Center, Denver, Colorado

JOEL N. LEFFLER, M.D.

Assistant Clinical Professor of Ophthalmology, University of Texas Southwestern Medical Center, Dallas, and Texas Tech University Health Science Center, Lubbock; Attending Physician, The Children's Hospital, Dallas, Texas

GARY M. LUM, M.D.

Professor of Pediatrics, University of Colorado School of Medicine; Section Head, Nephrology, and Director, Kidney Center, The Children's Hospital, Denver, Colorado

KATHLEEN A. MAMMEL, M.D.

Director, Adolescent Pediatrics, William Beaumont Hospital, Royal Oak, Michigan

JOSEPH MORELLI, M.D.

Associate Professor of Dermatology and Pediatrics, University of Colorado School of Medicine, Denver, Colorado

SUSAN NIERMEYER, M.D.

Associate Professor of Pediatrics, University of Colorado School of Medicine; Medical Director, Neonatal Education, The Children's Hospital, Denver, Colorado

RACHELLE NUSS, M.D.

Associate Professor of Pediatrics, University of Colorado School of Medicine, Denver, Colorado

PERLA SANTOS OCAMPO, M.D.

University Professor and Chancellor, University of the Philippines; Attending Pediatrician, Philippine General Hospital, St. Luke's Medical Center, Medical Center Manila, Capitol Medical Center, and Cardinal Santos Medical Center, Manila, Philippines

STEVEN R. POOLE, M.D.

Professor of Pediatrics, University of Colorado School of Medicine; Section Head, General Pediatrics and Pediatric Emergency Medicine, The Children's Hospital, Denver, Colorado

MICHAEL I. REIFF, M.D.

Assistant Professor of Pediatrics, University of Minnesota School of Medicine; Director, Learning and Behavior Problems Clinic, Children's Health Care Minneapolis, Minneapolis, Minnesota

BARTON D. SCHMITT, M.D.

Professor of Pediatrics, University of Colorado School of Medicine; Director of Consultative Services, The Children's Hospital, Denver, Colorado

JANET A. WESTON, M.D.

Associate Professor of Pediatrics, University of Colorado School of Medicine; Director of Growth and Parenting Clinic, Director of Resident Continuity Clinics, and Assistant Medical Director of Child Health Clinic, The Children's Hospital, Denver, Colorado

JAMES W. WIGGINS Jr., M.D.

Professor of Pediatrics, and Director, Pediatric Cardiology Fellowship Program, University of Colorado School of Medicine; Director, Cardiac Catheterization Laboratory, The Children's Hospital, Denver, Colorado

CONTENTS

Gastroenterologic Disorders

CLINICAL DECISION MAKING

CLINICAL DECISION MAKING

Stephen Berman, M.D.

Clinical decision making has three integrated phases: (1) diagnosis, (2) assessment of severity, and (3) management. Appropriate clinical decision making considers the need to make a precise diagnosis and the costs associated with indiscriminate use of diagnostic tests. It also assesses the risk of an adverse outcome because of inappropriate management and the costs and possible harmful effects of nonbeneficial therapeutic interventions. Clinical decision making is often difficult because of the overlap among many types of conditions. A single disorder can produce a wide spectrum of signs and symptoms, and many disorders can produce similar signs and symptoms.

A. All three phases of clinical decision making are based on a well-done history and physical examination. The pediatric history should include a review of the present illness. Identify the reasons for the visit and list the child's current problems. Evaluate the problems with respect to onset, duration, progression, precipitating or exacerbating factors, alleviating factors, and associations with other problems. Determine the functional impairment in relation to eating, play, sleep, other activities, and absence from school. Ask the patient or parents why they brought the child to see you. Does the patient have any allergies to drugs or foods? Is the patient taking any medications, up-to-date on immunizations? Has the patient ever been hospitalized or had any serious accidents? The medical history explores the general state of health. Review birth and developmental history. Elicit focused review of symptoms and a relevant family history and socioeconomic profile.

B. In the physical examination approach the child with gentleness, using a friendly manner and a quiet voice. First observe the child from a distance. If the child has a cold or cough, count respirations and assess the respiratory distress before removing the child's clothing. Note the general appearance. Is the child interactive and consolable? Note the level of activity and playfulness. Look at the skin and note any pallor, erythema, jaundice, cyanosis, and lesions. Check the lymph nodes for size, inflammation, and sensitivity. Examine the head, eyes, ears, nose, mouth, and throat. Use a pneumatic otoscope. Note abnormalities of the neck such as abnormal position, masses, and swelling of the thyroid glands. Examine the lungs for retractions and tachypnea, and listen for stridor, rhonchi, wheezing, and crepitations. When examining the heart, palpate for heaves or thrills and listen for murmurs, friction rubs, abnormal heart sounds, and uneven rhythm. During the abdominal examination note tympany, shifting dullness, tenderness, rebound tenderness, palpable organs or masses, fluid waves, and bowel sounds. Examine the male genitalia for hypospadias, phimosis, presence and size of the testes, and swellings or masses. Examine the female genitalia for vaginal discharge, adhesions, hypertrophy of the clitoris, and pubertal changes. Examine the rectum and anus, noting fissures, inflammation or irritation, prolapse, muscle tone, and imperforation of the anus. Examine the musculoskeletal system, noting limitations in full range of motion, point tenderness, any deformities or asymmetry, and gait disturbances. Examine the joints, hands, and feet. Assess the spine and back, noting posture, curvatures, rigidity, webbing of the neck, dimples, and cysts. The neurologic examination assesses cerebral function, cranial nerves, cerebellar function, the motor system, and the reflexes.

C. Initial nonspecific screening tests often include the CBC with differential and urinalysis. Subsequent laboratory tests and ancillary studies are based on the findings, history, and physical examination. These tests and studies should establish the pattern of involvement and extent of dysfunction. Information on the pattern of signs, symptoms, and findings from the ancillary tests is useful in identifying the cause of the disorder.

(Continued on page 4)

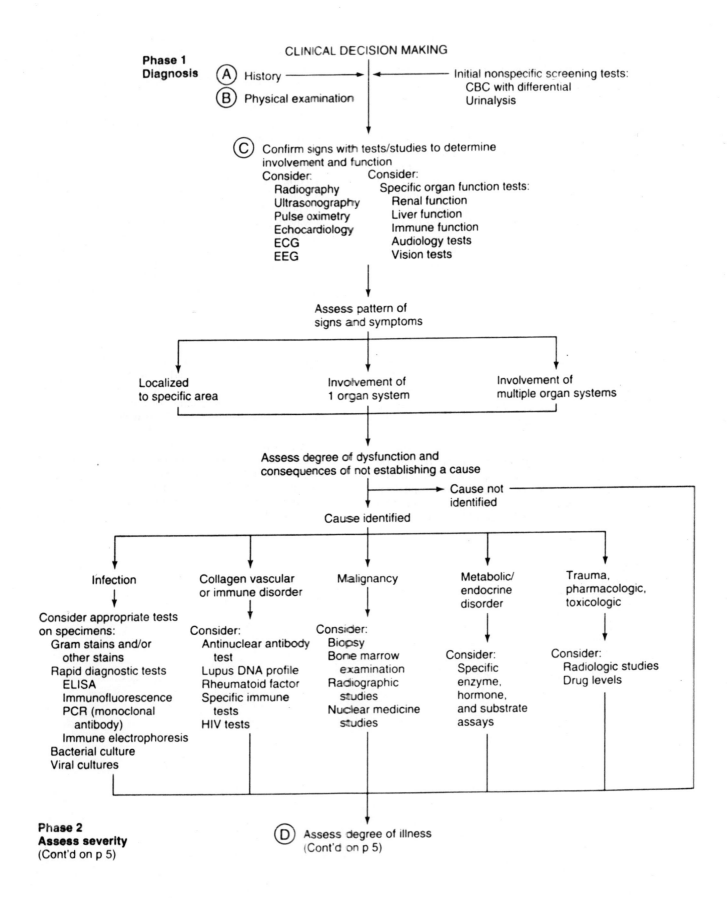

CLINICAL DECISION MAKING

**Phase 1
Diagnosis**

(A) History —————→ ←————— Initial nonspecific screening tests:
                                    CBC with differential
(B) Physical examination   Urinalysis

(C) Confirm signs with tests/studies to determine
    involvement and function
    Consider: Consider:
        Radiography   Specific organ function tests:
        Ultrasonography   Renal function
        Pulse oximetry   Liver function
        Echocardiology   Immune function
        ECG   Audiology tests
        EEG   Vision tests

Assess pattern of
signs and symptoms

| Localized to specific area | Involvement of 1 organ system | Involvement of multiple organ systems |

Assess degree of dysfunction and
consequences of not establishing a cause

→ Cause not identified

Cause identified

Infection

Consider appropriate tests
on specimens:
    Gram stains and/or
        other stains
    Rapid diagnostic tests
    ELISA
    Immunofluorescence
    PCR (monoclonal
        antibody)
    Immune electrophoresis
    Bacterial culture
    Viral cultures

**Collagen vascular
or immune disorder**

Consider:
    Antinuclear antibody
        test
    Lupus DNA profile
    Rheumatoid factor
    Specific immune
        tests
    HIV tests

Malignancy

Consider:
    Biopsy
    Bone marrow
        examination
    Radiographic
        studies
    Nuclear medicine
        studies

**Metabolic/
endocrine
disorder**

Consider:
    Specific
    enzyme,
    hormone,
    and substrate
    assays

**Trauma,
pharmacologic,
toxicologic**

Consider:
    Radiologic studies
    Drug levels

**Phase 2
Assess severity**
(Cont'd on p 5)

(D) Assess degree of illness
(Cont'd on p 5)

D. The clinical information obtained from the history, physical examination, and laboratory and ancillary tests is used to assess the degree of illness, which classifies patients into four categories. Very severely ill patients require immediate intervention and stabilization to prevent irreversible damage and death or severe morbidity. Severely ill patients require hospital admission (1) to receive therapy not usually available on an outpatient basis or (2) to have close observation and monitoring due to a high risk of a complication or rapid progression of the disease. The ability of parents and others to care for a child at home and the availability of a telephone and transportation, geographic isolation, and weather may also affect the decision for hospitalization. Moderately ill patients require specific treatment in an ambulatory setting. Mildly ill patients have a self-limited condition that will resolve spontaneously. This approach may require some modification to accommodate the substitution of home health care services for hospitalization. More often, however, home health care services allow patients to leave the hospital earlier than otherwise.

E. The assessment of severity (degree of illness) links diagnostic decision making with management. The management phase of clinical decision making addresses four questions: (1) Does the patient require immediate therapeutic intervention? (2) What specific therapy is indicated? (3) Where should the patient be managed: a hospital intensive care unit (ICU), a hospital ward, or at home? (4) How should the patient be monitored and what is the appropriate follow-up? The four management decisions—stabilization, hospitalization, specific treatment, and follow-up—are identified and boxed in each algorithm. In addition, the assessment of degree of illness may be presented in table form. A very severely ill patient should be hospitalized in an ICU. Stabilization should include respiratory, circulatory, and neurologic support. The goal of stabilization is to maintain tissue oxygenation, especially to the brain and other vital organs. Tissue oxygenation depends on the delivery of oxygen to the tissue. It requires a functioning respiratory system, including the airway and lungs, adequate circulatory blood volume, a functioning pump (heart), and adequate oxygen-carrying capacity (hemoglobin). It is therefore essential to maintain the ABCs (airway, breathing, and cardiac functions). In stabilizing a patient, establish an open airway, deliver oxygen, and assess air exchange (breathing). When exchange is inadequate, consider intubation and ventilation. Circulatory support is needed when hypotension or signs of poor perfusion are present. These signs include pale or mottled skin, coolness of the extremities, and capillary refill prolonged beyond 2 seconds. The initial phase of circulatory support is IV fluids. Additional pharmacologic treatment may be necessary. Some children with seizures or signs of neurologic dysfunction need neurologic support. This may include the administration of rapid-acting anticonvulsants and/or the rapid correction of any metabolic disturbance, such as hypoglycemia or electrolyte abnormalities. Severe anemia or hemorrhage requires the replacement of hemoglobin as well as volume with whole blood or packed blood cell transfusions. Always include a plan to monitor and assess the response to therapy. In many circumstances the follow-up is the most important part of the management plan. Proper education of the patient and family is the essential element in the follow-up plan. It must receive the attention that it deserves.

CLINICAL DECISION MAKING

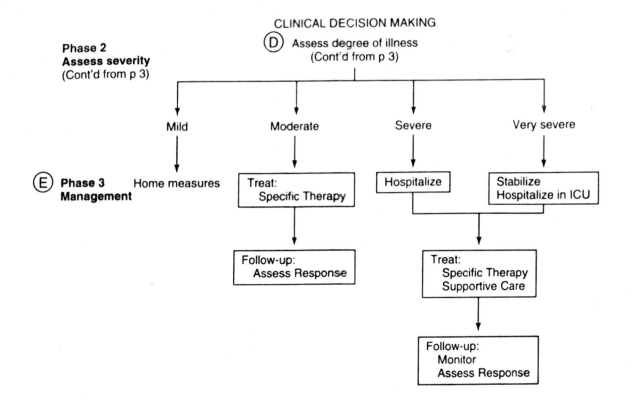

Phase 2
Assess severity
(Cont'd from p 3)

(D) Assess degree of illness
(Cont'd from p 3)

Mild | Moderate | Severe | Very severe

(E) **Phase 3**
Management
Home measures

Treat:
Specific Therapy

Hospitalize

Stabilize
Hospitalize in ICU

Follow-up:
Assess Response

Treat:
Specific Therapy
Supportive Care

Follow-up:
Monitor
Assess Response

BEHAVIORAL AND DEVELOPMENTAL DISORDERS

Evaluation of Psychogenic Symptoms
Attention Deficit Hyperactivity Disorder
Behavior Problems in School-Age Children
Child Abuse: Physical Abuse
Child Abuse: Sexual Abuse
Depression
Developmental Delay in Children Under 6
  Years of Age
Eating Disorders

Encopresis (Soiling)
Enuresis (Bedwetting)
Language Disorders
School Attendance Problems
School Learning Problems
Sleep Disturbances
Substance Abuse

EVALUATION OF PSYCHOGENIC SYMPTOMS

Stephen Berman, M.D.

A. Common psychogenic symptoms include recurrent or chronic abdominal pain, limb pain, vomiting, headache, chest pain, dizziness, syncope, hyperventilation, night terrors, enuresis, fighting, and phobias. Identify any evidence of psychosis as suggested by an altered sense of reality, delusions, or hallucinations. Serious psychiatric problems include autistic behavior, antisocial behavior, anorexia nervosa, severe depression, suicidal ideation, sexual identity disturbances, and substance abuse. Assess the patient's degree of self-esteem, self-confidence, anxiety level, and sense of security. Question the patient and family to learn how they deal with stressful situations, and identify the source of stress, including possible sexual abuse, recent serious illness, death of family members or friends, recent divorce or separation, change of residence, new school or teachers, or recent financial reverses, including unemployment. Assess family life for sustained mistreatment or unusual lifestyle. Obtain a family history of psychogenic illnesses such as headache, irritable bowel syndrome, peptic ulcer disease, and chronic abdominal pain and of psychiatric illnesses such as schizophrenia, depressive disorders, sociopathy, and substance abuse.

B. Perform a mental status examination and note orientation, memory, affect, and quality of thinking. Perform a careful, complete physical examination to identify any signs of underlying nonfunctional disease.

C. Mildly affected patients experience minimal disruption of normal activities. Moderately affected patients have symptoms that compromise their lifestyle, for example by resulting in school absences or failure or limitation of activity. Severely affected patients have evidence of psychopathology.

D. Consider school phobia as a common cause of pain in grade-school children, especially if the youngster has missed 5 or more days because of vague symptoms. Contact the child's teachers and school nurse. Identify any precipitating events in school, provide the child and family with reassurance regarding the child's physical health and have the child return to school immediately. Ask that the family contact you whenever the child misses any school days. High-school students who have school phobia are often either reacting to a significant life stress or have underlying psychopathology. When counseling and reassurance are not sufficient, refer these patients for family or individual therapy.

E. Counsel the child and family by explaining the mechanism of stress-related functional pain. Provide reassurance that the pain, although real, is not due to physical illness. When appropriate, suggest relaxation techniques such as deep, slow breathing, imagery, and self-induced hypnosis. When counseling fails to improve symptoms after two to four visits, refer to a psychiatrist or psychologist for individual and/or family therapy.

References

Schmitt BD. School phobia. The great imitator: A pediatric viewpoint. Pediatrics 1971; 48:433.

Schmitt BD. Time-out: Intervention of choice for the irrational years. Contemp Pediatr 1993; December:64.

PSYCHOGENIC ILLNESS Suspected

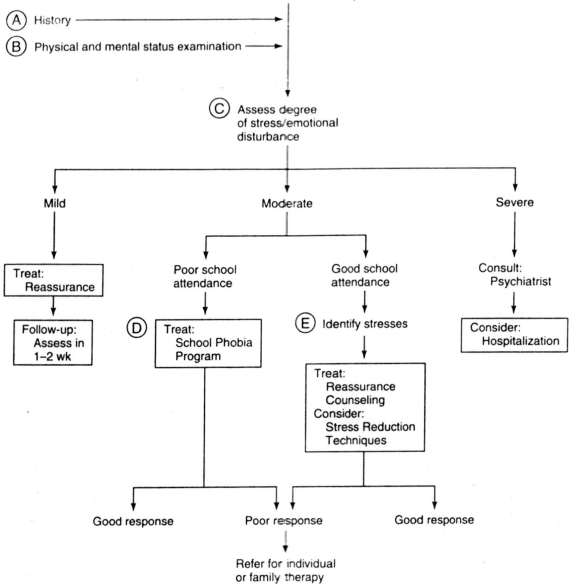

Ⓐ History

Ⓑ Physical and mental status examination

Ⓒ Assess degree of stress/emotional disturbance

Mild

Moderate

Severe

Treat:
Reassurance

Follow-up:
Assess in
1–2 wk

Poor school
attendance

Good school
attendance

Consult:
Psychiatrist

Ⓓ Treat:
School Phobia
Program

Ⓔ Identify stresses

Consider:
Hospitalization

Treat:
  Reassurance
  Counseling
Consider:
  Stress Reduction
  Techniques

Good response

Poor response

Good response

Refer for individual
or family therapy

ATTENTION DEFICIT HYPERACTIVITY DISORDER

Bonnie W. Camp, M.D., Ph.D.

Attention deficit hyperactivity disorder (ADHD) is the most common behavior problem that interferes with the child's functioning at school. Evidence of short attention span, hyperactivity, and other behavior problems are often present from an early age, but the problems usually do not become evident until the child is faced with the cognitive challenge of school. In addition, symptoms of ADHD may accompany and complicate developmental delay, learning disorders, family stress, conduct disorder, depression, and/or bipolar illness.

A. In the history determine signs of early childhood developmental delay, problems with growth or nutrition, sleeping disorders, difficulty toilet training, chronic illness, frequent hospitalizations, abuse, neglect, and family stress. Review any evaluations or therapies and obtain a comprehensive description of the child's current and past behavior and learning difficulties.

B. In the physical examination note physical, dysmorphic, or other characteristics of neurologic or genetic disorders (e.g., cerebral palsy), coordination problems, and neurologic soft signs. These soft signs probably reflect immaturity in neurologic development but are not diagnostic of a neurologic disorder. Along with clumsiness and awkwardness, they are common among children with ADHD.

C. Obtain the following directly from the school: information about intelligence and achievement status; a teacher's description of the child's behavior in the classroom; attendance information; a completed standard teacher rating scale for hyperactivity such as the ACTeRS scale; and a report of any sensory testing, individual educational plan placement (e.g., grade, special education), and of peer relations. A teacher's report of behavior in the classroom is essential; other testing can be performed independently.

D. Assess school behavior. Determine whether the core symptoms of ADHD are present (Table 1). Snap-IV is a convenient way of finding these symptoms. Teacher ratings on the attention and hyperactivity scale of the ACTeRS should be below the tenth percentile; ratings between the tenth and twentieth percentiles are considered borderline. The major differential diagnoses are depression, bipolar disorder, conduct disorder, and emotional reaction to learning disability. Symptoms of depression, including explosive outbursts and angry and frustrated interactions or a conduct disorder with fighting, stealing, lying, and malicious behavior, can be assessed through an interview and other standard instruments such as the Children's Depression Inventory, as well as school behavior checklists. Symptoms of ADHD can be present alone or in combination with other behavior and learning problems. Occasionally a child referred for behavior problems does not have behavior problems at school. This frequently appears as a discrepancy between reports from the school and complaints brought forth by the family. Unlike aggressive behavior at school, which usually reflects some disturbance at home, ADHD behavior at school is usually not a carryover of home problems. A good rule of thumb is that if symptoms of ADHD do not occur at school, the problem is not ADHD. New criteria for ADHD include symptoms in at least two settings (e.g., home and school).

E. Evaluate educational needs and services. Approximately 70% of children with ADHD have some problem processing information. Children who are functioning at least 20% below average in one or all academic areas need individual educational programming (IEP). Screening for discrepancies between IQ and achievement can often help determine educational needs. Screening tools to assess the degree of discrepancy include the Wide Range Achievement Test (WRAT) and the Kaufman Brief Intelligence Test (K-BIT). A detailed analysis of individual educational needs often requires the input of an educational specialist; however, simple analysis of the need for special education and the extent of its provision can often reveal areas in which the educational program is poorly adapted to the child's needs. If the educational program is inadequate, it is often impossible to assess the extent to which any behavior problems are an appropriate response to the educational environment. If the IEP appears to be questionable or inadequate, the final assessment of behavior problems should be delayed until adequate education evaluation is completed and the child is enrolled in an appropriate program.

(Continued on page 14)

ATTENTION DEFICIT HYPERACTIVITY DISORDER Suspected

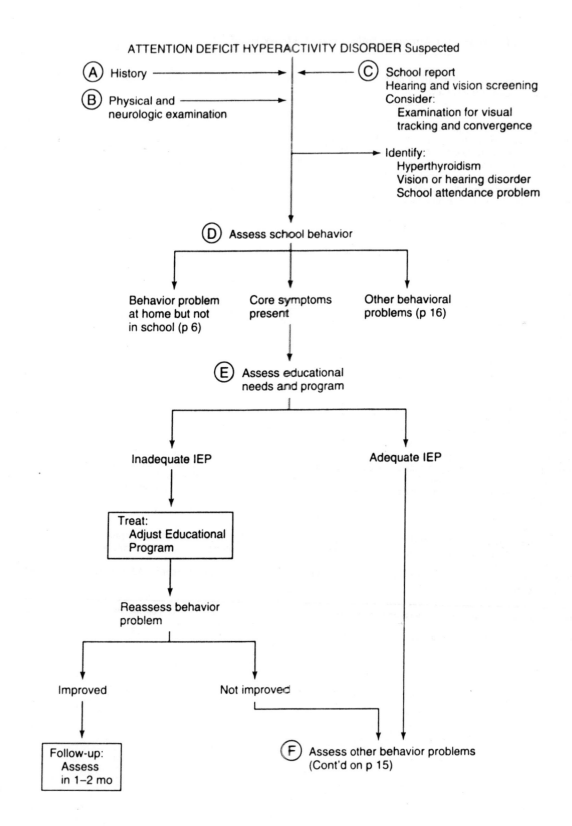

(A) History

(B) Physical and neurologic examination

(C) School report
Hearing and vision screening
Consider:
    Examination for visual
    tracking and convergence

Identify:
    Hyperthyroidism
    Vision or hearing disorder
    School attendance problem

(D) Assess school behavior

Behavior problem
at home but not
in school (p 6)

Core symptoms
present

Other behavioral
problems (p 16)

(E) Assess educational
needs and program

Inadequate IEP

Adequate IEP

Treat:
    Adjust Educational
    Program

Reassess behavior
problem

Improved

Not improved

Follow-up:
Assess
in 1–2 mo

(F) Assess other behavior problems
(Cont'd on p 15)

TABLE 1 Diagnostic Criteria for Attention Deficit Hyperactivity Disorder

A. Either 1 or 2:
   1. Six or more of the following symptoms of inattention have persisted for at least 6 months to a degree that is maladaptive and inconsistent with developmental level:

   Inattention
   a. Often fails to give close attention to details or makes careless mistakes in schoolwork, work, or other activities
   b. Often has difficulty sustaining attention in tasks or play activities
   c. Often does not seem to listen when spoken to directly
   d. Often does not follow through on instructions and fails to finish schoolwork, chores, or duties in the workplace not due to oppositional behavior or failure to understand instructions
   e. Often has difficulty organizing tasks and activities
   f. Often avoids, dislikes, or is reluctant to engage in tasks that require sustained mental effort, such as schoolwork or homework
   g. Often loses things necessary for tasks or activities (e.g., toys, school assignments, pencils, books, or tools)
   h. Is often easily distracted by extraneous stimuli
   i. Is often forgetful in daily activities

   2. Six or more of the following symptoms of hyperactivity-impulsivity have persisted for at least 6 months to a degree that is maladaptive and inconsistent with developmental level:

   Hyperactivity
   a. Often fidgets with hands or feet or squirms in seat
   b. Often leaves seat in classroom or in other situations in which remaining seated is expected
   c. Often runs about or climbs excessively in situations in which it is inappropriate (in adolescents or adults, may be limited to subjective feelings of restlessness)
   d. Often has difficulty playing or engaging in leisure activities quietly
   e. Is often on the go or often acts as if driven by a motor
   f. Often talks excessively

   Impulsivity
   g. Often blurts out answers before questions have been completed
   h. Often has difficulty awaiting turn
   i. Often interrupts or intrudes on others (e.g., butts into conversations or games)
B. Some hyperactive-impulsive or inattentive symptoms that cause impairment were present before age 7 years.
C. Some impairment from the symptoms is present in two or more settings (e.g., at school or work and at home).
D. There must be clear evidence of clinically significant impairment in social, academic, or occupational functioning.
E. The symptoms do not occur exclusively during the course of a pervasive developmental disorder, schizophrenia, or other psychotic disorder and are not better accounted for by another mental disorder (e.g., mood disorder, anxiety disorder, dissociative disorder, or a personality disorder).

Code based on type
314.01 Attention deficit hyperactivity disorder, combined type: if both criteria A1 and A2 are met for the past 6 months
314.00 Attention deficit hyperactivity disorder, predominantly inattentive type: if criterion A1 is met but criterion A2 is not met for the past 6 months
314.01 Attention deficit hyperactivity disorder, predominantly hyperactive-impulsive type: if criterion A2 is met but criterion A1 is not met for the past 6 months

Coding note: For individuals (especially adolescents and adults) who currently have symptoms that no longer meet full criteria, "in partial remission" should be specified.
Reproduced with permission of the American Psychiatric Association.

TABLE 2 Common Medications for Attention Deficit Hyperactivity Disorders

Medication	Indications	Contraindications	Dosage	Side Effects	Monitor
Methylphenidate (Ritalin)	ADHD	Tics, seizures	0.3 mg/kg/dose; maximum daily dose, 60 mg	Loss of appetite, insomnia, headaches, tics, rebound, other	School and home behavior, blood pressure
Dextroamphetamine (Dexedrine)	ADHD	Hypertension, hyperthyroidism	Age 6 and older, 5 mg qd or b.i.d.; increments of 2.5 mg; maximum daily dose, 40 mg/day	Loss of appetite, insomnia, headaches, tics, rebound, hypertension, other	School and home behavior, blood pressure
Pemoline (Cylert)	ADHD with attentional problems predominant	Abnormal liver studies	Age 6 and older, start with 37.5 mg qd; increments of 18.5 mg at qwk; maximum daily dose, 112.5 mg/day	Loss of appetite, insomnia, headaches, tics, rebound, hepatic dysfunction, other	School and home behavior, liver functions
Imipramine and Desipramine	ADHD with intolerance or ineffectiveness of stimulants	Concomitant use of monoamine oxidase inhibitor	1–2.5 mg/kg/day; maximum daily dose, 5 mg/kg/day	Nervousness, sleep disorders, tiredness, GI disturbance; other reactions observed in adults	School and home behavior, liver functions, ECG
Clonidine	ADHD with aggressive volatile behavior	ECG abnormality	3–4 μg/kg/day; start with 0.05 mg hs and increase by 0.05 mg every 3rd day to t.i.d.; maximum daily dose, 8 μg/kg or 0.5 mg/day	Sedation, dry mouth, constipation	ECG, school and home behavior

F. It is often difficult to distinguish between fighting and aggressive behavior resulting from the child's inability to keep his hands to himself, common among children with ADHD, and that arising from the complex symptoms of an oppositional or conduct disorder. Likewise, depression reflecting low self-esteem and a negative outlook based on failure to perform up to expectations because of ADHD may be confused with components of an endogenous bipolar disorder or reactive depression to significant loss. Once the core symptoms of ADHD have been established, estimate the degree of dominance of the ADHD symptoms. If ADHD appears to be dominant and other problems secondary, treat the ADHD and assess the effect on the other symptoms. If the other symptoms appear to be primary or out of control, refer the patient immediately to a psychologist or child psychiatrist.

G. Often children with ADHD need individual or family therapy as well as medication and educational programming. Medication, if successful, relieves some of the pressure; however, psychological treatment may be delayed or avoided to the detriment of the child. Referral of these patients for psychological services before introducing medication helps ensure that the emotional problems are not overlooked and promotes development of an appropriate multimodal treatment plan.

H. Stimulant medications (Table 2) have a long and well-established record of effectiveness in treating symptoms of ADHD. Methylphenidate (Ritalin) and dextroamphetamine (Dexedrine) are the most commonly used. Pemoline (Cylert) is also approved for use in ADHD but requires monitoring liver functions and gradually increasing the dose over 2 to 4 weeks. Another medicine approved for use in ADHD is thioridazine (Mellaril). Clonidine and imipramine are also used frequently.

I. Behavior modification contracts can often be developed in cooperation with the school, special services personnel, or a psychologist. Parent groups and reading materials can also be helpful.

J. Special educational needs must be met before a clear picture of the significance of ADHD can be elucidated. Some schools offer training in social skills and impulse control in the regular classroom or from a psychologist or social worker. Behavioral changes in children who are responding well to medication can often be traced to changes in the school or a breakdown of an otherwise well-functioning educational plan.

K. Family therapy and/or individual psychotherapy is often indicated as part of the treatment program when many unresolved emotional issues contribute to or exaggerate a primary attention deficit disorder. Children who have been abused or neglected have special needs for this form of therapy.

L. Often the efforts to improve the child's environment fail, and the situations causing problems are not well understood. A change of living circumstances or teacher can affect the child and alter the need for medication.

M. EEG biofeedback therapy is still a controversial approach to treatment of children with ADHD, but clinical reports indicate success in treating older children and adolescents, many of whom may not respond to other forms of treatment. Much is yet to be learned about this.

References

American Psychiatric Association. Diagnostic and statistical manual of mental disorders. 4th ed. Washington DC: American Psychiatric Association, 1994.

Bash MAS, Camp BW. Think aloud: Increasing social and cognitive skills—a problem solving program for children. Think aloud: Classroom programs, grades 1–2, grades 3–4, grades 5–6. Champaign, IL: Research Press, 1985.

Camp BW, Bash MAS. Think aloud: Increasing social and cognitive skills—a problem solving program for children. Think aloud: Primary level. Champaign, IL: Research Press, 1981.

Culbert TP, Banez GA, Reiff MI. Children who have attentional disorders: Interventions. Pediatr Rev 1994; 15:5.

Gittleman-Klein R. Prognosis of attention deficit disorder and its management in adolescence. Pediatr Rev 1987; 8:216.

Ingersol B. Your hyperactive child: A parent's guide to coping with attention deficit disorder. New York: Doubleday, 1988.

Kaufman AS, Kaufman NL. K-BIT: Kaufman Brief Intelligence Test. Circle Pines, MN: American Guidance Service, 1990.

Levine MD, Carey WB, Crocker AC, eds. Developmental-behavioral pediatrics. 2nd ed. Philadelphia: Saunders, 1992.

Reiff MI, Banez GA, Culbert TP. Children who have attentional disorders: Diagnosis and evaluation. Pediatr Rev 1993; 14:455.

Swanson JM. The SNAP-IVp rating scale. Department of Pediatrics, Division of Child Development, University of California, Irvine, Newport Beach, CA 92660.

Ullman RK, Sleator EK, Sprague RL. ADD-H: Comprehensive teacher's rating scale (ACTeRS). Champaign, IL: Metritech, 1988.

Wender PH. The hyperactive child, adolescent, and adult through the lifespan. New York: Oxford University Press, 1987.

Wilkinson GS. WRAT-3: Wide Range Achievement Test-3. Wilmington, DE: Jastak, 1993.

ATTENTION DEFICIT HYPERACTIVITY DISORDER Suspected
(F) Assess other behavior problems
(Cont'd from p 11)

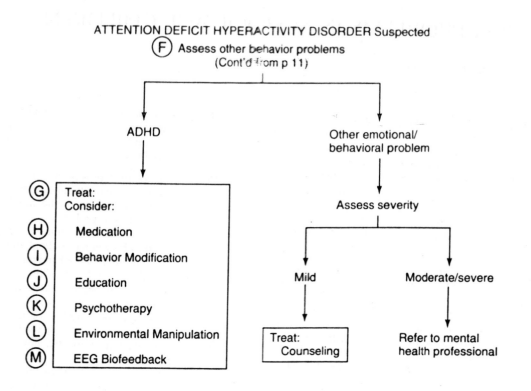

ADHD

(G) Treat:
Consider:

(H) Medication

(I) Behavior Modification

(J) Education

(K) Psychotherapy

(L) Environmental Manipulation

(M) EEG Biofeedback

Other emotional/
behavioral problem

Assess severity

Mild

Treat:
Counseling

Moderate/severe

Refer to mental
health professional

BEHAVIOR PROBLEMS IN SCHOOL-AGE CHILDREN

Bonnie W. Camp, M.D., Ph.D.

A. In the history determine signs of early childhood development delay, problems with growth or nutrition, sleeping disorders, difficulty with toilet training, chronic illness, frequent hospitalizations, abuse, neglect, and family stress. Review any evaluations or therapies and obtain a comprehensive description of any current or past behavior and learning problems. Many pediatricians use a 35-item checklist developed by Murphy and Jelenek to screen for psychosocial problems and psychiatric disorders.

B. In the physical examination note physical, dysmorphic, or other characteristics of neurologic or genetic disorders (e.g., cerebral palsy), coordination problems, and neurologic soft signs. These soft signs probably reflect immaturity in neurologic development but are not diagnostic of a neurologic disorder. Along with clumsiness and awkwardness, they are common among children with attention deficit hyperactivity disorder (ADHD).

C. Obtain directly from the school information about intelligence, achievement status, teacher's description of the child's behavior in the classroom, completion of a standard teacher rating scale for hyperactivity such as the ACTeRS scale; history of any sensory testing, attendance, individual educational plan and placement (grade, special education), and peer relations. A teacher's report of behavior in the classroom is essential; other testing can be performed independently.

D. The symptoms that describe ADHD commonly interfere with the child's functioning at school. Determine whether the core symptoms of ADHD are present (see p 10). The major differential diagnoses are depression, bipolar disorder, conduct disorder, and emotional reaction to learning disability. Symptoms of depression, including explosive outbursts, angry and frustrated interactions, and conduct disorder with fighting, stealing, lying, and malicious behavior, can be assessed through interviews and other standard instruments such as the Children's Depression Inventory and school behavior checklists. Symptoms of ADHD may be present alone or may accompany other behavior and learning problems.

E. Occasionally a child referred for behavior problems behaves well at school. This frequently appears as a discrepancy between reports from the school and complaints brought forth by the family. Unlike aggressive behavior at school, which usually reflects some disturbance at home, ADHD behavior at school is usually not a carryover of home problems. However, disruption at home is often manifested by aggressive behavior at school. Nevertheless, many children who live in the midst of conflict appear well-behaved in school or public.

F. When behavior problems occur only at home, evaluation should center on the family and the child's interaction with other members of the family. In some instances the behavior problems can be identified as transitional, i.e., occurring at transition phases in development, such as between preschool and regular school or between elementary school and middle school. Sleep problems, jealousy, and irritability often fall into this category. Typically reassurance regarding the transient nature of the problem is all that is required. Mildly dysfunctional families stimulate or maintain behavior problems. It is often useful to help the family understand that problems such as stomach aches occurring only on school days (usually Monday morning) or that a child's insistence that he is bad at school when indeed he is not may be a plea for attention. Signs of more severely dysfunctional families include physical, emotional, or sexual abuse, overprotectiveness, neglect, poor parenting practices, and overreliance on violence, coercion, or criticism in discipline. The assistance of a psychologist, psychiatrist, or social worker is needed in these circumstances.

G. If symptoms of ADHD are present, proceed by first evaluating ADHD. When core symptoms of ADHD are not present, determine the type of problem that is present. Common problems are encopresis, daytime wetting, conduct disorders, explosive outbursts, depression, and anxiety disorders. Habit disorders, such as encopresis and daytime wetting, that are not deeply entwined with family pathology often respond to the pediatrician's bowel or bladder regimen along with counseling. Refer the child to a mental health professional or team if the problem does not improve with appropriate counseling or the complexity of the problem necessitates additional help.

References

Clark RB. Psychosocial aspects of pediatric and psychiatric disorders. In: Hay WW Jr, Groothius JR, Hayward AR, Levin MJ, eds. Current pediatric diagnosis and treatment. 12th ed. Norwalk, CT: Appleton & Lange, 1995:154.

Levine MD, Carey WB, Crocker AC, Gross RT, eds. Developmental-behavioral pediatrics. Philadelphia: Saunders, 1983.

School-Age Child with BEHAVIOR PROBLEMS

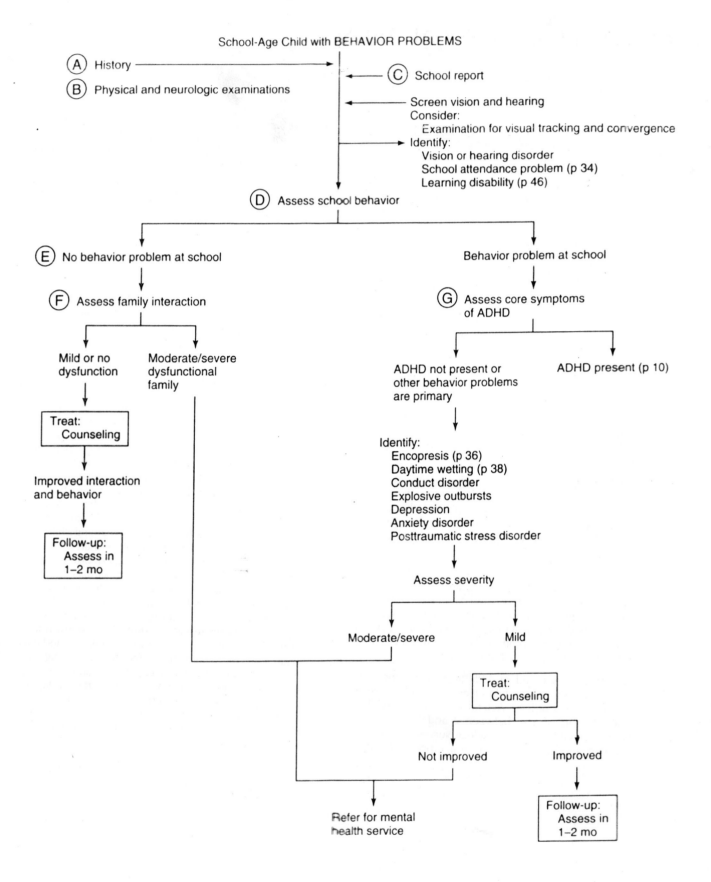

CHILD ABUSE: PHYSICAL ABUSE

Robert M. Brayden, M.D.

A. In the history ask how the injury happened, including sequence of events, people present, and delay before seeking medical attention. Record the parent's explanation of each positive physical finding. If the child is over age 2½ to 3 years, elicit the child's history in a private setting and compare it with the parent's version. Use adult translators who are not relatives or friends if there is a language barrier. Obtain a detailed 48-hour history of the feeding, sleeping, and behavior pattern. Check for growth failure, death of siblings, and the risk of abuse to siblings or the spouse.

B. In the physical examination document all bruises by site, size, shape, and color; note their resemblance to identifiable objects. Pay special attention to the scalp, retina, eardrums, pinnae, oral cavity, and genitals for signs of occult trauma. In severe cases color photographs are helpful records. Palpate all bones for tenderness and test joints for full range of motion. Unexplained change in level of consciousness or focal neurologic signs should prompt consideration of abusive head injury, even in infants without external signs of trauma (shaking-impact syndrome). Assess the child's medical and surgical problems appropriately, regardless of cause. Hospitalize children with severe injuries.

C. Systemic/organic diseases can mimic physical abuse. Consider diagnoses mimicking bone (osteogenesis imperfecta, congenital syphilis, metaphyseal chondrodysplasia), skin (bleeding diatheses, mongolian pigmentation, bullous impetigo, purpura), and intracranial (meningitis, sepsis) injuries.

D. Order a bleeding disorder screen in children with bruises if you suspect a bleeding disorder, if the case is expected to go to court, or if the parents deny inflicting the injuries and claim easy bruising. A bleeding disorder screen includes a platelet count, bleeding time, partial thromboplastin time, prothrombin time, thrombin time, and fibrinogen level (the last two are optional).

E. Bone trauma is found in 11% to 55% of physically abused children; young children are most vulnerable. In suspicious cases order a skeletal survey on every child under 2 years of age; between 2 and 5 years most children should receive a skeletal survey unless they have very mild injuries or are in a supervised setting (e.g., preschool); over age 5 years, obtain radiographs only if there is bone tenderness or limited range of motion. Ask the radiologist to date positive radiographic findings. Metaphyseal chip fractures or multiple body injuries at different stages of healing are highly suspicious. Always consider the possibility of head injury when children have suspicious fractures.

F. Evaluate intraabdominal injuries with laboratory tests of the pancreas, liver, and kidneys. Imaging studies of these organs and the spleen may also be indicated.

G. CT scanning is a good initial method to assess head injury; consider MRI when symptoms do not fit CT findings. Head-injured children may require emergent measures to control intracranial pressure and shock.

H. Many cases of physical abuse are first suspected because the injury is unexplained or the explanation is implausible and incompatible with the physical findings. A child over 3 or 4 years will often confirm that a particular adult hurt him or her. Note accusations of one parent by the other. Most diagnoses of physical abuse (nonaccidental trauma) can be based solely on the physical findings. Many bruises, burns, and scars are pathognomonic. Bruises on the buttocks and lower back are almost always related to spanking; fingerprints and thumbprints are found where a child has been forcefully grabbed; hard pinching leaves curvilinear bruises; slapping leaves a bruise with parallel lines running through it; attempts to silence a screaming child may bruise the upper lip and frenulum; human bite marks are distinctive paired crescent-shaped bruises facing each other; a bruise or welt often resembles the blunt instrument used. The most common sites of accidental bruises are the forehead, anterior tibia, and bony prominences. Suspect child abuse when life-threatening injuries result from reportedly short falls or stairway falls. Immersion burns usually produce a water line and may spare surfaces touching the porcelain surface (e.g., the buttocks) or flexed surfaces (e.g., intertriginous areas or the closed palm). Surface tension properties of liquids can help to explain patterns of scalds. Intentional cigarette burns should be distinguished from usually more superficial nonintentional burns and from skin trauma and infections.

(Continued on page 20)

CHILD ABUSE: PHYSICAL ABUSE Suspected

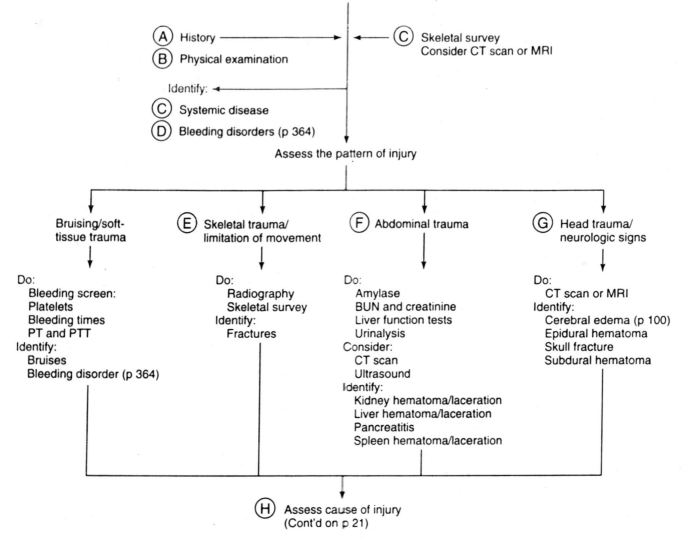

(A) History ———————→ ← (C) Skeletal survey
(B) Physical examination   Consider CT scan or MRI

Identify: ←
(C) Systemic disease
(D) Bleeding disorders (p 364)

Assess the pattern of injury

Bruising/soft-tissue trauma

(E) Skeletal trauma/limitation of movement

(F) Abdominal trauma

(G) Head trauma/neurologic signs

Do:
  Bleeding screen:
  Platelets
  Bleeding times
  PT and PTT
Identify:
  Bruises
  Bleeding disorder (p 364)

Do:
  Radiography
  Skeletal survey
Identify:
  Fractures

Do:
  Amylase
  BUN and creatinine
  Liver function tests
  Urinalysis
Consider:
  CT scan
  Ultrasound
Identify:
  Kidney hematoma/laceration
  Liver hematoma/laceration
  Pancreatitis
  Spleen hematoma/laceration

Do:
  CT scan or MRI
Identify:
  Cerebral edema (p 100)
  Epidural hematoma
  Skull fracture
  Subdural hematoma

(H) Assess cause of injury
(Cont'd on p 21)

I. Accidents are results of unexpected and unintentional forces. Reasonably prudent parents allow their children to be exposed to some risks that are generally low in injury potential or very low in frequency. Suspect a parent who has grossly failed to meet the safety needs of the child or whose child has had repeated serious injuries because of supervisory neglect.

J. Some cases are obvious; others are confusing. If you cannot decide whether the injuries are accidental or inflicted, seek immediate consultation. When in doubt, report suspicious injuries to the local child protection services (CPS) for investigation and follow-up observation. Pediatric orthopedists, radiologists, neurosurgeons, and forensic dentists may be helpful.

K. Immediately report to the local CPS. Include in the report evaluation treatment plans and recommendations for protection of the child and follow-up. Be available to the juvenile court when necessary. Report any concerns about the safety of siblings and the nonviolent spouse. For immersion burns many fire departments can measure the temperature of water in the home with properly standardized chemistry thermometers.

References

American Academy of Pediatrics, Section on Child Abuse and Neglect. A guide to references and resources in child abuse and neglect. Elk Grove Village, IL: American Academy of Pediatrics, 1994.

Kleinman PK. Diagnostic imaging of child abuse. Baltimore: Williams & Wilkins, 1987.

Ludwig S, Kornberg AE, eds. Child abuse: A medical reference. New York: Churchill Livingstone, 1992.

Schmitt BD. The child with non-accidental trauma. In: Kempe CH, Helfer RE, eds. The battered child. 4th ed. Chicago: University of Chicago Press, 1987:178.

Sirotnak AP, Krugman RD. Physical abuse of children: An update. Pediatr Rev 1994; 15:394.

CHILD ABUSE: PHYSICAL ABUSE Suspected

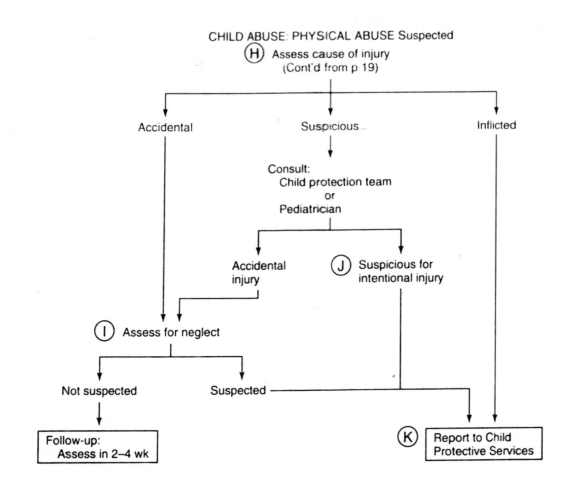

CHILD ABUSE: SEXUAL ABUSE

Robert M. Brayden, M.D.

Sexual mistreatment of children is conducted most commonly by family members, less frequently by friends and acquaintances, and least commonly by strangers. A detailed account of sexual experiences, unexplained vaginal bleeding, other genital symptoms, compulsive masturbation, precocious sexual behaviors, specific examination findings, sexually transmitted disease (STD), a rectal or vaginal foreign body, and/or proctitis should cause suspicion.

A. Take a careful history; fewer than 50% of abuse victims have physical or laboratory findings. Consider audio-taping interviews. Interview parents and children separately. Children older than 2½ to 3 years of age can provide an accurate description to a skillful interviewer. Enhance children's resistance to misleading or leading questions by being friendly rather than authoritarian, role-playing questions to which you know the answer to discourage guessing, encouraging admissions of lack of memory or confusion, indicating to the child that you weren't there, and allowing the child to stop the interview or disagree with or correct you. Ask open-ended questions if possible, and document all details concerning types and frequency of sexual activities. Note the child's special names for body parts. Document date, time, place, person, sites of sexual abuse, menstrual history, whether or not force was involved, the patient's concept of intercourse, and whether or not penetration or ejaculation occurred. Consider the possibility of unintentional or intentional suggestion (induced memory); refer the patient to a child psychiatrist or psychologist for additional evaluation if this is suspected.

B. Examine the body surface for signs of nongenital trauma. Assess the possibility of pregnancy. Examine the mouth and rectum for signs of acute trauma. Visually examine the external genitals for signs of trauma, laxity, or vaginal discharge. Use labial traction (grasp labia and protract them directly away from the child) and labial separation to examine the hymen and posterior fourchette areas. Although hymen width measurements in nonabused populations are published, the overall appearance of the tissue is more important than the horizontal measurement. Hymen width measurement is best done by colposcope with standardized optical measuring devices. In prepubertal children vaginal speculum examination and/or surgical exploration un-

der anesthesia is usually needed only when blood loss is unexplained or foreign body is expected. Consider magnification and photographic documentation of the genitalia using a colposcope if injuries are found. Most penetrating hymenal injuries occur posteriorly, between the 4 and 8 o'clock positions. Acute trauma of the genitals, rectum, or mouth usually has epithelial closure within 7 days and complete restoration of the tissues within 6 weeks. Acute injuries appear as lacerations, fissures, and abrasions. Anal laxity leading to dilation greater than 20 mm without stool present supports acute rectal penetration. Healed female genital injuries appear as clefts completely through the posterior hymen and hymenal attenuation. Healed anal injuries usually leave no discernible findings; however, scars or anal skin tags outside the midline suggest previous injury.

C. Consider consultation with a local child protection team or physician experienced in child sexual abuse evaluations. The female genitalia and anal examination have normal variability, and reliable evaluation requires some practiced skill. Some conditions can be misdiagnosed as resulting from trauma (e.g., lichen sclerosis, urethral prolapse).

D. Two categories of sexual abuse can be distinguished: (1) nonpenetrating contact (viewing or fondling the child's genitals, asking the child to fondle or masturbate the adult's genitals, exposure to pornography) and (2) penetrating sexual contact, including attempted and actual vaginal, oral, or rectal penetration. Evaluate each case individually for (1) degree of force, threat, or coercion; (2) the psychological response of the parent(s) and child; and (3) the need for laboratory investigation.

E. For nonpenetrating contact collect specimens as appropriate to test for semen on skin or clothing. Other specimens may be collected in some cases. Follow chain-of-possession procedures.

F. If penetration has occurred, collect specimens from the clothing and body (semen, pubic hair, scalp hair, fingernail and debris scrapings, saliva, blood samples) that help to identify the perpetrator. Use protocols to guide specimen collection. Adhere to chain-of-possession procedures. Consider having a pathologist or other laboratory expert confirm motile sperm identifi-

(Continued on page 24)

Patient with Suspected SEXUAL ABUSE

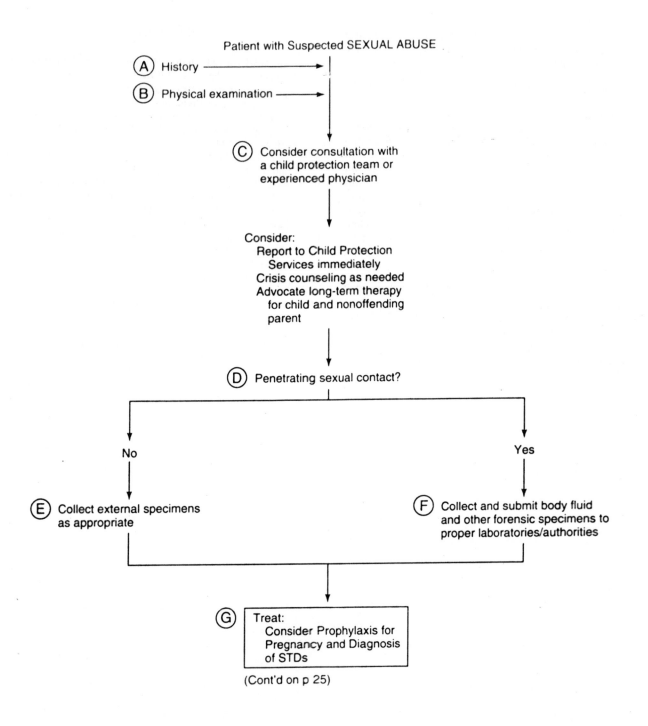

(A) History ───────────▶

(B) Physical examination ───────▶

(C) Consider consultation with
a child protection team or
experienced physician

Consider:
Report to Child Protection
Services immediately
Crisis counseling as needed
Advocate long-term therapy
for child and nonoffending
parent

(D) Penetrating sexual contact?

No

Yes

(E) Collect external specimens
as appropriate

(F) Collect and submit body fluid
and other forensic specimens to
proper laboratories/authorities

(G) Treat:
Consider Prophylaxis for
Pregnancy and Diagnosis
of STDs

(Cont'd on p 25)

cation. Consider forensic DNA testing. Collect a serum sample and save it to test in case subsequent serologic tests are positive.

G. Medication to prevent pregnancy can be given to girls who are postmenarchal and have had vaginal intercourse within 72 hours. If the pregnancy test is negative, consider giving norgestrel (Ovral) two tablets immediately, repeated once after 12 hours. Although this drug may have multiple mechanisms to prevent pregnancy, one established mechanism is as an abortifacient; get informed consent before taking this action. After obtaining initial culture and wet mount, treat adolescent victims of penetrating assault prophylactically with ceftriaxone (gonorrhea), doxycycline (Chlamydia), and metronidazole (Trichomonas). Make the decision to evaluate prepubertal children for STDs on an individual basis.

H. Follow-up examination for STDs should be done at 2 weeks after assault. Inquire about the effects of postcoital pregnancy prophylaxis. Repeat culture and wet mount tests. At 12 weeks, perform HIV, hepatitis B (unless vaccinated), and rapid plasma reagin (RPR) serologic testing. Obtain recent menstrual history.

References

American Academy of Pediatrics, Committee on Child Abuse and Neglect. Guidelines for the evaluation of sexual abuse of children. Pediatrics 1991; 87:254.

American Academy of Pediatrics, Section on Child Abuse and Neglect. A guide to references and resources in child abuse and neglect. Elk Grove Village, IL: American Academy of Pediatrics, 1994.

Bays J, Chadwick D. Medical diagnosis of the sexually abused child. Child Abuse Negl 1993; 17:91.

Brigham JC. Issues in the empirical study of the sexual abuse of children. In: Doris J, ed. The suggestibility of children's recollections. Washington, DC: American Psychological Association, 1991:110.

Centers for Disease Control and Prevention. 1993 sexually transmitted diseases treatment guidelines. MMWR 1993; 42 (No. RR-14):97.

Heger A, Emans SJ. Introital diameter as the criterion for sexual abuse. Pediatrics 1990; 85:222.

McCann J, Voris J. Perianal injuries resulting from sexual abuse: A longitudinal study. Pediatrics 1993; 91:390.

McCann J, Wells R, Simon M, Voris J. Genital findings in prepubertal girls selected for nonabuse: A descriptive study. Pediatrics 1990; 86:428.

Patient with Suspected SEXUAL ABUSE

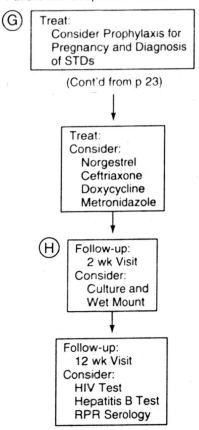

(G) Treat:
Consider Prophylaxis for
Pregnancy and Diagnosis
of STDs

(Cont'd from p 23)

Treat:
Consider:
Norgestrel
Ceftriaxone
Doxycycline
Metronidazole

(H) Follow-up:
2 wk Visit
Consider:
Culture and
Wet Mount

Follow-up:
12 wk Visit
Consider:
HIV Test
Hepatitis B Test
RPR Serology

DEPRESSION

Kathleen A. Mammel, M.D.

A. When depression is suspected, history should include presence of any vegetative symptoms such as depressive mood nearly every day, irritability, crying spells or inability to cry, sense of worthlessness or helplessness, isolation, diminished interest in usual activities, fatigue, poor concentration, change in appetite, loss or gain in weight, difficulty sleeping, or sleeping more. In children and adolescents, however, depression may be masked and may present instead as psychosomatic symptoms (headache, chest pain, abdominal pain, lethargy, syncope) or behavioral problems (self-destructive behavior, defiance, truancy, school failure, running away, substance abuse, sexual acting out, delinquent acts). The patient and parent should be directly questioned about the above symptoms. Patients should be asked privately about any thoughts of hurting themselves to assess suicidal ideation. A history of suicide gestures and any family history of psychiatric problems should be elicited.

B. In the physical examination rule out any contributing or underlying medical illness such as CNS process (closed-head injury, tumor, vascular lesion), metabolic or endocrine disorder (thyroid or parathyroid disorder, systemic lupus erythematosus, Wilson disease, Cushing or Addison disease, premenstrual syndrome, eating disorder), infection (mononucleosis, syphilis), mitral valve prolapse, or signs of medication toxicity or substance abuse.

C. The physician needs to assess whether this is an angry teenager, an acute depressive reaction with or without masking, or a serious psychiatric problem. *Mild* depression may result from an acute identifiable situation or personal loss. There should be no high-risk behaviors present. *Moderate* depression may have a longer history or mild behavior changes or dysfunction. *Severe* depression refers to psychotic thought processes or suicidal ideation with the inability to contract for safety. *Very severely* depressed is the patient who has gestured suicide or has a suicide plan.

D. The physician may feel comfortable counseling the patient with a mild reactive depression to enable him or her to verbalize and understand feelings and put things in perspective. The provider must remain available to the patient. Weekly follow-up visits are indicated to reassess the situation until it is resolved. At these visits the patient can be encouraged to express emotions, set realistic goals, and become more assertive.

E. Psychiatric referral is indicated for more prolonged symptoms, evidence of dysfunction, suspicion of bipolar disease, or other concerns. This may be referral to a psychiatrist, psychologist, or social worker skilled in working with children and adolescents and their families. If a medication evaluation is needed, a psychiatrist is most appropriate. Ongoing medical follow-up is important to be sure the referral was accomplished and to intervene in any medical consequences of acting-out behavior (e.g., substance abuse or sexual activity).

F. Emergency psychiatric consultation should be obtained for any patient who is severely depressed, psychotic, or acutely suicidal. It is the psychiatrist's responsibility to decide whether hospitalization or outpatient therapy is appropriate.

G. Patients who have just made gestures of suicide or have a delineated suicide plan should be hospitalized and in most states are psychiatrically holdable. Even if the patient appears not to be in acute medical danger, hospitalization is reasonable to ensure psychiatric evaluation and to establish a follow-up plan. The patient should not be released without psychiatric evaluation.

References

Brent DA. Suicide and suicidal behavior in children and adolescents. Pediatr Rev 1989; 10:269.

Committee on Adolescence, American Academy of Pediatrics. Suicide and suicide attempts in adolescents and young adults. Pediatrics 1988; 81:322.

Gourash L, Puig-Antich J. Medical and biologic aspects of adolescent depression. Semin Adolesc Med 1986; 2:299.

Greydanus DE. Depression in adolescence: A perspective. Adolesc Health Care 1986; 7(Suppl):S109.

Kaplan DW, Mammel KA. Adolescence. In: Hay WW, Groothuis JR, Hayward AR, Levin MJ, eds. Current pediatric diagnosis and treatment. 13th ed. Norwalk, CT: Appleton & Lange, 1996 (in press).

Patient with DEPRESSION

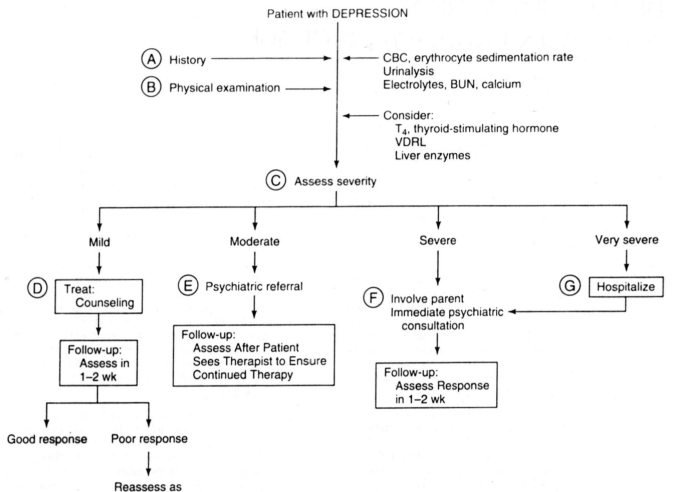

(A) History ⟶ ← CBC, erythrocyte sedimentation rate
Urinalysis
Electrolytes, BUN, calcium

(B) Physical examination ⟶

← Consider:
T₄, thyroid-stimulating hormone
VDRL
Liver enzymes

(C) Assess severity

Mild | Moderate | Severe | Very severe

(D) Treat:
Counseling

Follow-up:
Assess in
1–2 wk

Good response | Poor response

Reassess as
moderate

(E) Psychiatric referral

Follow-up:
Assess After Patient
Sees Therapist to Ensure
Continued Therapy

(F) Involve parent
Immediate psychiatric
consultation

Follow-up:
Assess Response
in 1–2 wk

(G) Hospitalize

DEVELOPMENTAL DELAY IN CHILDREN UNDER 6 YEARS OF AGE

Bonnie W. Camp, M.D., Ph.D.
Roxann Headley, M.D.

Mental retardation is both intellectual and adaptive functioning significantly below average (> 2 standard deviations) for chronologic age. By definition, this can be expected to characterize about 3% of the population. Delayed development is often the earliest sign of mental retardation. Whenever it is suspected, the work-up should include assessment for treatable causes of mental retardation as well as a description of functional limitations and recommendations for habilitation.

A. In the history note prenatal and perinatal information; illnesses; hospitalizations; developmental milestones; family history, especially of mental retardation and learning disabilities; growth; nutritional and social status. Identify any history of major anomalies or seizure disorders and ask the family whether there has been any regression in the child's development. Ask parents about their concerns, as these often are the key to developmental problems.

B. Include examination of growth (height, weight, and head circumference), dysmorphic features, evidence of genetic syndromes, and neurologic abnormality. Note any café-au-lait spots, neurofibromas, port-wine stains, and ash-leaf skin changes. Include a careful genital examination, since both small and enlarged gonads in boys can be associated with syndromes of developmental delay. Note evidence of autistic or strange behaviors such as hand flapping, toe walking, twirling, and perseveration. If neurologic abnormalities are not part of an identified syndrome, the child should be referred for complete neurologic examination, especially to rule out muscular dystrophy and CNS degenerative disorders.

C. Note the results of newborn screening (phenylketonuria [PKU], homocystinuria, galactosemia, maple syrup urine disease, thyroid disorder, and biotinidase deficiency). Screen for hearing, vision, and development. Vision screening can be performed reliably with the Allen picture cards beginning around 3 years of age, and most 4 year olds can respond to pure tone audiometry. If there are any questions about hearing or vision, refer infants for brain stem evoked response and/or an audiologic evaluation. Refer children with suspected vision or hearing problems for complete ophthalmologic evaluation or ENT and audiology evaluation.

D. Developmental screening will be most helpful in determining whether the child has delays in several areas or in a specific area only. Developmental surveillance or monitoring that does not rest on routine use of screening tests is an important means to encourage parents to raise concerns and to heighten the physician's awareness of possible problems. Selective use of screening tests to confirm suspicions is helpful, but monitoring should continue even if screening fails to confirm suspicions of delay in very young children. Screening tests such as the Denver II have been designed to describe as abnormal children below the third percentile. Educational standards commonly cite as evidence of global delay a 20% delay between chronologic age and mental age.

E. The most common specific delays without overall cognitive or global delay occur in speech and language, motor functioning, and emotional and behavioral development. Of these, speech and language delays are the most common. Among children under age 2 years, the most frequent presentation is a child who has few words, relies heavily on gestures, and/or has a sibling who talks for him or her. Often counseling with the parents to reduce their reliance on gestures and insistence on having the child make some sound to indicate what he or she wants is sufficient to bring language development to normal.

F. Motor delays in the very young child are usually first noted as gross motor delays. These are frequently accompanied by signs of cerebral palsy. Neuromotor development in children 6 months to 18 months can be assessed effectively with the infant neurologic international battery (Infanib), which sorts children into abnormal, transiently abnormal, and normal categories. All children who are clearly abnormal should be seen by rehabilitation services for occupational and physical therapy. Observation alone may be safe for many children with transient abnormalities if there are no signs of other delays.

G. Emotional and behavioral problems may decrease functioning, especially when they render the child (for example) fearful, withdrawn, oppositional, or bizarre. During developmental testing these characteristics may be demonstrated as poor cooperation, refusal, inattention, destructiveness, and similar problematic behaviors. Often a review of behavioral management styles within the family reveals specific areas that may yield to simple changes, such as the use of discipline or patterns of reinforcement. Distractibility and hyperactivity may present additional challenges to parents; however, in preschool children an appropriate behavior management program can usually manage these problems. Two factors that affect the success of such a program are the ability of both parent and child to make changes and the complexity of the problem. It is often possible to assess the responsiveness of a small child to a change in behavior management by assigning a task (e.g., sit in a chair) and noting the child's response to repeated praise for complying. Assess the parent's ability to change by observing how well he or she can carry out a suggestion.

(Continued on page 30)

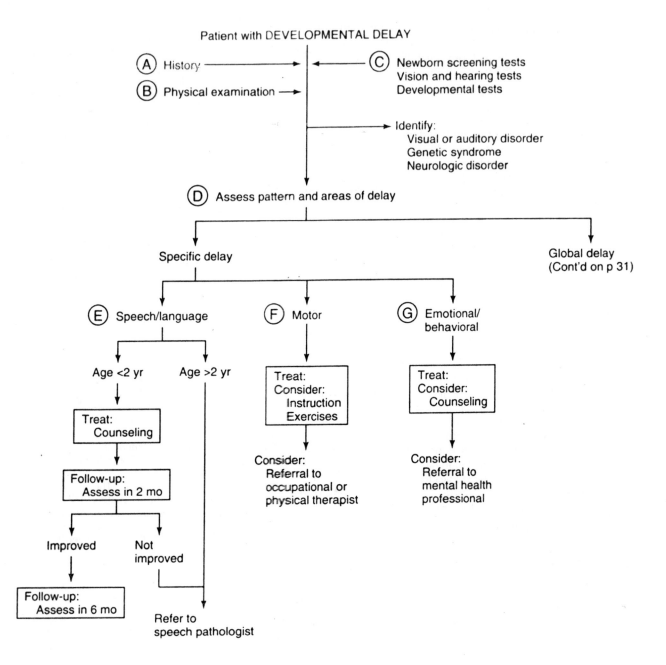

Patient with DEVELOPMENTAL DELAY

Ⓐ History

Ⓑ Physical examination

Ⓒ Newborn screening tests
Vision and hearing tests
Developmental tests

Identify:
Visual or auditory disorder
Genetic syndrome
Neurologic disorder

Ⓓ Assess pattern and areas of delay

Specific delay

Global delay
(Cont'd on p 31)

Ⓔ Speech/language

Ⓕ Motor

Ⓖ Emotional/
behavioral

Age <2 yr   Age >2 yr

Treat:
Counseling

Follow-up:
Assess in 2 mo

Improved   Not
improved

Follow-up:
Assess in 6 mo

Refer to
speech pathologist

Treat:
Consider:
Instruction
Exercises

Consider:
Referral to
occupational or
physical therapist

Treat:
Consider:
Counseling

Consider:
Referral to
mental health
professional

Be prepared to reassess and refer for counseling with a social worker, psychologist, or developmental pediatrician any family that does not show progress with counseling in the primary care setting.

H. Young children often fail to demonstrate their best functioning in a strange situation. Consider as mild delays those that appear to result from lack of appropriate activities or that are based on lack of opportunity or refusal to participate. Instructing the parent in activities to promote development with close follow-up and rescreening should reduce the number of false-positive responses referred for diagnostic evaluation; however, developmental monitoring may be necessary. Refusal to participate may be a sign of more extensive problems, including emotional disturbance, and should not be dismissed as inconsequential.

I. Laboratory studies may be ordered by the primary health care provider or left to the discretion of the specialist. The younger the child is when suspected of having a developmental disability, the more likely an identifiable basis for the disorder can be found. Chromosome studies, especially examining for fragile X, are likely to be the most fruitful tests performed at all ages. Analysis of the urine for organic and amino acids and serum for amino acids and electrolytes will rule out many metabolic causes of developmental delay. MRI or CT is useful to rule out intracranial anatomic abnormalities and evidence of disease (e.g., calcifications indicating congenital infection). Even if a newborn screen was reported as normal, rescreening for PKU, hypothyroidism, and biotinidase deficiency should be considered. Consider studies to identify prenatal infections (e.g., cytomegalovirus, toxoplasmosis) along with other indicated tests for specific syndromes.

J. Children with developmental disabilities and their families commonly have problems in several areas of functioning, including self-help, language, motor skills, social skills, and sensory functioning, along with social, financial, and emotional stresses. The multidisciplinary team approach to evaluation and program planning is the best way to identify all areas of concern and to avoid overlooking less salient issues. Integration of recommendations from all disciplines concerned with a child and family helps to reduce both fragmentation and duplication in care. The value of the team approach has recently been emphasized in passage of federal legislation PL99-457. That law provides for identification of infants who have or are at risk for disabilities, for a multidisciplinary team assessment, and for development of an individual family service plan (IFSP) emphasizing comprehensive early intervention services.

K. When a medical disorder is diagnosed, treatment for it should be coordinated with the appropriate specialist. Functional problems, which are often also present, are best approached by a multidisciplinary team.

References

American Psychiatric Association. Diagnostic and Statistical Manual of Mental Disorders. 4th ed. Washington, DC: American Psychiatric Association, 1994.

Camp BW. Developmental disabilities. In: Hay W, Groothius J, Hayward A, Levin M, eds. Current pediatric diagnosis and treatment. 12th ed. Norwalk, CT: Appleton & Lange, 1995:129.

Dworkin PH. British and American recommendation for developmental monitoring: The role of surveillance. Pediatrics 1989; 84:1000.

Ellison P, Horn J, Browning C. The construction of an infant neurologic international battery (INFANIB) for the assessment of neurologic integrity in infancy. Phys Ther 1985; 9:1326.

Frankenburg WK, Dodds JB. The Denver II. Denver: Developmental Materials, 1990.

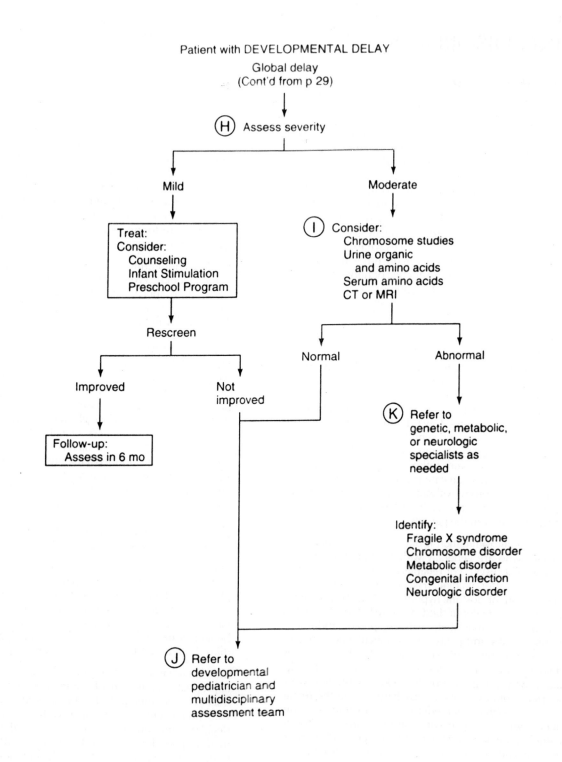

Patient with DEVELOPMENTAL DELAY
Global delay
(Cont'd from p 29)

(H) Assess severity

Mild

Moderate

Treat:
Consider:
  Counseling
  Infant Stimulation
  Preschool Program

(I) Consider:
  Chromosome studies
  Urine organic
    and amino acids
  Serum amino acids
  CT or MRI

Rescreen

Improved

Not
improved

Normal

Abnormal

Follow-up:
  Assess in 6 mo

(K) Refer to
genetic, metabolic,
or neurologic
specialists as
needed

Identify:
  Fragile X syndrome
  Chromosome disorder
  Metabolic disorder
  Congenital infection
  Neurologic disorder

(J) Refer to
developmental
pediatrician and
multidisciplinary
assessment team

EATING DISORDERS

Kathleen Mammel, M.D.

Anorexia nervosa is characterized by (1) weight 15% below expected for age and height, (2) fear of fatness or weight gain despite being underweight, (3) distorted body image, and (4) primary or secondary amenorrhea in women and girls.

Bulimia nervosa is diagnosed if the following are present: (1) repeated binging at least twice a week for 3 months or more, (2) patient perceiving eating to be out of control, (3) recurrent purging behavior to prevent weight gain (vomiting, use of laxatives, diuretics, emetics, excessive exercise, or severely restricted intake), and (4) overconcern with body image. Anorexia may be primarily restricting or purging. In some instances both diagnoses may be appropriate, or a patient may be anorexic at one point and turn bulimic later.

A. In the history ask about presenting symptoms, weight history (including maximum, minimum, and desired weight), dietary intake (including specifics of diets and binges, unusual eating behaviors, avoided foods), purging history (vomiting, diuretics, laxatives, emetics, excessive exercise), and menstrual history (irregular cycles, primary or secondary amenorrhea). In addition, direct the review of systems toward other diseases in the differential diagnosis and symptoms secondary to malnutrition or purging (dizziness, syncope, fatigue, muscle cramps, epigastric pain, reflux, hair loss, lanugo hair). The adolescent with an eating disorder often has one of these other symptoms without an overt complaint about weight. Obtain the history from the adolescent in private and then from the parents.

B. The physical examination is often normal, especially in bulimics who are generally within 10 pounds of ideal body weight (IBW). For reliability, weigh the patient in gown only after voiding. Hypothermia, bradycardia, hypotension, or postural hypotension may be present if the patient is malnourished or dehydrated. Anorexics may appear emaciated, with scaphoid abdomen, prominent ribs and joints, loss of subcutaneous tissue, and squaring off of the convergence of the thighs. In addition, there may be loss of shine and curl of scalp hair, downy lanugo hair on the body, excoriation over the spine from excessive sit-ups, hard stool in the rectal vault, and coldness and edema of the extremities. The patient who has been vomiting may have lost tooth enamel, particularly on the posterior aspect of the front teeth, or calluses on the dorsum of the index finger.

C. Teach the patient and family that the patient may be struggling with growing up or other emotional issues; the focus on eating and weight may be the patient's attempt to maintain a sense of control in life when feeling overwhelmed. The resulting physical symptoms are indicative of a psychiatric disorder. Psychotherapy involving the patient and family is necessary for a healthful outcome. The patient should be reassured that the aim is restoring health and regaining control, not gaining excess weight.

D. Medical monitoring must continue on a regular basis, initially weekly. Weights in gown only after voiding, vital signs, urine specific gravity, and specific questioning regarding dietary intake and physical symptoms must be done weekly until the patient is steadily gaining weight. Medical visits may then spread out to every 2 weeks until 90% of IBW is reached, then monthly until menses return. Bulimics should be monitored weekly until weight and electrolytes are stable and psychotherapy is under way. A behavioral contract signed by the patient, parents, and caregivers is useful. For anorexics, it might include long-term goal weight range, expected rate of weight gain, consequences of failure to meet weight goals, or even specifics of dietary intake. For bulimics, the contract might address a maintenance weight range, honesty regarding frequency of binging and purging, and gradually delaying purge behavior until more than an hour after meals. Antacids may be useful in preventing and treating reflux esophagitis and gastritis. Metoclopramide or cisapride may be helpful for delayed gastric emptying in early refeeding.

E. The dietitian can monitor intake, dispel food and calorie myths, and assist in developing well-balanced meal plans. The focus should be taken off of calories. A supplement such as Ensure or Carnation Instant Breakfast may be given if meals are not finished. Patients may benefit from a prenatal vitamin (containing multivitamins, iron, and folate) and a calcium supplement.

F. Individual, family, and/or group psychotherapy may be appropriate. Family involvement is critical with adolescents. The therapist should be skilled in working with adolescents and familiar with eating disorders. Regular communication between the therapist and medical provider is crucial to prevent splitting and to bring out discrepancies between the emotional and the physical level.

(Continued on page 34)

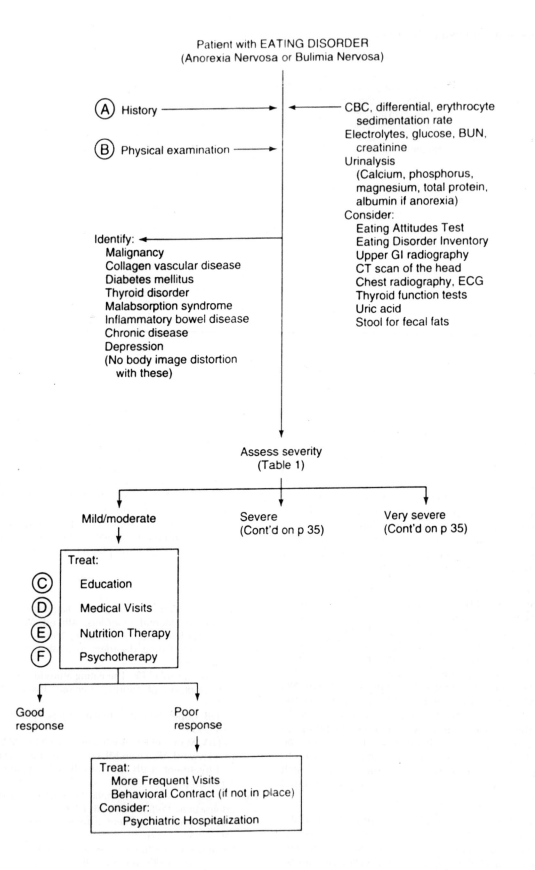

Patient with EATING DISORDER
(Anorexia Nervosa or Bulimia Nervosa)

(A) History

(B) Physical examination

CBC, differential, erythrocyte
   sedimentation rate
Electrolytes, glucose, BUN,
   creatinine
Urinalysis
   (Calcium, phosphorus,
   magnesium, total protein,
   albumin if anorexia)
Consider:
   Eating Attitudes Test
   Eating Disorder Inventory
   Upper GI radiography
   CT scan of the head
   Chest radiography, ECG
   Thyroid function tests
   Uric acid
   Stool for fecal fats

Identify:
   Malignancy
   Collagen vascular disease
   Diabetes mellitus
   Thyroid disorder
   Malabsorption syndrome
   Inflammatory bowel disease
   Chronic disease
   Depression
   (No body image distortion
      with these)

Assess severity
(Table 1)

Mild/moderate

Severe
(Cont'd on p 35)

Very severe
(Cont'd on p 35)

Treat:
(C) Education
(D) Medical Visits
(E) Nutrition Therapy
(F) Psychotherapy

Good
response

Poor
response

Treat:
   More Frequent Visits
   Behavioral Contract (if not in place)
Consider:
   Psychiatric Hospitalization

TABLE 1 Severity of Eating Disorders

Mild	Moderate	Severe	Very Severe
Recent onset of symptoms and Physiologically stable and No more than 15% < IBW and No severe psychiatric symptoms	Moderate physiologic abnormality, e.g., slight hypothermia or hypokalemia amenable to oral replacement and No more than 20% < IBW or Depression without suicidal ideation	30% < IBW or Evidence of metabolic disturbance: heart rate < 40, temperature < 36° C (96.8° F) systolic BP < 70, significant orthostatic hypotension, serum K⁺ < 2.5 despite oral replacement, severe dehydration or Severe binging and purging or Refusal of minimal oral intake or Severe depression or Family crisis or Inadequate response to outpatient treatment	40% < IBW or Severe dehydration or Severe electrolyte imbalance (depressed serum phosphorus or magnesium) or Constellation of bradycardia, hypothermia, hypotension or Arrhythmia or Decreased renal concentrating ability or Osteopenia or Suicidal ideation or psychosis

IBW, ideal body weight; BP, blood pressure.

G. Hospitalization may be necessary for medical or psychiatric reasons (see C). Short-term stays, for example, to correct electrolyte abnormalities, may be best accomplished on a pediatric or adolescent medical unit. Intermediate hospitalizations to establish weight gain and institute psychotherapy may also be accomplished on a medical unit with a team including physician, therapist, dietitian, and nursing staff. When a patient is expected to benefit from a longer stay with milieu therapy, adolescent psychiatric hospitalization is appropriate after medical stabilization. Eating disorder units may not be appropriate for adolescents if the population is largely adults or does not have a family emphasis.

H. Medical stabilization is the first goal. Fluid and electrolyte status should be corrected, with careful monitoring of vital signs. For anorexics, refeeding goes hand in hand with this. Rarely, nasogastric (NG) tube feedings or IV hyperalimentation is necessary for extremely malnourished or noncompliant patients. Most patients will finish meals or take an oral supplement when given the limited choices of oral refeeding or placement of an NG tube. All staff must remain firm in the goal to restore the patient to health. Often this requires supervising meals, use of the bathroom, and free time. Calcium, phosphorus, and magnesium should be closely monitored in the refeeding phase, as there may be a shift from serum to cells during conversion to anabolic metabolism. Watch for congestive heart failure during periods of rapid weight gain.

I. A thorough psychiatric evaluation can begin once the patient is medically stable. It may be necessary for patients with anorexia nervosa to gain weight before they can look at underlying issues. The psychologist can be instrumental in tailoring an individualized behavioral contract with the underlying principles of gradually reaching a goal weight range, interrupting binging and purging behaviors, developing more healthful coping strategies, understanding underlying issues, and restoring the appropriate level of control to the patient. The entire treatment team must support the contract. Weekly staff meetings are useful for discussing progress and plans, any splitting, and issues that arise in caring for difficult patients. When psychotherapy begins, family involvement is crucial. Group therapy may also be helpful, particularly for bulimic individuals. Antidepressants may be a useful adjunct, in particular the serotonin-reuptake inhibitors, which are believed to reduce intrusive food thoughts and play a role in appetite regulation.

References

American Psychiatric Association. Diagnostic and Statistical Manual of Mental Disorders. 4th ed. Washington, DC: American Psychiatric Association, 1994.

Commerci GD. Eating disorders in adolescents. Pediatr Rev 1988; 10:37.

Garner DM, Garfinkel PE. The eating attitudes test: An index of the symptoms of anorexia nervosa. Psychol Med 1979; 9:273.

Herzog DB, Copeland PM. Eating disorders. N Engl J Med 1985; 313:295.

Kaplan DW, Mammel KA. Adolescence. In: Hay WW, Groothuis JR, Hayward AR, Levin MJ, eds. Current pediatric diagnosis and treatment. 13th ed. Norwalk, CT: Appleton & Lange, 1996 (in press).

Palla B, Litt IF. Medical complications of eating disorders in adolescents. Pediatrics 1988; 81:613.

Powers PS. Inpatient treatment of anorexia nervosa. Pediatrician 1983–85; 12:126.

Vandereycken W. Outpatient management of anorexia nervosa. Pediatrician 1983–85; 12:118.

Williams RL. Use of the eating attitudes test and eating disorder inventory in adolescents. J Adolesc Health Care 1987; 8:266.

Patient with EATING DISORDER
Assess severity
(Cont'd from p 33)

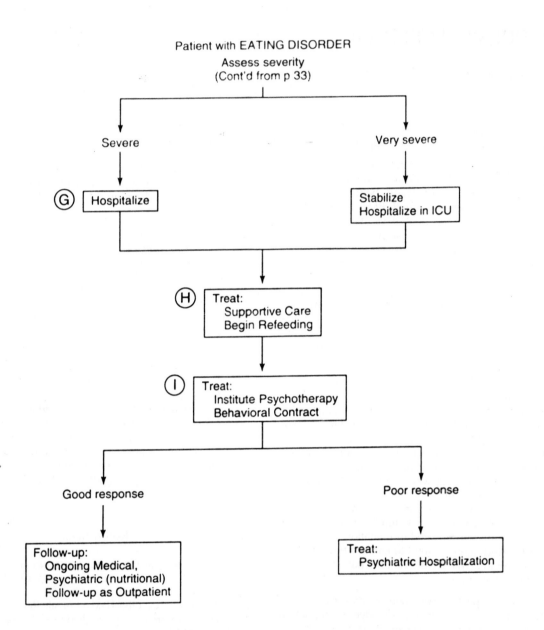

ENCOPRESIS (SOILING)

Barton D. Schmitt, M.D.

Encopresis, or soiling, is the voluntary or involuntary passing of feces into the underwear or other inappropriate site.

A. Most children with encopresis have severe constipation (impaction). They soil themselves several times a day with small amounts of stool. These children periodically have pain with bowel movements (BMs), blood on toilet tissue, and a huge stool that clogs the toilet. Some children hold back stools to avoid pain, others because they are locked in a power struggle with the parent. Determine if the patient uses the toilet for BMs and if public and school toilets are accepted. Since psychogenic factors are common, perform a psychosocial evaluation of all children with encopresis. Many have had punitive toilet training. Others have mild resistance as a result of too much punishment, lectures, or nagging. For intermittent encopresis of unknown origin, have the parents keep an encopresis diary to help determine the circumstances and triggers.

B. Differentiate retentive from nonretentive encopresis on the basis of impacted stool in the rectum. In impaction the rectum is distended and packed with claylike stool, and a midline suprapubic mass is usually palpable. Leakage of stool from the bottom of the impaction may occur several times a day (overflow diarrhea). Suspect nonimpacted encopresis when a normal BM is passed into the underwear once or twice a day without any history of constipation. A barium enema is indicated only if the anal canal will not admit a finger or if the rectum is empty on repeated examination. A flat-plate film of the abdomen is useful to confirm the diagnosis of impaction in atypical cases or if the patient refuses a rectal examination.

C. Remove the impaction with two or three hyperphosphate enemas. Another way to dislodge an impaction is to give 1 oz/year of age/day (8 oz maximum) of mineral oil by mouth for 3 or 4 days. Treat the child with a stool softener such as mineral oil, milk of magnesia, or lactulose for 3 months, until the diameter and tone of the bowel return to normal. Children who hold back because of pain or negativism need to be treated with a laxative (in addition to the stool softener, e.g., Dulcolax). Recommend a diet that includes increased amounts of bran, fresh fruits and vegetables, and decreased milk products. Instruct the parents that the older child should also sit on the toilet three times a day or the program will fail. Some children will not sit on the toilet unless offered incentives. The physician's continued involvement is critical even if the child needs referral to a psychologist or psychiatrist.

D. If the child has no evidence of constipation and the encopresis consists of a normal-sized BM into the underwear once or twice a day, the cause is almost always emotional. If there is no evidence of constipation and the soiling is a small amount, consider poor bowel habits such as postponing BMs (with partial leakage before reaching the toilet), small leakage with gas (e.g., lactose intolerance), partial emptying with sticky stools, or poor wiping.

E. Pediatric counseling, especially for nonimpacted soiling, involves setting up a new toileting program with the child's active participation, using a calendar, and stopping any reminders to sit on the toilet. The parents' main job is to detect any accidents and help the child change as soon as possible. Enemas and medications are not needed in nonretentive encopresis. Refer severely emotionally disturbed children (e.g., those who are depressed, acting out, or over the age of 6 and not impacted) for therapy.

References

Gleghorn EE, Heyman MB, Rudolph CD. No-enema therapy for idiopathic constipation and encopresis. Clin Pediatr 1991; 30:669.

Nolan T, Debelle G, Oberklaid F, et al. Randomised trial of laxatives in treatment of childhood encopresis. Lancet 1991; 338:523.

Pettei MJ. Chronic constipation. Pediatr Ann 1987; 16:796.

Rappaport LA, Levine MD. The prevention of constipation and encopresis: A developmental model and approach. Pediatr Clin North Am 1986; 33:856.

Schmitt BD. Toilet training refusal: Avoid the battle and win the war. Contemp Pediatr 1987; 4:32.

Schmitt BD, Mauro RD: 10 common errors in treating encopresis. Contemp Pediatr 1992; 9:47.

Patient with ENCOPRESIS (SOILING)

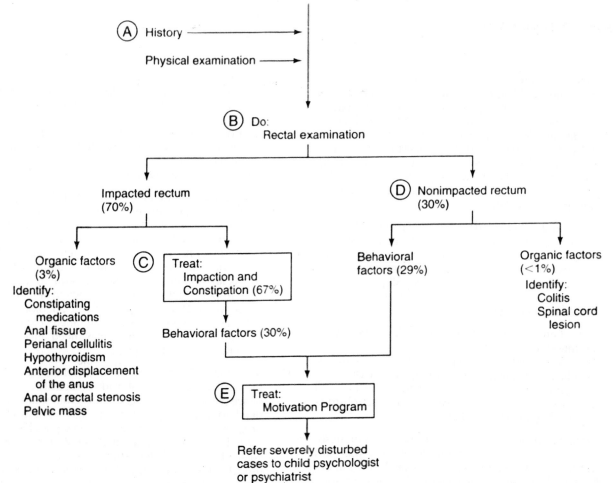

Ⓐ History

Physical examination

Ⓑ Do:
Rectal examination

Impacted rectum
(70%)

Ⓓ Nonimpacted rectum
(30%)

Organic factors
(3%)

Identify:
    Constipating
        medications
    Anal fissure
    Perianal cellulitis
    Hypothyroidism
    Anterior displacement
        of the anus
    Anal or rectal stenosis
    Pelvic mass

Ⓒ Treat:
    Impaction and
    Constipation (67%)

Behavioral factors (30%)

Behavioral
factors (29%)

Organic factors
(<1%)

Identify:
    Colitis
    Spinal cord
        lesion

Ⓔ Treat:
    Motivation Program

Refer severely disturbed
cases to child psychologist
or psychiatrist

ENURESIS (BEDWETTING)

Barton D. Schmitt, M.D.

A. Determine the age of onset, pattern (daytime vs. nighttime), and frequency of wetting. Note any dysuria, an abnormal urine stream (dribbling), constipation, soiling, polydipsia, and polyuria. Identify predisposing conditions such as frequent urinary tract infections (UTIs), fecal impaction, diabetes mellitus, CNS disease or trauma (diabetes insipidus), and severe emotional disturbance (deliberate wetting). Obtain a complete psychosocial history (see p 8) and identify children who appear severely disturbed.

B. Note a distended bladder or fecal impaction. Examine external genitals for vulvitis, adhesions, and signs of sexual abuse. Assess the anal sphincter wink, the child's gait, and the ankle deep tendon reflexes. Observe the urine stream. Perform a urinalysis for all patients, with special emphasis on the specific gravity, urine glucose, nitrite, and leukocytes.

C. Suspect an associated urinary tract malformation when an abnormal urine stream, constant wetness (dampness), or recurrent UTIs are present. Radiologic studies, including a voiding cystourethrogram (VCUG) and intravenous pyelography or renal ultrasonography, will identify ectopic ureters, a lower urinary tract obstruction, or a neurogenic bladder.

D. Categorize patients according to the pattern of enuresis. Nocturnal enuresis is common (>10% of 5 year olds wet their beds); diurnal enuresis is far less common. Nocturnal enuresis is involuntary; diurnal enuresis is commonly voluntary. When both forms are present, treat diurnal enuresis first.

E. Approximately one third of daytime wetters have urgency incontinence (unstable bladder). These children wet themselves while running to the toilet or while trying to undress; they do use the toilet, unlike those with behavioral problems; most are girls, and they may have a long history of intense bladder spasms; they are embarrassed by their problem; and the family history is commonly positive. Treat these children with stream-interruption exercises (counting to 10 before initiating the stream and while stopping at midstream); they should work up to interrupting for 3 minutes (use an egg timer). Oxybutynin (Ditropan) is also helpful for reducing bladder spasms. Bladder-stretching exercises are contraindicated; they lead to increased wetting.

F. Many daytime wetters deliberately wet themselves to retaliate for the pressures of toilet training. Some have been physically punished; others have been endlessly nagged and reminded. Most have mild oppositional problems and can be treated by the primary physician. Set up a new toilet-training program with the child's active participation using a calendar and incentive system. Have the parents discontinue any reminders to use the toilet but continue to remind the youngster to change to dry clothing when wet. Stream-interruption and bladder-stretching exercises are both counterproductive, as the child considers them an intrusion. Refer to the child psychiatrist or psychologist those who are depressed, overtly angry, or more than 8 years old. Also refer children with pervasive emotional problems.

G. A few children (infrequent voiders) hold back their urine for extended periods (e.g., >8 hours). Some become partial emptyers and have an increased risk of UTIs. Some develop trabeculated bladders, vesicoureteral reflux, hydronephrosis, and even renal failure. All of these children need VCUG and renal ultrasound. If the results are abnormal, they need referral to a urologist. Most respond to the motivation program described in F. Those with UTIs require prophylactic antibiotics. Those with vesicoureteral reflux require timed voidings every 3 hours. Younger children may need incentives to comply with timed voidings.

H. More than 75% of nighttime bed wetters have a small bladder capacity. Normal bladder capacity is 1 oz/year of age plus 2, or 10 ml/kg. Children with small bladders need to learn to awaken at night. Self-awakening programs are helpful, as are the new portable transistorized enuresis alarms (Potty Pager, Wet Stop, Nytone, Night Trainer). Bladder-stretching exercises can be used, but they cure only 35% of children and yield slow progress. Desmopressin is an effective, safe drug that can be used for special overnights, vacations, etc.

I. Children with an increased or normal bladder capacity respond to a program that helps them take responsibility for their symptoms. Have the family discontinue all punishment. Dry mornings should result in positive recognition (praise, a calendar, money). Wet mornings carry the natural consequence of changing the bed. Fluids are decreased during the 2 hours prior to bedtime, and the bladder is emptied at bedtime.

References

Crawford JD, ed. Treatment of nocturnal enuresis. J Pediatr 1989; 114 (Suppl):687.

Fernandes E. The unstable bladder in children. J Pediatr 1991; 118:831.

Forsythe WI, Butler RJ. Fifty years of enuretic alarms. Arch Dis Child 1989; 64:879.

Schmitt BD. Daytime wetting (diurnal enuresis). Pediatr Clin North Am 1982; 29:9.

Schmitt BD. Enuresis alarms. Contemp Pediatr 1986; 3:77.

Schmitt BD. Nocturnal enuresis: Finding the treatment that fits the child. Contemp Pediatr 1990; 7:70.

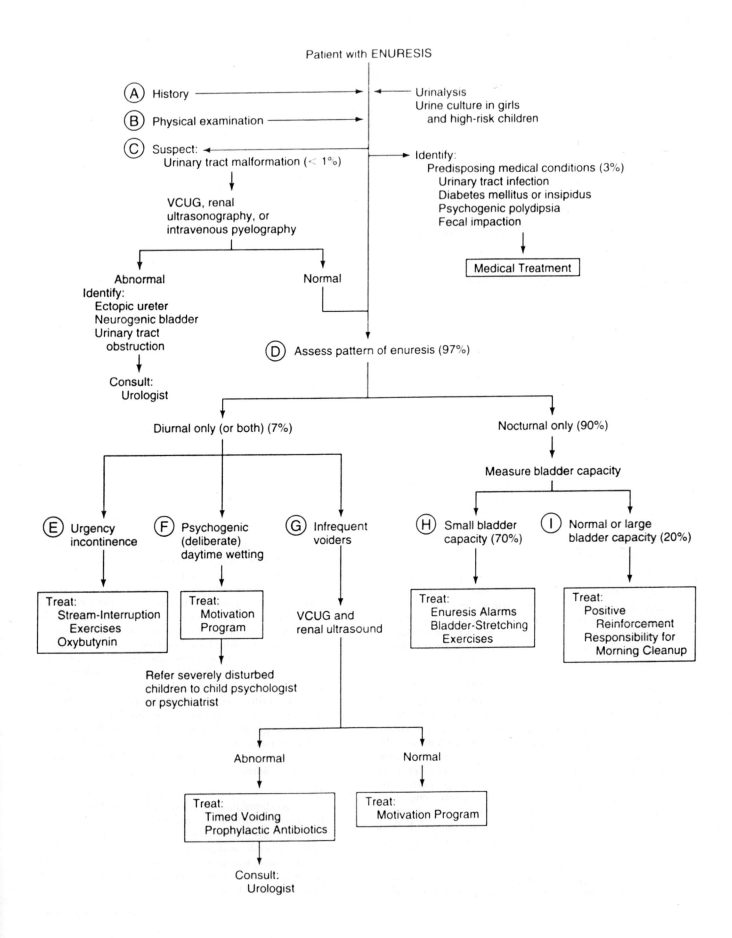

Patient with ENURESIS

(A) History

Urinalysis
Urine culture in girls
and high-risk children

(B) Physical examination

(C) Suspect:
Urinary tract malformation (< 1%)

Identify:
Predisposing medical conditions (3%)
Urinary tract infection
Diabetes mellitus or insipidus
Psychogenic polydipsia
Fecal impaction

Medical Treatment

VCUG, renal
ultrasonography, or
intravenous pyelography

Abnormal
Identify:
Ectopic ureter
Neurogenic bladder
Urinary tract
obstruction

Consult:
Urologist

Normal

(D) Assess pattern of enuresis (97%)

Diurnal only (or both) (7%)

Nocturnal only (90%)

Measure bladder capacity

(E) Urgency
incontinence

(F) Psychogenic
(deliberate)
daytime wetting

(G) Infrequent
voiders

(H) Small bladder
capacity (70%)

(I) Normal or large
bladder capacity (20%)

Treat:
Stream-Interruption
Exercises
Oxybutynin

Treat:
Motivation
Program

VCUG and
renal ultrasound

Treat:
Enuresis Alarms
Bladder-Stretching
Exercises

Treat:
Positive
Reinforcement
Responsibility for
Morning Cleanup

Refer severely disturbed
children to child psychologist
or psychiatrist

Abnormal

Normal

Treat:
Timed Voiding
Prophylactic Antibiotics

Treat:
Motivation Program

Consult:
Urologist

LANGUAGE DISORDERS

Stephen Berman, M.D.

DEFINITIONS

Developmental language disorder, affecting 5% to 10% of children, is a delay in the development of comprehension and the use of a spoken, written, or symbolic system of communication. **Receptive disorder** is an impairment in the ability to comprehend language. **Expressive disorder** is an impairment in the ability to express thoughts. **Dysarthria** is a control disorder of muscles used for articulation and phonation. **Dyspraxia** is an inability to use voluntarily the muscles needed for articulation. **Speech articulation disorder** is abnormal speech not caused by dysarthria, dyspraxia, or stuttering. **Stuttering,** a fluency disorder, is intermittent difficulty in producing a smooth flow of speech that is characterized by repetitions, hesitations, or blockages of speech.

A. If the child is older than 3 years, ask in the history whether he or she talks much spontaneously and if the speech is usually intelligible; becomes frustrated when asked questions and fails to ask many questions spontaneously; dislikes listening to stories, has difficulty understanding stories, and cannot relate events correctly; cannot learn simple songs and nursery rhymes; has difficulty playing with peers. In a younger child, when appropriate, ask how many words are spoken, about the ability to understand simple directions, and whether words are appropriately put together. Ask about the family history of disorders of hearing, language, attention deficit, learning, articulation, and stuttering.

B. In the physical examination perform pneumatic otoscopy to identify otitis and any middle ear effusion. Note any signs of a neurologic disorder, especially altered generalized muscle tone, any pathologic reflexes and any abnormality of muscle movement related to speaking, chewing, sucking, or swallowing. Note any abnormalities of the palate and oral structures.

C. The Early Language Milestone (ELM) is an excellent screening tool for identifying delayed language development in children younger than 3 years. Some physicians think that if the child fails the test, readministering it in 1 or 2 weeks improves the usefulness of the screening by decreasing unnecessary referrals. While the results of the ELM correlate well with more definitive testing in children 13 to 36 months of age, correlation is not so good for infants under 12 months. Physicians should not rely exclusively on the Denver Developmental Screening Test because it fails to identify 47% of children under 3 years who have delayed expressive language.

D. In many congenital disorders hearing loss is associated with mental retardation and produces marked language problems. These include Cockkayne, Down, Goldenhar, Herrmann, Hunter-Hurler, Klippel-Feil, Mobius, Pierre Robin, Treacher Collins, Waardenburg, and Wildervanck. In addition, sensorineural hearing loss caused by congenital infections (cytomegalovirus and rubella) or bacterial meningitis can produce a severe language delay.

E. The diagnostic criteria for a developmental language disorder are language test scores below nonverbal IQ test scores, interference with home and educational activities, and exclusion of global developmental delay, hearing loss, and neurologic disorder.

F. Repetition of words and phrases is common for children of 2 to 5 years age. A small proportion of these children progress to chronic stuttering. Characteristics that indicate a persistent problem include part-word repetition rather than full word or phrase, multiple rather than single repetitions, and irregular, abrupt (jerky) repetitions. Children with a severe problem appear to be under excessive tension and exhibit struggle and avoidance behavior. This leads to avoidance of speaking to strangers and of speaking in difficult situations. It is best to refer children to a speech language specialist when stuttering inhibits the child or continues longer than 6 months.

G. The effect of mild to moderate conductive hearing impairment related to persistent or recurrent otitis media is not clear. While the available data document a causal relationship between severe congenital or acquired hearing loss (usually sensorineural) and language development, they fail to establish a causal relationship between conductive hearing loss associated with otitis media and subsequent hearing-related development. Studies that link otitis media with hearing-related development have been reviewed in the Agency for Health Care Policy and Research publication *Clinical Practice Guideline: Otitis Media with Effusion in Young Children.* The report found "(1) a weak association between otitis media with effusion early in life and abnormal speech and language development in children younger than 4 years; and (2) a weak association between early otitis media with effusion and delay in expressive language development and behavior (attention) in children over 4 years."

H. The home environment is an important source of the language stimulation needed for normal development. Inadequate stimulation can be a result of insufficient care and attention or overprotection, especially from siblings who do and get everything for a younger child. Children who live in multilingual environments and are simultaneously learning more than one language may have transient delays.

(Continued on page 42)

Patient with LANGUAGE DISORDER

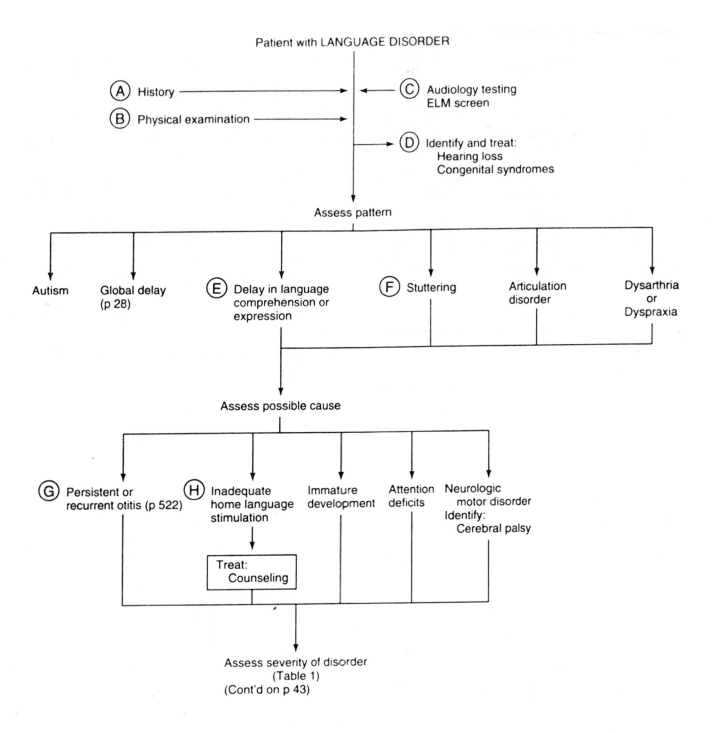

(A) History

(B) Physical examination

(C) Audiology testing
ELM screen

(D) Identify and treat:
Hearing loss
Congenital syndromes

Assess pattern

Autism

Global delay
(p 28)

(E) Delay in language
comprehension or
expression

(F) Stuttering

Articulation
disorder

Dysarthria
or
Dyspraxia

Assess possible cause

(G) Persistent or
recurrent otitis (p 522)

(H) Inadequate
home language
stimulation

Immature
development

Attention
deficits

Neurologic
motor disorder
Identify:
Cerebral palsy

Treat:
Counseling

Assess severity of disorder
(Table 1)
(Cont'd on p 43)

TABLE 1 Categories of Severity of Language Disorders

Mild	Moderate	Severe
Infant < 12 months without a hearing loss or other known cause of a language delay who fails to pass initial and repeat ELM tests Child < 2 years who is delayed 3 to 6 months in language development Mild stuttering consisting of repetitions in a child unaware of any difficulty	Child > 3 years who is hard to understand Child 12 months to 3 years who fails to pass initial and repeat ELM screening tests or is delayed more than 6 months in language development Moderate stuttering with prolongations and blockages but no verbal inhibition	Child > 5 years of age with delayed or abnormal language development Severe stuttering that is consistent and associated with fear and avoidance of speaking Global delay (mental retardation), autism, neurologic disorder

References

American Speech/Language/Hearing Association: Definition: Communication disorders and variations. ASHA Reports 1982; 24:949.

Coplan J, Gleason JR. Unclear speech: Recognition and significance of unintelligible speech in preschool children. Pediatrics 1988; 82:447.

Fischel JE, Whitehurst GJ, Caulfield MB, et al. Language growth in children with expressive language delay. Pediatrics 1989; 82:218.

Guitar BE. Stuttering and stammering. Pediatr Rev 1985; 7:163.

Klein S. Evaluation for suspected language disorders in preschool children. Pediatr Clin North Am 1991; 38:1455.

Montgomery TR. When "not talking" is the chief complaint. Contemp Pediatr 1994; 11:49.

Richardson SO. The child with "delayed speech." Contemp Pediatr 1992; September:55.

Stool SE, Berg AO, Berman S, et al. Otitis media with effusion in young children: Clinical practice guideline. Number 12. AHCPR Publication No. 94-0622. Rockville, MD: Agency for Health Care Policy and Research, Public Health Service, U.S. Department of Health and Human Services. July 1994.

Walker D, Gugenheim S, Downs MP, et al. Early Language Milestone Scale and language screening of young children. Pediatrics 1992; 83:284.

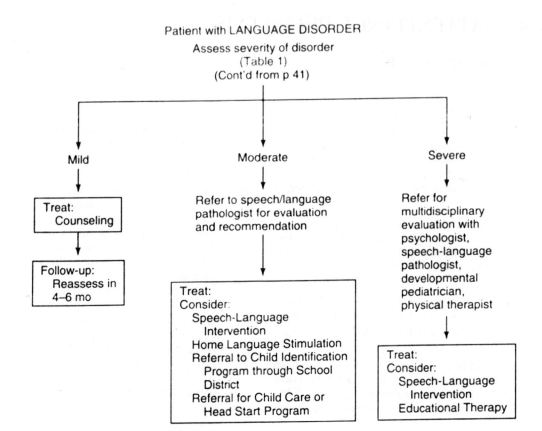

Patient with LANGUAGE DISORDER
Assess severity of disorder
(Table 1)
(Cont'd from p 41)

Mild

Treat:
Counseling

Follow-up:
Reassess in
4–6 mo

Moderate

Refer to speech/language
pathologist for evaluation
and recommendation

Treat:
Consider:
  Speech-Language
   Intervention
  Home Language Stimulation
  Referral to Child Identification
   Program through School
   District
  Referral for Child Care or
   Head Start Program

Severe

Refer for
multidisciplinary
evaluation with
psychologist,
speech-language
pathologist,
developmental
pediatrician,
physical therapist

Treat:
Consider:
  Speech-Language
   Intervention
  Educational Therapy

SCHOOL ATTENDANCE PROBLEMS

Bonnie W. Camp, M.D., Ph.D.

A. School attendance, regardless of performance, is one of the best predictors of mental health in adulthood. In the history obtain a thorough description of the pattern of the attendance problem. Note psychogenic complaints, the parents' method of managing attendance issues, behavior problems at home or at school, and drug or alcohol abuse.

B. Perform a complete physical and neurologic examination. Identify any chronic illness or disorder contributing to poor school attendance (e.g., asthma, severe acne, other disfiguring condition) and treat any medical condition.

C. Find out about intelligence, achievement, school performance and grades, educational history, signs of stress or school problems, and changes in behavior management at school.

D. Assess vision and hearing if screening information from school is not available. Consider examining visual tracking and convergence problems, especially if behavior problems involve resistance about doing schoolwork.

E. The family's contribution, particularly the mother's, is a crucial determinant of the type of problem. Determine whether the mother encourages the child to go to school, monitors attendance, and remains in touch with the school, rather than allowing the child to stay home with minor complaints, having a hard time letting the child go off to school, and/or transferring her own anxiety to the child. Some parents actively discourage attendance because of distrust or disagreement, and others make no effort to see that the child goes to school out of disinterest or neglect.

F. When the family appears to encourage attendance yet the child attends irregularly, consider poor supervision and avoidance syndromes as the most likely source of difficulty. Separation anxiety may be an important part of the problem. A major mental disorder in an adolescent, e.g., paranoia or psychosis, may induce school avoidance.

G. School avoidance is used here to identify attendance problems associated with stress from difficulty at school but not usually intertwined with the family's encouragement of the child to stay home. The stress may be caused by painful or humiliating experiences in the classroom, poor performance, panic attacks, or influence of older siblings or peers. A major task of school for every child every day is to avoid humiliation. Common humiliations include teasing, disrobing in gym, bullying,

and inability to perform. Differentiate mild problems that are highly circumscribed or acute and seem amenable to environmental manipulation from more severe disorders that are complex and/or chronic, including frank paranoia.

H. Avoidance syndromes usually represent some form of agoraphobia and/or personality characteristics of withdrawal. See DSM-IV-R (American Psychiatric Association) for a full discussion of avoidance disorders of childhood and adolescence, avoidant personality syndrome, and panic disorder. The acute onset of school attendance problems in adolescence with a significant component of separation anxiety may be an early sign of psychosis.

I. Parents may encourage attendance but fail to provide enough supervision to see that the child arrives at school. Truancy and involvement with gangs, drugs, and delinquency are often associated with poor supervision, lack of positive involvement with the child, and discipline that is too lax or too harsh.

J. Separation anxiety may appear in a family that is encouraging attendance. Sometimes this surfaces as a control issue, as when a young boy objects to his mother going to work while he is at school.

K. In folie à deux there is very little differentiation between mother and child, and the child's symptoms mirror those of the mother. A very disruptive form of the disorder may be seen when the mother's intense anxiety is transferred to the child and interferes with school attendance and performance.

L. Children with significant chronic diseases (e.g., pulmonary, cardiac) may be treated as unnecessarily vulnerable by the family. In this situation families often treat the child as less capable than he or she really is. They may make unnecessary demands for home teaching on the basis that the child is too sick to go to school. These problems are best handled by a multidisciplinary team that can offer an integrated and coordinated approach to the child and family problems.

M. Classic school phobia is based on separation anxiety and is commonly manifested by psychogenic symptoms (e.g., stomachaches, headaches) that appear only on school days and strike a ready response in the parent who is not too interested in separating from the child. Supporting the parent to insist on attendance unless the physician or nurse specifies otherwise is usually sufficient to deal with the problem. More severe problems that do not respond to this management may require referral to a mental health professional.

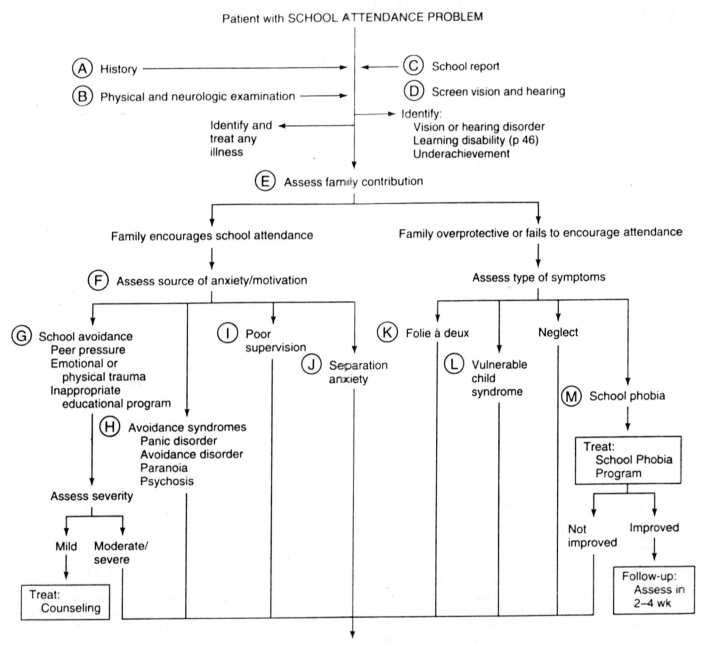

Patient with SCHOOL ATTENDANCE PROBLEM

(A) History ⟶ (C) School report

(B) Physical and neurologic examination ⟶ (D) Screen vision and hearing

Identify and treat any illness ⟵ Identify:
Vision or hearing disorder
Learning disability (p 46)
Underachievement

(E) Assess family contribution

Family encourages school attendance

(F) Assess source of anxiety/motivation

(G) School avoidance
Peer pressure
Emotional or
physical trauma
Inappropriate
educational program

(I) Poor supervision

(J) Separation anxiety

(H) Avoidance syndromes
Panic disorder
Avoidance disorder
Paranoia
Psychosis

Assess severity

Mild   Moderate/ severe

Treat: Counseling

Family overprotective or fails to encourage attendance

Assess type of symptoms

(K) Folie à deux   Neglect

(L) Vulnerable child syndrome

(M) School phobia

Treat:
School Phobia
Program

Not improved   Improved

Follow-up:
Assess in
2–4 wk

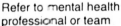

Refer to mental health professional or team

References

American Psychiatric Association. Diagnostic and statistical manual of mental disorders. 4th ed. Washington, DC: American Psychiatric Association, 1994.

Levine MD, Carey WB, Crocker AC, eds. Developmental-behavioral pediatrics. 2nd ed. Philadelphia: Saunders, 1992.

Schmitt BD. School avoidance. In: Parker S, Zuckerman B, eds. Behavioral and developmental pediatrics: A handbook for primary care. Boston: Little, Brown, 1995.

SCHOOL LEARNING PROBLEMS

Bonnie W. Camp, M.D., Ph.D.

School learning problems are present in an estimated 12% to 26% of schoolchildren, depending on the criteria and definition used and the population under study.

A. In the history determine signs of early childhood developmental delay, problems with growth or nutrition, sleeping disorders, toilet training, chronic illness, frequent hospitalizations, abuse, neglect, and family stress. Review any evaluations or therapies and obtain a comprehensive description of the child's behavior and learning from early infancy on. Pay particular attention to the history of speech and language development, as delay in this area is often present in the mentally retarded, slow learners, and children with specific learning disabilities as well as in those who have speech and language deficits.

B. In the physical examination note physical, dysmorphic, and other characteristics of neurologic or genetic disorders (e.g., cerebral palsy); coordination problems and neurologic soft signs; the latter probably reflect immaturity in neurologic development but are not diagnostic of a neurologic disorder.

C. Obtain directly from the school information about intelligence, achievement status, teacher's description of the child's behavior in the classroom, completion of a standard teacher rating scale for hyperactivity such as the ACTeRS scale, history of any sensory testing, attendance, individual educational plan, educational placement (grade, special education), and peer relations. A teacher's report of behavior in the classroom is essential; other testing can be performed independently.

D. A discrepancy of more than 20 points between IQ and standard scores of achievement or a difference of 35 or more percentile points almost always indicates some learning disability. For smaller differences see specific formulas (e.g., Camp). Differentiate among the mentally retarded child (achievement and IQ consistent and both more than two standard deviations below average), the slow learner (IQ and achievement both below average but consistent), and the child with specific learning disability (significant discrepancy between IQ and achievement). Screening tools for this assessment include the Wide Range Achievement Test (WRAT) and Kaufman Brief Intelligence Test (K-BIT).

E. Children who are functioning close to expectancy may have learning problems associated with mental retardation or low-normal functioning. Treatment of these problems is educational, and usually the pediatrician's role is to help the family ensure that the child has an appropriate educational program and to monitor progress. The child of average or above-average intelligence whose achievement is appropriate for IQ level but who fails to perform in school may present as having learning problems. Often, however, these children have attention deficit hyperactivity disorder (ADHD) or other behavioral problems that interfere with performance at school.

F. Children who are functioning at least 20% below average in one or all academic areas need individual educational programming (IEP). Detailed analysis of individual educational needs often requires the input of an educational specialist; however, simple analysis of the need for special education and the extent to which it is being provided can often reveal areas where the educational program is poorly adapted to the child's needs. A review of educational history often reveals major gaps in educational experience, numerous changes of school, and other disruptive experiences.

G. When the educational history and experience have been adequate and there is a significant difference between IQ and achievement in one or more areas, attempt to distinguish among specific and general learning disabilities, those with a genetic or neurologic basis, those that appear to be secondary to emotional problems or psychiatric disorder, and underachievement associated with weak motivation, family and cultural influences, or program failures.

H. Under Public Law 94-142 all children are entitled to a free and appropriate public education, including a variety of special education services. A common description of such services includes programs for blind, hearing-impaired, physically disabled, mentally retarded, and emotionally disturbed children and for those with behavior disorders and specific learning disabilities. Slow learners often do not meet criteria for special services, and thus it may be a problem to obtain adequate help. Any child can be referred for evaluation by the school staffing team. This team writes an IEP for each child and tries to implement it. Often the physician's role is to assist the family in making sure that appropriate services are received, to monitor progress, and to assist in obtaining private tutoring when necessary.

References

Camp BW. Developmental disorders. In: Hay W, Groothuis JR, Hayward AR, Levin MJ, eds. Current pediatric diagnosis and treatment. 12th ed. Norwalk, CT: Appleton & Lange, 1995.

Kaufman AS, Kaufman NS. Kaufman Brief Intelligence Test. Circles Pines, MN: American Guidance Service, 1990.

Levine MD, Carey WB, Crocker AC. Developmental and behavioral pediatrics. 2nd ed. Philadelphia: Saunders, 1992.

McLoughlin JA. Learning disabilities. In: Reynolds CR, Mann L, eds. Encyclopedia of special education. New York: Wiley, 1987.

Patient with SCHOOL LEARNING PROBLEM

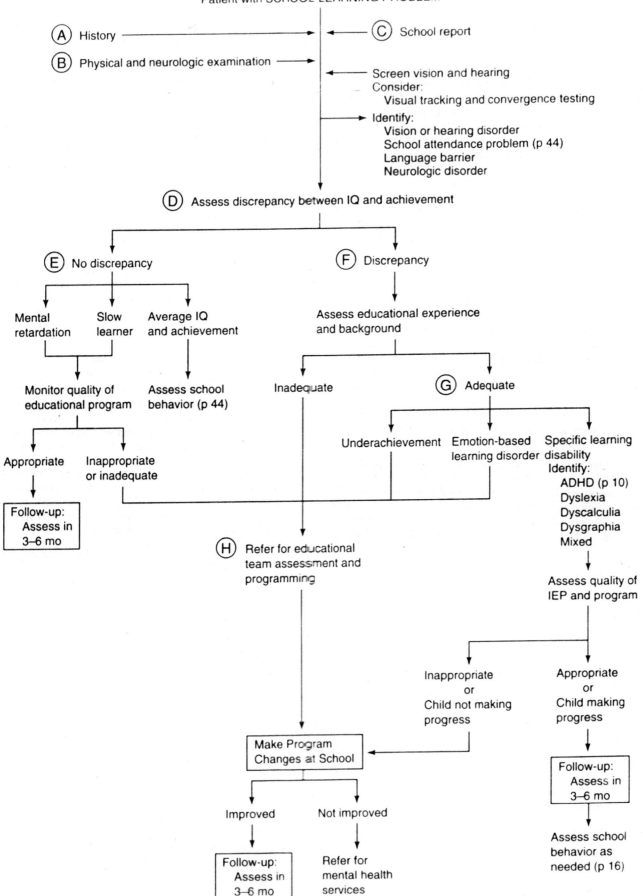

SLEEP DISTURBANCES

Michael I. Reiff, M.D.

Sleep problems occur in 20% to 30% of infants and children of preschool age. Problems include difficulty falling asleep, night waking, sleepwalking and talking, and night terrors. Infants usually develop a diurnal/nocturnal sleeping pattern by 6 weeks, and by 9 months most infants have developed patterns of well-consolidated nighttime sleep. Sleep problems in infants and children are generally filtered through parents' perceptions. Infants and children may remain undisturbed by their sleep patterns. Parental attitudes, expectations, and sleep habits as well as environmental factors, parent-child interactions, and general parenting skills must be considered. There is evidence that helping poor sleepers with their nighttime behavior also benefits their daytime interactions with key caregivers.

A. Bedtime rituals should be consistently reinforced. This may include establishing a routine bedtime: initiating developmentally appropriate routines such as regular attention to hygiene (washing, brushing teeth) and transitional routines (stories, books, prayers, "goodnights") and the introduction of transitional objects such as blankets or stuffed animals (*avoid* bottles and pacifiers). Children and infants should be put to bed while awake to avoid the necessity for other parental interventions during the night. Contingency charts can be used to reinforce these activities where developmentally appropriate.

B. There are three types of sleep regulation problems. *Delayed sleep phase* is the inability to go to sleep at a proposed bedtime, which results in delayed early morning awakening that may be perceived as behavior problems, struggles at bedtime, or lazy morning behavior. *Advanced sleep phase* is early nighttime sleep or difficulty staying awake until a proposed bedtime and early morning awakening (usually presents as parental complaints about early morning awakening). *Inappropriate sleep patterns* are regular late afternoon naps, early morning naps, or early morning feedings, which reinforce late bedtimes or interfere with reasonable early morning waking schedules.

C. *Phase delays* (1 to 3 hours) may be treated by putting the child to bed late (at the natural sleep time) — thus avoiding nighttime sleep struggles — then gradually awaken the child earlier and follow this by gradually earlier bedtimes. *Advanced sleep phases* can be treated with gradually later bedtimes and similar delays in naps and mealtimes. *Inappropriate sleep schedules* may be treated by carefully attending to nap times, early morning feeding patterns, and interactions or feedings during the night in conjunction with establishing regular and developmentally appropriate sleep schedules.

D. Encourage open communications about fears. Accommodations such as night lights and other changes in the sleep environment may be made. Children should be directly reassured about fears, and regular bedtime routines should be enforced (see A). Contingency charts can reinforce staying in bed and limiting verbal requests. A program for the gradual and staged withdrawal of attention around bedtime may be necessary and may include measures like a parent sleeping on a mattress in the child's room, progressively restricting physical and verbal attention, and gradually moving back to the parent's room. Relaxation and mental imagery may be used if developmentally appropriate.

(Continued on page 50)

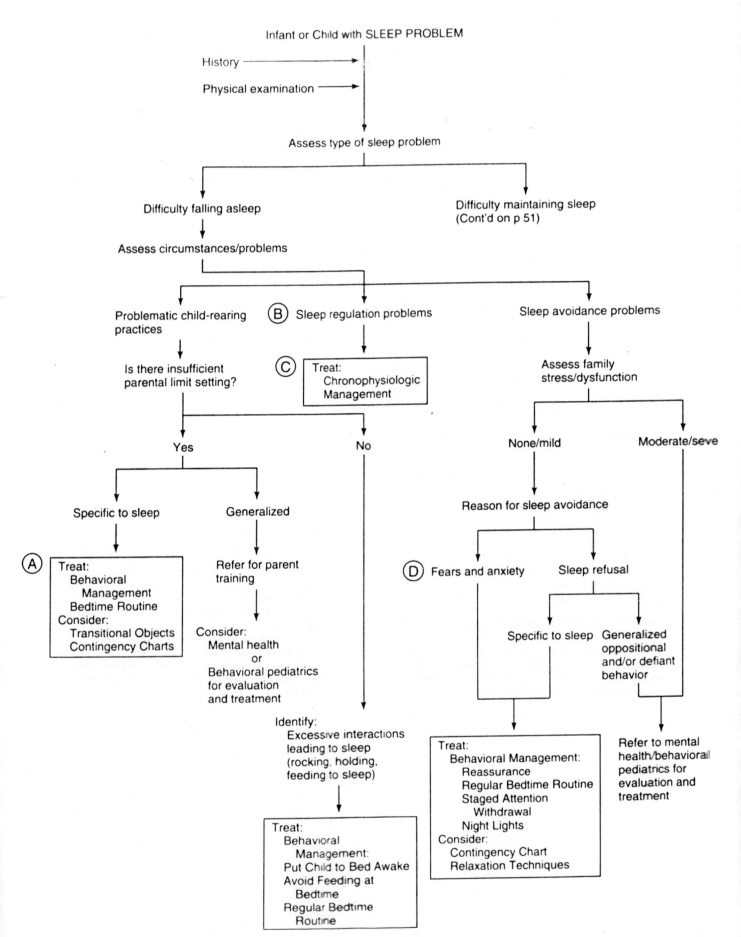

Infant or Child with SLEEP PROBLEM

History ⟶

Physical examination ⟶

Assess type of sleep problem

Difficulty falling asleep

Difficulty maintaining sleep
(Cont'd on p 51)

Assess circumstances/problems

Problematic child-rearing practices

(B) Sleep regulation problems

Sleep avoidance problems

Is there insufficient parental limit setting?

(C) Treat:
Chronophysiologic Management

Assess family stress/dysfunction

None/mild

Moderate/severe

Yes

No

Reason for sleep avoidance

Specific to sleep

Generalized

(D) Fears and anxiety

Sleep refusal

(A) Treat:
Behavioral
    Management
Bedtime Routine
Consider:
Transitional Objects
Contingency Charts

Refer for parent training

Specific to sleep

Generalized oppositional and/or defiant behavior

Consider:
Mental health
    or
Behavioral pediatrics
for evaluation
and treatment

Identify:
Excessive interactions
leading to sleep
(rocking. holding,
feeding to sleep)

Treat:
Behavioral Management:
    Reassurance
    Regular Bedtime Routine
    Staged Attention
        Withdrawal
    Night Lights
Consider:
    Contingency Chart
    Relaxation Techniques

Refer to mental
health/behavioral
pediatrics for
evaluation and
treatment

Treat:
Behavioral
    Management:
Put Child to Bed Awake
Avoid Feeding at
    Bedtime
Regular Bedtime
    Routine

E. Settling is an infant's ability to consolidate long, sustained sleep periods; e.g., the ability to sleep uninterrupted from midnight until 5:00 AM for 4 weeks, waking up less often than once a week.

F. Delayed settling is commonly seen in low birth weight premature infants, infants in whom there have been medical complications during pregnancy, and perinatally brain-damaged infants. Colic may also alter sleep schedules longer than the observed fussiness and irritability.

G. Certain feeding patterns tend to be associated with later settling. These include breast-feeding versus bottle-feeding, infants nursing constantly throughout the day for pacification, and infants fed large quantities at night. The early introduction of rice cereal does not affect sleeping through the night.

H. Transient disruptions of sleep may occur around times of acute family stress, with nightmares during vacations, or accompanying illness. Parents should respond appropriately to these awakenings but be cautious not to reinforce undesirable sleep patterns.

I. Infants and children should, ideally, be put to bed awake. All children may awaken several times during the night, but most can self-regulate a return to sleep. Infants who have learned to associate falling asleep with feeding will demand this upon night awakening. This problem can be managed by discontinuing bottles left in the bed, by phasing out night feedings, and by increasing intervals between daytime feedings. Some parents respond to nighttime crying by soothing, rocking, or comforting. Infants can become trained to expect this when they awaken. This situation can be managed by responding only briefly to periods of crying and increasing the intervals between responses.

J. Some parents are hypersensitive to children's night awakenings. Before responding they should give children sufficient time to self-regulate back to sleep rather than changing diapers or engaging in activities that lead to increased arousal.

K. Examine issues related to separation anxiety. Provide an optimal sleep environment, which may include night lights and open bedroom doors, and provide transitional objects. Parents may need to comfort children but should provide minimal stimulation. Consider closer monitoring of television and movie violence.

L. Night terrors occur in 5% of young children and present as screaming, talking, agitation, and thrashing or running. The child often cries out about dangers in the room. The child is actually still in a sleep state and cannot be comforted. This may be accompanied with autonomic signs including sweating and increased heart rate. Episodes last 5 to 30 minutes and end with the child quietly returning to calm sleep. Multiple episodes during the night are uncommon, and there is no recall of the episode. Night terrors are not associated with any psychological disorder. Interactions, like attempts to comfort and fully awaken the child, may lead to prolongation of symptoms or may complicate sleep problems.

M. Increased night awakenings can occur with conditions causing pain, cow's milk allergy, gastroesophageal reflux, persistent otitis media, or respiratory difficulties. Methylxanthines, stimulant medications, some anticonvulsants and antibiotics, as well as street drugs, can also lead to sleep disruption. Children who are mentally retarded or brain-damaged may not respond to behavioral management. Consider a trial of cow's milk exclusion when infant sleep problems persist despite appropriate changes in bedtime routine and other behavioral approaches.

N. When transitioning from crib to bed, reinforce healthy sleep initiation habits and consider behavior modification programs.

O. Examine issues of family functioning as well as cultural and socioeconomic issues when co-sleeping is associated with a sleep problem.

References

Adair R, Bauchner H. Sleep problems in childhood. Curr Probl Pediatrics 1993;147.

Edwards K, Christophersen E. Treating common sleep problems of young children. J Devel Behav Pediatr 1994; 15:207.

Fuchs-Schacter F, Fuchs M, Bijur PE, et al. Cosleeping and sleep problems in Hispanic-American urban young children. Pediatrics 1989; 84:522.

Lozoff B, Zuckerman B. Sleep problems in children. Pediatr Rev 1988; 10:17.

Macknin ML, VanderBrug Medendorp S, Maier MC. Infant sleep and bedtime cereal. Am J Dis Child 1989; 143:1066.

Minde K, Faucon A, Faulkner S. Sleep problems in toddlers: Effects on their daytime behavior. J Am Acad Adolesc Psychiatry 1994; 33, 8:1114.

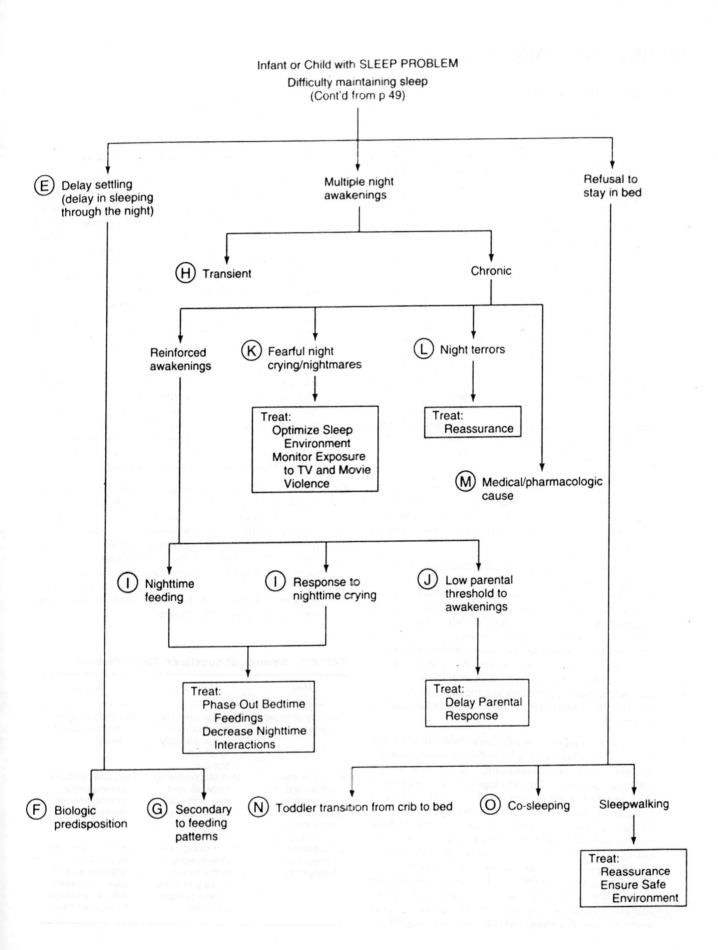

Infant or Child with SLEEP PROBLEM

Difficulty maintaining sleep
(Cont'd from p 49)

(E) Delay settling
(delay in sleeping
through the night)

Multiple night
awakenings

Refusal to
stay in bed

(H) Transient

Chronic

Reinforced
awakenings

(K) Fearful night
crying/nightmares

(L) Night terrors

Treat:
Optimize Sleep
Environment
Monitor Exposure
to TV and Movie
Violence

Treat:
Reassurance

(M) Medical/pharmacologic
cause

(I) Nighttime
feeding

(I) Response to
nighttime crying

(J) Low parental
threshold to
awakenings

Treat:
Phase Out Bedtime
Feedings
Decrease Nighttime
Interactions

Treat:
Delay Parental
Response

(F) Biologic
predisposition

(G) Secondary
to feeding
patterns

(N) Toddler transition from crib to bed

(O) Co-sleeping

Sleepwalking

Treat:
Reassurance
Ensure Safe
Environment

SUBSTANCE ABUSE

Kathleen A. Mammel, M.D.

A. Most of the clues to the diagnosis of substance abuse will be obtained from the history if it is obtained in a nonjudgmental fashion. Denial may cause the adolescent to minimize use, however. Speaking to the adolescent in a direct but supportive fashion may elicit more information. A history of acute drug abuse (overdose or suicide gesture), faltering school performance, mood swings, poor motivation, family conflict, change of peer groups, or trouble with the law is a red flag. Inquire about substances used, duration and frequency of use, amount used, and attitude toward use. Assuming the adolescent uses a substance gives him or her permission to discuss it; for example, ask "How much do you drink?" rather than "Do you drink?" Ask about peers, family relationships, school performance, and any pre-existing emotional or educational difficulties. Alcohol, marijuana, cocaine, and LSD are the drugs most commonly used by adolescents. Risk factors for substance abuse include characteristics of normal adolescence (love of danger, impulsiveness, need for immediate gratification), low self-esteem, poor coping skills, family history of substance abuse, parental modeling of smoking, drinking, or other drug use, family attitudes toward drugs, and drug-using peers.

B. Physical findings of substance abuse are minimal and nonspecific, such as injected sclera, signs of trauma, upper respiratory symptoms. Cocaine may cause episodic hypertension and tachycardia or nasal septum changes.

C. Drug screens are appropriate at the time of acute abuse or intoxication. Since substances may be misrepresented or adulterated, a drug screen should be done even if the adolescent can tell you what he or she used. Drug screens should not be done merely at the parent's or school's request. Their concern reveals that a problem exists. Separate interviews with the adolescent and parents is likely to identify the nature of the problem. Drug screening outside of an acute situation or monitoring during a treatment program may interfere with the physician-patient rapport and preclude further treatment.

D. Anticipatory guidance on substance abuse should begin during grade school and include discussions of situations the teenager is likely to encounter, such as how to deal with peer pressure. The development of good coping skills and strong self-esteem are also important. Education about the physical and psychological effects of various substances should be made available to both parents and adolescents. Families and physicians should give clear drug-free messages and encourage discussion. For the experimental user, a contract between patient and physician is often effective, but ongoing monitoring is necessary. During monitoring the physician should address school performance, family relations, peer relations, sexual activity, and substance use. Continued difficulties in school or home life or ongoing use requires further involvement of the parents and referral.

E. It is important to convince the parents of the severity of the situation before making a referral to therapy. Alleviating parental guilt may reduce enabling behavior and ensure follow-through. Self-help groups offer a drug-free peer group and support. This might include Alcoholics Anonymous or Narcotics Anonymous, which have teen groups in many locations, or a school group. Know whether the group provides support or treatment. Individual or family psychotherapy is indicated if it is unclear whether family dysfunction preceded or followed the substance abuse or when other issues are identified. A therapist who is skilled in working with adolescents and their families is needed.

F. The primary physician should see the patient again after referral to be sure that it was helpful and to let the adolescent know that the physician is still interested. Additional concerns, e.g., the need for contraception, may necessitate medical intervention. The physician may obtain urine drug screens for periodic monitoring, with the patient's knowledge and consent, and should be in frequent contact with the therapist.

G. Severe substance abuse requires removing the adolescent from drugs and a drug-using peer group, even if the substance abuse is considered to be a maladaptive coping pattern of other problems. This may be accomplished through a residential drug treatment center or adolescent inpatient psychiatric hospitalization. Treatment must require drug-free status, explore associated psychological issues, and require family involvement. Sufficient duration of treatment and aftercare are necessary to prevent recidivism.

TABLE 1 Severity of Substance Abuse Problem

Mild	Moderate	Severe
Curiosity or experimentation	Regular use of alcohol or marijuana, possibly other substances	Psychological or chemical dependency
Alcohol or marijuana used occasionally on weekends for recreation or social purposes	Use progresses to midweek and may occur before or during school	Daily use, difficulty achieving euphoria, frequent depression
Little change in behavior or functioning	Mood swings, decline in school performance, truancy, change of peer groups common	School failure, family conflicts, trouble with law evident; user may prostitute or sell drugs to support habit

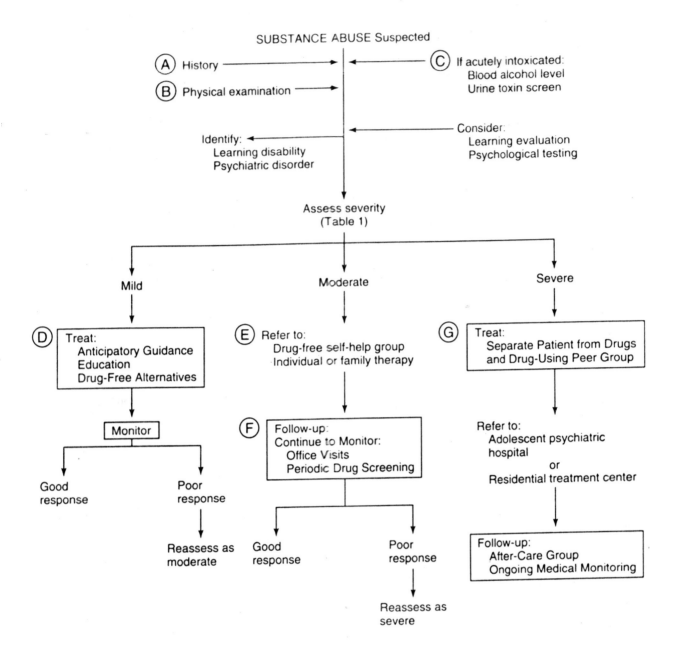

SUBSTANCE ABUSE Suspected

(A) History ——————→

(B) Physical examination ——————→

(C) If acutely intoxicated:
Blood alcohol level
Urine toxin screen

Identify: ←——————
Learning disability
Psychiatric disorder

Consider:
Learning evaluation
Psychological testing

Assess severity
(Table 1)

Mild

Moderate

Severe

(D) Treat:
Anticipatory Guidance
Education
Drug-Free Alternatives

(E) Refer to:
Drug-free self-help group
Individual or family therapy

(G) Treat:
Separate Patient from Drugs
and Drug-Using Peer Group

Monitor

(F) Follow-up:
Continue to Monitor:
Office Visits
Periodic Drug Screening

Refer to:
Adolescent psychiatric
hospital
or
Residential treatment center

Good
response

Poor
response

Good
response

Poor
response

Follow-up:
After-Care Group
Ongoing Medical Monitoring

Reassess as
moderate

Reassess as
severe

References

American Academy of Pediatrics Policy Statement. Screening for drugs of abuse in children and adolescents. AAP News. March 1989:9.

Anglin TM. Adolescent substance abuse. In: Hay WW, Groothuis JR, Hayward AR, Levin MJ, eds. Current pediatric diagnosis and treatment. 12th ed. Norwalk, CT: Appleton & Lange, 1995:210.

Hawkins JD, Lishner DM, Catalano RF Jr. Childhood predictors of adolescent substance abuse: Towards an empirically grounded theory. J Child Contemp Soc 1986; 18:1.

Kandel DB, Logan JA. Patterns of drug use from adolescence to young adulthood: I. Periods of risk for initiation, continued use, and discontinuation. Am J Pub Health 1984; 74:660.

Macdonald DI. Substance abuse. Pediatr Rev 1988; 10:89.

Schonberg SK, ed. Substance abuse: A guide for health professionals. American Academy of Pediatrics, 1988.

Smith DE, Schwartz RH, Martin DM. Heavy cocaine use by adolescents. Pediatrics 1989; 83:539.

CARDIOVASCULAR DISORDERS

Evaluation of Heart Disease/Cyanotic Heart
    Disease
Bradyarrhythmias
Congestive Heart Failure

Hypertension
Rheumatic Fever
Supraventricular Tachycardias

EVALUATION OF HEART DISEASE/CYANOTIC HEART DISEASE

James W. Wiggins, Jr., M.D.
Stephen Berman, M.D.

Central cyanosis is produced by 3 g or more of reduced hemoglobin per 100 ml of blood. This may be caused by one or more of the following physiologic abnormalities: (1) alveolar hypoventilation, (2) right-to-left shunt, (3) ventilation perfusion inequality, (4) impairment of diffusion in the lung, and (5) decreased affinity of hemoglobin for oxygen. Peripheral cyanosis is caused by vasomotor instability or a normal vasoconstrictive response to cold that causes decreased blood flow in the hands and feet. Abnormalities such as those described with central cyanosis are not present.

A. In the history document frequency, onset, and duration of cyanosis. Note precipitating factors such as feeding, exercise, respiratory infection, apnea, and seizures. Note associated symptoms such as cough, dyspnea, orthopnea, poor feeding, sweating, fatigue, squatting, weight loss, and failure to thrive. Note family history of congenital heart disease, history of acquired heart disease (rheumatic fever, Kawasaki syndrome), or pulmonary disease.

B. In the physical examination differentiate central from peripheral cyanosis. Central cyanosis is best visualized in the tongue and mucous membranes. Peripheral cyanosis associated with cool and sweaty extremities does not necessarily indicate central cyanosis. Assess the circulatory status, including blood pressure, heart rate, core temperature, capillary refill, pulses, and skin color. Assess presence and type of heart murmur (Tables 1 to 4). Note signs of heart disease, hyperdynamic precordium, single S_2, S_3-S_4 gallop, arrhythmia, clicks, friction rub, rales, wheezes, retractions, hepatomegaly, peripheral edema, and ascites. Look for signs of pulmonary, neurologic, or infectious disease.

C. The arterial blood gas (ABG) measures the partial pressure of dissolved oxygen in blood. Perform the ABG by obtaining a blood gas in room air (if possible) and 100% Fio_2. Suspect a fixed right-to-left shunt when 100% oxygen fails to increase the Pao_2 substantially. Cyanosis can be present with significant congestive heart failure because of pulmonary edema but should respond appropriately to oxygen. Cardiology consultation is necessary in all forms of symptomatic cardiac problems. Echocardiography is usually diagnostic and can often differentiate secondary pulmonary hypertension in the newborn from congenital heart disease.

D. Cardiac catheterization, medication (such as prostaglandin E_1), and surgical palliation or correction are often required shortly after diagnosis.

(Continued on page 59)

TABLE 1   Innocent Murmurs

Defect	Diagrammatic Representation	Chief Murmur Characteristics	Associated Findings
Carotid bruit		Systolic murmur near the clavicles or over the carotids; soft; faint thrill	Present at any age; murmur disappears on supination
Venous hum		Continuous murmur at clavicles	Detected during early school years; murmur disappears on supination, compression of jugular vein, turning head
Pulmonary flow murmur		Systolic murmur at ULSB; soft; in infants, transmits to back and axillae	Present in infants or adolescents; murmur dissipates on supination
Vibratory murmur (Still's)		Systolic murmur between LLSB and apex; musical	Detected during early school years; murmur intensifies on supination

A_2, aortic component of second heart sound; P_2, pulmonary component of heart sound; LLSB, lower left sternal border; LSB, left sternal border; ULSB, upper left sternal border; URSB, upper right sternal border.
Adapted from Park MK. Pediatric cardiology for practitioners. 2nd ed. Chicago: Year Book Medical Publishers, 1988. In Allen HD, Golinko RJ, Williams RG. Heart murmurs in children: When is a workup needed? Contemp Pediatr 1994; 11:29.

TABLE 2 Left-to-Right Shunts

Defect	Diagrammatic Representation	Chief Murmur Characteristics	Associated Findings
Ventricular septal defect		Well-localized holosystolic murmur usually at LLSB; thrill may be present; soft	Congenital lesion; common in fetal alcohol syndrome; Down syndrome; precordial hyperactivity may be present
Atrial septal defect		Ejection murmur at ULSB; loud S_1; widely split, fixed S_2; middiastolic murmur may be present	Congenital lesion; common in fetal alcohol syndrome; left chest may be enlarged
Patent ductus arteriosus		Continuous murmur along ULSB (seldom continuous in neonates); thrill; grade 1–4; machinery-like	Congenital lesion; often detected at birth, especially in preterm infants; bounding pulses, precordial hyperactivity may be present; murmur intensifies on supination
Acyanotic tetralogy of Fallot		Ejection murmur along LSB; usually no P component in S_2; thrill may be present	Congenital lesion; can be confused with ventricular septal defect
Coarctation of the aorta		Sometimes heard in back; thrill; soft; ejection clicks, early diastolic murmurs may be present if associated with bicuspid aortic valve	Arm pulses stronger and earlier than leg pulses; heaving apical impulse may be present

A_2, aortic component of second heart sound; P_2, pulmonary component of second heart sound; EC, ejection click; LLSB, lower left sternal border; LSB, left sternal border; ULSB, upper left sternal border; URSB, upper right sternal border.
Adapted from Park MK. Pediatric cardiology for practitioners. 2nd ed. Chicago: Year Book Medical Publishers, 1988. In Allen HD, Golinko RJ, Williams RG. Heart murmurs in children: When is a workup needed? Contemp Pediatr 1994; 11:29.

TABLE 3 Obstructive Lesions

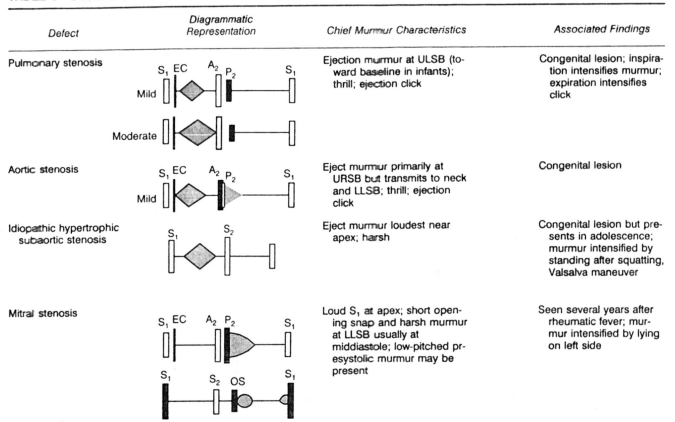

Defect	Diagrammatic Representation	Chief Murmur Characteristics	Associated Findings
Pulmonary stenosis	Mild / Moderate	Ejection murmur at ULSB (toward baseline in infants); thrill; ejection click	Congenital lesion; inspiration intensifies murmur; expiration intensifies click
Aortic stenosis	Mild	Eject murmur primarily at URSB but transmits to neck and LLSB; thrill; ejection click	Congenital lesion
Idiopathic hypertrophic subaortic stenosis		Eject murmur loudest near apex; harsh	Congenital lesion but presents in adolescence; murmur intensified by standing after squatting, Valsalva maneuver
Mitral stenosis		Loud S_1 at apex; short opening snap and harsh murmur at LLSB usually at middiastole; low-pitched presystolic murmur may be present	Seen several years after rheumatic fever; murmur intensified by lying on left side

A_2, aortic component of second heart sound; P_2, pulmonary component of second heart sound; EC, ejection click; OS, opening snap; LLSB, lower left sternal border; LSB, left sternal border; ULSB, upper left sternal border; URSB, upper right sternal border.
Adapted from Park MK. Pediatric cardiology for practitioners. 2nd ed. Chicago: Year Book Medical Publishers, 1988. In Allen HD, Golinko RJ, Williams RG. Heart murmurs in children: When is a workup needed? Contemp Pediatr 1994; 11:29.

TABLE 4 Regurgitant Lesions

Defect	Diagrammatic Representation	Chief Murmur Characteristics	Associated Findings
Aortic regurgitation		Early diastolic decrescendo murmur at or left of sternum; blowing; thrill, secondary midsystolic murmur due to increased flow may be present	May occur in Marfan syndrome; bounding pulses and precordial noise may be present; murmur intensified by sitting, leaning forward, and holding breath
Pulmonary regurgitation		Short, early diastolic murmur and secondary midsystolic murmur due to increased flow along LSB	Usually congenital lesion
Mitral regurgitation		Holosystolic murmur at apex, transmits to left axilla; grade 3–4; wide splitting of S_2; short rumbles after loud S_3	May occur in Marfan syndrome; precordial noise may be present; murmur heard at left axilla when lying on left side
Tricuspid regurgitation		Holosystolic murmur to immediate right or left of sternum; grade 2–3; wide splitting of S_2; short rumbles after loud S_3	Seen more often in infants, toddlers; inspiration intensifies murmur and S_3

A_2, aortic component of second heart sound; P_2, pulmonary component of second heart sound; LLSB, lower left sternal border; LSB, left sternal border; ULSB, upper left sternal border; URSB, upper right sternal border.
Adapted from Park MK. Pediatric cardiology for practitioners. 2nd ed. Chicago: Year Book Medical Publishers, 1988. In Allen HD, Golinko RJ, Williams RG. Heart murmurs in children: When is a workup needed? Contemp Pediatr 1994; 11:29.

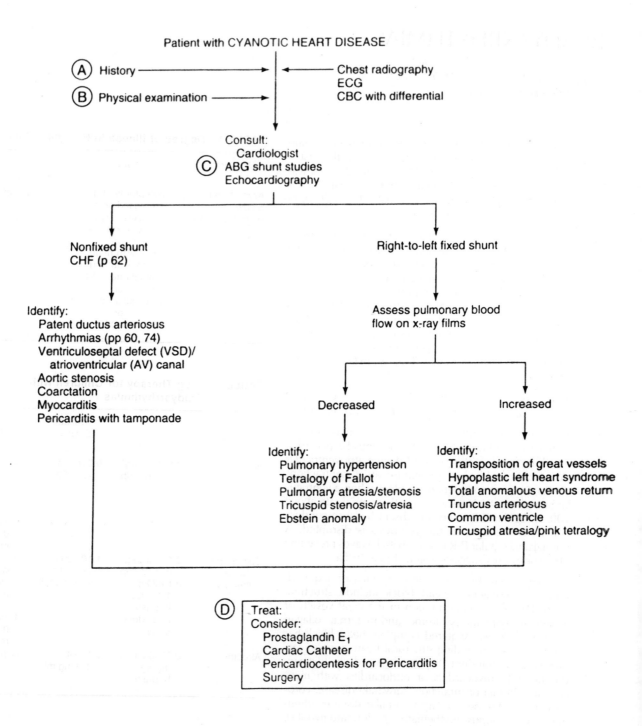

Patient with CYANOTIC HEART DISEASE

(A) History ⟶ ⟵ Chest radiography
ECG
(B) Physical examination ⟶ CBC with differential

Consult:
Cardiologist
(C) ABG shunt studies
Echocardiography

Nonfixed shunt
CHF (p 62)

Right-to-left fixed shunt

Identify:
Patent ductus arteriosus
Arrhythmias (pp 60, 74)
Ventriculoseptal defect (VSD)/
atrioventricular (AV) canal
Aortic stenosis
Coarctation
Myocarditis
Pericarditis with tamponade

Assess pulmonary blood
flow on x-ray films

Decreased

Increased

Identify:
Pulmonary hypertension
Tetralogy of Fallot
Pulmonary atresia/stenosis
Tricuspid stenosis/atresia
Ebstein anomaly

Identify:
Transposition of great vessels
Hypoplastic left heart syndrome
Total anomalous venous return
Truncus arteriosus
Common ventricle
Tricuspid atresia/pink tetralogy

(D) Treat:
Consider:
Prostaglandin E$_1$
Cardiac Catheter
Pericardiocentesis for Pericarditis
Surgery

References

Allen HD, Golinko RJ, Williams, RG. Heart murmurs in children: When is a workup needed? Contemp Pediatr 1994; 11:29.

Guntheroth WG. Initial evaluation of child for heart disease. Pediatr Clin North Am 1978; 25:657.

Kawabori I. Cyanotic congenital heart defects with decreased pulmonary blood flow. Pediatr Clin North Am 1978; 25:759.

Kawabori I. Cyanotic congenital heart defects with increased pulmonary blood flow. Pediatr Clin North Am 1978; 25:777.

Morray JP, Lynn AM, Mansfield PB. Effect of pH and Pco$_2$ on pulmonary and systemic hemodynamics after surgery in children with congenital heart disease and pulmonary hypertension. J Pediatr 1988; 113:474.

Rudolph AM. Causes of cyanosis in newborn infants. Pediatrics, 18th ed. New York: Appleton & Lange, 1987:1306.

Shannon DC, Lasser M, Goldbatt A, et al. The cyanotic infant: Heart disease or lung disease. N Engl J Med 1972; 287:951.

BRADYARRHYTHMIAS

James W. Wiggins, Jr., M.D.
Stephen Berman, M.D.

Suspect a bradyarrhythmia when the resting awake heart rate is less than 100 beats per minute (bpm) during the first 3 months of life, less than 80 for children under 2 years, less than 70 for children 2 to 10 years, and less than 55 for adolescents. A sleeping heart rate is usually 10 to 20 bpm lower in infants and young children.

A. Determine the onset, duration, and severity of the slow heart rate. Note symptoms related to decreased cerebral flow such as syncope, dizziness, and confusion. Symptoms of congestive heart failure (CHF) include poor feeding, irritability, sweating, puffiness, cyanotic spells, and symptoms of respiratory distress. Chest pain and angina suggest decreased coronary artery blood flow. Identify predisposing conditions such as structural heart disease, prior cardiac surgery, medications or drug ingestions, collagen vascular diseases, hypothyroidism, CNS disorders, and recent viral illness.

B. Assess the cardiac status. Note signs of CHF and underlying structural heart disease (see pp 56 to 62).

C. The ECG will identify most bradyarrhythmias as complete or second-degree heart block, sinus bradycardia, slow junctional rhythm, second-degree atrioventricular (AV) block or blocked premature atrial contractions (PACs). Suspect complete heart block when a ventricular rate of 4 to 80 is associated with an atrial rate above 100. A regular P-R interval is absent because conduction from the atria to the ventricles is disrupted. A normal and regular P-R interval with P waves preceding QRS complexes suggests a sinus bradycardia.

D. Complete heart block can be congenital or acquired. Causes of congenital heart block include structural heart disease (levotransposition of the great vessels or asplenia-polysplenia syndrome) and maternal collagen vascular diseases. Acquired complete heart block has several causes, including structural heart disease, cardiac surgery (transient or permanent), drugs (digoxin, propranolol), myocarditis or endocarditis with myocardial ischemia or infarction (Kawasaki disease, coronary artery disease), collagen vascular diseases (rheumatic fever, lupus erythematosus, dermatomyositis), glycogen storage diseases (Pompe disease), and cardiac tumors.

E. Causes of sinus pauses (sick sinus syndrome) include drugs (digoxin, propranolol), myocarditis or endocarditis, cardiac surgery, structural heart disease, hypothyroidism, and conditions associated with elevated intracranial pressure (meningoencephalitis, brain tumor).

F. Treat severely ill patients who have a complete AV block with isoproterenol or epinephrine 0.1 to 1 µg/kg/minute. If bradycardia persists, institute emergency transvenous pacing. Consider a trial of atropine (Table 2) in patients with sinus bradycardia (avoid with blocked PACs). Close monitoring is essential, since

TABLE 1   Degree of Illness in Bradyarrhythmia

Moderate	Severe	Very Severe
Asymptomatic Stable Heart rate ≥ 45	Symptoms of decreased cerebral or coronary artery blood flow *or* Infant with heart rate ≤ 50 and atrial rate > 140 *or* Ventricular rate < 45 *or* Widened QRS	Signs of shock, congestive heart failure, or altered mental status

TABLE 2   Drug Therapy for Children with Bradyarrhythmias

Drug	Dosage	Available Solutions	Remarks
Isoproterenol	0.1–1 µg/kg/min IV drip	0.2 mg/ml (1:5000)	0.6 × body weight in kilograms = mg dose in 100 ml 1 ml/hr = 0.1 µg/kg/min
Epinephrine Acute therapy	0.1–1 µg/kg/min IV drip 0.1 ml/kg 1:10,000 IV push (max dose 5 ml)	1:10,000 concentration (0.1 mg/ml)	0.6 × body weight in kilograms = mg dose in 100 ml 1 ml/hr = 0.1 µg/kg/min
Atropine	0.02–0.04 mg/kg IV push	0.1, 0.4, 1.0 mg/ml	IV push

pharmacologic therapy may be complicated by a tachyarrhythmia.

G. Refer for a permanent pacemaker patients at high risk of developing a tachyarrhythmia, CHF, or episodes of decreased cerebral or coronary blood flow.

References

Chameides L, ed. Textbook of advanced life support. Dallas: American Heart Association; 1989.

Fish F, Benson DW. Disorders of cardiac rhythm and conduction. In: Emmanouilides GC, Riemenschneider TA, Allen HD,

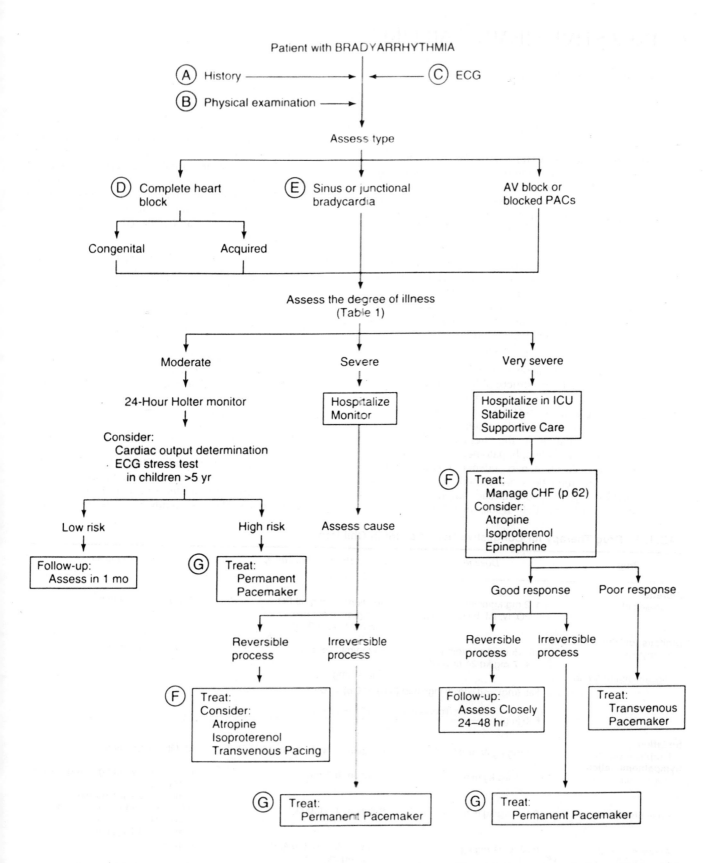

Patient with BRADYARRHYTHMIA

(A) History ──────────→ ←────── (C) ECG

(B) Physical examination ──→

Assess type

(D) Complete heart block

(E) Sinus or junctional bradycardia

AV block or blocked PACs

Congenital   Acquired

Assess the degree of illness
(Table 1)

Moderate   Severe   Very severe

24-Hour Holter monitor

Hospitalize
Monitor

Hospitalize in ICU
Stabilize
Supportive Care

Consider:
Cardiac output determination
ECG stress test
in children >5 yr

(F) Treat:
Manage CHF (p 62)
Consider:
Atropine
Isoproterenol
Epinephrine

Low risk   High risk   Assess cause

Good response   Poor response

Follow-up:
Assess in 1 mo

(G) Treat:
Permanent
Pacemaker

Reversible
process

Irreversible
process

Reversible
process

Irreversible
process

Treat:
Transvenous
Pacemaker

(F) Treat:
Consider:
Atropine
Isoproterenol
Transvenous Pacing

Follow-up:
Assess Closely
24–48 hr

(G) Treat:
Permanent Pacemaker

(G) Treat:
Permanent Pacemaker

Gutgesell HP, eds. Heart disease in infants, children and adolescents. 5th ed. Baltimore: Williams & Wilkins, 1995:1555.

Garson G, Gillette PC, McNamara DG. A guide to cardiac dysrhythmias in children. New York: Grune & Stratton, 1980

Karpawich PP, Gillette PC, Garson A, et al. Congenital complete atrioventricular block: Clinical and electrophysiologic predictors of need for pacemaker insertion. Am J Cardiol 1981, 48:1098.

CONGESTIVE HEART FAILURE

James W. Wiggins Jr., M.D.

DEFINITION

Congestive heart failure (CHF) is a failure of the heart to keep up with the demands of the body. This may result from pressure overload (outflow or inflow obstructions), volume overload (left-to-right shunts, valve regurgitation, severe anemia), depressed myocardial function (cardiomyopathy, myocarditis, ischemia, toxins, hypoglycemia, hypocalcemia, sepsis), and arrhythmias.

A. In the history note symptoms such as feeding difficulties, sweating, cough, dyspnea, orthopnea, wheezing, and puffiness. Identify predisposing conditions such as congenital heart disease, acquired heart disease (rheumatic fever, cor pulmonale, endocarditis, storage diseases), medications and drugs, and hematologic disorders (hemolytic anemia, thalassemia, sickle cell disease).

B. In the physical examination assess the circulatory status: note signs of CHF and structural heart disease. These signs include tachycardia (>160 beats per minute [bpm] during infancy, >100 bpm in older children), heart murmurs, clicks, S_3-S_4 gallop, pulsus alterans (beat-to-beat variation in the strength of the pulse), jugular venous distention, hepatomegaly, cyanosis, and edema. Suspect pulmonary edema if cough, rales, wheezes, and retractions are present. Cool, mottled extremities suggest poor cardiac output and vasoconstriction. Chronic CHF results in failure to thrive.

C. On the chest radiograph note any cardiomegaly or pulmonary congestion. Cardiomegaly can be caused by ventricular dilation secondary to volume overload, myocardial function abnormalities, or a pericardial effusion. On electrocardiography note arrhythmias, cardiac ischemia, and ventricular hypertrophy. An echocardiogram will identify a pericardial effusion and underlying structural heart disease and assess cardiac contractility and performance.

D. Treat arrhythmias associated with digitalis toxicity with phenytoin, pacemaker, and/or digoxin-immune Fab (antigen-binding fragments). Perform pericardiocentesis when a pericardial effusion produces tamponade. Correct electrolyte abnormalities that impair cardiac function such as hypokalemia or hyperkalemia, hypercalcemia, or hyponatremia. Correct a severe anemia with a slow packed red blood cell transfusion (consider a partial exchange transfusion). Treat underlying primary pulmonary disease such as pneumonia, which contributes to CHF by causing hypoxia and/or pulmonary vasoconstriction.

E. Hospitalize in an ICU very severely ill patients with shock, marked respiratory distress, or altered mental status. Monitor continuously arterial blood pressure, central venous pressure or pulmonary wedge pressures, and urine output. Administer oxygen and monitor arterial blood gases (ABG) frequently. Intubate and ventilate

TABLE 1 Drug Therapy for Congestive Heart Failure in Children

Drug	Dosage	Product Availability	Remarks
Diuretic			
Furosemide	1–2 mg/kg/dose PO, IV, IM, b.i.d. or t.i.d.	Solution: 10 mg/ml PO 10 mg/ml injectable Tabs: 20, 40, 80 mg	IV push <4 mg/min
Digitalis toxicity			
Phenytoin	10–15 mg/kg loading 4–7 mg/kg/24 hr b.i.d.	50 mg/ml injectable	Slow push over 20 min
Digoxin-immune Fab		Vial: 40 mg	
	Fab (mg) = (Digoxin ingested [mg] × 0.8) × **66.7**		
	$$\text{Fab (mg)} = \frac{\text{Serum digoxin (ng/ml)} \times \text{BW (kg)} \times 5.6}{1000} \times 66.7$$		
Sedation			
Morphine sulfate	0.1 mg/kg IV or IM	Solution: 2, 4, 5, 8, 10, 15 mg/ml	Monitor respirations
Sympathomimetics			
Isoproterenol	0.1–1 μg/kg/min	Solution: 0.2 mg/ml	0.6 × body wt in kg = mg dose in 100 ml 1 ml/hr = 0.1 μg/kg/min
Epinephrine	0.1–1 μg/kg/min	Solution: 1:10,000	0.6 × body wt in kg = mg dose in 100 ml 1 ml/hr = 0.1 μg/kg/min
Atropine	0.02–0.04 mg/kg	Solution: 0.1, 0.3, 0.4, 0.5, 1, 1.2 mg/ml	IV push
Dopamine	5–20 μg/kg/min	Solution: 40, 80, 160 mg/ml	6 × body wt in kg = mg dose in 100 ml 1 ml/hr = 1 μg/kg/min
Dobutamine	2–15 μg/kg/min	Solution: 12.5 mg/ml	6 × body wt kg = mg dose in 100 ml 1 ml/hr = 1 μg/kg/min

(Continued on page 64)

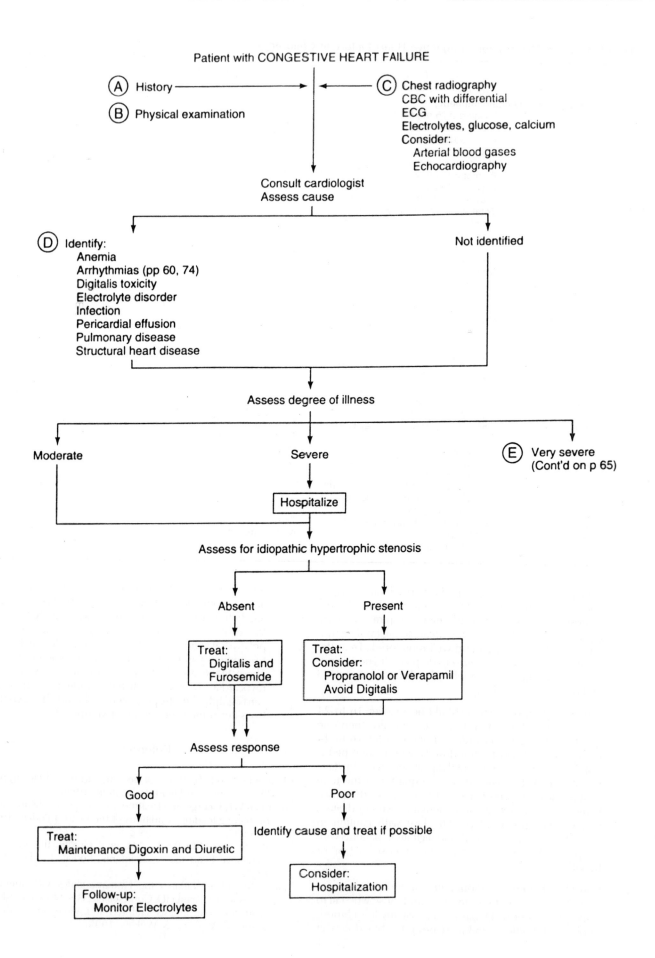

Patient with CONGESTIVE HEART FAILURE

Ⓐ History

Ⓑ Physical examination

Ⓒ Chest radiography
CBC with differential
ECG
Electrolytes, glucose, calcium
Consider:
    Arterial blood gases
    Echocardiography

Consult cardiologist
Assess cause

Ⓓ Identify:
    Anemia
    Arrhythmias (pp 60, 74)
    Digitalis toxicity
    Electrolyte disorder
    Infection
    Pericardial effusion
    Pulmonary disease
    Structural heart disease

Not identified

Assess degree of illness

Moderate

Severe

Ⓔ Very severe
(Cont'd on p 65)

Hospitalize

Assess for idiopathic hypertrophic stenosis

Absent

Present

Treat:
Digitalis and
Furosemide

Treat:
Consider:
    Propranolol or Verapamil
    Avoid Digitalis

Assess response

Good

Poor

Treat:
    Maintenance Digoxin and Diuretic

Identify cause and treat if possible

Follow-up:
    Monitor Electrolytes

Consider:
    Hospitalization

Drug	Dosage	Product Availability	Remarks
Inotropic agents (nonsympathomimetic)			
Amirone lactate	Loading 0.75 mg/kg/dose over 2–3 min Continuous infusion 5–10 μg/kg/min Max 10 mg/kg/24 hr	Solution: 5 mg/ml IV	
Digoxin	Premature or newborn Loading doses: give ½ total loading dose initially and ¼ q6h × 2 **Total** dose 30 μg/kg IV/24 hr Infant, child 40 μg/kg/24 hr b.i.d. IV or PO; max depends on serum digoxin level (therapeutic range 0.8–2 ng/ml) Maintenance all 10 μg/kg/24 hr given b.i.d.	Tabs: 0.125, 0.25, 0.5 mg Solution: 50 μg/ml PO liquid 100 μg/ml IV	
Vasodilators			
Hydralazine	0.1–0.2 mg/kg/dose IM or IV q4–6h PO: 0.75–1 mg/kg/day; max 7.5 mg/kg/day	Solution: 20 mg/ml injectable Tabs: 10, 25, 50, 100 mg	
Sodium nitroprusside	0.5–1 μg/kg/min Begin 0.5–1 μg/kg/min and titrate to desired effect	Vial: 50 mg/vial	0.6 × body wt kg = mg dose in 100 ml 1 ml/hr = 1 μg/kg/min
Propranolol	IV 0.01–0.1 mg/kg/dose slow push over 5 min (max 1 mg) PO 0.5–1 mg/kg/dose q6h	Liquid: 1 mg/ml Tabs: 10, 20, 40, 60, 80, 90 mg SR caps: 80, 120, 160 mg	
Verapamil	Children: PO 4–8 mg/kg/day t.i.d.-q.i.d. IV 100–300 μg/kg (max 5 mg)	Tabs: 40, 80, 120 mg SR tabs: 120, 180, 240 mg IV: 2.5 mg/ml	
Captopril	Infants <2 mo: 0.1–0.25 mg/kg/dose q8–24h Infants >2 mo, children: 0.3–0.5 mg/kg/24 hr in 1–4 divided doses, max 6 mg/kg/day	Tabs: 12.5, 25, 50 mg	
Enalapril	PO 0.1 mg/kg/day qd or b.i.d. (titrate up) IV 5–10 μg/kg/dose q8–24h	Tabs: 2.5, 5, 10 mg IV: 1.25 mg/ml	

SR, sustained release.

if the patient is severely agitated with borderline oxygenation or evidence of pending respiratory failure. Correct acidosis; avoid sodium bicarbonate if respiratory failure is present. Consider morphine sulfate for agitation only if the patient is intubated and well monitored. Treat the patient initially with IV furosemide push. If good urine-flow is not established, double the dose of furosemide and repeat it after 1 hour.

F. Administration of digitalis should occur over 16 to 24 hours: give half of the total dosage initially, then one quarter 8 to 12 hours later and one quarter 16 to 24 hours later. Administer the dose IV when tissue perfusion is poor at 80% of the total digitalis dosage. The daily maintenance dose should be one quarter of the total digitalis dosage given twice a day. Consider the possibility of digitalis toxicity or inadequate levels of digitalis in patients who develop CHF. Use with caution in patients with myocarditis. Avoid digitalis in patients with idiopathic hypertrophic subaortic stenosis (IHSS) or hypokalemia.

G. Consider dopamine, dobutamine, amirone lactate, or isoproterenol for patients in shock and those who fail to respond to therapy. Dopamine has slightly less chronotropic cardiac effects and increases renal blood flow at infusion rates less than 20 mg/kg/minute. Dobutamine and amirone lactate have mostly inotropic effects and are better agents for severe myocardial dysfunction. Vasodilators (afterload-reducing agents), such as captopril, hydralazine, and sodium nitroprusside, can be used to produce vasodilation and improve cardiac output. These agents are most effective in patients with severe myocardial dysfunction. If IHSS is identified by echocardiography, inotropic agents should be avoided. Consider using propranolol or verapamil.

References

Chameides L, ed. Textbook of pediatric advanced life support. Dallas: American Heart Association, 1989.

Friedman WF, George BL. Treatment of congestive heart failure by altering loading conditions of the heart. J Pediatr 1985; 106:697.

Ross RD, Bollinger RO, Pinsky WW, et al. Grading the severity of congestive heart failure in infants. Pediatr Cardiol 1992; 13:72.

Talner NS. Heart failure. In: Emmanouilides GC, Riemenschneider TA, Allen HD, Gutgesell HP, eds. Moss and Adams heart disease in infants, children and adolescents. 5th ed. Baltimore: Williams & Wilkins, 1995.

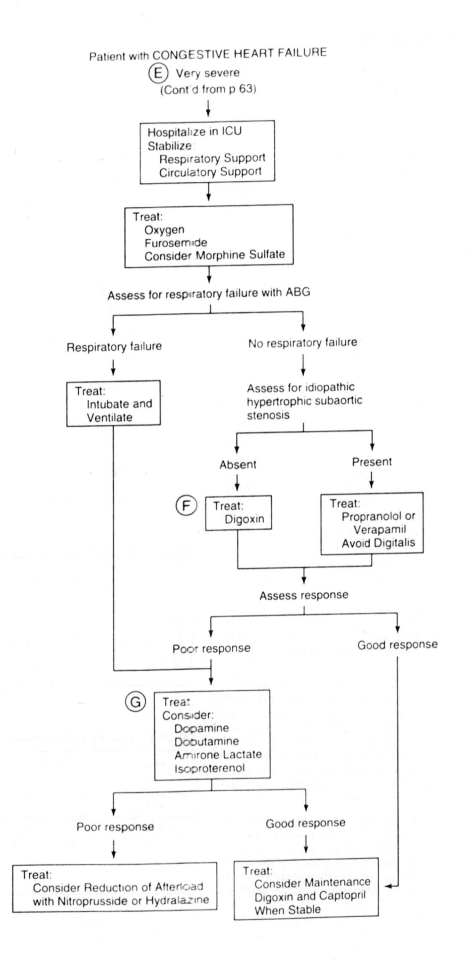

Patient with CONGESTIVE HEART FAILURE
(E) Very severe
(Cont'd from p 63)

Hospitalize in ICU
Stabilize:
    Respiratory Support
    Circulatory Support

Treat:
    Oxygen
    Furosemide
    Consider Morphine Sulfate

Assess for respiratory failure with ABG

Respiratory failure

Treat:
    Intubate and
    Ventilate

No respiratory failure

Assess for idiopathic
hypertrophic subaortic
stenosis

Absent

(F) Treat:
    Digoxin

Present

Treat:
    Propranolol or
    Verapamil
    Avoid Digitalis

Assess response

Poor response

Good response

(G) Treat:
Consider:
    Dopamine
    Dobutamine
    Amirone Lactate
    Isoproterenol

Poor response

Good response

Treat:
    Consider Reduction of Afterload
    with Nitroprusside or Hydralazine

Treat:
    Consider Maintenance
    Digoxin and Captopril
    When Stable

HYPERTENSION

James W. Wiggins Jr., M.D.
Stephen Berman, M.D.

DEFINITION

Hypertension is blood pressure exceeding the 90th percentile for age, height, and weight of the patient (Table 1). Blood pressures should be taken with an appropriate-sized blood pressure cuff. The bladder should be wide enough to equal or exceed two thirds of the length of the upper arm and should completely encircle the arm. The muffling of the pulse should be taken as diastolic blood pressure.

A. In the history ask about family history of hypertension, heart disease, stroke and symptoms of nausea, headache, irritability, failure to thrive, and deteriorating school performance. Ask about use of an umbilical artery catheter in the newborn. Note full review of systems, including renal and metabolic, and current medications.

B. Blood pressure and pulses should be taken in all four extremities. Differential pulses or differences in blood pressures between upper and lower extremities suggest coarctation of the aorta. Perform a thorough funduscopic examination, looking for arteriovenous nicking, tortuosity, hemorrhage, and papilledema. Note signs of hypertensive encephalopathy such as seizures, stroke, altered mental status, focal neurologic defects. In the abdominal examination note presence and size of both kidneys. An abdominal bruit suggests renal artery stenosis. Note edema, thyroid size, hirsutism, striae, and other signs of endocrine disorder.

C. Assess the severity of hypertension (Table 2). Severely ill patients may have signs of congestive heart failure (infants), hypertensive encephalopathy, or accelerated hypertension. Moderate hypertension may have mild or no symptoms and diastolic pressures 10 to 15 mm Hg above normal. Mild hypertension is usually asymptomatic, with mild diastolic pressure elevation.

D. Perform a basic diagnostic evaluation in patients with documented blood pressures above the 95th percentile and in those with blood pressures between the 90th and 95th percentiles who have elevation documented weekly for 4 weeks. The evaluation includes CBC, urinalysis and urine culture, serum sodium, potassium, chloride, carbon dioxide, BUN, creatinine, and echocardiogram (for baseline left ventricular mass). Add a lipid profile if patient has essential hypertension or if the family has a history of hypertension.

E. Nonpharmacologic therapy includes reduced sodium intake, weight reduction for obese patients, exercise, change in lifestyle, and decreased stress. Avoid stimulant medications, sympathomimetic amines, amphetamines, steroids, oral contraceptives, and decongestants, which may elevate pressures. Discourage cigarette smoking.

An exercise stress test perhaps should precede an exercise program.

F. First-line medications for hypertension include β-blockers (such as propranolol) and/or a diuretic (such as hydrochlorothiazide). For dosages, see Table 3. Both drug groups may be lipogenic, and serum lipids must be followed.

G. For severe hypertension, diazoxide given as an IV push followed by diuretics (unless volume contracted) and other parenteral antihypertensives (β-blockers, diuretics, vasodilators) should be used. Patients must be monitored closely during administration.

H. Patients unresponsive to diazoxide may be treated with a continuous infusion of sodium nitroprusside. When used longer than 48 hours and/or in high dosages, monitor for cyanide toxicity.

I. For moderately ill patients, parenteral β-blockers, diuretics, or vasodilators (hydralazine) may be indicated.

J. An extensive diagnostic evaluation includes chest radiography, ECG, creatinine clearance, renal ultrasonography, renal scan, intravenous pyelography, vesicoureterography, and renal angiography.

(Continued on page 68)

TABLE 1 Blood Pressures Indicating Hypertension

Age	Systolic (mm Hg) >90%	Diastolic (mm Hg) >90%
Newborn–7 days	>100	—
8–30 days	>110	—
1 month–2 years	>124	>74
3–12 years	>130	>86
>12 years	>144	>90

TABLE 2 Severity of Hypertension

Mild	Moderate	Severe
Asymptomatic and	Mild symptoms or	Signs of congestive heart failure or
Diastolic pressure <15 mm Hg above normal	Diastolic pressure ≥15 mm Hg above normal	Hypertensive encephalopathy or Accelerated hypertension

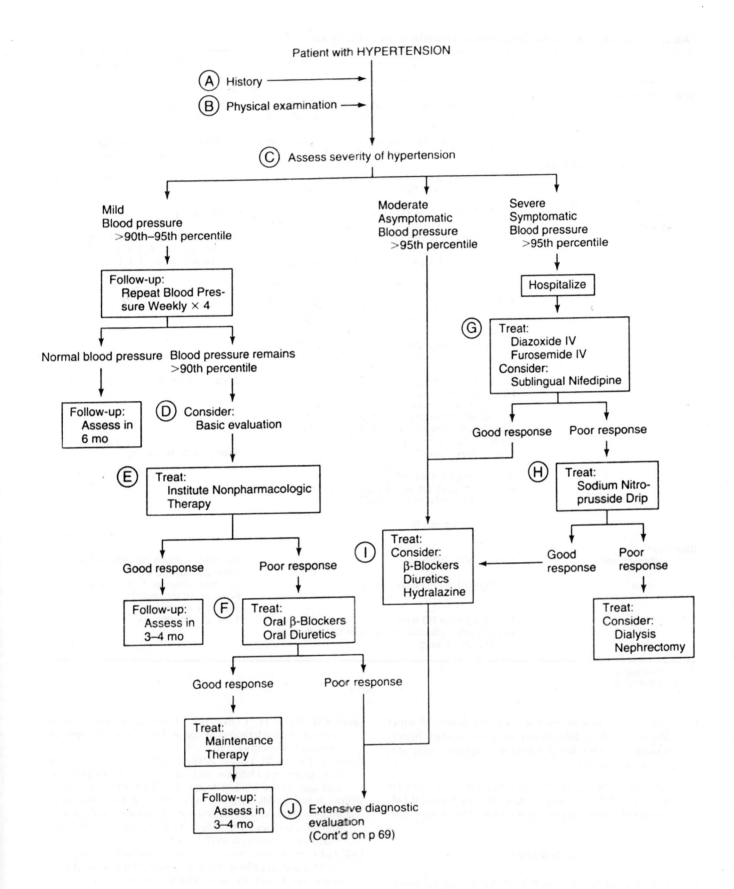

Patient with HYPERTENSION

(A) History ──────────→
(B) Physical examination ──→

(C) Assess severity of hypertension

Mild
Blood pressure
>90th–95th percentile

Moderate
Asymptomatic
Blood pressure
>95th percentile

Severe
Symptomatic
Blood pressure
>95th percentile

Follow-up:
Repeat Blood Pres-
sure Weekly × 4

Hospitalize

(G) Treat:
Diazoxide IV
Furosemide IV
Consider:
Sublingual Nifedipine

Normal blood pressure

Blood pressure remains
>90th percentile

Follow-up:
Assess in
6 mo

(D) Consider:
Basic evaluation

Good response

Poor response

(E) Treat:
Institute Nonpharmacologic
Therapy

(H) Treat:
Sodium Nitro-
prusside Drip

Good response

Poor response

Good response

Poor
response

Follow-up:
Assess in
3–4 mo

(F) Treat:
Oral β-Blockers
Oral Diuretics

(I) Treat:
Consider:
β-Blockers
Diuretics
Hydralazine

Treat:
Consider:
Dialysis
Nephrectomy

Good response

Poor response

Treat:
Maintenance
Therapy

Follow-up:
Assess in
3–4 mo

(J) Extensive diagnostic
evaluation
(Cont'd on p 69)

TABLE 3 Drugs Used in the Treatment of Hypertension in Children

Drug	Dosage	Product Availability
Severe hypertension		
Diazoxide	1–3 mg/kg/dose rapid IV push up to 150 mg/dose Repeat in 5–15 min until good reduction in BP, then q4–24h p.r.n.	Injectable solution: 15 mg/5 ml
Sodium nitroprusside	0.5–10 µg/kg/min IV drip (titrate up) (avoid exposure to light)	50 mg vial 0.6 × body wt kg = mg dose in 100 ml 1 ml/hr = 0.1 µg/kg/min
Moderate to severe hypertension		
Hydralazine	0.1–0.2 mg/kg/dose IM or IV q4–6h 0.75–3 mg/kg/24 hr PO q6–12h (max 7.5 mg/kg/day)	Injectable solution: 20 mg/ml Tabs: 10, 25, 50, 100 mg
Calcium channel blocker Nifedipine	0.25–0.5 mg/kg/dose PO t.i.d. or q.i.d.	Caps: 10 mg
β-Blocker Propranolol	0.01–0.1 mg/kg/dose slow IV push over 5 min Begin 0.5–1 mg/kg/24 hr PO q6–12h, then increase at 3–5 day intervals to maximum 2 mg/kg/24 hr p.r.n. Infants <2 mo: 0.05–0.1 mg/kg/dose PO t.i.d. or q.i.d. Infants >2 mo and children: Begin 0.15 mg/kg/dose IV given over 5 min, double at 2 hr intervals until hypertension is controlled; maximum dose 6 mg/kg/24 hr Adolescents: Begin 25 mg PO b.i.d. or t.i.d., then increase at 1–2 wk intervals to maximum 150 mg t.i.d.	Tabs: 10, 20, 40, 60, 80, 90 mg SR cap: 80, 120, 160 mg Injectable solution: 1 mg/ml
Captopril	Child: Begin 0.15 mg/kg/dose Double at 2 hr intervals until hypertension is controlled; maximum dosage 6 mg/kg/24 hr Adolescent: Begin 25 mg b.i.d. or t.i.d. Increase at 1–2 wk intervals to maximum 150 mg t.i.d.	Tabs: 12.5, 25, 50, 100 mg
Enalapril maleate	Children: 0.05–0.15 mg/kg/dose PO qd or b.i.d., maximum 40 mg/24 hr or 0.05–0.1 mg/kg/dose q6h IV Adolescent/adult: 2.5–5 mg/day PO increase to 10–40 mg/day in 1–2 divided doses or 0.625–1.25 mg q6h IV	Injectable solution: 1.25 mg/ml Tabs: 2.5, 5, 10, 20 mg
Diuretics*		
Hydrochlorothiazide	1 mg/kg/dose PO b.i.d.	Injectable solution: 50 mg/5 ml Tabs: 25, 50, 100 mg
Furosemide	1–2 mg/kg/dose PO b.i.d. or t.i.d.	Injectable solution: 10 mg/ml IV Solution: 10 mg/ml PO Tabs: 20, 40, 80 mg
Spironolactone	1–2 mg/kg/dose PO b.i.d. May use with hydrochlorothiazide or furosemide for potassium sparing	Tabs: 25, 50, 100 mg

*Monitor electrolytes.
SR, sustained release.

K. Captopril, enalapril maleate, or a calcium channel blocker can be administered for more resistant hypertension. Monitor renal functions; captopril may decrease renal function.

L. Ultimately, the cause of severe hypertension must be dealt with. Choices may include therapy for renal failure, renal artery stenosis, or removal of the endocrine-secreting tumor.

References

Gillman MW, Cook NR, Rosner B, et al. Identifying children at high risk for the development of essential hypertension. J Pediatr 1993; 122:837.

Lauer RM, Burns TL, Clarke WR. Assessing children's blood pressure: Considerations of age and body size. The muscatine study. Pediatrics 1987; 75:1081.

Rosner B, Prineas RJ, Loggie JMH, Daniels SR. Blood pressure nomograms for children and adolescents, by height, sex, and age, in the United States. J Pediatr 1993; 123:871.

Shalma A, Sinaiko AR. Systemic hypertension in heart disease in infants, children and adolescents. In: Emmanuoilides GC, Riemenschneider TA, Allen HD, Gutgesell HP, eds. Baltimore: Williams & Wilkins, 1995:1641.

Task Force on Blood Pressure Control in Children. National Heart, Lung and Blood Institute Report on the Second Task Force on Blood Pressure Control in Children—1987. Pediatrics 1987; 79:1.

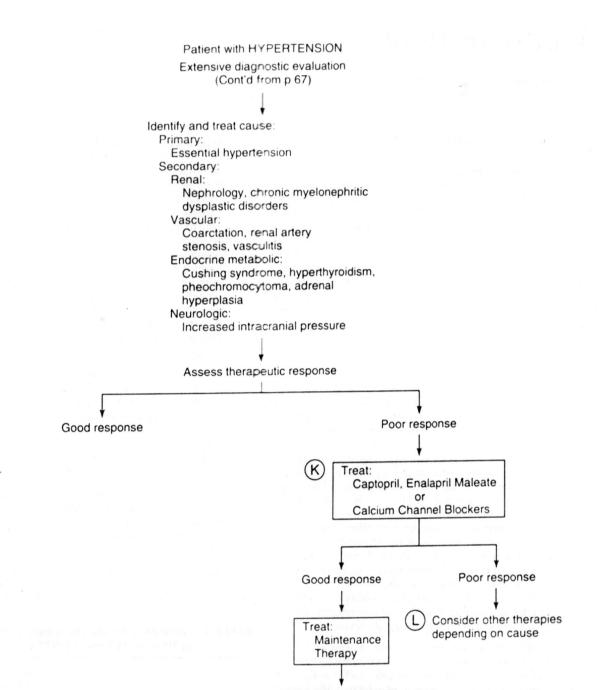

Patient with HYPERTENSION

Extensive diagnostic evaluation
(Cont'd from p 67)

Identify and treat cause:
  Primary:
    Essential hypertension
  Secondary:
    Renal:
      Nephrology, chronic myelonephritic
      dysplastic disorders
    Vascular:
      Coarctation, renal artery
      stenosis, vasculitis
    Endocrine metabolic:
      Cushing syndrome, hyperthyroidism,
      pheochromocytoma, adrenal
      hyperplasia
    Neurologic:
      Increased intracranial pressure

Assess therapeutic response

Good response

Poor response

(K) Treat:
    Captopril, Enalapril Maleate
    or
    Calcium Channel Blockers

Good response

Poor response

Treat:
Maintenance
Therapy

(L) Consider other therapies
    depending on cause

Follow-up:
Assess Monthly

RHEUMATIC FEVER

Perla Santos Ocampo, M.D.
Stephen Berman, M.D.

DEFINITION

Acute rheumatic fever (ARF) is an immune-mediated inflammation to a group A streptococcal infection with *S. pyogenes*. It remains unclear whether the development of ARF is related to a genetic susceptibility, a more virulent mucoid streptococcal strain, or other cofactors. The clinical criteria used to diagnose ARF are two major or one major and two minor criteria with supporting evidence of a preceding streptococcal infection, based on the revised Jones criteria (Table 1). Incidence varies considerably over time, between different areas, and in different ethnic groups. In the United States incidence rates for 5 to 17 year olds between 1935 and 1960 reached 40 to 65 per 100,000 and then dropped to 0.5 to 1.88 per 100,000 between 1977 and 1981. In developing countries the incidence remains about 20 to 25 per 100,000 population.

A. Ask for a history of sore throat and streptococcal infection about 2 weeks (range 1 to 5 weeks) before the onset of rheumatic fever symptoms. However, many patients have subclinical infections without any indication of a prior streptococcal infection. Ask about fever and painful, swollen joints. If they are present, determine the pattern of involvement. In migratory arthritis the disease resolves after 2 to 4 days in the initial joints and develops in new joints. In rapidly additive arthritis new joints become involved before resolution in the initial joints. Ask about the use of salicylates or other nonsteroidal antiinflammatory drugs. Juvenile rheumatoid arthritis (JRA) often responds quickly to this therapy. Ask about symptoms of congestive heart failure such as increased sweating, poor feeding, cyanosis, shortness of breath, dyspnea, fast or difficult breathing, ability to sleep flat, and edema. Facial grimacing, odd movements, and/or unusual emotional outbursts suggest chorea.

B. On physical examination note any swollen or tender joints. Knees, ankles, elbows, and wrists are commonly affected. Cardiac findings include tachycardia and murmurs, the most common of which is the apical high-pitched, blowing, holosystolic, grade II murmur of mitral valvulitis. Random, rapid, involuntary, purposeless, nonrhythmic movements (usually the face and upper extremities) indicate chorea. Look for subcutaneous nodules that are movable, hard, round, painless swellings over bony prominences. Erythema marginatum is a fine lacy erythematous rash found mainly over the trunk and inner surfaces of the arms and legs.

C. Obtain a throat culture. When negative, test for streptococcal antibodies. Only 80% of infected patients have an elevated antistreptolysin O (ASO) titer. Request other streptococcal antibodies, e.g., anti-DNase B and antihyaluronidase (AH) titer, for patients suspected for rheumatic fever who have a normal ASO titer. Remember that streptococcal antibodies may begin to decline after 2 months. Erythrocyte sedimentation rate (ESR) and C-reactive protein (CRP) are not specific for rheumatic fever but are useful for determining activity. Take a chest film to detect cardiac enlargement and pericardial effusion. Electrocardiographic changes are prolongation of the P-R interval, flattened or inverted T waves due to myocarditis, and/or elevation of the ST segment in pericarditis. Findings of left atrial enlargement associated with mitral insufficiency include a terminal-negative P in V1 greater than 1 mm deep and 0.04 second wide and a prolonged duration or bifid P wave. A prolonged P-R interval may be nonspecific and should not be the sole criterion used to diagnose carditis. In patients with suspected ARF presenting with chorea and/or polyarthritis but without a murmur, Doppler echocardiography often detects mitral regurgitation and cardiac involvement. The mitral valve is most often involved, followed by the tricuspid and aortic valves.

D. Treat all patients with benzathine penicillin to eradicate group A streptococcus (Table 2). Subsequently start a prophylaxis program for prevention of recurrent rheumatic fever with intramuscular benzathine penicillin every 21 to 28 days, depending on the risk of recurrence. An oral alternative is penicillin V. Prophylaxis is the most important aspect of disease management. For penicillin-allergic patients, use erythromycin or a cephalosporin.

E. Patients with severe or very severe carditis with ARF should be hospitalized. The need for bed rest is unclear, but it is probably not necessary for all hospitalized patients. Daily examination should emphasize the cardiac findings.

F. Aspirin is effective for arthritis and mild carditis.

(Continued on page 72)

TABLE 1 Guidelines for the Diagnosis of Initial Attack of Rheumatic Fever* (1992 Jones Criteria)

Major Manifestations	Minor Manifestations	Supporting Evidence of Antecedent Group A Streptococcal Infection
Carditis	Clinical	Positive throat culture or rapid streptococcal antigen test
Polyarthritis	Arthralgia	
Chorea	Fever	
Erythema marginatum	Laboratory	
Subcutaneous nodules	Elevated acute phase reactants	Elevated or rising streptococcal antibody titer
	Erythrocyte sedimentation rate	
	C-reactive protein	
	Prolonged P-R interval	

*If supported by evidence of preceding group A streptococcal infection, the presence of two major manifestations or of one major and two minor manifestations indicates a high probability of acute rheumatic fever.
Adapted from Special Writing Group of the Committee on Rheumatic Fever, Endocarditis, and Kawasaki Disease of the Council on Cardiovascular Disease in the Young of the American Heart Association. Guidelines for the diagnosis of rheumatic fever: Jones Criteria, updated 1992. JAMA 1992; 268:2069.

Patient with RHEUMATIC FEVER

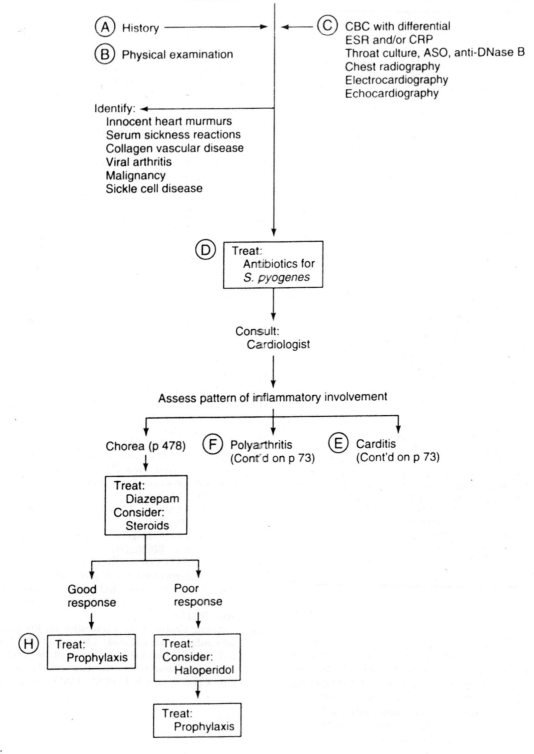

(A) History

(B) Physical examination

(C) CBC with differential
ESR and/or CRP
Throat culture, ASO, anti-DNase B
Chest radiography
Electrocardiography
Echocardiography

Identify:
Innocent heart murmurs
Serum sickness reactions
Collagen vascular disease
Viral arthritis
Malignancy
Sickle cell disease

(D) Treat:
Antibiotics for
S. pyogenes

Consult:
Cardiologist

Assess pattern of inflammatory involvement

Chorea (p 478)

(F) Polyarthritis
(Cont'd on p 73)

(E) Carditis
(Cont'd on p 73)

Treat:
Diazepam
Consider:
Steroids

Good
response

Poor
response

(H) Treat:
Prophylaxis

Treat:
Consider:
Haloperidol

Treat:
Prophylaxis

TABLE 2 Drugs Used in the Treatment of Rheumatic Fever in Children

Drug	Dosage	Product Availability
Benzathine Penicillin G	< 60 lb (27 kg) 600,000 U ≥ 60 lb (27 kg) 1.2 million U every 21–28	300,000 U/ml (10 ml) days 600,000 U/ml (1, 2, 4 ml)
Penicillin V	< 60 lb (27 kg) 125 mg b.i.d. ≥ 60 lb (27 kg) 250 mg b.i.d.	Susp: 125 and 250/5 ml Tabs: 125, 250, 500 mg
Drugs for ARF Salicylates (Aspirin)	Initial 60 mg/kg/24 hr PO q6–8h. If needed, increase 10 mg/kg/24 hr at 5-day intervals to maximum 100 mg/kg/24 hr	Tabs: 65, 81, 325, 500, 650 mg
Prednisone	1 mg/kg/dose PO b.i.d.	Solution: 5 mg/5 ml Tabs: 1, 2.5, 5, 10, 20, 50 mg
Diazepam (Valium)	0.12–0.8 mg/kg/24 hr PO divided t.i.d. or q.i.d.	Tabs: 2, 5, 10 mg
Haloperidol (Haldol)	Children 3–6 yr: PO 0.01–0.03 mg/kg/24 hr Children 6–12 yr: Begin 0.5 mg/24 hr and increase by 0.5 mg/24 hr each day if needed (maximum, 15 mg or adverse reaction) Children > 12 yr: Begin 6 mg/24 hr (usual maintenance 9 mg/24 hr)	Tabs: 0.5, 1, 2, 5, 10 mg
Digoxin	Digitalization Premature or newborn: Total dose 30 μg/kg IV Infant/child: 40 μg/kg/24 hr b.i.d. IV or PO; maximum depends on serum digoxin level (therapeutic range 0.8–2 ng/ml) Maintenance all: 10 μg/24 hr b.i.d.	Tabs: 0.125, 0.25, 0.5 mg Oral solution: 50 μg/ml IV solution: 100 μg/ml

ARF, acute rheumatic fever.

G. The use of steroids in these patients is controversial. Put patients with carditis and cardiomegaly on a regimen of prednisone for 2 weeks; decrease the daily dose by 5 mg every 2 to 3 days over another 2 weeks. When tapering, add salicylates. Continue salicylates for 1 month after prednisone. Digoxin must be used with caution in patients with heart failure due to myocarditis because many have a low tolerance for digoxin (Table 2).

H. The duration of prophylaxis is controversial. Maintain prophylaxis for life in patients with valvular insufficiency. Those with transient valvular insufficiency should receive prophylaxis through adolescence, and those without valvulitis or carditis should receive prophylaxis for at least 2 years after their rheumatic episode if there is no recurrence. Benzathine penicillin should be given every 3 rather than 4 weeks.

References

Alves Meira ZM, Mota CCC, Tonelli E, et al. Evaluation of secondary prophylactic schemes, based on benzathine penicillin G, for rheumatic fever in children. J Pediatr 1993; 123:156.

Ayoub EM. Acute rheumatic fever. In: Adams FH, ed. Moss heart disease in infants, children and adolescents. 4th ed. Baltimore: Williams & Wilkins, 1989:692.

Ayoub EM. Prophylaxis in patients with rheumatic fever: Every three or every four weeks? J Pediatr 1989; 115:89.

Ayoub EM, Hakim AZ. Rheumatic fever. In: Kaplan SL, ed. Current therapy in pediatric infectious disease. St. Louis: Mosby, 1993:237.

Dajani A, Taubert K, Ferrieri P, et al. Treatment of acute streptococcal pharyngitis and prevention of rheumatic fever: A statement for health professionals. Pediatrics 1995; 96:758.

Foster J. Rheumatic fever: Keeping up with the Jones criteria. Contemp Pediatr 1993; March:51.

Lue H-C, Wu M-H, Wang J-K, et al. Long-term outcome of patients with rheumatic fever receiving benzathine penicillin G prophylaxis every 3 weeks versus every 4 weeks. J Pediatr 1994; 125:812.

Martin DR, Voss LM, Walker SJ, Lennon D. Acute rheumatic fever in Auckland, New Zealand: Spectrum of associated group A streptococci different from expected. Pediatr Infect Dis J 1994; 13:264.

Rathmore MH, Barton LL: Acute rheumatic pericarditis. Pediatr Infect Dis J 1989; 8:183.

Shields WD, Bray PF. A danger of haloperidol therapy in children. J Pediatr 1976; 88(2):301.

Shulman ST, Amren DP, Bisno AL, et al. Prevention of rheumatic fever: A statement for health professionals by the Committee on Rheumatic Fever and Infective Endocarditis of the Council on Cardiovascular Disease in the Young. Circulation 1984; 70:1118A.

Special Writing Group of the Committee on Rheumatic Fever, Endocarditis, and Kawasaki Disease of the Council on Cardiovascular Disease in the Young of the American Heart Association. Guidelines for the diagnosis of rheumatic fever: Jones Criteria updated 1992. JAMA 1992; 268:2069.

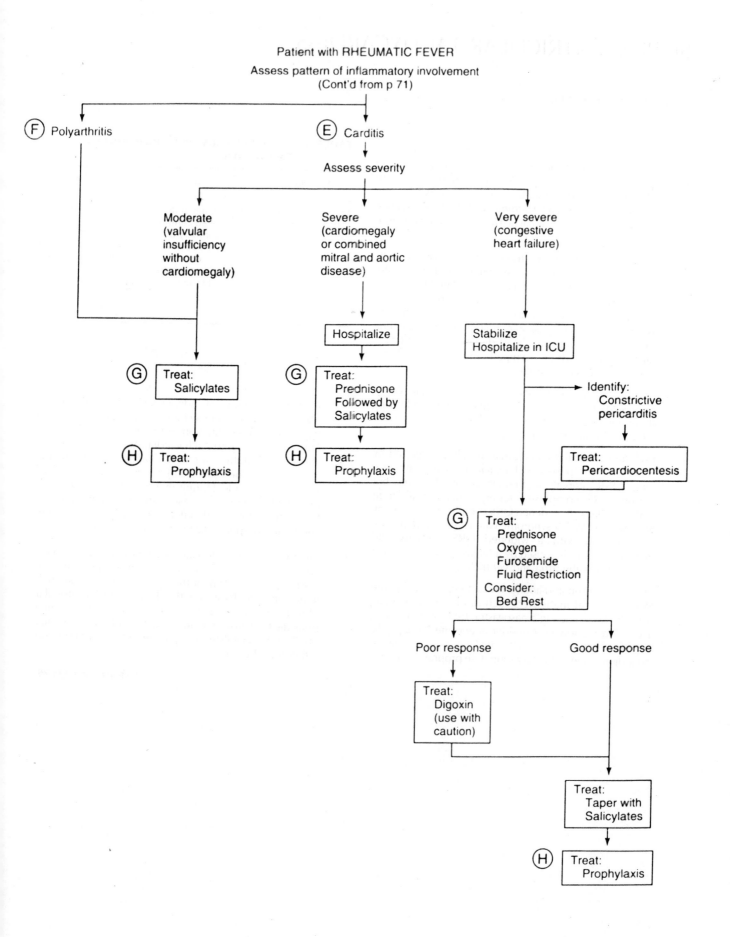

Patient with RHEUMATIC FEVER
Assess pattern of inflammatory involvement
(Cont'd from p 71)

Ⓕ Polyarthritis

Ⓔ Carditis

Assess severity

Moderate
(valvular
insufficiency
without
cardiomegaly)

Severe
(cardiomegaly
or combined
mitral and aortic
disease)

Very severe
(congestive
heart failure)

Hospitalize

Stabilize
Hospitalize in ICU

Ⓖ Treat:
Salicylates

Ⓖ Treat:
Prednisone
Followed by
Salicylates

Identify:
Constrictive
pericarditis

Ⓗ Treat:
Prophylaxis

Ⓗ Treat:
Prophylaxis

Treat:
Pericardiocentesis

Ⓖ Treat:
Prednisone
Oxygen
Furosemide
Fluid Restriction
Consider:
Bed Rest

Poor response

Good response

Treat:
Digoxin
(use with
caution)

Treat:
Taper with
Salicylates

Ⓗ Treat:
Prophylaxis

SUPRAVENTRICULAR TACHYCARDIAS

James W. Wiggins, Jr., M.D.
Stephen Berman, M.D.

Supraventricular tachycardia (SVT) is most common during early infancy; the heart rate in infants is usually 200 to 300 beats per minute (bpm). In older children the rates are generally between 150 and 250. The majority of SVT is some form of reentry tachycardia (including Wolff-Parkinson-White [WPW] syndrome). Ectopic atrial tachycardia is rare and more difficult to treat.

A. In the history determine the onset, duration, severity, and frequency of recurrence of the rapid heart rate. Note any palpitations and symptoms related to congestive heart failure (poor feeding, rapid breathing) and decreased coronary blood flow (chest pain or angina). Identify any predisposing condition or precipitating factor such as congenital heart disease, infection (myocarditis), fever, drugs (sympathomimetics, amphetamines), or WPW syndrome.

B. In the physical examination assess the cardiac status. Note signs of congestive heart failure and underlying structural heart disease such as Ebstein's anomaly or L-transposition (see p 62).

C. Exclude ventricular tachycardia, which is suggested by wide QRS complexes. SVT usually presents with prolonged P-R intervals, abnormally shaped P waves, but narrow QRS complexes. Rarely, when an aberrant pattern is present, widened QRS complexes accompany SVT. Suspect WPW syndrome when a short P-R interval is associated with a widened QRS complex and delta-wave. This is caused by a bypass conduction tract that connects the atria and ventricles.

D. In older children and adolescents attempt to disrupt the SVT with vagal maneuvers such as placing an ice bag over the face, passing a nasogastric tube or performing a Valsalva maneuver. Consider adenosine 75 μg/kg IV bolus or verapamil 0.05 to 0.1 mg/kg IV as an alternative to cardioversion or digitalization. Use propranolol rather than digoxin in patients with WPW syndrome, atrial flutter, or atrial fibrillation.

E. When vagal maneuvers have failed, use adenosine to treat children with SVT. Adenosine binds to receptors of AV nodal cells to alter calcium or potassium channels so that antegrade conduction in the AV node is blocked. This prevents reentry tachycardia. Adenosine does not affect atrial flutter, atrial fibrillation, or ventricular tachycardia. When successful, the tachycardia resolves within 20 seconds. During therapy, monitor the heart rate and blood pressure. Asthmatics may suffer respiratory distress. Other side effects are flushing, headache, chest pain, dyspnea, dizziness, and rarely hypotension.

F. Treat very severely ill patients with direct current (DC) synchronized cardioversion. Synchronization of the discharge to the peak of the QRS complex is essential; it prevents discharge on the T wave and ventricular fibrillation. Use ¼ and ½ watts/second/pound. Since prior digitalization may increase the risk of ventricular fibrillation, digitalize the patient after cardioversion rather than before.

(Continued on page 76)

TABLE 1 Degree of Illness in Supraventricular Tachycardia

Moderate	Severe	Very Severe
Asymptomatic and stable	Symptoms of decreased cerebral or coronary artery blood flow or Signs of congestive heart failure	Shock or hypotension or Moderate to severe congestive heart failure or Altered mental status

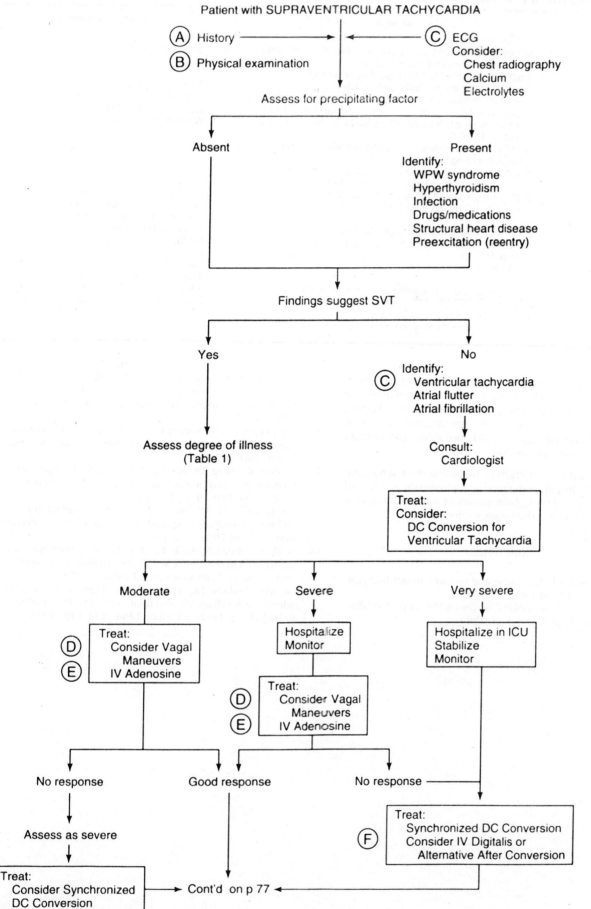

Patient with SUPRAVENTRICULAR TACHYCARDIA

(A) History ————————→ ←———— (C) ECG
(B) Physical examination   Consider:
                                        Chest radiography
                                        Calcium
                                        Electrolytes

Assess for precipitating factor

Absent   Present
                                         Identify:
                                           WPW syndrome
                                           Hyperthyroidism
                                           Infection
                                           Drugs/medications
                                           Structural heart disease
                                           Preexcitation (reentry)

Findings suggest SVT

Yes   No
                                    (C) Identify:
                                           Ventricular tachycardia
                                           Atrial flutter
                                           Atrial fibrillation

Assess degree of illness   Consult:
(Table 1)   Cardiologist

                                    Treat:
                                    Consider:
                                      DC Conversion for
                                      Ventricular Tachycardia

Moderate   Severe   Very severe

Treat: Hospitalize   Hospitalize in ICU
(D) Consider Vagal   Monitor   Stabilize
    Maneuvers   Monitor
(E) IV Adenosine
                      Treat:
                        Consider Vagal
                  (D)   Maneuvers
                  (E)   IV Adenosine

No response   Good response   No response ———————

Assess as severe   Treat:
                                              Synchronized DC Conversion
Treat: (F)   Consider IV Digitalis or
  Consider Synchronized   → Cont'd on p 77 ←   Alternative After Conversion
  DC Conversion

75

TABLE 2 Drug Therapy for Supraventricular Tachycardia in Children

Drug	Dosage	Product Availability
Adenosine	IV rapid push 75–250 µg/kg over 1–2 sec; if no response double dose and repeat in 1–2 min Adult 6 mg, then 12 mg IV bolus if no response	Solution: 3 mg/ml
Digoxin	Digitalization: give ½ initially and ¼ 6qh × 2 Premature or newborn: Total dose 15–30 µg/kg/24 hr IV given in 3 doses (½ dose, ¼ dose, ¼ dose) over 24 hr Infant or child up to 5 yr: 20–50 µg/kg/24 hr; give ½ initially and ¼ q6h × 2 IV or PO max depends on serum digoxin level (therapeutic range 0.8–2 ng/ml) Maintenance: 5–10 µg/kg/24 hr PO b.i.d.; for premature babies or infants, 5 µg/kg; for children > 1 mo, 10 µg/kg	Tabs: 0.125, 0.25, 0.5 mg Liquid: 50 µg/ml PO IV solution: 100 µg/ml
Propranolol	0.01–0.1 mg/kg/dose IV slow push over 5 min; 0.5–4 mg/kg/24 hr PO q6–8h (max 60 mg/24 hr)	Injectable solution: 1 mg/ml Tabs: 10, 20, 40, 60, 80, 90 mg SR caps: 80, 120, 160 mg
Verapamil	Children: PO 4–8 mg/kg/day divided t.i.d. IV dosing: 100–300 µg/kg (max 5 mg/dose); repeat q15min (max 15 mg)	Tabs: 40, 80,120 mg SR tabs: 120, 180, 240 mg IV: 2.5 mg/ml
Quinidine sulfate	20–40 mg/kg/24 hr q4–6h	Caps: 200, 300 mg Tabs: 100, 200, 300 mg
Procainamide	Children: IV load 3–6 mg/kg over 5 min (max 100 mg/dose; may repeat × 2) Continuous drip IV 20–80 µg/kg min PO 15–50 mg/kg/24 hr given q3–6h up to max 4 g/24 hr	Injectable solution: 100 mg/ml, 500 mg/ml Caps, tabs: 250, 375, 500 mg

G. Treat infants after an initial episode and older children with recurrent SVT episodes with maintenance oral therapy (Table 2). The oral regimen may be digoxin, propranolol, quinidine sulfate, procainamide, or verapamil. Avoid the use of cold medicines that contain sympathomimetic amines.

H. Patients who are refractory to treatment or who have syncope should undergo electrophysiologic study and be considered for radiofrequency or surgical ablation of bypass tract or arrhythmogenic focus.

References

Camm AJ, Garratt CJ. Adenosine and supraventricular tachycardia. N Engl J Med 1991; 325:1621.

Chameides L, ed. Textbook of advanced life support. Dallas: American Heart Association, 1989.

Deal BJ, Keane JF, Gillette PC, Garson A. Wolff-Parkinson-White syndrome and supraventricular tachycardia during infancy: Management and followup. J Am Coll Cardiol 1985; 1:130.

Dick M, O'Connor BK, Serwer GA, et al. Use of radiofrequency current to ablate accessory connections in children. Circulation 1991; 84:2318.

Donnerstein RL, Berg RA, Shehab Z, Ovadia M. Complex atrial tachycardias and respiratory syncytial virus infections in infants. J Pediatr 1994; 125:23.

Frassica JJ, Orav EJ, Walsh EP, Lipshultz SE. Arrhythmias in children prenatally exposed to cocaine. Arch Pediatr Adolesc Med 1994; 148:1163.

Melita AV, Sanchez GR, Sacks EJ, et al. Ectopic automatic atrial tachycardia in children: Clinical characteristic, management and followup. J Am Coll Cardiol 1988; 2:379.

Ralston MA, Knilans TK, Hannon DW, Daniels SR. Use of adenosine for diagnosis and treatment of tachyarrhythmias in pediatric patients. J Pediatr 1994; 124:139. 1993.

Patient with SUPRAVENTRICULAR TACHYCARDIA
Good response
(Cont'd from p 75)

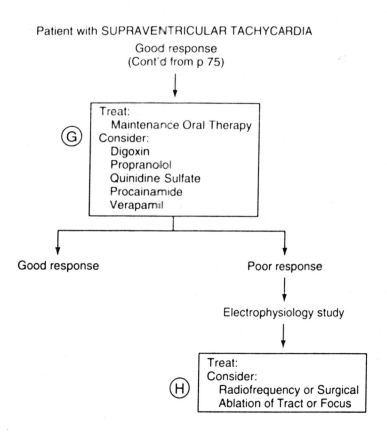

Good response

Poor response

Electrophysiology study

DERMATOLOGIC DISORDERS

EVALUATION OF SKIN LESIONS

Stephen Berman, M.D.
Joseph Morelli, M.D.

A. In the history determine the onset, progression, distribution, duration, and recurrence of the lesions. Note the presence of prodromal and associated symptoms, including pruritus, fever, cough, coryza, vomiting, diarrhea, jaundice, lymphadenopathy, altered mental status, arthritis, and failure to thrive. Identify any precipitating factor or agent, including infection, drugs or medications, trauma, sunburn, frostbite, water immersion, foods, and soaps. Note predisposing conditions such as atopic disease (atopic dermatitis, allergic rhinitis, asthma), malignancy, collagen vascular disease, liver disease, renal disease, and mucocutaneous diseases.

B. In the physical examination recognize primary lesions, including macules, papules, plaques, nodules, wheals, vesicles, and cysts. According to accepted definitions, a macule is a color change in the skin that is flat to the surface and not palpable. A papule is a firm, raised lesion with distinct borders 1 cm or less in diameter. A plaque is a firm, raised, flat-topped lesion with distinct borders and an epidermal change larger than 1 cm in diameter. A nodule is a raised lesion with indistinct borders and a deep palpable portion. A large nodule is called a tumor. A wheal is an area of tense edema within the upper dermis producing a flat-topped, slightly raised lesion. A vesicle is a papule filled with clear fluid. A bulla is a lesion larger than 1 cm in diameter filled with clear fluid. A cyst is a raised lesion containing a sac filled with liquid or semisolid material. Recognize secondary changes such as pustules, oozing and erosions, crusting, and scaling. With any rash determine its distribution, arrangement, and color. Note the specific location of the rash (generalized, truncal, flexural creases, extremities, hands, and feet). Lesions occurring in a straight line are called linear. Lesions arranged in a circular configuration are annular. Note associated signs of infection or systemic disease such as lymphadenopathy, hepatomegaly, splenomegaly, arthritis, jaundice, and heart murmur.

C. Common laboratory procedures related to dermatologic conditions include potassium hydroxide (KOH) preparations to identify fungal infections, scabies prep, exfoliative cytology, and skin biopsy. To perform a KOH prep, scrape scale from the lesion onto a glass slide and add a drop of 10% KOH to dissolve the stratum corneum cells. Heat gently to dissolve the cells more quickly. Cover the slide with a cover slip and examine for branching hyphae. A scabies prep should be performed if scabies is suspected (see p 96). Perform exfoliative cytology by breaking the blister and scraping its base. Place the scrapings on a glass slide. After drying, stain the slide with Wright's or Giemsa stain and examine for the presence of epidermal giant cells (herpes simplex or herpes zoster) or acantholytic cells (pemphigus).

D. Suspect acne when pustules and white papules (closed comedones) are located on the face, upper back, and upper chest in adolescents. Drug-induced acne can be produced by glucocorticosteroids, androgens, adrenocorticotropic hormone, diphenylhydantoin, or isoniazid. In bacterial or chemical folliculitis all lesions are in the same stage at the same time. Suspect candidiasis when satellite papulopustular lesions are present around a central, raised erythematous area. Suspect bacteremia with gonococcus or meningococcus when the patient presents with fever, signs of toxicity, and an acral distribution of pustules.

Reference

Weston WL, Lane AT, Morelli JG. A color textbook of pediatric dermatology. 2nd ed. St. Louis: Mosby, 1995.

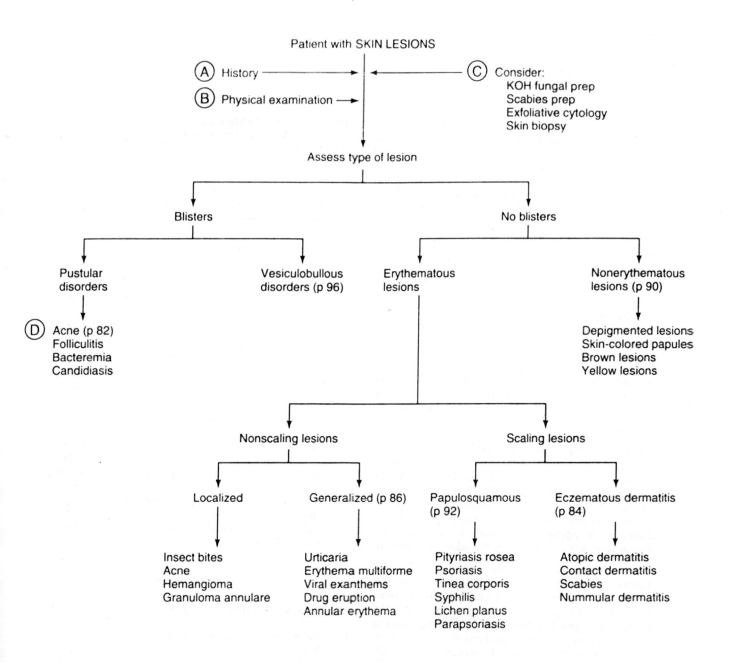

Patient with SKIN LESIONS

(A) History

(B) Physical examination

(C) Consider:
KOH fungal prep
Scabies prep
Exfoliative cytology
Skin biopsy

Assess type of lesion

Blisters

No blisters

Pustular
disorders

Vesiculobullous
disorders (p 96)

Erythematous
lesions

Nonerythematous
lesions (p 90)

(D) Acne (p 82)
Folliculitis
Bacteremia
Candidiasis

Depigmented lesions
Skin-colored papules
Brown lesions
Yellow lesions

Nonscaling lesions

Scaling lesions

Localized

Generalized (p 86)

Papulosquamous
(p 92)

Eczematous dermatitis
(p 84)

Insect bites
Acne
Hemangioma
Granuloma annulare

Urticaria
Erythema multiforme
Viral exanthems
Drug eruption
Annular erythema

Pityriasis rosea
Psoriasis
Tinea corporis
Syphilis
Lichen planus
Parapsoriasis

Atopic dermatitis
Contact dermatitis
Scabies
Nummular dermatitis

ACNE

Stephen Berman, M.D.

Acne vulgaris occurs when hormonal changes of puberty stimulate increased sebum production and hyperkeratinization of the pilosebaceous duct. The hyperkeratinization and excess sebum production lead to obstruction of the follicular opening. Noninflammatory acne includes open comedones (blackheads) and closed comedones (whiteheads). The hair follicle becomes colonized by bacteria *(Propionibacterium acnes).* The bacteria initiate an inflammatory response that ruptures the canal wall and produces a papulopustule. Inflammatory acne presents with raised red papules, pustules, or cystic lesions. Cystic acne develops when pustules rupture under the skin and become lined with epithelium. This process produces permanent scarring.

A. Educate the patient about proper washing with mild soap and avoiding excessive scrubbing. Use of oil-based cosmetics and lubricants should be limited or avoided. Diet usually does not affect acne.

B. Benzoyl peroxide has antibacterial action, reduces free fatty acid concentrations, and has comedolytic activity. Use a 5% gel. It is as effective as 10% gel but less irritating. Although the liquid and cream forms are less irritating, they are much less effective. Treat noninflammatory acne initially with daily application and increase to twice daily if needed. A thin layer should be applied to the entire face when completely dry, avoiding the areas around the eyes and mouth. The layer is left on all day. Oil-free or water-based moisturizers help skin dryness and irritation. If side effects persist, consider alternate-day application. Failure to improve over several weeks is an indication for additional therapy.

C. Retin-A, or tretinoin, available in gel (0.025% and 0.01%) and cream (0.05% and 0.1%), acts by preventing comedone formation and opening closed comedones. Retin-A is quite drying and irritating to the skin. It should be applied to the face in the evening, avoiding areas around the eyes, nose, and mouth. It is important to use a sunscreen (protective factor of at least 15) while outdoors. Use of Retin-A can worsen acne initially because of irritation of small comedones. A 6 to 12 week course may be necessary before a good response becomes apparent. Resistant cases can be treated with Retin-A in the evening and benzoyl peroxide or a topical antibiotic during the day.

D. Failure to respond to benzoyl peroxide within 6 to 8 weeks is an indication for topical antibiotic therapy with

TABLE 1 Oral Antibiotics Used in the Treatment of Acne in Adolescents

Drug	Dosage	Product Availability
Erythromycin	500 mg b.i.d. PO	Tabs: 250, 500 mg
Tetracycline	500 mg b.i.d. PO	Tabs: 250, 500 mg

erythromycin (1.5% to 3%), tetracycline (0.22%), clindamycin (1%), or meclocycline (1%).

E. Treat inflammatory acne that fails to respond to topical therapy with oral tetracycline or erythromycin for 1 to 3 months (Table 1). If inflammation improves, reduce the dose. Erythromycin should be given with food, and tetracycline should be given on an empty stomach. Avoid tetracycline in pregnancy.

F. Consider referral to a dermatologist for isotretinoin (Accutane) treatment of patients who have cystic acne with scarring that fails to respond to topical therapy plus oral antibiotics. Isotretinoin should not be used by pregnant or nursing mothers (causes severe birth defects) and should be used with caution by sexually active women and girls (only when an acceptable contraceptive method is being used). Side effects include cheilitis, dry skin, epistaxis, conjunctivitis, arthralgias, headache, fatigue, photosensitivity, hepatitis, depression, and elevation of triglycerides. Monitor fasting triglycerides, cholesterol, CBC, and liver function tests every 4 weeks.

References

Hurwitz S. Acne treatment for the 90's. Contemp Pediatr 1995; 12:19.

Hurwitz S. Acne vulgaris: Pathogenesis and management. Pediatr Rev 1994; 15:47.

Layton AM, Cunliffe WJ. Guidelines for optimal use of isotretinoin in acne. J Am Acad Dermatol 1992; 27:S2.

Pochi PE, Shalita AR, Strauss JS, et al. Classification of acne: Report of the consensus conference on acne classification. J Am Acad Dermatol 1991; 24:495.

Weston WL, Lane AT, Morelli JG. A color textbook of pediatric dermatology. 2nd ed. St. Louis: Mosby, 1995.

Winston MH, Shalita AR. Acne vulgaris: Pathogenesis and treatment. Pediatr Clin North Am 1991; 38:889.

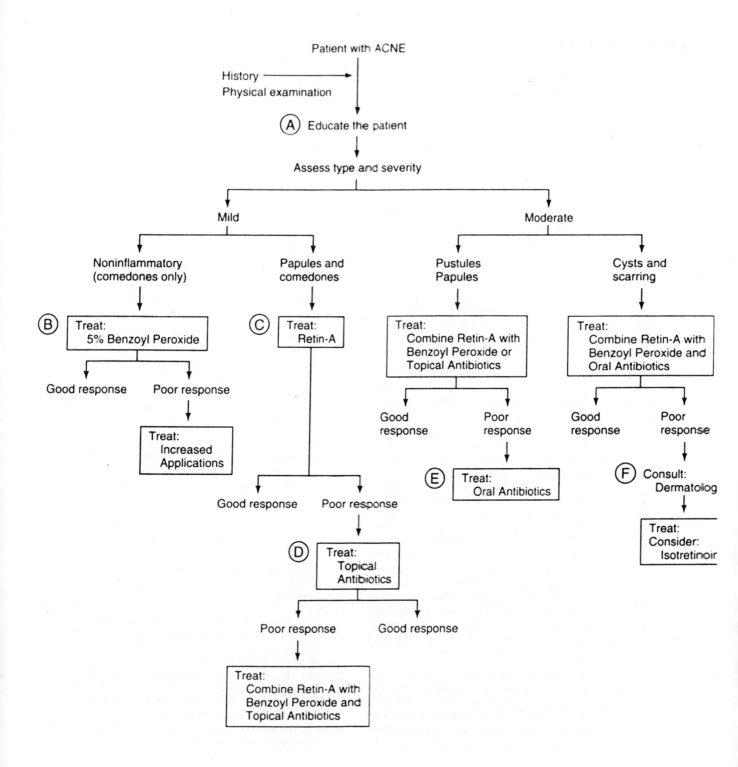

Patient with ACNE

History ——→
Physical examination

(A) Educate the patient

Assess type and severity

Mild

Noninflammatory
(comedones only)

(B) Treat:
5% Benzoyl Peroxide

Good response   Poor response

Treat:
Increased
Applications

Papules and
comedones

(C) Treat:
Retin-A

Good response   Poor response

(D) Treat:
Topical
Antibiotics

Poor response   Good response

Treat:
Combine Retin-A with
Benzoyl Peroxide and
Topical Antibiotics

Moderate

Pustules
Papules

Treat:
Combine Retin-A with
Benzoyl Peroxide or
Topical Antibiotics

Good
response   Poor
response

(E) Treat:
Oral Antibiotics

Cysts and
scarring

Treat:
Combine Retin-A with
Benzoyl Peroxide and
Oral Antibiotics

Good
response   Poor
response

(F) Consult:
Dermatolog

Treat:
Consider:
Isotretinoir

DERMATITIS

Stephen Berman, M.D.
Joseph Morelli, M.D.

Eczematous dermatitis, or inflammation of the epidermis and superficial dermis, causes pruritus and secondary skin changes of marked dryness, oozing, crusting, erosions, vesiculations, and epidermal thickening.

A. Identify substances that cause contact dermatitis by direct irritation or an allergic mechanism. An underlying skin disorder such as severe dryness or atopic dermatitis disrupts the normal epidermal barrier and increases susceptibility to irritants and infection. The most common form of irritant dermatitis is diaper rash, which is related to prolonged contact with urine and feces. The presence of satellite lesions or erosions suggests secondary infection with *Candida*. Treat diaper rash by frequent dry diaper changes, minimal washing of the diaper area, and either mycostatin or an imidazole cream.

B. Suspect allergic contact dermatitis when the rash has a local distribution, especially on the hands or feet. Secondary changes of vesiculation, oozing, and excoriation are common. A linear arrangement on the arms or legs suggests contact with a plant such as poison ivy or poison oak. Allergic contact dermatitis is related to cell-mediated immunity. Common allergens that act as haptenes include pentadecacatechol found in poison oak and poison ivy, nickel in jewelry and zippers, dichromates in tanned leather, and several chemicals in glues, rubber, dyes, cosmetics, shampoos, and topical medications. When appropriate, consider patch testing to identify a specific allergen. Treatment consists of topical steroids for 2 to 3 weeks. Use wet dressings for severe generalized pruritus; water evaporation relieves the pruritus, causes vasoconstriction, and debrides crusting. Instruct the parent to place cotton pajamas in tepid water and wring out the excess water. Have the child wear dry pajamas over the damp ones. Consider oral prednisone 1 mg/kg once daily for 14 to 21 days when allergic contact dermatitis is severe.

C. Suspect atopic dermatitis when its characteristic age-dependent distribution is seen. Involvement of the feet is especially common is school-age children and adolescents and is called juvenile plantar dermatosis; eyebrows may be involved at any age. Approximately half of the children with atopic dermatitis have an associated history of allergic rhinitis or asthma. Treat acute exacerbations with topical steroids and antihistamines. Recognize and treat secondary infections with *Staphylococcus aureus* and *Streptococcus pyogenes*. Consider wet dressings when oozing, excoriations, and crusting are marked. Avoid using fluorinated steroids on the face because of dermal atrophy, telangiectasia, hypopigmentation, and acne. Maintain adequate skin hydration with routine use of lubricant creams (Eucerin) and cetaphil lotions. Use antihistamines when necessary for pruritus. Avoid occlusive clothing, frequent soaping, wool clothes, and cleaning agents and chemicals.

D. Suspect nummular eczema when coinlike lesions 1 to 10 cm in diameter are distributed symmetrically on the extremities or trunk. The lesions can be dry and scaly or wet and oozing. Dry lesions can be confused with tinea corporis and wet lesions with impetigo. Treat both lesions with topical steroids three times daily for 1 to 2 weeks.

E. Greasy scale on the face and scalp of infants and also in the nasolabial folds of the face, posterior auricular areas, scalp, or chest of adolescents suggests seborrheic dermatitis. Treat these cases with nonfluorinated topical steroids three times daily for 1 to 2 weeks.

References

Kay J, Gawkrodger DJ, Marek MD, Jaron AJ. The prevalence of childhood atopic eczema in a general population. J Am Acad Dermatol 1994; 30:35.

Weston WL, Lane AT, Morelli JG. A color textbook of pediatric dermatology. 2nd ed. St. Louis: Mosby, 1995.

Weston WL, Weston JA, Kinoshita J, et al. Prevalence of positive epicutaneous tests among infants, children and adolescents. Pediatrics 1986; 78:1070.

Williams HC, Burney PG, Pembroke AC, Hay RJ. The U.K. working party's diagnostic criteria for atopic dermatitis. I. Derivation of a minimum set of discriminators for atopic dermatitis. Br J Derm 1994; 131:383.

Yohn JJ, Weston WL. Topical glucocorticosteroids. Curr Prob Dermatol 1990; II:Mar/April.

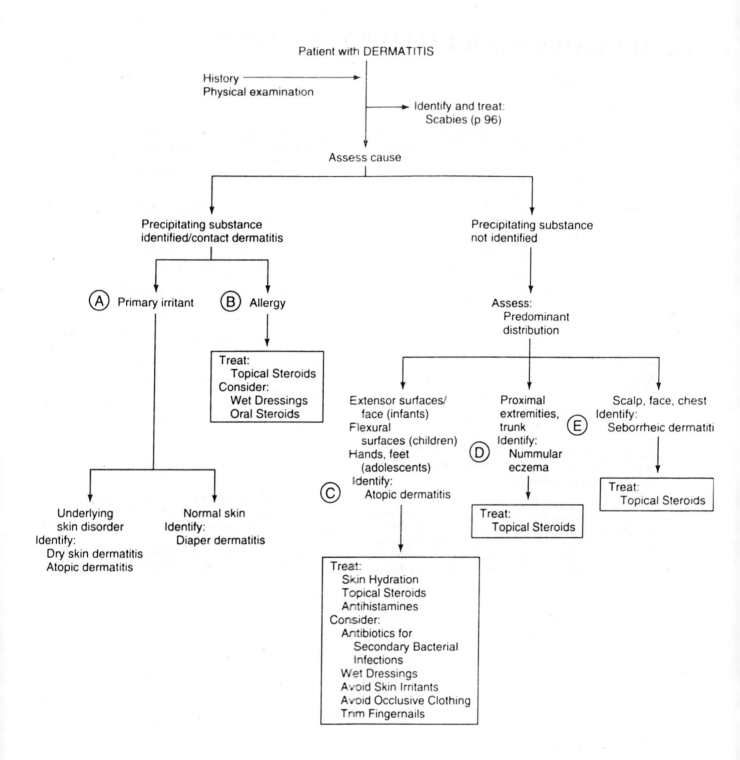

Patient with DERMATITIS

History
Physical examination

Identify and treat:
Scabies (p 96)

Assess cause

Precipitating substance
identified/contact dermatitis

Precipitating substance
not identified

(A) Primary irritant   (B) Allergy

Treat:
 Topical Steroids
Consider:
 Wet Dressings
 Oral Steroids

Assess:
 Predominant
 distribution

Extensor surfaces/
face (infants)
Flexural
 surfaces (children)
Hands, feet
 (adolescents)
Identify:
 Atopic dermatitis
(C)

Proximal
extremities,
trunk
Identify:
 Nummular
 eczema
(D)

Scalp, face, chest
Identify:
 Seborrheic dermatiti
(E)

Treat:
 Topical Steroids

Underlying
skin disorder
Identify:
 Dry skin dermatitis
 Atopic dermatitis

Normal skin
Identify:
 Diaper dermatitis

Treat:
 Skin Hydration
 Topical Steroids
 Antihistamines
Consider:
 Antibiotics for
  Secondary Bacterial
  Infections
 Wet Dressings
 Avoid Skin Irritants
 Avoid Occlusive Clothing
 Trim Fingernails

Treat:
 Topical Steroids

ERYTHEMATOUS MACULOPAPULAR LESIONS

Stephen Berman, M.D.

A. Insect bite reactions generally occur in bunches and are usually few in number. Observe for signs of secondary infection. Urticaria lesions are transient and usually last less than 1 hour. Lesions of erythema multiforme have a symmetric distribution, begin as red papules, and progress over 7 to 10 days to lesions with a dusky center and a red border. They may form blisters. Prescribe a trial of oral antihistamines such as hydroxyzine hydrochloride 2 to 4 mg/kg/day in four divided doses or diphenhydramine hydrochloride 5 mg/kg/day in four divided doses for urticaria or erythema multiforme. Erythema infectiosum (fifth disease) presents in childhood without systemic symptoms. The rash first appears on the face as a bright red erythema, then evolves into an erythematous maculopapular rash distributed primarily over the extremities. As the rash fades, it develops a lacelike appearance.

B. The presence of high fever of unknown origin over 3 to 4 days followed by development of a rash suggests roseola. The rash usually appears first on the trunk, then spreads to involve the neck, upper extremities, face, and lower extremities. The rash lasts 1 to 2 days. Roseola occurs most frequently in children between 6 months and 3 years of age. Consider enterovirus in cases with an associated aseptic meningitis.

C. Mononucleosis presents with a rash in 10% to 15% of cases. The rash is most commonly an erythematous maculopapular eruption but can appear scarlatiniform, urticarial, or hemorrhagic. Associated findings may include pharyngitis, lymphadenopathy, splenomegaly, hepatitis, pneumonitis, and CNS involvement (meningitis, encephalitis, or Guillain-Barré syndrome). Follow patients for the development of severe complications such as acute airway obstruction, ruptured spleen, hemolytic anemia, thrombocytopenia, carditis, and orchitis.

D. Suspect scarlet fever when pharyngitis, fever, abdominal pain, and malaise are associated with an erythematous, punctiform (sandpaper) rash. Associated findings include circumoral pallor, flushed cheeks, a strawberry tongue, and Pastia's sign (transverse lines in antecubital fossae). The rash often desquamates. At least three types of erythrogenic toxin have been identified. Treat scarlet fever patients under 30 lb with 10 days of 125 mg penicillin V potassium (Pen-Vee K) four times daily or 300,000 U benzathine penicillin IM; patients between 30 and 60 lb with 250 mg Pen-Vee K four times daily or 600,000 U benzathine penicillin IM; patients between 60 and 90 lb with 500 mg Pen-Vee K four times daily or 900,000 U with benzathine penicillin IM; and patients over 90 lb with 500 mg Pen-Vee K four times daily or 1,200,000 U benzathine penicillin IM.

References

Breathnach SM, Hintner H. Adverse drug reactions in the skin. Oxford: Blackwell Scientific Publications, 1992.

Hogan PA, Morelli JG, Weston WL. Viral exanthems. Curr Probl Dermatol 1992; 4:35.

Weston WL, Lane AT, Morelli JG. A color textbook of pediatric dermatology. 2nd ed. St. Louis: Mosby, 1995.

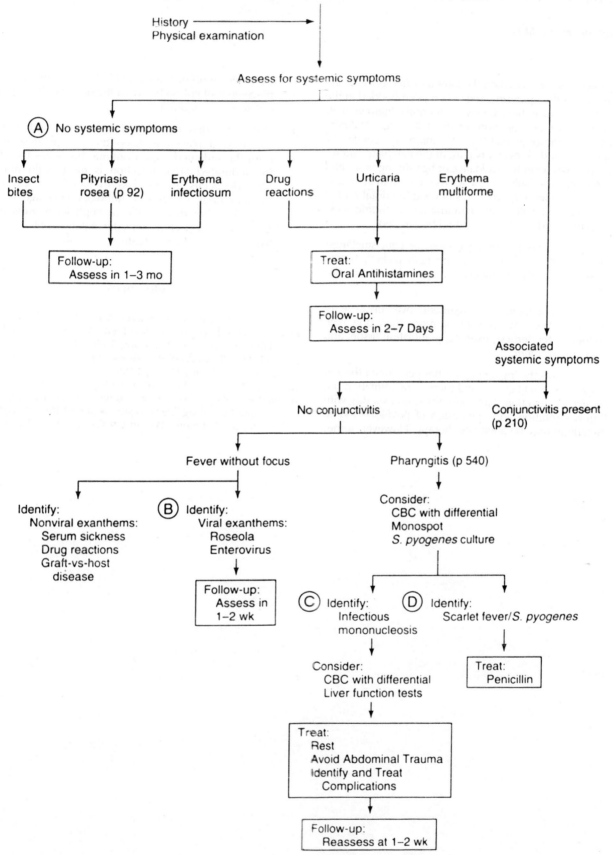

Patient with ERYTHEMATOUS MACULOPAPULAR LESIONS

History ⎯⎯⎯⎯⎯→
Physical examination

Assess for systemic symptoms

(A) No systemic symptoms

Insect bites | Pityriasis rosea (p 92) | Erythema infectiosum | Drug reactions | Urticaria | Erythema multiforme

Follow-up:
Assess in 1–3 mo

Treat:
Oral Antihistamines

Follow-up:
Assess in 2–7 Days

Associated systemic symptoms

No conjunctivitis

Conjunctivitis present (p 210)

Fever without focus

Pharyngitis (p 540)

Identify:
Nonviral exanthems:
Serum sickness
Drug reactions
Graft-vs-host disease

(B) Identify:
Viral exanthems:
Roseola
Enterovirus

Follow-up:
Assess in 1–2 wk

Consider:
CBC with differential
Monospot
S. pyogenes culture

(C) Identify:
Infectious mononucleosis

(D) Identify:
Scarlet fever/S. pyogenes

Treat:
Penicillin

Consider:
CBC with differential
Liver function tests

Treat:
Rest
Avoid Abdominal Trauma
Identify and Treat Complications

Follow-up:
Reassess at 1–2 wk

INGROWN NAILS

Rachelle Nuss, M.D.

An ingrown nail occurs when the lateral or free edge of the nail penetrates the epidermis and becomes embedded in the adjacent soft-tissue either laterally or anteriorly. Ingrown nails are the result of one or more of the following: (1) faulty footwear, (2) improper nail care, (3) injury, (4) congenital malalignment, and (5) overcurvature of the nail plate. Therefore, prophylaxis includes avoidance of tight-fitting shoes and socks, trimming the nails straight across rather than in an arc, and cutting the nail only when it is beyond the distal end of the lateral nail fold. Self-induced trauma such as thumb sucking, nail biting, and nail picking should be avoided.

A. Does the patient wear tight shoes or tight stockings? How are the nails cut? Are the nails picked, bitten, or sucked? Is there any erythema, tenderness, or discharge?

B. Look for congenital malalignment, overcurvature of the nail plate, involvement of more than one nail, erythema, tenderness, exudate, granulation tissue, and joint involvement.

C. In mild cases the ingrowing nail has penetrated the soft tissues of the nail groove and there is inflammation but no sign of infection. Hot soaks three times a day with Burow's solution and application of povidone iodine (Betadine) may be adequate therapy. However, some-times elevation of the embedded area of the nail with placement of cotton between the nail and the adjacent soft-tissue is required.

D. The embedded nail should be excised and a small cotton wad placed to keep the nail plate separate from the inflamed area. Continue hot soaks to soften the indurated area. Infection is most often due to *Stephylococcus aureus*, less frequently to *Candida*, *Pseudomonas*, or *Proteus*. Antibiotic coverage should be with either dicloxacillin or cephalexin (Keflex). If *Candida* is suspected, consider nightly application of nystatin (Mycostatin) cream.

References

Gould J. The foot book. Baltimore: Williams & Wilkins, 1988.

Krausz C. Onychopathy. In: Pine J, ed. Podiatric dermatology. Baltimore: Williams & Wilkins, 1986:74.

Lane AT, Morelli JG. A color textbook of pediatric dermatology. 2nd ed. St. Louis: Mosby, 1995.

Tachdjian M. The child's foot. Philadelphia: Saunders, 1985.

Templeton J, Ziegler M. Minor trauma and minor lesions. In: Fleisher G, Ludwig S, eds. Textbook of pediatric emergency medicine. Baltimore: Williams & Wilkins, 1993:1299.

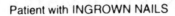

Patient with INGROWN NAILS

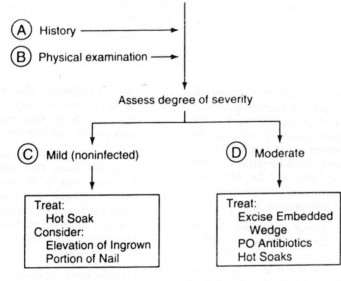

Ⓐ History ────────────▶

Ⓑ Physical examination ──▶

Assess degree of severity

Ⓒ Mild (noninfected)

Treat:
    Hot Soak
Consider:
    Elevation of Ingrown
    Portion of Nail

Ⓓ Moderate

Treat:
    Excise Embedded
    Wedge
    PO Antibiotics
    Hot Soaks

NONBLISTERING, NONERYTHEMATOUS SKIN LESIONS

Stephen Berman, M.D.
Joseph Morelli, M.D.

A. Warts usually appear on the extremities, especially hands and feet, as solitary papules with an irregular scaly surface. Keratosis pilaris is a follicular plug of scale within a body hair opening. Lesions usually develop on the extensor surfaces of the extremities and on the cheeks in children between 18 months and 3 years of age. The lesions are rarely erythematous or pustular. Epidermal nevi have a warty appearance and are arranged in a linear pattern. They are usually present at birth.

B. Microcomedones of acne appear as solitary, discrete dome-shaped papules that are skin colored or slightly whitish in appearance. They first appear over the forehead and cheeks when the child is 8 to 10 years old. Treat with topical keratolytic agents, retinoic acid cream 0.05%, or benzoyl peroxide gel 5%. Flat warts are broad, skin-colored papules, usually grouped together and found on the face and extremities. Flat warts have a smooth surface that is flat or planar rather than dome shaped as seen in microcomedones. Molluscum contagiosum, dome-shaped solitary papules with central umbilication, may be grouped together anywhere on the skin surface. The lesions, which are produced by a DNA virus (pox virus), may be passed from person to person by skin-to-skin contact. They are larger than microcomedones and have a central plug.

C. Pityriasis alba usually presents in childhood as multiple oval, scaly, flat, hypopigmented patches on the face, extensor surface of the arms, and upper trunk. The lesions have indistinct borders, do not itch, and are usually distributed symmetrically. Lesions of tinea versicolor are smaller and have distinct borders and a fine scale. They are distributed most often on the upper chest and back. Diagnose these cases with a KOH examination of a lesion, which will show short, curved hyphae and numerous spores. Vitiligo is associated with complete depigmentation rather than the hypopigmentation of pityriasis alba or tinea versicolor. A Wood's lamp examination will reveal a dramatic porcelain-white change in vitiligo but only subtle changes in color with pityriasis alba or tinea versicolor.

D. Café-au-lait spots are tan and are usually in sun-protected areas. They are larger than freckles and are not sun responsive. Suspect neurofibromatosis when six café-au-lait spots are present or multiple café-au-lait spots are found in the axilla or groin area. Junctional nevi are usually dark brown or black rather than tan. Mongolian spots are blue or blue-black and have indistinct borders.

E. Juvenile xanthogranulomas commonly present as yellow papules or nodules on the head or neck. Juvenile xanthogranuloma may have associated eye lesions that can be misdiagnosed as retinoblastoma. A nevus sebaceous (a hamartoma of the sebaceous glands) appears as a yellow linear plaque on the face or scalp. At puberty the lesion develops a warty appearance and has a cancerous predisposition.

References

Ceballos PI, Ruiz-Maldonado R, Mihm MC Jr. Current concepts: Melanoma in children. N Engl J Med 1995; 332:656.

Huson SM. Recent developments in the diagnosis and management of neurofibromatosis. Arch Dis Child 1989; 64:745.

Jaisankar TJ, Baruah MC, Garg BR. Vitiligo in children. Int J Dermatol 1992; 31:621.

Orlow SJ. Melanomas in children. Pediatr Rev 1995; 16:365.

Weston WL, Lane AT, Morelli JG. A color textbook of pediatric dermatology. 2nd ed. St. Louis: Mosby, 1995.

Williams H, Pottier A, Strachan D. The descriptive epidemiology of warts in British schoolchildren. Br J Dermatol 1993; 128:504.

Patient with NONBLISTERING, NONERYTHEMATOUS SKIN LESIONS

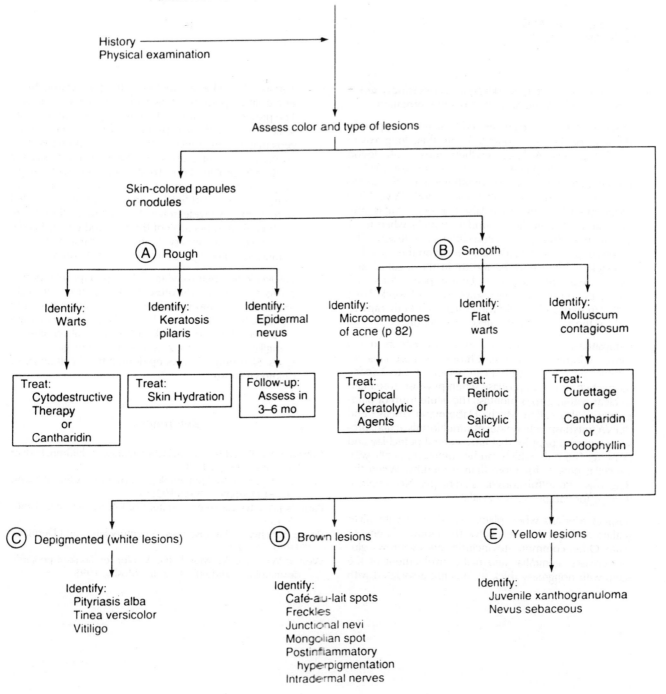

History ——————→
Physical examination

Assess color and type of lesions

Skin-colored papules
or nodules

(A) Rough

Identify:
Warts

Identify:
Keratosis
pilaris

Identify:
Epidermal
nevus

Treat:
Cytodestructive
Therapy
or
Cantharidin

Treat:
Skin Hydration

Follow-up:
Assess in
3–6 mo

(B) Smooth

Identify:
Microcomedones
of acne (p 82)

Identify:
Flat
warts

Identify:
Molluscum
contagiosum

Treat:
Topical
Keratolytic
Agents

Treat:
Retinoic
or
Salicylic
Acid

Treat:
Curettage
or
Cantharidin
or
Podophyllin

(C) Depigmented (white lesions)

Identify:
Pityriasis alba
Tinea versicolor
Vitiligo

(D) Brown lesions

Identify:
Café-au-lait spots
Freckles
Junctional nevi
Mongolian spot
Postinflammatory
  hyperpigmentation
Intradermal nerves

(E) Yellow lesions

Identify:
Juvenile xanthogranuloma
Nevus sebaceous

PAPULOSQUAMOUS DISORDERS

Stephen Berman, M.D.
Joseph Morelli, M.D.

Papulosquamous disorders are skin lesions consisting of red or purple papules with scale and often plaque formation.

A. Suspect pityriasis rosea when red oval lesions appear in the lines of skin stress oriented with their long axis in parallel planes. A large, erythematous, scaly lesion called the herald patch occurs in 80% of cases. When present before the outbreak of other lesions, the herald patch is easily confused with tinea corporis. A viral-like prodrome with fever and malaise may occur but is rare. In adolescents consider secondary syphilis when fever and adenopathy are associated with palmar lesions. The lesions of pityriasis rosea usually occur on the trunk but in black children may be mostly in the inguinal and axillary areas and extremities. Lesions persist for 4 to 8 weeks, but pruritus usually resolves within 1 week. Treat with sun exposure or ultraviolet light (UVL) therapy to reduce the pruritus and quicken resolution.

B. Parapsoriasis, a rare type of skin disease, occurs in two forms: chronic and acute. Chronic parapsoriasis resembles pityriasis rosea but can persist for 2 to 3 years. Suspect chronic parapsoriasis when pityriasis rosea fails to clear within 2 to 3 months. The acute form of parapsoriasis, also called Mucha-Habermann disease and PLEVA (pityriasis lichenoides et varioliformis acuta), presents with red papules that have central petechiae and crusting. The rash, which can be confused initially with varicella, persists for more than 9 months. When the diagnosis is doubtful, consider skin biopsy. No definitive therapy for parapsoriasis is available.

C. Suspect psoriasis when plaques associated with silver scaling and a red base involve the elbows, knees, or scalp. Other common sites include ears, eyebrows, gluteal creases, genitalia, and nails. Involvement of the scalp with nongreasy thick scale is not associated with hair loss. Nail changes include pitting, yellowing, thickening, and separation of the nail plate from the nail bed. The presence of multiple discrete droplike papules with scales suggests chronic psoriasis, which is seen in approximately one third of the cases of psoriasis. Skin biopsy in cases of psoriasis is characterized by signs of epidermal proliferation. Treat mild cases with tar gel preparations twice a day for 1 to 3 months and UVL from natural or artificial sources. Topical fluorinated steroids may provide relief, but systemic steroids are contraindicated because of the rebound effect. Recognize and treat secondary staphylococcal infection of the lesions. Avoid using antimetabolites in children.

D. Suspect lichen planus when flat-topped, pruritic purple polygonal papules are present. Oral, penile, and scalp lesions are common. Scalp lesions are associated with hair loss. Nail involvement is rare. Treat cases with topical steroids for 4 to 8 weeks. Consider oral prednisone 1 mg/kg/day for 1 to 2 weeks in severe generalized cases. Skin biopsy shows epidermal basal cell injury of unknown cause.

References

Cottoni F, Ena P, Tedde G, et al. Lichen planus in children. Pediatr Dermatol 1993; 10:132.

Krueger GG, Duvic M. Epidemiology of psoriasis: Clinical issues. J Invest Dermatol 1994; 102:14.

Parsons JM. Pityriasis rosea update. J Am Acad Dermatol 1986; 15:159.

Ross S, Sanchez JL. Parapsoriasis: A century later. Int J Dermatol 1990; 29:329.

Weston WL, Lane AT, Morelli JG. A color textbook of pediatric dermatology. 2nd ed. St. Louis: Mosby, 1995.

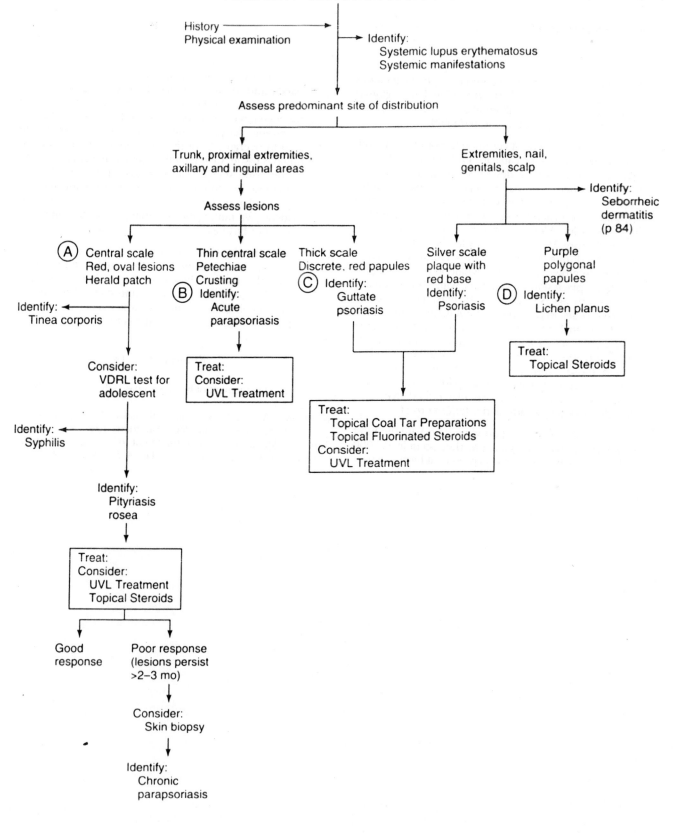

Patient with PAPULOSQUAMOUS LESIONS

History
Physical examination → Identify:
Systemic lupus erythematosus
Systemic manifestations

Assess predominant site of distribution

Trunk, proximal extremities, axillary and inguinal areas

Assess lesions

(A) Central scale
Red, oval lesions
Herald patch

Identify: ←
Tinea corporis

Consider:
VDRL test for
adolescent

Identify: ←
Syphilis

Identify:
Pityriasis
rosea

Treat:
Consider:
UVL Treatment
Topical Steroids

Good
response

Poor response
(lesions persist
>2–3 mo)

Consider:
Skin biopsy

Identify:
Chronic
parapsoriasis

(B) Thin central scale
Petechiae
Crusting
Identify:
Acute
parapsoriasis

Treat:
Consider:
UVL Treatment

Thick scale
Discrete, red papules
(C) Identify:
Guttate
psoriasis

Treat:
Topical Coal Tar Preparations
Topical Fluorinated Steroids
Consider:
UVL Treatment

Extremities, nail,
genitals, scalp

→ Identify:
Seborrheic
dermatitis
(p 84)

Silver scale
plaque with
red base
Identify:
Psoriasis

Purple
polygonal
papules
(D) Identify:
Lichen planus

Treat:
Topical Steroids

VASCULAR BIRTHMARKS

Joseph Morelli, M.D.

Vascular birthmarks are the most common type of cutaneous birth defect. They should be classified as either hemangiomas or malformations. Vascular malformations are defined by the predominant vessel type within the birthmark.

A. Hemangiomas, the most common tumor of childhood, are benign tumors of capillary endothelium. Hemangiomas should not be described as capillary or cavernous; all hemangiomas are capillary, and the terms superficial, deep, and mixed should be used. Some 20% are present at birth and the rest arise during the first 8 weeks of life. Hemangiomas have a very predictable natural history. They grow rapidly for the first year of life, especially during the first 6 months. During the second year of life growth stops and involution begins. Regression takes place slowly over years, with 50% maximally regressed by age 5 years and 90% maximally regressed by age 9 years. Regression does not define return of the skin to normal. Most hemangiomas are not associated with complications and do not require treatment. Any facial or diaper area hemangioma should be treated, as should those causing high-output cardiac failure or platelet trapping with consumption coagulopathy. Treatment options include vascular pulsed dye laser, oral glucocorticosteroids, and interferon α-2a.

B. Capillary malformations (port wine stains) are the most common vascular malformation. They occur in 3:1000 births. Port wine stains, always present at birth, are usually flat and light pink at birth and become progressively darker and thicker with age. Port wine stains covering a large portion of the face including the first division of the trigeminal nerve are associated with Sturge-Weber syndrome. All port wine stains have the potential to lead to overgrowth of the underlying skin and subcutaneous tissue. Overgrowth of an extremity covered by a port wine stain is called Klippel-Trenaunay-Weber syndrome. Treatment of choice for port wine stains is the vascular pulsed dye laser. There is considerable evidence warranting the beginning of laser treatments as soon after birth as possible.

C. Other vascular malformations, including lymphangiomas, should be defined by the predominant vessel within the lesion. These vascular malformations are much less common than port wine stains. They are all very difficult to treat and are best managed with the input of a specialized vascular malformation clinic.

References

Morelli JG. Management of hemangiomas. Adv Dermatol 1993; 8:327.

Mulliken JB, Young AY. Vascular birthmarks: Hemangiomas and malformations. Philadelphia: Saunders, 1988.

Tan OT. Management and treatment of benign cutaneous vascular lesions. Philadelphia: Lea & Febiger, 1992.

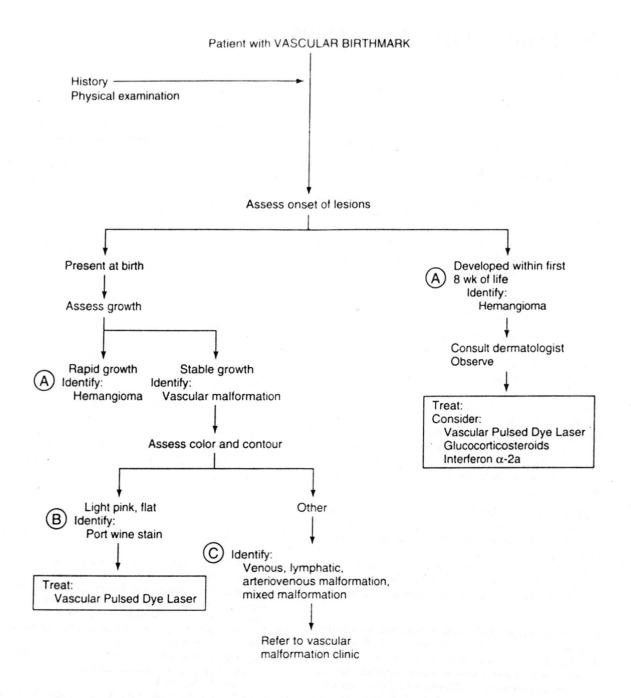

Patient with VASCULAR BIRTHMARK

History ———————————————→
Physical examination

Assess onset of lesions

Present at birth

Assess growth

Rapid growth
(A) Identify:
   Hemangioma

Stable growth
Identify:
Vascular malformation

Assess color and contour

Light pink, flat
(B) Identify:
   Port wine stain

Treat:
   Vascular Pulsed Dye Laser

Other

(C) Identify:
   Venous, lymphatic,
   arteriovenous malformation,
   mixed malformation

Refer to vascular
malformation clinic

(A) Developed within first
   8 wk of life
   Identify:
      Hemangioma

Consult dermatologist
Observe

Treat:
Consider:
   Vascular Pulsed Dye Laser
   Glucocorticosteroids
   Interferon α-2a

VESICULOBULLOUS DISORDERS

Stephen Berman, M.D.

A. Epidermolysis bullosa has 17 separate types. They can be subdivided into three types: epidermal, junctional, and dermal. The epidermal and junctional types are nonscarring, and the dermal forms are scarring. Epidermolysis bullosa simplex (autosomal dominant, nonscarring), junctional epidermolysis bullosa (autosomal recessive, nonscarring), and recessive dystrophic epidermolysis bullosa (autosomal recessive, scarring) present in the newborn period. Forms that begin in infancy and childhood include dominant dystrophic epidermolysis bullosa (autosomal dominant, scarring) and epidermolysis bullosa simplex. Children with hereditary mechanobullous disorders should be referred to a regional epidermolysis bullosa center.

B. Urticaria pigmentosa (mastocytosis) is a disease with macular and nodular pigmented lesions affecting newborns and infants. The disease is characterized by urticaria formed by gentle stroking of the lesions (Darier sign). In some cases the inflammation in response to mild trauma is so intense that blistering occurs. Systemic symptoms such as flushing, wheezing, diarrhea, and syncope occur infrequently. When necessary, treat patients with hydroxyzine hydrochloride 2 to 4 mg/kg/day divided in four doses. If symptoms are not controlled by antihistamines, refer the patient to a dermatologist.

C. Epidermolytic hyperkeratosis (congenital bullous ichthyosiform erythroderma) is a blistering disorder associated with erythroderma and thickened, scaling skin lesions. Originally considered a variant of ichthyosis, epidermolytic hyperkeratosis is now categorized as a mechanobullous disease. It is caused by abnormal keratin formation. The mode of inheritance is autosomal dominant.

D. Incontinentia pigmenti usually occurs in girls as blisters arranged in a linear pattern on extremities. The lesions develop a warty appearance and last until approximately 1 year of age. Swirls of brown pigmentation can also be found on the trunk. Mental retardation, seizures, microcephaly, and ocular and skeletal abnormalities are associated with this disorder.

E. Suspect bacterial impetigo when moist, honey-colored crusts on each lesion cover an area of skin greater than 1 cm. Early bullous impetigo looks like an acute burn, contact dermatitis, or a friction blister. Viral infections that present with a vesicular eruption include varicella, herpes zoster, hand-foot-mouth disease (Coxsackie), enteroviral infections, and herpes simplex. Grouped vesicles with a dry crust suggest herpes simplex. Consider obtaining bacterial and/or viral cultures and staining a smear of the blister's contents with Wright's stain to identify epidermal giant cells associated with viral infections.

F. Lesions on the palms and soles suggest scabies. Search the interdigital webs, palms, and soles. Diagnostic S-shaped burrows are observed in most infants and young children. Scrape several lesions to identify the scabies mite, feces, or ova under the microscope. If present, treat with lindane (Kwell) lotion or permethrin (Elimite) cream.

G. When acquired blistering lesions persist for longer than 1 month, obtain a skin biopsy for routine histopathology and immunofluorescence to clarify the diagnosis. Treat linear IgA dermatoses and dermatitis herpetiformis with sulfapyridine or dapsone; treat bullous pemphigoid disease with systemic corticosteroids.

References

Burton JL. Keratin genes and epidermolytic hyperkeratosis. Lancet 1993; 344:1103.

Calvelli CF, Gaspari AA. When the vesicles aren't chickenpox. Contemp Pediatr 1993; December:48.

Fine J-D, Bauer EA, Briggamon RA, et al. Revised clinical and laboratory criteria for subtypes of inherited epidermolysis bullosa. J Am Acad Dermatol 1991; 24:119.

Gorski JI, Burright EN. The molecular genetics of incontinentia pigmenti. Semin Dermatol 1993; 12:255.

Kirtschig H, Wojnarowska F. Autoimmune blistering diseases: An update of diagnostic methods and investigations. Clin Exp Dermatol 1994; 19:97.

Weston WL, Lane AT, Morelli JG. A color textbook of pediatric dermatology. 2nd ed. St. Louis: Mosby, 1995.

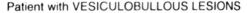

Patient with VESICULOBULLOUS LESIONS

History
Physical examination

Assess onset and precipitating factors

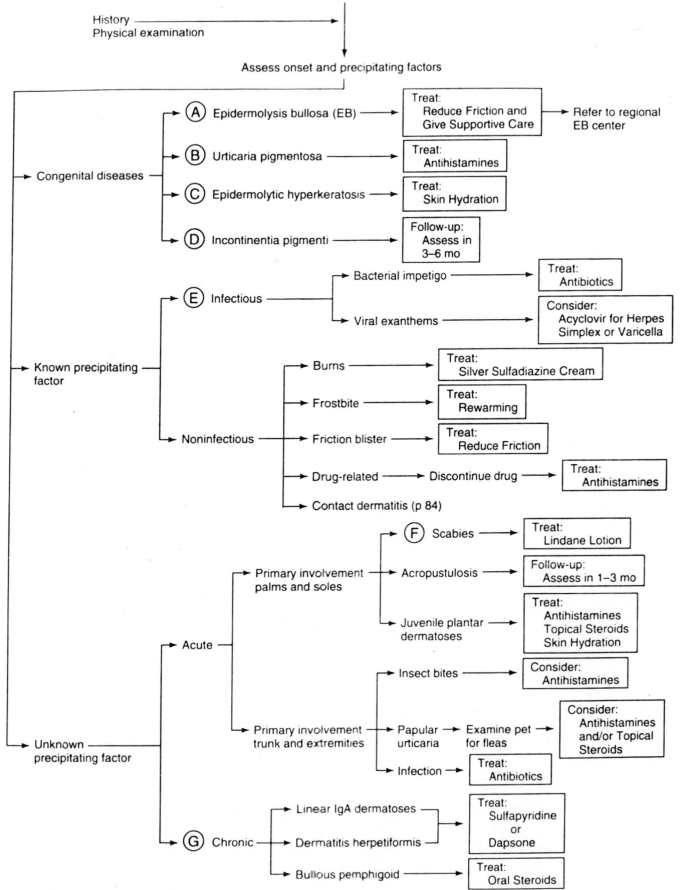

Congenital diseases

- (A) Epidermolysis bullosa (EB) → Treat: Reduce Friction and Give Supportive Care → Refer to regional EB center
- (B) Urticaria pigmentosa → Treat: Antihistamines
- (C) Epidermolytic hyperkeratosis → Treat: Skin Hydration
- (D) Incontinentia pigmenti → Follow-up: Assess in 3–6 mo

Known precipitating factor

- (E) Infectious
  - Bacterial impetigo → Treat: Antibiotics
  - Viral exanthems → Consider: Acyclovir for Herpes Simplex or Varicella
- Noninfectious
  - Burns → Treat: Silver Sulfadiazine Cream
  - Frostbite → Treat: Rewarming
  - Friction blister → Treat: Reduce Friction
  - Drug-related → Discontinue drug → Treat: Antihistamines
  - Contact dermatitis (p 84)

Unknown precipitating factor

- Acute
  - Primary involvement palms and soles
    - (F) Scabies → Treat: Lindane Lotion
    - Acropustulosis → Follow-up: Assess in 1–3 mo
    - Juvenile plantar dermatoses → Treat: Antihistamines Topical Steroids Skin Hydration
  - Primary involvement trunk and extremities
    - Insect bites → Consider: Antihistamines
    - Papular urticaria → Examine pet for fleas → Consider: Antihistamines and/or Topical Steroids
    - Infection → Treat: Antibiotics
- (G) Chronic
  - Linear IgA dermatoses → Treat: Sulfapyridine or Dapsone
  - Dermatitis herpetiformis
  - Bullous pemphigoid → Treat: Oral Steroids

EMERGENCIES

Cerebral Edema
Coma
Fever or Acute Illness in a
 Child with Sickle Cell Disease
Meningitis

Prehospital Basic Life Support
Respiratory Distress/Cyanosis
Shock/Hypotension
Status Epilepticus

CEREBRAL EDEMA

Stephen Berman, M.D.

Cerebral edema, or brain swelling, is categorized as cytotoxic, vasogenic, or interstitial. Cytotoxic edema is produced by conditions that disrupt intracellular metabolism and allow sodium and water to accumulate intracellularly. Causes include Reye syndrome, viral encephalitis, hypoxic or ischemic insult, lead intoxication, syndrome of inappropriate diuretic hormone, and hexachlorophene toxicity. Vasogenic or extracellular edema occurs with capillary leakage through a disrupted blood-brain barrier. Causes include tumors, hematomas, trauma, abscess, cerebritis, and infarction. In interstitial edema acute hydrocephalus forces CSF to pass through the ependymal lining of the ventricles.

A. Note symptoms of cerebral edema and increased intracranial pressure such as persistent vomiting, severe headache, irritability, confusion, and altered mental status.

B. Visualize the fundi for venous pulsations, papilledema, hemorrhage, and exudates, and assess the level of brain dysfunction (see p 104). Note any focal neurologic signs, seizure activity, and abnormal reflexes. Severe bradycardia suggests increased intracranial pressure.

C. The Glasgow Coma Score is a useful guide in management and prognosis. Sum the score of each of the three categories to give a total score. *Eye opening:* 4 spontaneous, 3 to speech, 2 to pain, and 1 none. *Verbal response:* 5 oriented, 4 confused, 3 inappropriate, 2 incomprehensible, 1 none. *Motor response:* 6 obeys commands, 5 localizes pain, 4 withdraws, 3 flexion to pain, 2 extension to pain, 1 none. Patients with scores of 3 or 4 have a poor prognosis and if they survive, often suffer severe sequelae.

(Continued on page 102)

TABLE 1   Drugs Used in the Treatment of Cerebral Edema in Children

Drug	Dosage	Product Availability
Mannitol	Loading 0.5–1 g/kg/dose; then 0.25 g/kg/dose IV push repeated at 5-min intervals p.r.n.; dose may if necessary be increased to 1 g/kg/dose Preoperative neurosurgical dose 1.5–2 g/kg/dose q30–60min	IV solution: 5%, 10%, 15%, 25%
Furosemide (Lasix)	1–2 mg/kg/dose to maximum 6 mg/kg/day	IV solution: 10 mg/ml (2, 4, 10 ml)
Dexamethasone (Decadron)	Loading 1.5 mg/kg/dose Maintenance: 1.5 mg/kg/24 hours divided q4–6h for 5 days, then taper over 5 days	IV solution: 4, 10, 24 mg/ml
Morphine	0.1–0.2 mg/kg/dose q2–4h to maximum of 15 mg/dose	IV solution: 2, 4, 8, 10, 15 mg/ml
Pancuronium (Pavulon)	Infants > 1 mo and children: Initial 0.06–0.1 mg/kg/dose Maintenance: 0.02–0.1 mg/kg/dose q30–60min p.r.n.	IV solution: 1, 2 mg/ml
Pentobarbital	Initial 3–5 mg/kg/dose IV Maintenance: 2–3.5 mg/kg/dose IV every hour as needed to maintain level between 25 and 40 μg/ml	IV solution: 50 mg/ml

Patient with CEREBRAL EDEMA

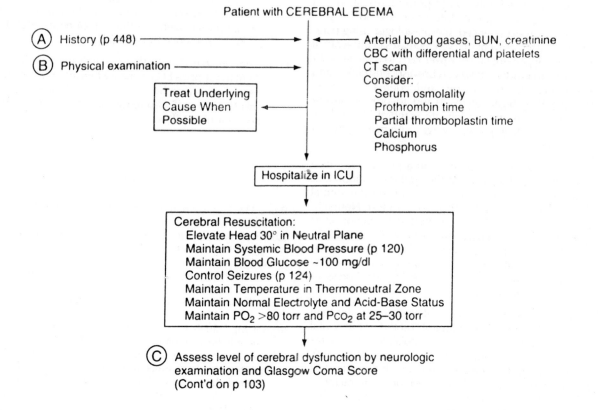

(A) History (p 448) ————————————→ ←——— Arterial blood gases, BUN, creatinine
                                                  CBC with differential and platelets
(B) Physical examination ————————→   CT scan
                                                  Consider:
                                                      Serum osmolality
Treat Underlying   Prothrombin time
Cause When ←   Partial thromboplastin time
Possible   Calcium
                                                      Phosphorus

Hospitalize in ICU

Cerebral Resuscitation:
  Elevate Head 30° in Neutral Plane
  Maintain Systemic Blood Pressure (p 120)
  Maintain Blood Glucose ~100 mg/dl
  Control Seizures (p 124)
  Maintain Temperature in Thermoneutral Zone
  Maintain Normal Electrolyte and Acid-Base Status
  Maintain PO_2 >80 torr and Pco_2 at 25–30 torr

(C) Assess level of cerebral dysfunction by neurologic
examination and Glasgow Coma Score
(Cont'd on p 103)

D. Consider elective intubation to prevent aspiration and sudden respiratory arrest. Intubation should be performed by an experienced anesthesiologist using paralyzing agents to prevent marked increases in intracranial pressure. Hyperventilate to lower Pco_2 to a range of 25 to 30 torr to produce mild cerebrovasoconstriction and reduce cerebral blood flow and edema formation. Maintain Pco_2 higher than 20 torr to prevent severe vasoconstriction and inadequate cerebral blood flow. Manage acute high pressure waves with manual hyperventilation.

E. Monitor intracranial pressure with a pressure-sensitive device that can be placed in the epidural, subdural, or subarachnoid spaces or the lateral ventricle. The normal intracranial pressure is less than 10 to 15 torr. Normally, the cerebral blood flow is unaffected by minor alterations in systemic arterial pressures between 50 and 150 torr. When cerebral dysfunction disrupts autoregulation, the cerebral perfusion pressure is determined by the difference between mean systemic arterial pressure and intracranial pressure.

F. Treat an elevation of intracranial pressure greater than 15 torr with intravenous mannitol (Table 1). Follow vital signs and urine output, serum osmolality, and electrolytes closely. Avoid serum osmolalities greater than 300. Consider using furosemide 5 minutes before the first dose to reduce a paradoxic elevation in intracranial pressure. The efficacy of steroids (dexamethasone) has been demonstrated for vasogenic edema but not for cytotoxic edema. Consider using morphine and pancuronium to reduce increased intracranial pressure secondary to agitation and muscle spasm. Osmotic agents remove fluid only from uninjured brain tissue. Avoid using osmotic agents in the first 24 hours after trauma or in the presence of renal failure.

G. Consider barbiturate therapy with pentobarbital sufficient to suppress EEG activity when intracranial pressure cannot otherwise be adequately controlled. Hypothermia to 32° C will also reduce cerebral metabolism and cerebral blood flow.

References

Bruce DA. Management of cerebral edema. Pediatr Rev 1983; 4:217.

Griffith JF, Brassfield JC. Increased intracranial pressure. Pediatr Rev 1981; 2:269.

Mickell JJ, Reigel DH, Cook DR, et al. Intracranial pressure monitoring in normalization therapy in children. Pediatrics 1977; 59:606.

Miller JD. Barbiturates in raised intracranial pressure. Ann Neurol 1979; 6:189.

Rosner MJ, Daughian S. Cerebral perfusion pressure management in head trauma. J Trauma 1990; 30:933.

Schaible DH, Cupit GC, Swedlow DB, Rocci ML Jr. High-dose pentobarbital pharmacokinetics in hypothermic brain-injured children. J Pediatr 1982; 100:655.

Trauner DA. Barbiturate therapy in acute brain injury. J Pediatr 1986; 109:742.

White BC, Wiegenstein JG, Winegar CD. Brain ischemic anoxia. JAMA 1984; 251:1586.

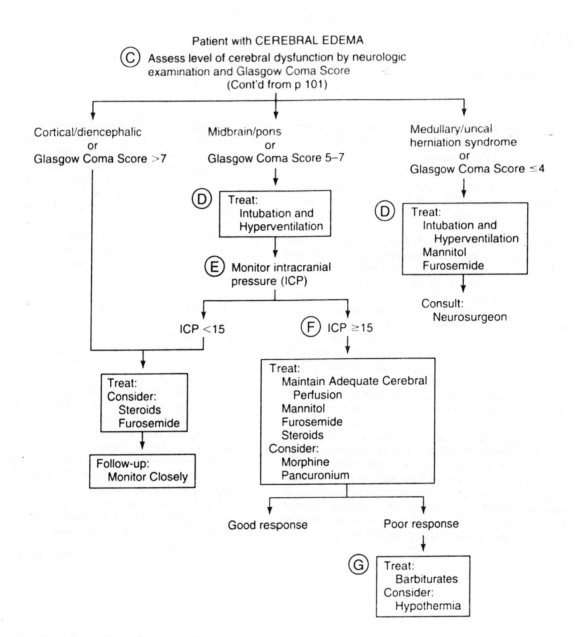

Patient with CEREBRAL EDEMA

(C) Assess level of cerebral dysfunction by neurologic examination and Glasgow Coma Score (Cont'd from p 101)

Cortical/diencephalic or Glasgow Coma Score >7

Midbrain/pons or Glasgow Coma Score 5–7

Medullary/uncal herniation syndrome or Glasgow Coma Score ≤4

(D) Treat:
Intubation and Hyperventilation

(E) Monitor intracranial pressure (ICP)

ICP <15

(F) ICP ≥15

(D) Treat:
Intubation and Hyperventilation
Mannitol
Furosemide

Consult:
Neurosurgeon

Treat:
Consider:
Steroids
Furosemide

Follow-up:
Monitor Closely

Treat:
Maintain Adequate Cerebral Perfusion
Mannitol
Furosemide
Steroids
Consider:
Morphine
Pancuronium

Good response

Poor response

(G) Treat:
Barbiturates
Consider:
Hypothermia

COMA

Stephen Berman, M.D.

Coma results from brain dysfunction, i.e., inadequate interaction between the cerebral hemispheres and the reticular activating systems of the diencephalon, midbrain, and pons.

A. Brain stem auditory-evoked responses and visual-evoked potentials may be useful predictors of brain stem function and outcome.

B. Assess the level of brain dysfunction by evaluating consciousness, pattern of breathing, pupil size and reflexes, oculomotor function, and motor responses. Involvement limited to the cerebral hemispheres and basal ganglia causes confusion or delirium associated with a normal breathing pattern, normal-sized or small reactive pupils, roving eye movements, and spontaneous movements of the extremities. Diencephalic dysfunction causes stupor and unresponsiveness, periodic or Cheyne-Stokes breathing, small reactive pupils, positive oculocephalic (doll's eye movements) and oculovestibular reflexes, and decorticate posturing. Signs of midbrain and upper pons dysfunction include hyperventilation, moderate pupillary dilation (3 to 5 mm), dysconjugate gaze with loss of oculocephalic and oculovestibular reflexes, and decerebrate posturing. Dysfunction of the lower pons and medullary level causes a shallow and irregular breathing pattern, fixed and dilated pupils, absent eye movements, and flaccid paralysis. Rapid rostro-caudal deterioration suggests herniation through the tentorial notch (central herniation syndrome). Unilateral pupillary dilation associated with signs of midbrain dysfunction is caused by compression of the third nerve with displacement of the temporal lobe through the tentorial notch (uncal herniation syndrome). Both herniation syndromes can be associated with bradycardia, hypertension, and an irregular breathing pattern. The duration of coma and the Glasgow Coma Scale (Tables 1 and 2) are useful in determining the severity and outcome in posttraumatic coma (see p 652). Patients with scores of 3 or 4 have a poor prognosis, and if they survive often suffer severe sequelae. Guidelines for determination of brain death in children with coma remain controversial. The American Academy of Pediatrics guidelines are as follows: (1) coma, apnea, *and* flaccid tone; (2) documentation of no brain stem function, including nonresponsive pupils, absence of eye movements (spontaneous or stimulated), absence of corneal, gag, cough, sucking, rooting reflexes, and movement of bulbar muscles; (3) absence of associated hypothermia or hypotension; and (4) no spontaneous or induced movement. Additional laboratory tests are an EEG to demonstrate absence of electrocerebral activity and a cerebral radionuclide angiogram that fails to show intracranial arterial circulation. Brain deaths for infants 7 days to 2 months requires two confirmatory examinations and EEGs separated by at least 48 hours. For infants 2 months to 1 year, two examinations and EEGs separated by 24 hours or a confirmatory radionuclide angiographic study at the initial examination are required. Children older than 1 year with an irreversible

(Continued on page 106)

TABLE 1 Glasgow Coma Score

Activity	Best Response	Score
Eye opening	Spontaneous	4
	To verbal stimuli	3
	To pain	2
	None	1
Verbal	Oriented	5
	Confused	4
	Inappropriate words	3
	Nonspecific sounds	2
	None	1
Motor	Follows commands	6
	Localizes pain	5
	Withdraws to pain	4
	Flexion response to pain	3
	Extension response to pain	2
	None	1

From Packer RJ, Berman PH. Coma. In: Fleisher GR, Ludwig S, eds. Textbook of pediatric emergency medicine. 3rd ed. Baltimore: Williams & Wilkins, 1993:122.

TABLE 2 Modified Coma Score for Infants

Activity	Best Response	Score
Eye opening	Spontaneous	4
	To speech	3
	To pain	2
	None	1
Verbal	Coos, babbles	5
	Irritable, cries	4
	Cries to pain	3
	Moans to pain	2
	None	1
Motor	Normal spontaneous movements	6
	Withdraws to touch	5
	Withdraws to pain	4
	Abnormal flexion	3
	Abnormal extension	2
	None	1

From Packer RJ, Berman PH. Coma. In: Fleisher GR, Ludwig S, eds. Textbook of pediatric emergency medicine. 3rd ed. Baltimore: Williams & Wilkins, 1993:122.

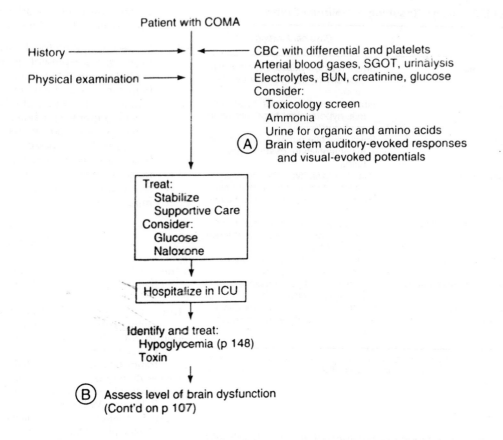

Patient with COMA

History ──────────────→ | ←──── CBC with differential and platelets
                          Arterial blood gases, SGOT, urinalysis
Physical examination ───→ Electrolytes, BUN, creatinine, glucose
                          Consider:
                              Toxicology screen
                              Ammonia
                              Urine for organic and amino acids
                    (A)   Brain stem auditory-evoked responses
                              and visual-evoked potentials

Treat:
    Stabilize
    Supportive Care
Consider:
    Glucose
    Naloxone

Hospitalize in ICU

Identify and treat:
    Hypoglycemia (p 148)
    Toxin

(B) Assess level of brain dysfunction
(Cont'd on p 107)

TABLE 3 Drugs Resulting in Delirium/Coma

Drug	Physical Findings
Barbiturates	Small, reactive pupils, hypothermia, flaccidity (doll's eye may be absent)
Opiates	Pinpoint, reactive pupils, hypothermia, hypotension, hypoventilation, bradycardia
Psychedelics	Small, reactive pupils, hypertension, hyperventilation, dystonic posturing
Amphetamines	Dilated pupils, hyperthermia, hypertension, tachycardia, arrhythmia
Cocaine	Dilated pupils, hyperthermia, tachycardia
Atropine-scopolamine	Dilated pupils, hyperthermia, flushing, hot, dry skin, supraventricular tachycardia
Glutethimide	Midposition, irregular fixed pupils, hypothermia, flaccidity
Tricyclic antidepressants	Hyperthermia, hypotension, supraventricular tachycardia
Phenothiazines	Hypotension, arrhythmia, dystonia
Methaqualone	As barbiturates, if severe tachycardia, dystonia

From Packer RJ, Berman PH. Coma. In: Fleisher GR, Ludwig S, eds. Textbook of pediatric emergency medicine. 3rd ed. Baltimore: Williams & Wilkins, 1993:122.

cause do not require laboratory confirmation but should have confirmatory examinations separated by at least 12 hours.

C. Suspect a toxic metabolic disease when the neurologic assessment demonstrates inconsistencies in the level of dysfunction among breathing pattern, pupillary reflexes, eye movements, and motor responses.

D. Suspect a supratentorial mass lesion when focal neurologic signs are present or the clinical course suggests central or uncal heriation. Causes include intracranial hematomas (subdural, epidural, intracerebral), brain tumors, contusions, and infarctions. Subtentorial mass lesions present with brain stem signs such as cranial nerve palsies and altered oculovestibular reflexes. Causes include a posterior fossa hematoma or tumor, basilar aneurysm, and brain stem or pontine hemorrhage. Hypoglycemia and herpes simplex encephalitis may cause focal neurologic signs that suggest structural mass lesions.

References

Annas GJ, Bray PF, Bennett DR, et al. Guidelines for the determination of brain death in children. Pediatrics 1987; 80:298.

Freeman JM, Ferry PC. New brain death guidelines in children: Further confusion. Pediatrics 1988; 81:301.

Lieh-Lai MW, Theodorou AA, Sarnaik AP, et al. Limitations of the Glasgow Coma Scale in predicting outcome in children with traumatic brain injury. J Pediatr 1992; 120:195.

Packer RJ, Berman PH. Coma. In: Fleisher GR, Ludwig S, eds. Textbook of pediatric emergency medicine. 3rd ed. Baltimore: Williams & Wilkins, 1993:122.

Plum F, Posner JB. The diagnosis of stupor and coma. Philadelphia: Davis, 1972.

Strickbine-Van Reet P, Glaze DG, Hrachovy RA. A preliminary prospective neurophysiological study of coma in children. Am J Dis Child 1984; 138:492.

Yager JY, Johnston B, Seshia SS. Coma scales in pediatric practice. Am J Dis Child 1990; 144:1088.

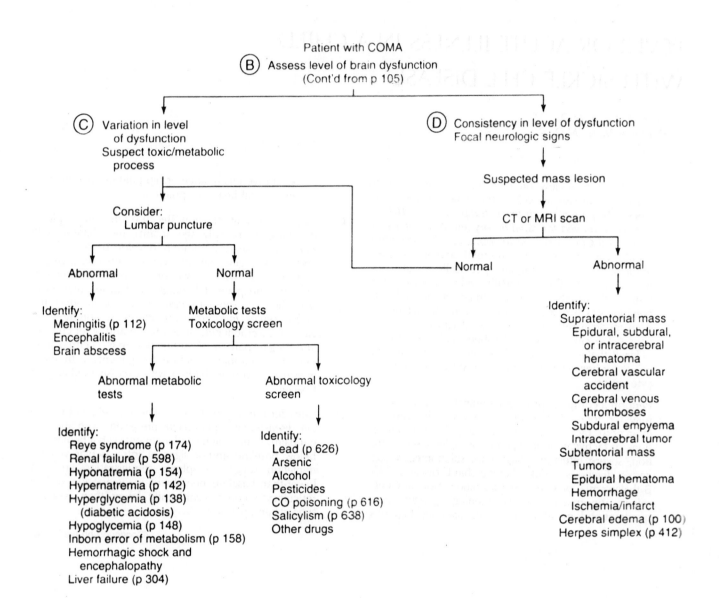

Patient with COMA

(B) Assess level of brain dysfunction
(Cont'd from p 105)

(C) Variation in level
of dysfunction
Suspect toxic/metabolic
process

(D) Consistency in level of dysfunction
Focal neurologic signs

Consider:
Lumbar puncture

Suspected mass lesion

CT or MRI scan

Abnormal

Normal

Normal

Abnormal

Identify:
Meningitis (p 112)
Encephalitis
Brain abscess

Metabolic tests
Toxicology screen

Abnormal metabolic
tests

Abnormal toxicology
screen

Identify:
Reye syndrome (p 174)
Renal failure (p 598)
Hyponatremia (p 154)
Hypernatremia (p 142)
Hyperglycemia (p 138)
(diabetic acidosis)
Hypoglycemia (p 148)
Inborn error of metabolism (p 158)
Hemorrhagic shock and
encephalopathy
Liver failure (p 304)

Identify:
Lead (p 626)
Arsenic
Alcohol
Pesticides
CO poisoning (p 616)
Salicylism (p 638)
Other drugs

Identify:
Supratentorial mass
Epidural, subdural,
or intracerebral
hematoma
Cerebral vascular
accident
Cerebral venous
thromboses
Subdural empyema
Intracerebral tumor
Subtentorial mass
Tumors
Epidural hematoma
Hemorrhage
Ischemia/infarct
Cerebral edema (p 100)
Herpes simplex (p 412)

FEVER OR ACUTE ILLNESS IN A CHILD WITH SICKLE CELL DISEASE

Peter A. Lane, M.D.
Rachelle Nuss, M.D.

A. In the history review prior problems associated with sickle cell disease as well as the details of the acute illness. *All patients with fever (temperature > 101° F) should be triaged for rapid history and physical assessment, and CBC, reticulocyte count, and blood culture should be drawn and parenteral antibiotics given immediately (see C).* Inquire specifically about fever, pain, cough, shortness of breath, and neurologic symptoms. Ask whether pain is similar or dissimilar to previous sickle pains. Determine from the patient or from medical records the precise diagnosis (homozygous sickle cell anemia, sickle-hemoglobin C disease, sickle β-thalassemia) as well as the patient's baseline values for hemoglobin, hematocrit, WBC, and reticulocyte count.

B. Perform a complete physical examination; search carefully for foci of infection. Note fever (infection or infarction), tachypnea (pneumonia, pulmonary infarction), or tachycardia or hypotension (splenic sequestration, severe infection). Significant splenomegaly suggests a diagnosis of sickle-hemoglobin C disease, sickle β-thalassemia, or splenic sequestration. Note any neurologic abnormalities (stroke, meningitis), right upper quadrant abdominal tenderness (biliary colic, hepatitis, vasoocclusive crisis), knee or hip pain (aseptic necrosis of the femoral head), or priapism.

C. Assess the risk of infection. Because functional asplenia develops at an early age, infants and children with sickle cell disease commonly develop bacterial sepsis and/or meningitis. Patients with a temperature greater than 101° F (with or without a focus of infection) or with unexplained lethargy or diarrhea may have overwhelming sepsis (*Streptococcus pneumoniae* and *Haemophilus influenzae* are the most common organisms). Immediately obtain blood and other cultures and begin parenteral antibiotics (e.g., ceftriaxone). Perform a lumbar puncture for patients with meningismus or young children with excessive lethargy or toxicity.

D. Consider the possibility of an illness unrelated to sickle cell disease (e.g., appendicitis presenting with abdominal pain). Acute splenic enlargement with a hematocrit below baseline and/or signs of intravascular volume depletion suggest a splenic sequestration crisis. A lower-than-baseline hematocrit in association with a reticulocyte count significantly lower than baseline suggests an aplastic crisis.

(Continued on page 110)

Patient with ACUTE ILLNESS ASSOCIATED WITH SICKLE CELL DISEASE

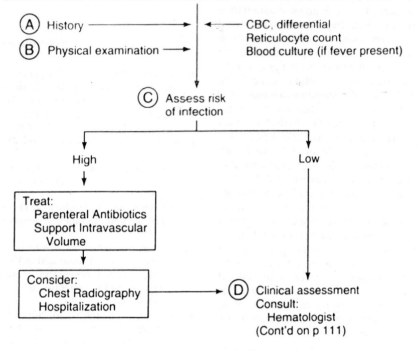

E. Vasoocclusive crises with severe pain secondary to ischemia may occur in any part of the body. Treatment includes hydration with 1 to 1½ times maintenance fluids (sickle cell patients have hyposthenuria but avoid excessive hydration) and adequate analgesia (codeine for mild pain, morphine or hydromorphone for severe pain). Nonsteroidal antiinflammatory analgesics (e.g., ibuprofen, ketoralac) may also be useful in some cases. Do *not* use repeated doses of meperidine because it has the potential to induce seizures. Indications for hospitalization include inability to maintain hydration orally and the failure of oral analgesics to control pain. It is sometimes difficult to differentiate an abdominal crisis from cholecystitis. Imaging studies, surgical consultation, and comparison of liver function tests with baseline values may be helpful. Consider the possibility of acute osteomyelitis *(Staphylococcus aureus, Salmonella)* in patients thought to have bone infarctions, but infarction is far more common. Pulmonary infarction is difficult to differentiate from bacterial pneumonia *(S. pneumoniae, H. influenzae, S. aureus, Mycoplasma)*; thus, antibiotic coverage should be provided if fever is present. A cerebrovascular accident is indication for exchange transfusion and subsequent chronic transfusions. Boys with priapism may benefit from exchange transfusion and may require surgical drainage.

F. Aplastic crises, which are common in association with viral illness, especially human parvovirus, represent a transient inability of erythropoiesis to keep pace with chronic hemolysis. The rapidly falling hemoglobin may result in congestive heart failure; red cell transfusions are sometimes needed to support the patient until adequate red cell production resumes.

G. Splenic sequestration can be a life-threatening emergency requiring prompt red cell transfusions to maintain intravascular volume. Such episodes, often triggered by infection, tend to recur.

H. Sickle cell patients who require general anesthesia for surgical procedures should be first transfused to reduce the risk of perioperative sickling complications.

References

Emond AM, Collis R, Darvill D, et al. Acute splenic sequestration in homozygous sickle cell disease: Natural history and management. J Pediatr 1985; 107:201.

Grundy R, Howard R, Evans J. Practical management of pain in sickling disorders. Arch Dis Child 1993; 69:256.

Lane PA. Sickle cell disease. Pediatr Clin North Am 1996 (in press).

Lane PA, Rogers ZR, Woods GM, et al. Fatal pneumococcal septicemia in hemoglobin SC disease. J Pediatr 1994; 124:859.

Ohene-Frempong K. Stroke in sickle cell disease: Demographic, clinical, and therapeutic considerations. Semin Hematol 1991; 28:213.

Rogers ZR, Buchanan GR. Bacteremia in childhood with sickle hemoglobin C disease and sickle β-thalassemia: Is prophylactic penicillin necessary? J Pediatr 1995; 127:348.

Serjeant GR. Sickle cell disease. 3rd ed. New York: Oxford University Press, 1992.

Vichinsky EP, Haberkern CM, Neumayr L, et al. A comparison of conservative and aggressive transfusion regimens in the perioperative management of sickle cell disease. N Engl J Med 1995; 333:206.

Vichinsky EP, Lubin BH. Suggested guidelines for the treatment of children with sickle cell anemia. Hematol Oncol Clin North Am 1987; 1:483.

Vichinsky E, Williams R, Das M, et al. Pulmonary fat embolism: A distinct cause of severe acute chest syndrome in sickle cell anemia. Blood 1994; 83:3107.

Wilimas JA, Flynn PM, Harris S, et al. A randomized study of outpatient treatment with ceftriaxone for selected febrile children with sickle cell disease. N Engl J Med 1993; 329:472.

Zarkowsky HS, Gallagher D, Gill FM, et al. Bacteremia in sickle hemoglobinopathy. J Pediatr 1986; 109:579.

Patient with ACUTE ILLNESS ASSOCIATED WITH SICKLE CELL DISEASE

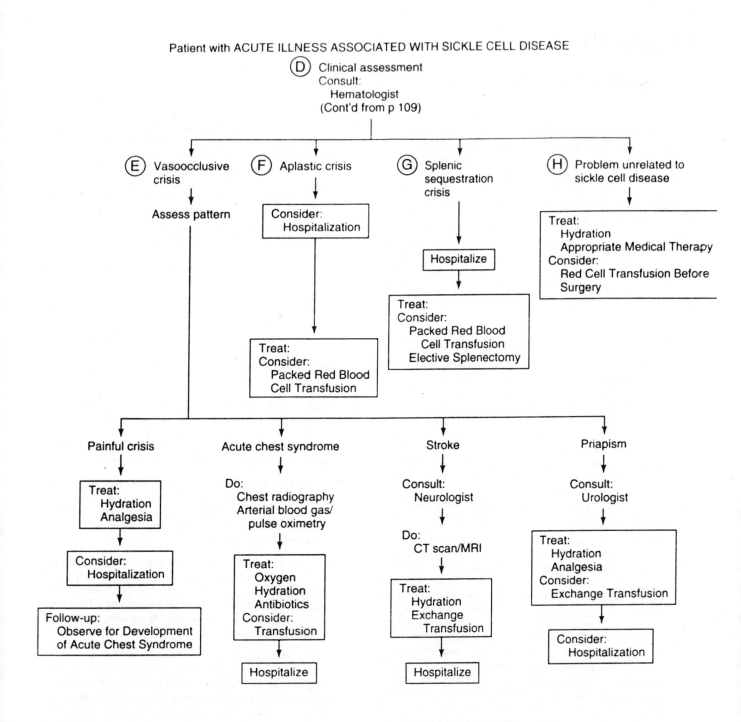

MENINGITIS

Stephen Berman, M.D.

Meningitis (inflammation of the meninges) is caused by viral or bacterial infections. Approximately two thirds of diagnosed cases are viral and one third bacterial. The most common viral infections are enteroviruses (coxsackievirus, echovirus, and mumps virus) and herpes simplex virus. The bacterial pathogens that cause neonatal meningitis include group B streptococcus (GBS), gram-negative enteric organisms, *Staphylococcus aureus, Listeria monocytogenes,* and enterococci. The pathogens of infants more than 3 months of age and children are *Haemophilus influenzae* type B (HIB), *Streptococcus pneumoniae, Neisseria meningitidis,* and *Salmonella.* The frequency of HIB infection has decreased dramatically with immunization. There is an overlap of pathogens at ages 1 to 3 months.

A. In the history ask about the onset, pattern, and degree of fever. Risk factors include immunization status, current medications, allergies, underlying conditions such as cardiopulmonary, GI or renal disease, sickle cell disease, central venous catheter, other indwelling lines, and conditions and therapy that compromise immunity, especially HIV infection. Look for alterations in the mental status and normal level of activity, including playfulness, irritability, feeding and sleeping patterns, responsiveness, and seizures. Ask about respiratory symptoms (cough, congestion, coryza, sore throat, earache, fast or difficult breathing, chest indrawing [retractions]) and GI symptoms (vomiting, diarrhea, abdominal distention, abdominal pain, blood in stools).

B. On physical examination look, listen, and feel for findings that suggest meningitis. Note signs of meningeal irritation, altered mental status, nuchal rigidity, a bulging fontanelle, paradoxic irritability, and Brudzinski and Kernig signs. In Brudzinski sign the knees flex in response to rapid flexion of the neck. Kernig sign is resistance to extension of the leg. Evaluate hydration status and note signs of shock such as mottled skin color, slow capillary refill, increased pulse, and decreased blood pressure. Perform a neurologic examination and document focal neurologic signs, weakness, or ataxia. Measure the head circumference. Note any exanthem, purpura or petechiae and soft-tissue, bone, or joint infection. Patients with *N. meningitidis* or *H. influenzae* bacteremia should have a lumbar puncture regardless of their clinical appearance. The incidence of *H. influenzae* meningitis in patients with occult bacteremia is 15%, and with facial or periorbital cellulitis, 9%. One fourth of these patients lack clinical findings of meningitis.

C. The initial diagnosis of meningitis is based on examination of the CSF. After the neonatal period a normal CSF should have no more than 10 white blood cells per cubic millimeter, a glucose level above 50% of the serum concentration, a protein level less than 45 mg/dl, and a negative Gram stain. The Gram stain is positive in 85% to 99% of patients without pretreatment and in 79% of pretreated patients with culture-proven bacterial meningitis. The risk of bacterial meningitis is low regardless of prior antibiotic therapy in a stable patient when the Gram stain is negative, the CSF cell count is less than 200 cells with less than 50% polymorphonuclear leukocytes, and glucose is above 40 mg/dl. CSF cell counts above 500/mm^3 are suggestive but not diagnostic of bacterial infection, as 45% of patients with enteroviral meningitis have CSF counts above 500/mm^3. Consider preoxygenation to reduce hypoxemia during a lumbar puncture for infants. Anemia is common in *H. influenzae* infection because of acute hemolysis with an impaired bone marrow response. Thrombocytopenia and anemia suggest disseminated intravascular coagulation (DIC), which can be confirmed with a prothrombin time (PT), partial thromboplastin time (PTT), fibrinogen, and fibrin split products.

D. Obtain a cranial CT or MRI before performing lumbar puncture when focal neurologic signs, papilledema, or cardiovascular instability suggests generalized cerebral edema or a brain abscess. However, do not delay antibiotic therapy until the CSF is obtained.

E. Assess the degree of illness. Very severely ill patients have signs of severe dehydration, shock, respiratory distress, DIC, electrolyte abnormalities, hypoglycemia, markedly altered mental status, prolonged seizures, or focal neurologic signs.

F. For the initial 24 to 48 hours patients with bacterial meningitis should be monitored for hemodynamic stability, neurologic status, urine output, electrolytes, glucose, and calcium. Maintain the patient's hydration in the normal range. Correct significant dehydration and avoid overhydration.

G. Initial antibiotic therapy is based on the age of the patient. Treat neonates with ampicillin and an aminoglycoside (gentamicin) or cefotaxime. Ampicillin is needed to cover *Listeria* and enterococci. Treat infants 1 to 3 months of age with ampicillin and ceftriaxone to broaden the coverage for resistant *H. influenzae.* Treat older infants and children with ampicillin and ceftriaxone or chloramphenicol. Cefotaxime can be substituted for ceftriaxone. Switch to the single best antibiotic when culture and sensitivity results are available. Use penicillin G or ampicillin for GBS, *N. meningitidis,* and sensitive *S. pneumoniae;* ampicillin for *Listeria* and susceptible *H. influenzae;* ceftriaxone or chloramphenicol for β-lactamase–positive *H. influenzae.* Consider adding vancomycin to the initial therapy if penicillin-resistant *S. pneumoniae* is present in the area (Table 1). The duration of IV therapy varies with the pathogen. Treat gram-negative enterics

(Continued on page 114)

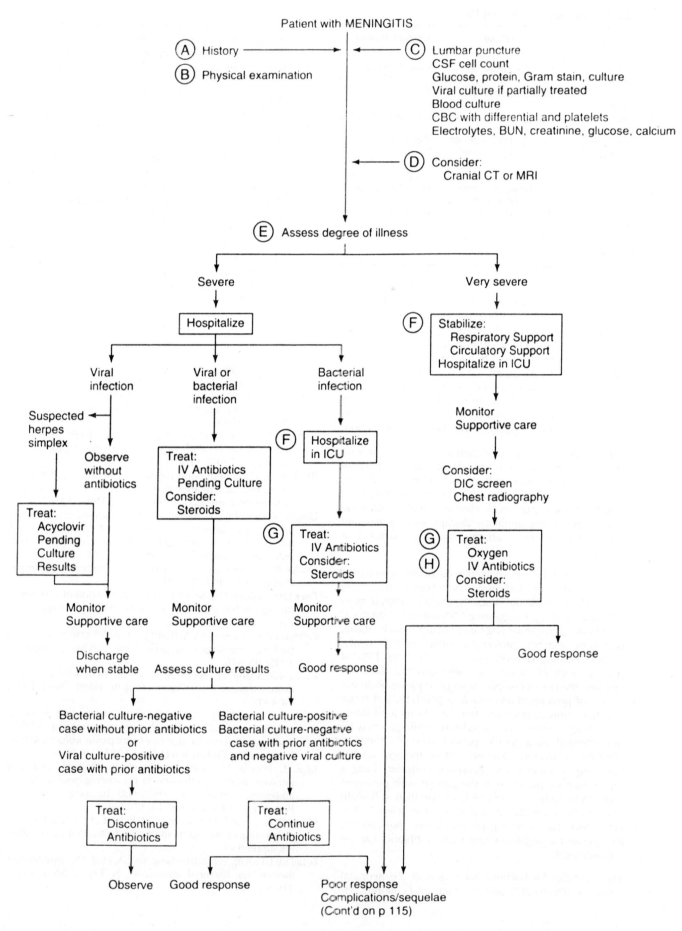

Patient with MENINGITIS

Ⓐ History
Ⓑ Physical examination

Ⓒ Lumbar puncture
CSF cell count
Glucose, protein, Gram stain, culture
Viral culture if partially treated
Blood culture
CBC with differential and platelets
Electrolytes, BUN, creatinine, glucose, calcium

Ⓓ Consider:
Cranial CT or MRI

Ⓔ Assess degree of illness

Severe

Hospitalize

Viral infection

Viral or bacterial infection

Bacterial infection

Suspected herpes simplex

Observe without antibiotics

Treat:
IV Antibiotics
Pending Culture
Consider:
Steroids

Ⓕ Hospitalize in ICU

Treat:
Acyclovir
Pending Culture Results

Ⓖ Treat:
IV Antibiotics
Consider:
Steroids

Monitor
Supportive care

Monitor
Supportive care

Monitor
Supportive care

Discharge when stable

Assess culture results

Good response

Bacterial culture-negative case without prior antibiotics
or
Viral culture-positive case with prior antibiotics

Bacterial culture-positive
Bacterial culture-negative case with prior antibiotics and negative viral culture

Treat:
Discontinue Antibiotics

Treat:
Continue Antibiotics

Observe

Good response

Poor response
Complications/sequelae
(Cont'd on p 115)

Very severe

Ⓕ Stabilize:
Respiratory Support
Circulatory Support
Hospitalize in ICU

Monitor
Supportive care

Consider:
DIC screen
Chest radiography

Ⓖ
Ⓗ Treat:
Oxygen
IV Antibiotics
Consider:
Steroids

Good response

TABLE 1 Therapy for Meningitis

Drug	IV Dose	Product Availability
Ampicillin sodium	50 mg/kg/dose q6h	Vials: 0.125, 0.25, 0.5, 1, 2, 4 g
Cefotaxime (Claforan)	50 mg/kg/dose q6h	Vials: 0.5, 1, 2 g
Ceftriaxone (Rocephin)	50 mg/kg/dose q12h	Vials: 0.25, 0.5, 1 g
Chloramphenicol	25 mg/kg/dose q6–8h	Vial: 1 g
Dexamethasone	0.15 mg/kg/dose q6h IV × 4 days	Solution: 4 mg/ml (1, 5, 10, 25 ml) 10 mg/ml (10 ml)
Gentamicin	2.5 mg/kg/dose q8h (neonates q12h)	Vials: 20, 80 mg
Penicillin G sodium	40–50,000 U/kg/dose q4h	Vial: 5 million unit
Vancomycin (Vancocin)	10–15 mg/kg/dose q6h	Vials: 500 mg, 10 g

fo 21 days; GBS, 14 days; *S. pneumoniae*, 10 to 14 days; *H. influenzae*, 7 to 10 days; and *N. meningitidis*, 7 days. When using aminoglycosides or chloramphenicol, monitor blood levels (therapeutic levels for gentamicin or tobramycin are 4 to 8 μg/ml; for kanamycin or amikacin, 15 to 25 μg/ml; for chloramphenicol, 10 to 20 μg/ml). Adequate blood chloramphenicol levels can be achieved with oral administration. If possible, avoid aminoglycosides in patients with renal disease and chloramphenicol in patients with hepatic dysfunction.

H. The administration of dexamethasone before or with antibiotics appears to reduce the incidence of sensorineural hearing loss without increasing mortality or other complications. The antiinflammatory effects of dexamethasone may mask clinical conditions that fail to respond to the antibiotic therapy such as resistant *S. pneumoniae*, brain abscess, and mycobacterial or fungal infection.

I. Patients should improve within 48 hours of initiating antibiotic therapy. Indications of a poor response are persistent opisthotonos, seizures, coma or altered mental status, and signs suggesting CNS complication (focal neurologic signs, enlarging head circumference, ataxia, persistent seizures, prolonged coma, altered mental status). Prolonged fever occurs in 10% to 15% of patients with *H. influenzae* meningitis but does not increase the risk of complications or sequelae. Rule out causes of prolonged fever such as phlebitis, soft-tissue infection, urinary tract infection, and bone joint infection. Drug fever must be considered. Antibiotics may be discontinued in a febrile patient who is otherwise clinically recovered. Routine end of therapy lumbar puncture is unnecessary; however, consider doing a repeat lumbar puncture in the patient with persistent fever. When a deciliter of CSF has fewer than 300 white blood cells, fewer than 25% polymorphonuclear leukocytes, less than 100 mg protein, more than 30 mg glucose and a negative Gram stain, antibiotics can be discontinued.

J. The mortality for bacterial meningitis in the neonatal period is 10% to 20% and in infants and children, 3% to 10%. Sequelae are present in 25% to 50% of survivors: language disorders, 15%; sensorineural hearing loss, 10%; mental retardation, 10%; and seizures, 3% to 8%. Sequelae are more likely in patients with delayed sterilization of CSF and complications. The sequelae of enteroviral meningitis in the first year of life vary. A recent study found that survivors had no major impairments. An earlier study reported that 58% are normal, 15% have significant handicaps, and 26% have possible impairments.

K. Signs of CNS complications are focal neurologic findings, prolonged seizures, persistent alterations in mental status, enlarging head circumferences, and ataxia. A CT scan will identify significant CNS pathology: subdural effusion or empyema, cerebral edema, cerebral abscess, cerebral infarction, or hydrocephalus. Small subdural effusions are common and should not be drained. Aspirate an effusion or empyema if it is large and associated with ventricular displacement, focal neurologic signs, signs of increased intracranial pressure, or deterioration in the patient's condition.

References

Baker RC, Bausher JC. Meningitis complicating acute bacterial facial cellulitis. Pediatr Infect Dis J 1986; 5:421.

Bergman I, Painter MJ, Wald ER, et al. Outcome in children with enteroviral meningitis during the first year of life. J Pediatr 1987; 110:705.

Bonadio WA. The cerebrospinal fluid: Physiologic aspects and alterations associated with bacterial meningitis. Pediatr Infect Dis J 1992; 11:423.

Bradley JS. Dexamethasone therapy in meningitis: Potentially misleading antiinflammatory effects in central nervous system infections. Pediatr Infect Dis J 1994; 13:823.

Dagan R, Jenista JA, Menegus MA. Association of clinical presentation, laboratory findings, and virus serotypes with the presence of meningitis in hospitalized infants with enterovirus infection. J Pediatr 1988; 113:975.

Dodge PR. Neurological sequelae of acute bacterial meningitis. Pediatr Ann 1994; 23:101.

Fiser DH, Grobier GA, Smith CE, et al. Prevention of hypoxemia during lumbar puncture in infancy with preoxygenation. Pediatr Emerg Care 1993; 9:81.

Grimwood K, Anderson VA, Bond L, et al. Adverse outcomes of bacterial meningitis in school-age survivors. Pediatrics 1995; 95:646.

Kanra GY, Ozen H, Secmeer G, et al. Beneficial effects of dexamethasone in children. Pediatr Infect Dis J 1995; 14:490.

Kaplan SL, Smith EO, Willis C, et al. Association between preadmission oral antibiotic therapy and cerebrospinal fluid findings and sequelae due to *Haemophilus influenzae* type B meningitis. Pediatr Infect Dis J 1985; 5:626.

Kilpi T, Peltola H, Jauhianen T, et al. Oral glycerol and intravenous dexamethasone in preventing neurologic and audiologic sequelae of childhood bacterial meningitis. Pediatr Infect Dis J 1995; 14:270.

Klein JO, Feigin RD, McCracken GH. Report of the task force on diagnosis and management of meningitis. Pediatrics 1986; 78(Suppl):959.

Lebel MH, Frei BJ, Syrogiannopoulous GA, et al. Dexamethasone therapy for bacterial meningitis. N Engl J Med 1988; 319:964.

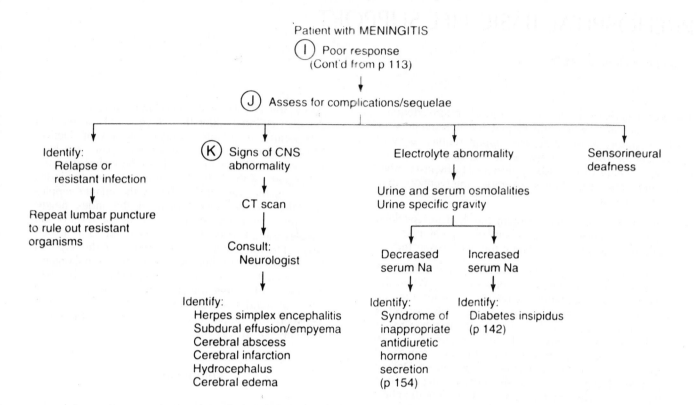

Patient with MENINGITIS

(I) Poor response
(Cont'd from p 113)

(J) Assess for complications/sequelae

Identify:
Relapse or
resistant infection

Repeat lumbar puncture
to rule out resistant
organisms

(K) Signs of CNS
abnormality

CT scan

Consult:
Neurologist

Identify:
Herpes simplex encephalitis
Subdural effusion/empyema
Cerebral abscess
Cerebral infarction
Hydrocephalus
Cerebral edema

Electrolyte abnormality

Urine and serum osmolalities
Urine specific gravity

Decreased
serum Na

Identify:
Syndrome of
inappropriate
antidiuretic
hormone
secretion
(p 154)

Increased
serum Na

Identify:
Diabetes insipidus
(p 142)

Sensorineural
deafness

.... dio CM, Faingezicht I, Paris M, et al. The beneficial effects of early dexamethasone administration on infants and children with bacterial meningitis. N Engl J Med 1991; 324:1525.

Sloas MM, Barrett FF, Chesney PJ, et al. Cephalosporin treatment failure in penicillin- and cephalosporin-resistant *Streptococcus pneumoniae* meningitis. Pediatr Infect Dis J 1992; 11:662.

Snedeker JD, Kaplan SL, Dodge PR, et al. Subdural effusion and its relationship with neurologic sequelae of bacterial meningitis in infancy: A prospective study. Pediatrics 1990; 86:163.

Syrogiannopoulos GA, Nelson JD, McCracken GH. Subdural collections of fluid in acute bacterial meningitis: A review of 136 cases. Pediatr Infect Dis J 1986; 5:343.

Waler JA, Rathore MH. Outpatient management of pediatric bacterial meningitis. Pediatr Infect Dis J 1995; 14:89.

PREHOSPITAL BASIC LIFE SUPPORT

Stephen Berman, M.D.

The goal of pediatric basic life support is to restore adequate tissue oxygenation when the patient has a respiratory or cardiorespiratory arrest. Basic life support requires a rapid assessment of responsiveness, breathing, and circulation. Cardiopulmonary arrest is usually produced by hypoxia rather than ventricular arrhythmias, so rapid intervention may prevent cardiac arrest.

A. Assess responsiveness by tapping the child and speaking loudly. Because of the possibility of a spinal injury, do not move or shake the child if trauma is suspected.

B. Open the airway with the head tilt–chin lift maneuver (Fig. 1) or the jaw-thrust maneuver (Fig. 2). When the patient is not spontaneously breathing, perform rescue breathing. If a mask with a one-way valve or other device is available, use it. If the patient is less than 1 year old, place your mouth over the infant's nose and mouth to create a seal. In an older patient make a mouth-to-mouth seal and pinch the patient's nose closed. Deliver two slow breaths of 1 to 1.5 seconds, pausing between the breaths. The chest should rise. Failure of the chest to rise after repositioning a nonbreathing unconscious patient suggests a foreign body obstruction.

C. Assess the circulation by checking the carotid artery pulse in children older than 1 year and the brachial artery pulse in infants younger than 1 year. Deliver chest compressions with the patient supine on a hard flat surface. The head should not be higher than the other parts of the body. For an infant place the index finger on the sternum just below the infant's nipples and the middle fingers next to the index finger. Compress the chest one finger below the level of the nipples using two or three fingers about ½ to 1 inch apart. Do not compress the chest over the xyphoid process because of the risk of injury to internal organs. For a child 1 to 8 years of age identify the notch where the lower ribs meet the sternum and place the heel of your hand over the lower half of the sternum between the nipple line and the notch. Compress the chest 1 to 1½ inches.

References

Chameides L, Hazinski MF, eds. Textbook of pediatric advanced life support. Chicago: American Heart Association, 1994.

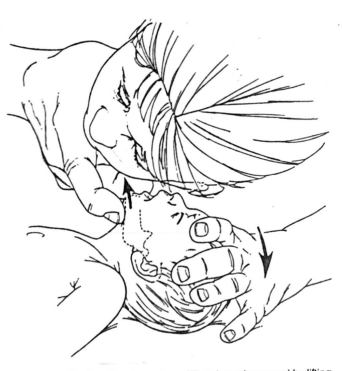

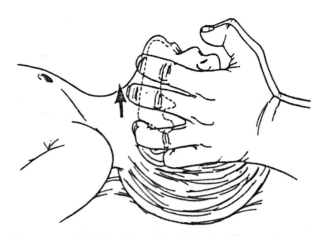

Figure 1 The head tilt–chin lift maneuver. One hand is used to tilt the head, extending the neck. The index finger of the rescuer's other hand lifts the mandible outward by lifting on the chin. Head tilt should not be performed if cervical spine injury is suspected. (From Chameides L, Hazinski MF, eds. Textbook of pediatric advanced life support. Chicago: American Heart Association, 1994:3-4; with permission.)

Figure 2 The jaw-thrust maneuver. The airway is opened by lifting the angle of the mandible. The rescuer uses two or three fingers of each hand to lift the jaw while the remaining fingers guide the jaw upward and outward. (From Chameides L, Hazinski MF, eds. Textbook of pediatric advanced life support. Chicago: American Heart Association, 1994:3-5; with permission.)

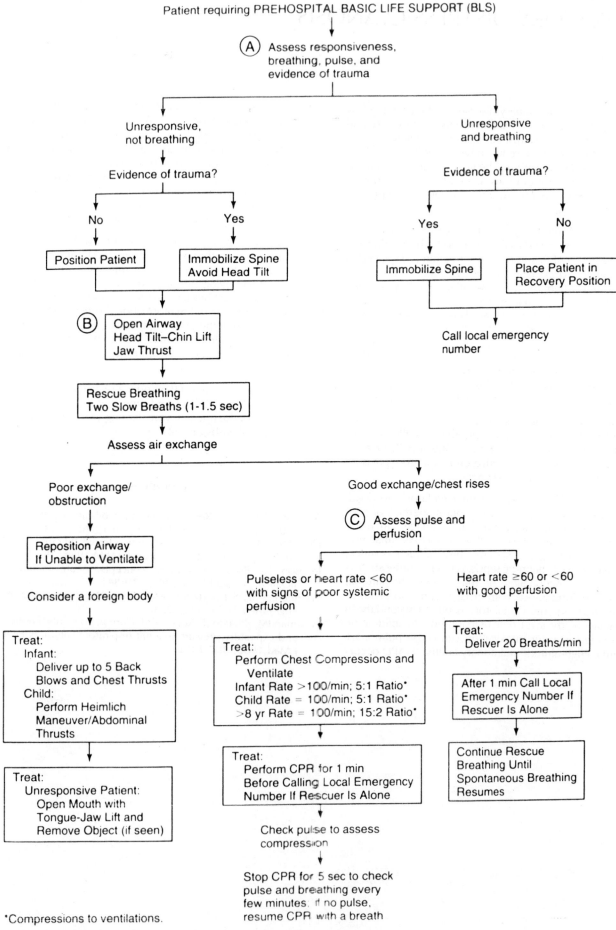

Patient requiring PREHOSPITAL BASIC LIFE SUPPORT (BLS)

(A) Assess responsiveness, breathing, pulse, and evidence of trauma

Unresponsive, not breathing

Evidence of trauma?

No → Position Patient

Yes → Immobilize Spine Avoid Head Tilt

(B) Open Airway Head Tilt–Chin Lift Jaw Thrust

Rescue Breathing Two Slow Breaths (1-1.5 sec)

Assess air exchange

Poor exchange/obstruction

Reposition Airway If Unable to Ventilate

Consider a foreign body

Treat:
  Infant:
    Deliver up to 5 Back Blows and Chest Thrusts
  Child:
    Perform Heimlich Maneuver/Abdominal Thrusts

Treat:
  Unresponsive Patient:
    Open Mouth with Tongue-Jaw Lift and Remove Object (if seen)

Good exchange/chest rises

(C) Assess pulse and perfusion

Pulseless or heart rate <60 with signs of poor systemic perfusion

Treat:
  Perform Chest Compressions and Ventilate
  Infant Rate >100/min; 5:1 Ratio*
  Child Rate = 100/min; 5:1 Ratio*
  >8 yr Rate = 100/min; 15:2 Ratio*

Treat:
  Perform CPR for 1 min Before Calling Local Emergency Number If Rescuer Is Alone

Check pulse to assess compression

Stop CPR for 5 sec to check pulse and breathing every few minutes. If no pulse, resume CPR with a breath

Heart rate ≥60 or <60 with good perfusion

Treat:
  Deliver 20 Breaths/min

After 1 min Call Local Emergency Number If Rescuer Is Alone

Continue Rescue Breathing Until Spontaneous Breathing Resumes

Unresponsive and breathing

Evidence of trauma?

Yes → Immobilize Spine

No → Place Patient in Recovery Position

Call local emergency number

*Compressions to ventilations.

117

RESPIRATORY DISTRESS/CYANOSIS

Stephen Berman, M.D.

Cyanosis related to pulmonary disease can be produced by alveolar hypoventilation, ventilation profusion inequality, and impairment of oxygen diffusion. Cyanosis is related to the presence of 3 g or more of reduced hemoglobin per 100 ml. It is best detected by examining the lips, tongue, and mucous membranes. Peripheral cyanosis related to slow blood flow and large differences in arteriovenous oxygen is often present in the hands, feet, and circumoral areas.

A. The arterial blood gas (ABG) measures the partial pressure of dissolved oxygen in blood. The relationship between the ABG and oxygen saturation is displayed in the oxygen dissociation curve. Pulmonary disease is suggested when the administration of 100% oxygen results in a substantial increase in the Pao_2 compared with a gas obtained in room air. The shunt study is useful in identifying fixed right-to-left shunts that suggest cardiac disease or marked pulmonary hypertension. A Pao_2 less than 55 torr on 80% to 100% oxygen or a Pco_2 over 50 torr suggests respiratory failure. Intubate and ventilate these children. Consider the use of sedation/paralysis when the patient is fighting the ventilator.

B. Adult respiratory distress syndrome results when severe damage to the capillary endothelial cells reduces surfactant levels, causing massive atelectasis. Use assisted ventilation with positive end-expiratory pressure to maintain adequate oxygenation.

C. Pulmonary edema results from circulatory overload, decreased oncotic pressure (hypoproteinemia), or capillary damage and leak. Capillary damage can result from a direct pulmonary insult such as a toxic inhalation or near drowning or a systemic process such as shock, anoxia, or overwhelming sepsis. A CNS disorder such as meningitis, encephalitis, or mass lesion (hematoma, tumor, or intracranial hemorrhage) can also produce pulmonary edema. Circulatory overload secondary to renal failure, the syndrome of inappropriate antidiuretic hormone, or water intoxication can cause pulmonary edema. High-altitude pulmonary edema (HAPE) occurs in children and adolescents who live at low altitude and travel above 8500 feet, in residents of high-altitude areas who return home from low altitudes, and in residents of high-altitude areas who develop a viral upper respiratory infection. Clinical signs include dyspnea, cough, periodic breathing, and frothy sputum. Pulmonary edema seen on the x-ray film may be only right-sided with basilar involvement. Manage cases with oxygen and return patients to a lower altitude.

D. Space-occupying pulmonary lesions with air leak include pneumothorax, pneumomediastinum, pneumopericardium, and pulmonary interstitial emphysema. Space-occupying lesions without air leaks include diaphragmatic hernia, congenital lobar emphysema, cystic adenomatoid malformation, bronchiogenic cysts, eventration of the diaphragm, lung abscess, and tumor. Work up a pulmonary mass with tomograms and a CT scan. Consider fluoroscopy, bronchoscopy, and angiography.

E. Obstructive lesions of the upper airway include choanal atresia, Pierre Robin syndrome, vocal cord paralysis, stenosis of the trachea, vascular rings, foreign body, and congenital webs or cysts.

References

Anas NG, Perkin RM. Resuscitation and stabilization of the child with respiratory disease. Pediatr Ann 1986; 15:43.

Flick MR, Murray JF. High-dose corticosteroid therapy in the adult respiratory distress syndrome. JAMA 1984; 251:1054.

Johnson TS, Rock PB. Current concepts: Acute mountain sickness. N Engl J Med 1988; 319:841.

Weinberger SE, Schwartzstein RM, Weiss JW. Hypercapnia. N Engl J Med 1989; 321:1223.

Weisman IM, Rinaldo JE, Rogers RM. Current concepts: Positive end-expiratory pressure in adult respiratory failure. N Engl J Med 1982; 307:1381.

Patient with RESPIRATORY DISTRESS/CYANOSIS

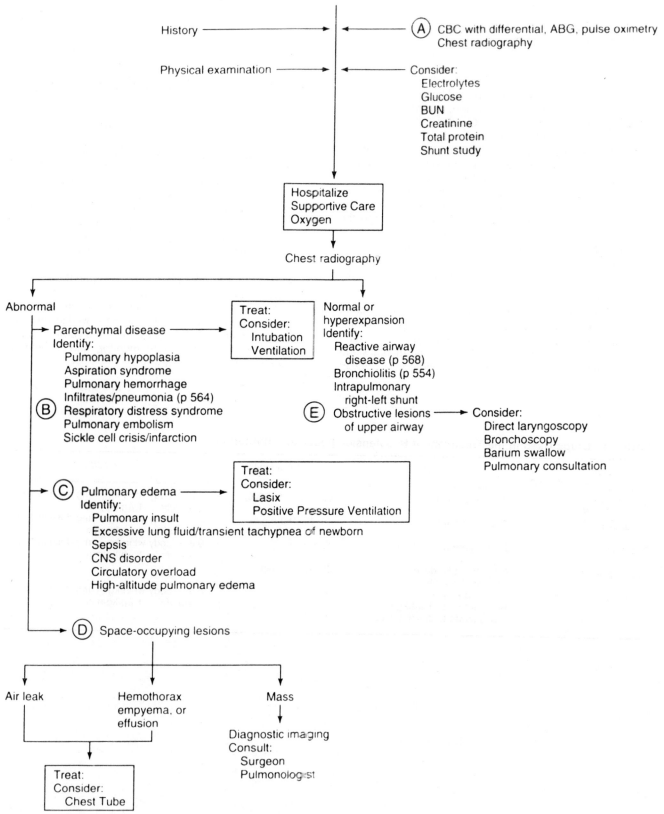

History ⟶ ⟵ Ⓐ CBC with differential, ABG, pulse oximetry
Chest radiography

Physical examination ⟶ ⟵ Consider:
Electrolytes
Glucose
BUN
Creatinine
Total protein
Shunt study

Hospitalize
Supportive Care
Oxygen

Chest radiography

Abnormal

⟶ Parenchymal disease
Identify:
Pulmonary hypoplasia
Aspiration syndrome
Pulmonary hemorrhage
Infiltrates/pneumonia (p 564)
Ⓑ Respiratory distress syndrome
Pulmonary embolism
Sickle cell crisis/infarction

Treat:
Consider:
Intubation
Ventilation

Normal or
hyperexpansion
Identify:
Reactive airway
disease (p 568)
Bronchiolitis (p 554)
Intrapulmonary
right-left shunt
Ⓔ Obstructive lesions ⟶ Consider:
of upper airway   Direct laryngoscopy
Bronchoscopy
Barium swallow
Pulmonary consultation

⟶ Ⓒ Pulmonary edema
Identify:
Pulmonary insult
Excessive lung fluid/transient tachypnea of newborn
Sepsis
CNS disorder
Circulatory overload
High-altitude pulmonary edema

Treat:
Consider:
Lasix
Positive Pressure Ventilation

⟶ Ⓓ Space-occupying lesions

Air leak

Hemothorax
empyema, or
effusion

Mass

Diagnostic imaging
Consult:
Surgeon
Pulmonologist

Treat:
Consider:
Chest Tube

SHOCK/HYPOTENSION

James W. Wiggins Jr., M.D.
Stephen Berman, M.D.

In shock, tissue oxygenation is impaired because of hypoperfusion related to poor cardiac function, hypovolemia, or loss of vascular tone (septic shock). Cardiac failure may be a primary and/or secondary abnormality. Possible mechanisms adversely affecting cardiac function in shock include decreased coronary blood flow, marked acidosis, high levels of myocardial depressant factor, and increased peripheral vasoconstriction (afterload). Hypovolemia may be related to an obvious event such as acute external hemorrhage, vomiting, diarrhea, diuresis, or extensive burns. Occult loss into the third space occurs with peritonitis, pulmonary edema, and intracranial or internal hemorrhage. Vasodilation produced by sepsis, spinal cord injuries, anaphylaxis, or drugs produces a relative hypovolemia without fluid loss from the vascular space.

A. In the physical examination assess the circulatory status. Note the blood pressure, heart rate, respiratory rate, capillary refill (normal, < 2 seconds), skin color, temperature, and urine output. Evaluate the mental status and note signs of CNS disease. Also note signs of heart failure such as gallop rhythm, hepatomegaly, peripheral edema, and distended neck veins.

B. The objective in the treatment of shock is the reestablishment of adequate tissue perfusion and oxygenation. This requires monitoring of ventilation (Pa_{O_2}, P_{CO_2}, pH), blood pressure, cardiac function (cardiac output), circulatory blood volume (central venous pressure [CVP], wedge pressure) and oxygen-carrying capacity (hemoglobin). A systemic arterial catheter allows continuous monitoring of systemic arterial pressure as well as access for blood sampling and blood gas determinations. Other venous lines should include a CVP line in the right atrium and a large-bore venous line for infusion of fluids and drugs. Consider placing a balloon-tip flow-directed Swan-Ganz catheter, preferably a thermodilution cardiac output catheter. This allows measurement of right atrial pressures, pulmonary capillary wedge pressures (approximates left atrial pressures), and cardiac output. Place an ECG, heart rate monitor, and catheter to document urine output.

(Continued on page 122)

TABLE 1 Drugs Used in the Treatment of Hypotension/Reduction of Afterload

Drug	Dosage	Product Availability	Remarks
Isoproterenol	0.1–1 µg/kg/min	0.2 mg/ml (1:5000)	0.6 × body wt in kg = mg dose in 100 ml 1 ml/hr = 1 µg/kg/min
Dopamine	5–20 µg/kg/min	40, 80, 160 mg/ml	0.6 × body wt in kg = mg dose in 100 ml 1 ml/hr = 1 µg/kg/min
Dobutamine	2–15 µg/kg/min	12.5 mg/ml	0.6 × body wt in kg = mg dose in 100 ml 1 ml/hr = 1 µg/kg/min
Hydralazine	0.1–0.2 mg/kg/dose IM or IV q4–6h	20 mg/ml inject	
Sodium nitroprusside	0.5–1 µg/kg/min Begin with 0.5–1 µg/kg/min and titrate to desired effect	50 mg/vial	0.6 × body wt in kg = mg dose in 100 ml 1 ml/hr = 1 µg/kg/min

Patient with SHOCK/HYPOTENSION

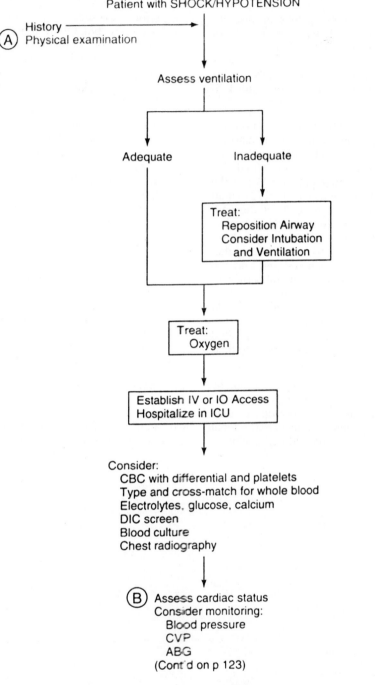

(Cont'd on p 123)

C. After establishing adequate ventilation, stabilize the circulation with an isotonic fluid infusion of 10 to 20 ml/kg as rapidly as the degree of hypotension warrants. Treat severe acidosis (pH < 7.2, base deficit − 10 or greater) with an infusion of sodium bicarbonate; initially administer half of the dose calculated by the body weight (kg) × the base deficit × 0.4 (usually 2 to 3 mEq/kg). Consider antibiotics when septic shock is suspected.

D. If possible, restore the circulatory blood volume using the CVP as a guide. In patients with a low hematocrit, fluids should include either whole blood or packed red blood cells and fresh frozen plasma; use colloid (5% albumin or plasminate) for other patients. When the CVP is less than 6 torr, administer at least 4 ml/kg of fluid over 10 minutes, and monitor the CVP. If the CVP changes by less than 2 torr, administer another 4 ml/kg bolus over 10 minutes. Continue administering boluses of fluid until the CVP rises to 5 to 10 torr, indicating that circulatory blood volume has been restored and the patient is normotensive with good peripheral perfusion. When using wedge pressures, levels less than 10 torr in the first 24 to 48 hours are considered low and should be increased to 15 torr during this time. In patients in cardiogenic shock, this value may be already elevated with a normal CVP. If cardiomegaly exists prior to fluid administration, use all fluids with caution.

E. Sympathomimetic amines increase cardiac output by improving myocardial contractility and increasing heart rate. Dopamine has slightly fewer chronotropic cardiac effects compared with isoproterenol and increases renal blood flow at infusion rates less than 20 μg/kg/minute.

When 150 mg is added to 250 ml of D_5W or normal saline, 1 ml/kg/hour equals 10 μg/kg/minute. Isoproterenol infusions can be started at 0.1 μg/kg/minute if necessary, but follow the patient closely for tachyarrhythmias or ischemia. Add 1.5 mg to 250 ml of D_5W so that 1 ml/kg/hour equals 0.1 μg/kg/minute. Dobutamine is very effective in cardiogenic shock in doses of 2.5 to 15 μg/kg/minute.

F. The goal of vasodilator therapy is to reduce the resistance to left ventricular ejection (afterload). Consider using a short-acting vasodilator such as sodium nitroprusside at 1 μg/kg/minute. The maximum dosage of nitroprusside is 8 to 10 μg/kg/minute. Cyanide may accumulate at higher infusion rates, causing acidosis. Check cyanide levels if used at higher doses for more than 48 hours. An alternative is hydralazine 0.1 to 0.2 mg/kg intravenously every 4 to 6 hours.

References

Chameides L. Textbook of advanced pediatric life support. Dallas: American Heart Association, 1989.

Perkin RM, Levin DL. Shock in the pediatric patient. Part 1. J Pediatr 1982; 101:163.

Perkin RM, Levin DL. Shock in the pediatric patient. Part 2. J Pediatr 1982; 101:319.

Saez-Llorens X, McCracken GH. Sepsis syndrome and septic shock in pediatrics: Current concepts of terminology, pathophysiology, and management. J Pediatr 1993; 123:497.

Seri I. Cardiovascular, renal, and endocrine actions of dopamine in neonates and children. J Pediatr 1995; 126:333.

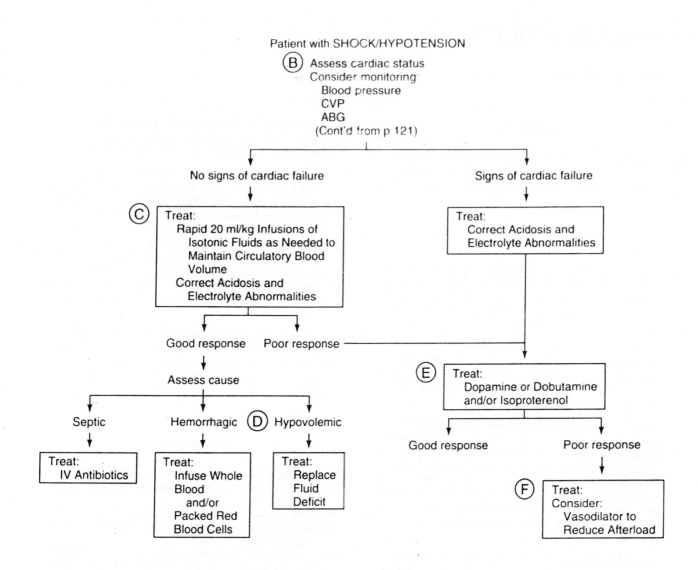

Patient with SHOCK/HYPOTENSION

(B) Assess cardiac status
Consider monitoring:
Blood pressure
CVP
ABG
(Cont'd from p 121)

No signs of cardiac failure   Signs of cardiac failure

(C) Treat:
Rapid 20 ml/kg Infusions of
Isotonic Fluids as Needed to
Maintain Circulatory Blood
Volume
Correct Acidosis and
Electrolyte Abnormalities

Treat:
Correct Acidosis and
Electrolyte Abnormalities

Good response   Poor response

Assess cause

Septic   Hemorrhagic   (D) Hypovolemic

Treat:
IV Antibiotics

Treat:
Infuse Whole
Blood
and/or
Packed Red
Blood Cells

Treat:
Replace
Fluid
Deficit

(E) Treat:
Dopamine or Dobutamine
and/or Isoproterenol

Good response   Poor response

(F) Treat:
Consider:
Vasodilator to
Reduce Afterload

STATUS EPILEPTICUS

Stephen Berman, M.D.

DEFINITION

Status epilepticus is generalized tonic-clonic seizures lasting longer than 20 minutes or recurrent seizures with failure to regain consciousness for longer than 30 minutes. Mortality is 6% to 18%.

ETIOLOGY

Status epilepticus has many causes, including infection (meningitis and encephalitis), anoxia, metabolic and electrolyte disorders, toxins, encephalopathies, malignancies, vascular disorders, and head trauma. However, no cause can be identified in about half of children.

A. In the history ask about a trigger or precipitating cause such as a head injury, prior neurologic condition, or drug ingestion. Determine whether the child has any acute or chronic illness, especially diabetes, renal, or metabolic disease.

B. Stabilize the patient to maintain adequate tissue oxygenation. Respiratory support includes establishing an adequate airway by repositioning the child's head and if necessary placing an oral or nasopharyngeal airway. Administer oxygen by mask to all patients. If air exchange is poor, institute bag mask ventilation, and if necessary intubate. Circulatory support with IV fluids may be necessary if signs of shock or hypotension are present.

C. Protect the patient from injury by placing the child on a soft flat area free of hard or sharp objects. If the child is on a bed, table, or stretcher, prevent the child from falling. Consider quickly placing a nasogastric tube to empty the stomach to prevent aspiration of vomitus.

D. Rapidly obtain IV access, draw blood for the initial laboratory studies, and administer a rapid-acting anticonvulsant, preferably lorazepam (Table 1). Lorazepam has a longer duration of action than diazepam and is less likely to result in respiratory depression or hypotension when additional drugs are given. If seizures are not controlled, begin an IV infusion of phenytoin and monitor for cardiac arrhythmia. Treat continuing seizures with an IV infusion of phenobarbital. Repeat phenobarbital every 30 minutes as needed to control seizures.

E. Consider administering IV glucose if a Dextrostix test or the clinical situation indicates hypoglycemia. Infuse a bolus of 25% dextrose (4 ml/kg) followed by 10% dextrose in quarter normal saline at a maintenance volume infusion rate (see p 148).

References

Lacey DJ, Singer WD, Horwitz SJ, et al. Lorazepam therapy of status epilepticus in children and adolescents. J Pediatr 1986; 108:771.

McBride MC. Status epilepticus. Pediatr Rev 1995; 16:386.

Selbst SM. Office management of status epilepticus. Pediatr Emerg Care 1991; 7:106.

Snead OC, Miles MV. Treatment of status epilepticus in children with rectal sodium valproate. J Pediatr 1985; 106:323.

TABLE 1   Drug Therapy of Status Epilepticus in Children and Adolescents

Drug	Dosage	Rate of Infusion	Repeat Instructions
Diazepam (Valium)	0.3 mg/kg IV (max 4 mg for infant, 10 mg older child)	Dose over 2 min	May repeat q10min × 2
Lorazepam (Ativan, Alzapam)	0.1 mg/kg IV (max 4 mg)	<2 mg/min	May repeat q10min × 3
Phenytoin (Dilantin)	15–20 mg/kg IV (1 mg/kg/min/load)	<50 mg/min	Do not repeat Monitor blood level
Phenobarbital	Infants/small child: 10–20 mg/kg IV Older child/adult: 5–10 mg/kg IV	<30 mg/min	Repeat as needed

Patient with STATUS EPILEPTICUS

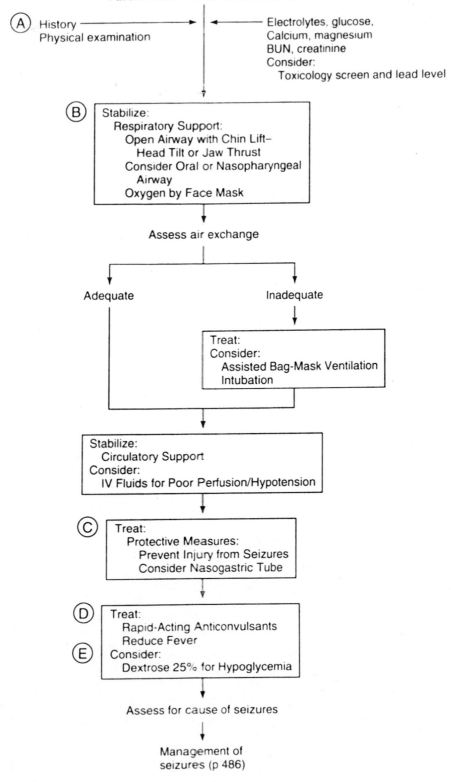

(A) History ————————————→ | ←——— Electrolytes, glucose,
Physical examination .... Calcium, magnesium
BUN, creatinine
Consider:
Toxicology screen and lead level

(B) Stabilize:
Respiratory Support:
Open Airway with Chin Lift–
Head Tilt or Jaw Thrust
Consider Oral or Nasopharyngeal
Airway
Oxygen by Face Mask

Assess air exchange

Adequate   Inadequate

Treat:
Consider:
Assisted Bag-Mask Ventilation
Intubation

Stabilize:
Circulatory Support
Consider:
IV Fluids for Poor Perfusion/Hypotension

(C) Treat:
Protective Measures:
Prevent Injury from Seizures
Consider Nasogastric Tube

(D) Treat:
Rapid-Acting Anticonvulsants
Reduce Fever
(E) Consider:
Dextrose 25% for Hypoglycemia

Assess for cause of seizures

Management of
seizures (p 486)

ENDOCRINE AND METABOLIC DISORDERS

Ambiguous Genitalia
Delayed Puberty
Hypercalcemia
Hyperglycemia
Hyperkalemia
Hypernatremia
Hypocalcemia
Hypoglycemia
Hypokalemia

Hyponatremia
Inborn Errors of Metabolism
Metabolic Acidosis
Obesity
Precocious Puberty in Boys
Precocious Puberty in Girls
Reye-Like Syndrome
Short Stature

AMBIGUOUS GENITALIA

Michael S. Kappy, M.D., Ph.D.
Carrie A. Ganong, M.D.

A. Note predisposing factors and conditions such as a family history of ambiguous genitalia, congenital adrenal hyperplasia (CAH), infant deaths, or maternal virilization.

B. Accurately describe the infant's phallus and the relationship of the urethral opening to the glans. Presence of at least one testis suggests the Y chromosome in the karyotype. Absence of palpable testes in the scrotal, labial, or inguinal region implies that *the child is a girl with salt-losing congenital adrenal hyperplasia until proven otherwise.* Associated abnormalities in the genitourinary system suggest a dysmorphic syndrome as opposed to an inherited metabolic disorder.

C. Much information can be gained about internal anatomy with the use of pelvic ultrasonography and a genitogram (i.e., a contrast study delineating the extent of the posterior vagina) to help identify the gonads and uterus if present.

D. Definitive karyotyping should be done in all cases, in contrast to screening tests, such as Y fluorescence and buccal smear. The results of karyotyping separate cases into genetic males (XY) with incomplete virilization, genetic females (XX) with excessive virilization, and chromosomal aberrations fitting neither genotype.

E. The evaluation of incomplete virilization in a genetic male may be most readily accomplished by measuring serum luteinizing hormone (LH), testosterone (T), and dihydrotestosterone (DHT). This enables the physician to distinguish between defects of the hypothalamopituitary axis and those of the testes. In addition, it helps identify defects in the androgen receptor causing end-organ insensitivity to androgens. It is imperative that age-appropriate norms be used to interpret these results, since the normal serum concentrations of LH, T, and DHT change considerably over the first 3 months of life. In most cases it is better to wait 2 to 4 weeks before measuring these hormones if there is no suggestion that an enzymatic disorder of the adrenal gland is present (i.e., normal plasma renin activity and no evidence of hypoglycemia). Gender assignment, usually based on the size of the infant's phallus, should be made as soon as possible, even before a definitive endocrine cause is identified. Consider an exploratory laparotomy and gonadal biopsy when the metabolic work-up is negative. Examine internal structures, including the gonads and the Wolffian duct derivatives (seminal vesicles, ejaculatory ducts, epididymis, and vas deferens) to identify XY gonadal dysgenesis, true hermaphroditism, and idiopathic ambiguity. Normal testicular tissue with reduced or absent Wolffian structures associated with normal circulating T and DHT indicates a receptor defect (androgen insensitivity).

F. The combination of low levels of LH and T and DHT suggests a hypothalamopituitary defect. Ordinarily these defects do not cause ambiguity per se, but they do cause micropenis. The degree of incompleteness of virilization is not nearly as severe as with either testicular or end-organ (receptor) defects. Assessment of hypothalamopituitary function should be done with the help of an endocrinologist, as described in the chapter "Short Stature" (see p 178).

G. High LH and normal to high T and DHT levels usually suggest end-organ insensitivity to androgens. In these patients testes are present, but external and internal virilization are defective, resulting in ambiguous genitalia on physical examination and absent or severely compromised Wolffian duct development. This includes the epididymis, vas deferens, seminal vesicles, and ejaculatory ducts. Müllerian derivatives (cervix, uterus, and oviducts) are absent, since the testes produce normal amounts of Müllerian inhibitory factor in utero.

H. The management of ambiguous genitalia may include surgery. Assignment of gender should be made soon after birth with consultations of both surgical and endocrine subspecialists. Even if the karyotype indicates a genetic male, incomplete virilization that compromises the size of the phallus to less than 1.5 cm stretched length in the term newborn often necessitates raising the child as a girl. Thus, reconstructive surgery, including vaginoplasty and gonadectomy, is often indicated. The latter is particularly important in infants born with mixed karyotypes containing Y chromosomal material, since their gonads are much more susceptible to the development of neoplasia than are those with a uniform sex chromosome karyotype.

I. A high level of LH with low T and DHT levels suggests an inborn error of androgen and/or T biosynthesis (Fig. 1). Because errors of androgen biosynthesis may also

(Continued on page 130)

TABLE 1 Drug Therapy for Congenital Adrenal Hyperplasia

Glucocorticoid replacement: Cortisol (hydrocortisone) (Cortef) PO 10–25 mg/m²/day divided into 2 doses (older children) or 3 doses (infants)
Mineralocorticoid replacement: 9-fludrocortisol (Florinef) PO 0.05–0.2 mg daily

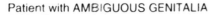

Patient with AMBIGUOUS GENITALIA

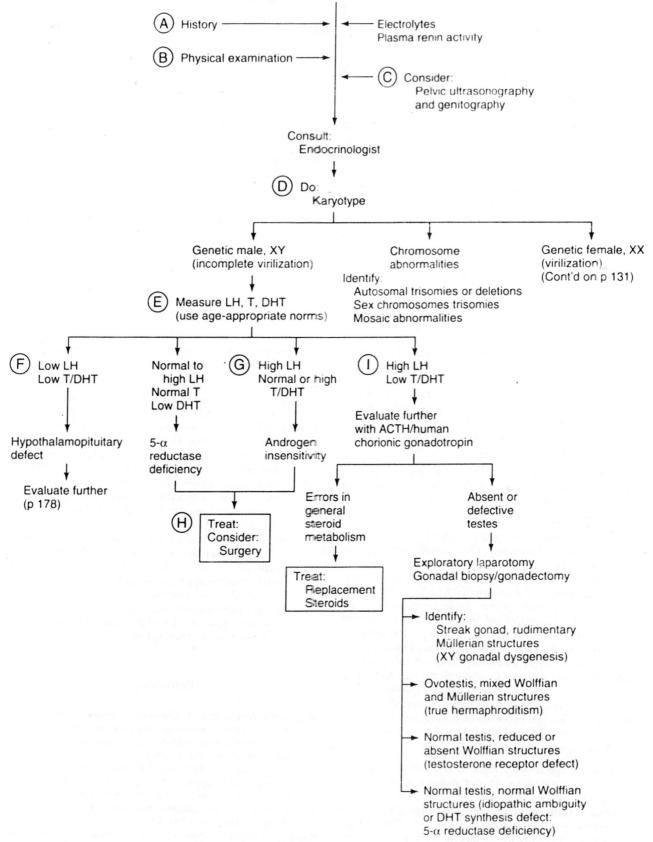

(A) History ⟶ ⟵ Electrolytes
Plasma renin activity

(B) Physical examination ⟶

⟵ (C) Consider:
Pelvic ultrasonography
and genitography

Consult:
Endocrinologist

(D) Do:
Karyotype

Genetic male, XY
(incomplete virilization)

Chromosome
abnormalities
Identify:
Autosomal trisomies or deletions
Sex chromosomes trisomies
Mosaic abnormalities

Genetic female, XX
(virilization)
(Cont'd on p 131)

(E) Measure LH, T, DHT
(use age-appropriate norms)

(F) Low LH
Low T/DHT

Normal to
high LH
Normal T
Low DHT

(G) High LH
Normal or high
T/DHT

(I) High LH
Low T/DHT

Hypothalamopituitary
defect

5-α
reductase
deficiency

Androgen
insensitivity

Evaluate further
with ACTH/human
chorionic gonadotropin

Evaluate further
(p 178)

(H) Treat:
Consider:
Surgery

Errors in
general
steroid
metabolism

Absent or
defective
testes

Treat:
Replacement
Steroids

Exploratory laparotomy
Gonadal biopsy/gonadectomy

➤ Identify:
Streak gonad, rudimentary
Müllerian structures
(XY gonadal dysgenesis)

➤ Ovotestis, mixed Wolffian
and Müllerian structures
(true hermaphroditism)

➤ Normal testis, reduced or
absent Wolffian structures
(testosterone receptor defect)

➤ Normal testis, normal Wolffian
structures (idiopathic ambiguity
or DHT synthesis defect:
5-α reductase deficiency)

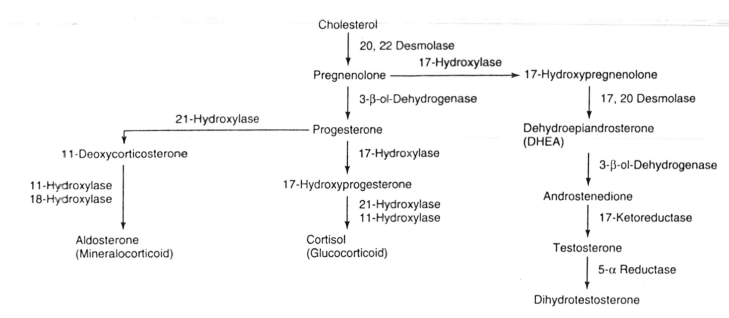

Figure 1 Steroid hormone biosynthesis.

involve enzymes necessary for the production of cortisol and aldosterone (viz., 17-hydroxylase and 3-β-oldehydrogenase), these infants should have an assessment of adrenocortical metabolism using an adrenocorticotropic hormone (ACTH; Cortrosyn) stimulation test. Babies with a more distal metabolic defect (e.g., 17-ketosteroid reductase or 5-α reductase) do not have other clinically significant adrenal metabolic defects. A deficiency of 5-α reductase is characterized by normal plasma T but low plasma DHT levels.

J. Maternal virilization, which is not always obvious, should be pursued, particularly if the evaluation of a genetically female infant is unproductive.

K. The absence of both maternal virilization and elevated androgens suggests idiopathic ambiguity (dysmorphia) or true hermaphroditism. Occasionally infants with CAH do not have elevations of 17-hydroxyprogesterone or androstenedione compared with normals for age, especially if they are studied in the first day or two of life. Thus, normal findings for these hormones in the presence of a virilized girl should not be considered conclusive and should probably be repeated after the first week or 10 days while the clinician continues to monitor electrolytes and await the results of measured plasma renin activity. Continued normal tests may prompt the need for an exploratory laparotomy and gonadal biopsy, especially if the diagnosis of true hermaphroditism is entertained. Karyotyping of gonadal cells may show a mixed XX and XY despite a peripheral XX karyotype.

L. Monitoring electrolytes alone is not sufficient for the diagnosis of mineralocorticoid deficiency in cases of CAH, since babies who are salt losers often maintain normal serum concentrations of electrolytes at the expense of elevated plasma renin activity. Thus, a high plasma renin activity in the face of normal electrolytes indicates compensated salt losing and may be more

common than overt salt loss manifested by hyponatremia and hyperkalemia. Both degrees of salt-losing tendency are generally treated with mineralocorticoid replacement (fludrocortisone acetate, or Florinef).

M. Since most babies with CAH (21-hydroxylase deficiency) are salt losers, even though some may be able to compensate temporarily, it is preferable to treat with a combination of mineralocorticoid and glucocorticoid replacement (Table 1). The usual mineralocorticoid is fludrocortisone. Glucocorticoid replacement is provided with hydrocortisone, using the lowest possible dose that suppresses adrenal androgen secretion and allows for normal growth and development. A replacement dose of 25 mg/m²/day orally in three divided doses is begun, but it may inhibit normal growth. For this reason the dose is usually reduced to approximately 15 mg/m²/day after the first 2 or 3 months. The infant's growth velocity and skeletal maturation must be monitored so that the appropriate glucocorticoid dose can be maintained. Fludrocortisone is less effective in infants than in older children, and it is not uncommon to see babies on a dose of 0.1 to 0.2 mg/day, whereas an adult rarely needs more than 0.1 mg daily.

References

Migeon CJ, Berkovitz GD. Congenital defects of the external genitalia in the newborn and prepubertal child. In: Carpenter SE, Rock J, eds. Pediatric and adolescent gynecology. New York: Raven Press, 1992:77.

Migeon CJ, Berkovitz GD, Brown TR. Sexual differentiation and ambiguity. In: Kappy MS, Blizzard RM, Migeon CJ, eds. Wilkins: The diagnosis and treatment of endocrine disorders in childhood and adolescence 4th ed. Springfield, IL: Charles C. Thomas, 1994:573.

Pagon RA. Diagnostic approach to the newborn with ambiguous genitalia. Pediatr Clin North Am 1987; 34:1019.

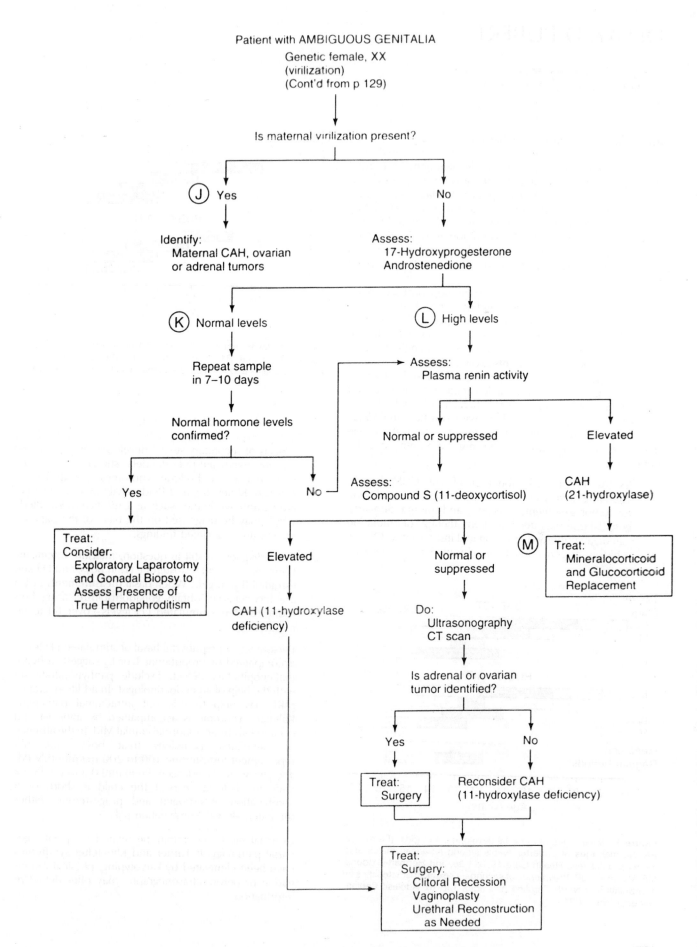

Patient with AMBIGUOUS GENITALIA
Genetic female, XX
(virilization)
(Cont'd from p 129)

Is maternal virilization present?

(J) Yes

Identify:
Maternal CAH, ovarian
or adrenal tumors

No

Assess:
17-Hydroxyprogesterone
Androstenedione

(K) Normal levels

Repeat sample
in 7–10 days

Normal hormone levels
confirmed?

Yes

No

Treat:
Consider:
    Exploratory Laparotomy
    and Gonadal Biopsy to
    Assess Presence of
    True Hermaphroditism

(L) High levels

Assess:
Plasma renin activity

Normal or suppressed

Assess:
Compound S (11-deoxycortisol)

Elevated

CAH (11-hydroxylase
deficiency)

Normal or
suppressed

Do:
Ultrasonography
CT scan

Is adrenal or ovarian
tumor identified?

Yes

Treat:
Surgery

No

Reconsider CAH
(11-hydroxylase deficiency)

Elevated

CAH
(21-hydroxylase)

(M) Treat:
    Mineralocorticoid
    and Glucocorticoid
    Replacement

Treat:
Surgery:
    Clitoral Recession
    Vaginoplasty
    Urethral Reconstruction
    as Needed

DELAYED PUBERTY

Carrie A. Ganong, M.D.
Michael S. Kappy, M.D., Ph.D.

An evaluation of delayed puberty in a child of either sex depends on the judgment of the physician, who is guided by the upper limits of ages for the development of normal pubertal events. For example, if there is no breast development in a girl by age 14 years, pubertal delay is significant. Likewise, if no testicular or penile enlargement occurs in a boy by age 14 years, puberty is significantly delayed and further evaluation is warranted. The condition most likely to be confused with pathologically delayed pubertal maturation is constitutional delay, and often it is not easy to differentiate the two at the first visit.

Constitutional delay is the most common form of delayed pubertal maturation. In this condition the child's rate of physical maturation is slower than that of peers. The bone age is usually delayed for chronologic age but is equal to the height age. Pubertal maturation is correspondingly delayed, and often one or both parents gives a similar history, i.e., delayed menarche in the mother or growth after high school in the father. There is considerable variation in the onset and development of secondary sexual characteristics in both boys and girls (Figs. 1 and 2). In boys with constitutional delay short-term (4 to 6 months) treatment with testosterone (Depo-Testosterone) 25 to 100 mg IM/month may be beneficial.

A. In the history ask about significant CNS disease, including surgery, chemotherapy, and cranial irradiation for tumor treatment; infection; and trauma. Similarly, gonadal trauma, infection, chemotherapy, or irradiation can delay puberty due to gonadal insufficiency. Obtain a history of general systemic chronic illness, anorexia,

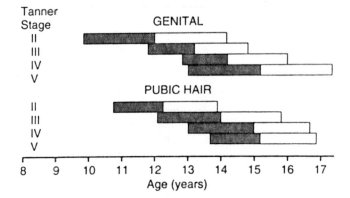

Figure 2 Mean ages of pubertal development in boys. (Data derived from Lee PA. Normal ages of pubertal events among American males and females. J Adolesc Health Care 1980; 1:26.)

and stress. A careful Tanner staging is necessary, as is a comparison with age-specific norms for the various aspects of secondary sexual development (Figs. 1 and 2). Only significant pubertal delay should be evaluated comprehensively. Exclude syndromes such as Turner, Noonan, Klinefelter, and Prader-Willi by formal karyotyping and syndromes such as Laurence-Moon-Biedl, which may be diagnosed on the basis of the patient's obesity and associated findings.

B. If the diagnosis is still in question, measure luteinizing hormone (LH) and testosterone (T) in boys, and LH and estradiol (E_2) in girls. When basal measurements of LH are inconclusive, obtain gonadotropin-releasing hormone (GnRH)—stimulated LH levels—over 60 to 90 minutes.

C. Persistence of prepubertal basal or stimulated LH levels accompanied by prepubertal T or E_2 suggests a hypothalamopituitary defect. Exclude panhypopituitarism with the help of an endocrinologist. In addition, cranial MRI may help to rule out intracranial pathology. Kallman syndrome is accompanied by anosmia and occasionally by an abnormal cranial MRI. In the absence of identifiable pathology treat boys with full-replacement testosterone 100 to 200 mg monthly IM, and girls with oral estrogen (Premarin) 0.3 to 0.625 mg daily for 1 to 2 years if the child is short, or a combination of estrogen and progesterone, either separately or with combination pills.

D. Gonadal insufficiency may be related to specific gonadal pathology. If Turner and Klinefelter syndromes have been eliminated by karyotyping, physical examination or pelvic ultrasonography may offer definitive information.

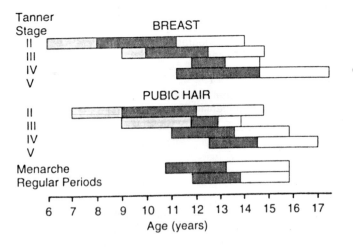

Figure 1 Mean ages of pubertal development in girls. (From Lee PA. Normal ages of pubertal events among American males and females. J Adolesc Health Care 1980; 1:26; and Herman-Giddons ME, Macmillan JP. Prevalence of secondary sexual characteristics in a population of North Carolina girls ages 3 to 10. Adolesc Pediatr Gynecol 1991; 4:21.)

Patient with DELAYED PUBERTY

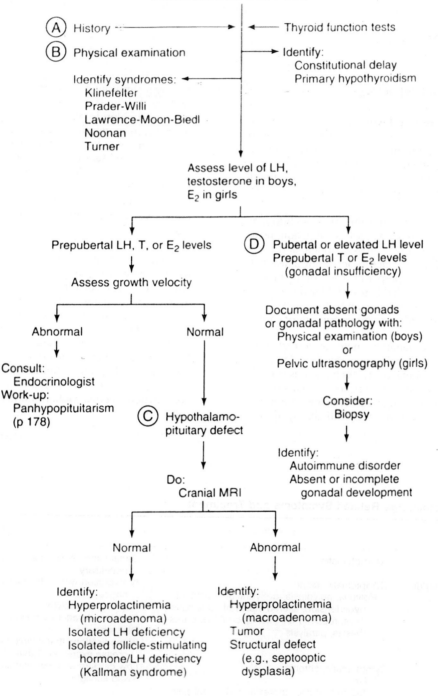

(A) History

Thyroid function tests

(B) Physical examination

Identify:
  Constitutional delay
  Primary hypothyroidism

Identify syndromes:
  Klinefelter
  Prader-Willi
  Lawrence-Moon-Biedl
  Noonan
  Turner

Assess level of LH,
testosterone in boys,
E₂ in girls

Prepubertal LH, T, or E₂ levels

(D) Pubertal or elevated LH level
Prepubertal T or E₂ levels
(gonadal insufficiency)

Assess growth velocity

Document absent gonads
or gonadal pathology with:
  Physical examination (boys)
    or
  Pelvic ultrasonography (girls)

Abnormal

Normal

Consult:
  Endocrinologist
Work-up:
  Panhypopituitarism
  (p 178)

(C) Hypothalamo-
pituitary defect

Consider:
  Biopsy

Identify:
  Autoimmune disorder
  Absent or incomplete
    gonadal development

Do:
Cranial MRI

Normal

Abnormal

Identify:
  Hyperprolactinemia
    (microadenoma)
  Isolated LH deficiency
  Isolated follicle-stimulating
    hormone/LH deficiency
    (Kallman syndrome)

Identify:
  Hyperprolactinemia
    (macroadenoma)
  Tumor
  Structural defect
    (e.g., septooptic
    dysplasia)

References

Heinze HJ. Ovarian function in adolescents with Turner syndrome. Adolesc Pediatr Gynecol 1994; 7:3.
Herman-Giddens ME, MacMillan JP. Prevalence of secondary sexual characteristics in a population of North Carolina girls ages 3 to 10. Adolesc Pediatr Gynecol 1991; 4:21.
Lee P. Normal ages of pubertal events among American males and females. J Adol Health Care 1980; 1:26.
Saenger P. Clinical review 48: The current status of diagnosis and therapeutic intervention in Turner's syndrome. J Clin Endocrinol Metab 1993; 77:297.

HYPERCALCEMIA

Carrie A. Ganong, M.D.
Michael S. Kappy, M.D., Ph.D.

DEFINITIONS

A normal serum calcium (Ca) level is 8.9 to 10.1 mg/dl or an ionized Ca of 4.5 to 5.1 mg/dl. Levels in normal newborns are slightly lower. Premature newborns may have levels as low as 7 mg/dl. **Hypercalcemia** is a serum level greater than 10.5 to 11 mg/dl or ionized level above 5 to 5.5 mg/dl. Symptoms may not correspond to serum levels.

A. In the history ask about symptoms such as abdominal pain, anorexia, behavioral changes, constipation, headache, polyuria, respiratory distress or apnea, and weakness. Identify predisposing factors, including a history of treated renal disease, hyperparathyroidism, dietary excess of vitamin D or A (fish oil), use of thiazide diuretics, and immobilization of a major limb. Note any family history of calcium disorders, seizures, tumors, or cancer.

B. In the physical examination note abnormal deep tendon reflexes, bone pain, hypertension, failure to thrive, and developmental delay. A characteristic elflike face with hypertelorism and large, low-set ears with or without craniostenosis suggests Williams syndrome. Note cardiac findings associated with this syndrome.

C. Manage symptomatic hypercalcemia initially with hydration. Infuse 0.9% normal saline with 40 mEq/L potassium chloride at 1.5 times maintenance, adding magnesium as needed. When hydration is complete, furosemide may be added to increase Ca and sodium (Na) excretion. Avoid thiazide diuretics, which increase Ca retention. Consider oral phosphorus supplementation if the child is hypophosphatemic. Phosphate cannot be given IV with Ca because calcium phosphate complexes can precipitate into soft-tissues with fatal results (Table 1).

D. Table 2 lists drug therapies. Prednisone 2 mg/kg up to 60 mg/day can be given for vitamin D–dependent causes of hypercalcemia. Prednisone decreases Ca absorption from the gut and blocks bone resorption of Ca. Corticosteroids work by blocking extrarenal hydroxylation of vitamin D. This may be particularly helpful when hypercalcemia results from bone or hematologic cancer. Calcitonin, bisphosphonates, plicomycin, and gallium nitrate block bone resorption of Ca. Calcitonin also increases Ca excretion. In severe hypercalcemia obtain immediate surgical consultation.

(Continued on page 136)

TABLE 1 Hypercalcemia: Age-Related Symptoms and Treatment

Serum Calcium Level	Symptoms	Treatment
11–12 mg/dl	Asymptomatic	Dietary intervention can be used but may not be necessary
>12 mg/dl (levels >14 mg/dl are frequently life-threatening)	Symptomatic, acute Polyuria, polydipsia, dehydration, vomiting, hypertension, altered states of consciousness, reduced QT interval on ECG, paresthesias, paralysis	IV hydration with 0.9% saline at 1.5 × maintenance Replace electrolytes Furosemide after hydration Dialysis IV medications that inhibit osteoclasts and/or increase excretion (Table 2)
	Symptomatic, chronic Infants: failure to thrive, anorexia, abdominal pain, irritability, dysuria	Low calcium and low vitamin D diet Avoid sunlight
	Older child: nephrocalcinosis, osteopenia, impaired concentrating ability, emotional lability, pruritus, joint pain, growth failure	Low calcium diet (<100 mg/day; aim for 25–35 mg/day)

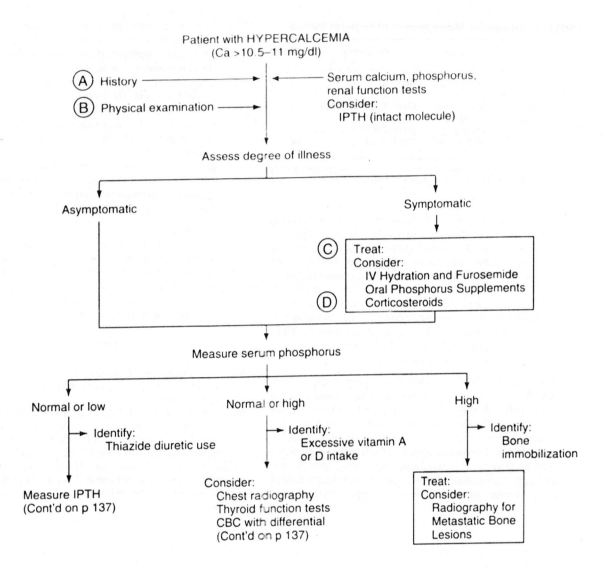

Patient with HYPERCALCEMIA
(Ca >10.5–11 mg/dl)

(A) History —————————— Serum calcium, phosphorus,
renal function tests
(B) Physical examination ————— Consider:
IPTH (intact molecule)

Assess degree of illness

Asymptomatic   Symptomatic

(C) Treat:
Consider:
IV Hydration and Furosemide
Oral Phosphorus Supplements
(D) Corticosteroids

Measure serum phosphorus

Normal or low   Normal or high   High

Identify: Identify: Identify:
Thiazide diuretic use Excessive vitamin A   Bone
or D intake   immobilization

Measure IPTH   Consider: Treat:
(Cont'd on p 137)   Chest radiography   Consider:
Thyroid function tests   Radiography for
CBC with differential   Metastatic Bone
(Cont'd on p 137)   Lesions

TABLE 2 Drugs for Management of Hypercalcemia

Generic	Dose	Frequency	Route
Calcitonin	4–8 U/kg	q6–12h	SC, IM
Bisphosphonates			
etidronate	7.5 mg/kg	Over 4 hr (3–7 days)	IV
pamidronate	1 mg/kg	Over 24 hr	IV
Plicamycin	25 μg/kg	Over 4–6 hr	IV
Gallium nitrate	200 mg/m²	For 5 days	IV

Adapted from Allen SH, Goldstein DE, Miles JH, et al. Hypercalcemia in the pediatric patient: A review and case reports. Int Pediatr 1993; 8:409.

E. Williams syndrome is characterized by poor feeding, failure to thrive, elfin face, heart defects (e.g., supravalvular aortic stenosis), and hypercalcemia with a normal immunoreactive parathyroid hormone (IPTH) level. Hypercalcemia may result from excessive maternal intake of vitamin D or unusual sensitivity to vitamin D; treatment consists of decreasing intake of vitamin D and Ca. Familial benign hypercalcemia, an autosomal dominant disorder, results in mildly elevated Ca levels (12 to 13 mg/dl with normal IPTH levels). Urinary Ca excretion is low, and treatment is often unnecessary.

F. Elevation of IPTH levels identifies hyperparathyroidism, which is usually due to generalized hyperplasia of the chief cells of the parathyroid glands. Other causes include parathyroid adenoma and two forms of autosomal dominant multiple endocrine neoplasia (MEN). In MEN type I, hyperparathyroidism is associated with a nonfunctioning chromophobe adenoma, insulinoma, and peptic ulceration due to a gastrin-secreting tumor of the pancreas. In MEN type II, hyperparathyroidism is associated with medullary carcinoma of the thyroid, pheochromocytoma, and mucosal neuromas (type IIb). Secondary hyperparathyroidism may be associated with renal disease, since defective renal excretion of phosphate leads to hyperphosphatemia and decreased serum Ca levels. The hypocalcemia stimulates parathormone secretion secondarily so that normal serum Ca is maintained. This hyperparathyroidism may persist even after treatment of renal disease by dialysis or transplantation, and hypercalcemia with variable serum phosphorus levels ensues. This autonomous hyperfunctioning of the parathyroid glands has been termed tertiary hyperparathyroidism and is treated by removal of one or more of the parathyroid glands.

G. Hypercalcemia is also seen in a variety of conditions, including sarcoidosis, hyperthyroidism and hypothyroidism, and a variety of tumors, particularly leukemias. Some of these tumors secrete hormones that are immunologically similar to parathormone; in other tumors prostaglandins or unknown factors are thought to cause the hypercalcemia.

References

Allen SH, Goldstein DE, Miles JH, et al. Hypercalcemia in the pediatric patient: A review and case reports. Int Pediatr 1993; 8:409.

McMurtry CT, Schranck FW, Walkenhorst DA, et al. Significant developmental elevation in serum parathyroid hormone levels in a large kindred with familial benign (hypocalciuric) hypercalcemia. Am J Med 1992; 93:247.

Pollack MR, Chou YHW, Marx SJ, et al. Familial hypocalciuric hypercalcemia and neonatal severe hyperparathyroidism. J Clin Invest 1994; 93:1108.

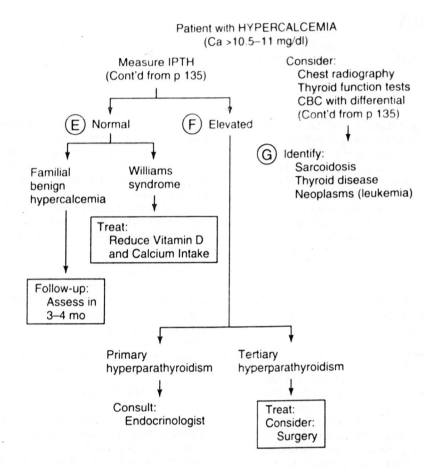

Patient with HYPERCALCEMIA
(Ca >10.5–11 mg/dl)

Measure IPTH
(Cont'd from p 135)

Consider:
  Chest radiography
  Thyroid function tests
  CBC with differential
  (Cont'd from p 135)

Ⓔ Normal   Ⓕ Elevated

Ⓖ Identify:
  Sarcoidosis
  Thyroid disease
  Neoplasms (leukemia)

Familial
benign
hypercalcemia

Williams
syndrome

Treat:
  Reduce Vitamin D
  and Calcium Intake

Follow-up:
Assess in
3–4 mo

Primary
hyperparathyroidism

Tertiary
hyperparathyroidism

Consult:
  Endocrinologist

Treat:
Consider:
  Surgery

HYPERGLYCEMIA

Michael S. Kappy, M.D., Ph.D.
Carrie A. Ganong, M.D.

A. Note symptoms that suggest diabetes mellitus such as polyuria, polydipsia, and weight loss despite polyphagia. Identify predisposing conditions or factors such as known diabetes, steroid medications, recent head injury, and excessive IV glucose administration. This is especially pertinent in premature infants, whose ability to maintain normal blood glucose concentrations in the face of IV glucose is less than that of full term infants or older children. In patients with insulin-dependent diabetes, note symptoms and signs of infection, and obtain history of any missed insulin doses.

B. Assess vital signs, circulatory status, and state of hydration. Note alterations in mental status and abnormal neurologic signs, particularly focal signs. Assess growth and pubertal development.

C. The management of diabetic ketoacidosis includes the correction of dehydration, restoration of adequate circulation and renal function, replacement of electrolyte losses (sodium, potassium, and phosphorus), correction of metabolic acidosis, lowering of hyperglycemia without causing hypoglycemia or cerebral edema, and stopping ketogenesis. Initiate therapy during the first hour with 10 to 20 ml normal saline or Ringer's lactate/kg body weight. Calculated fluid deficits should be replaced slowly, over 36 to 48 hours, to prevent cerebral edema. When the initial venous pH is below 7 and the patient has cardiac or pulmonary depression resulting from the acidosis, consider giving 1 to 2 mEq sodium bicarbonate/kg body weight as an isotonic solution (1 : 6 dilution) during the first hour or two of intravenous therapy. Discontinue bicarbonate therapy when the venous pH reaches 7.1. Begin an IV insulin infusion after the first hour (in most cases) or sooner if the patient is severely acidotic (pH < 7). Start with 0.1 U/kg/hour of regular insulin IV and adjust the rate according to the responses observed in blood glucose and bicarbonate content. Monitor blood glucose concentrations hourly at first and then every 2 hours after a response pattern is documented. Electrolytes, including bicarbonate concentration, should be monitored every 2 hours at first and less frequently as the patient recovers. The blood glucose should decrease approximately 75 mg/dl/hour on this regimen, but individual responses vary considerably. Add glucose as 5% or 10% to the IV fluids when the blood glucose decreases to 250 to 300 mg/dl to prevent hypoglycemia and possibly cerebral edema. IV fluids should contain potassium (after documenting patient's urine output) in a concentration of 40 mEq/L (20 mEq/L each of potassium chloride and potassium phosphate).

When the venous bicarbonate concentration is above 15 mEq/L, consider beginning subcutaneous regular insulin therapy (0.1 to 0.2 U/kg/dose) and discontinuing the IV insulin infusion. Repeat insulin doses before meals and before bedtime in amounts based on the blood glucose concentration as determined using a chemical strip. Gradually establish a split mixed insulin regimen (two daily doses, each containing regular and isophane [NPH] insulin) before discharging the patient from the hospital.

D. Nonketotic hyperosmolar coma occurs when changes in sensorium are associated with blood glucose concentrations above 800 mg/dl in the absence of significant metabolic acidosis. Hospitalize the patient and begin a regular insulin infusion of 0.05 to 0.10 U/kg/hour to lower blood glucose slowly. Replace calculated fluid deficits slowly, over 36 to 48 hours, to prevent cerebral edema. Monitor blood glucose every hour.

E. Institute insulin therapy for a new diabetic as an outpatient when no significant ketoacidosis is present. Initiate insulin therapy using short-acting and intermediate-acting insulin such as Regular insulin and NPH insulin. Begin with 0.5 to 1.0 U/kg/day with two thirds of the dose in the morning and one third of the dose at night. The morning dose is usually one third Regular insulin and two thirds NPH insulin, while the evening dose is usually half Regular insulin and half NPH insulin. Have the parents monitor the patient's blood glucose concentration with a reagent strip such as Chemstrip that can be read directly or with an electronic metering device. Adjust the insulin doses on the basis of these determinations, particularly before the three major meals of the day and at bedtime. Supplement each dose with Regular insulin as necessary. In addition to insulin therapy, implement a complete educational program for the patient and his or her parents, including the role of nutrition and exercise in the total care of the child with diabetes.

References

Arslanian S, Becker D, Drash A. Diabetes mellitus in the child and adolescent. In: Kappy MS, Blizzard RM, Migeon CJ, eds. The diagnosis and treatment of endocrine disorders in childhood and adolescence. 4th ed. Springfield, IL: Charles C. Thomas, 1994:961.

Santiago JV. Lessons from the diabetes control and complications trial. Diabetes 1993; 42:1549.

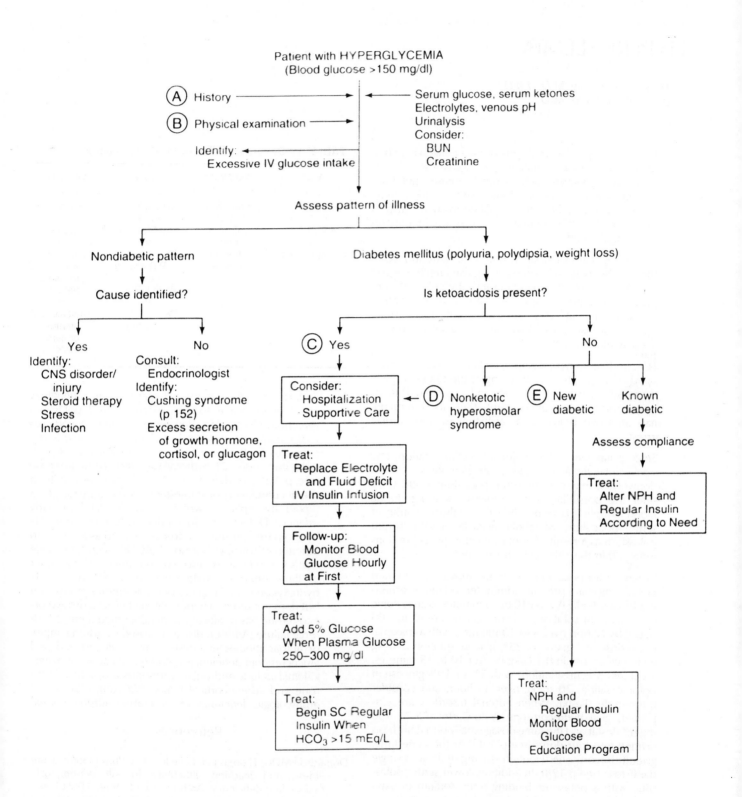

Patient with HYPERGLYCEMIA
(Blood glucose >150 mg/dl)

(A) History

(B) Physical examination

Identify:
Excessive IV glucose intake

Serum glucose, serum ketones
Electrolytes, venous pH
Urinalysis
Consider:
BUN
Creatinine

Assess pattern of illness

Nondiabetic pattern

Cause identified?

Yes

Identify:
CNS disorder/
injury
Steroid therapy
Stress
Infection

No

Consult:
Endocrinologist
Identify:
Cushing syndrome
(p 152)
Excess secretion
of growth hormone,
cortisol, or glucagon

Diabetes mellitus (polyuria, polydipsia, weight loss)

Is ketoacidosis present?

(C) Yes

Consider:
Hospitalization
Supportive Care

(D) Nonketotic
hyperosmolar
syndrome

Treat:
Replace Electrolyte
and Fluid Deficit
IV Insulin Infusion

Follow-up:
Monitor Blood
Glucose Hourly
at First

Treat:
Add 5% Glucose
When Plasma Glucose
250–300 mg/dl

Treat:
Begin SC Regular
Insulin When
HCO₃ >15 mEq/L

No

(E) New
diabetic

Known
diabetic

Assess compliance

Treat:
Alter NPH and
Regular Insulin
According to Need

Treat:
NPH and
Regular Insulin
Monitor Blood
Glucose
Education Program

139

HYPERKALEMIA

Michael S. Kappy, M.D., Ph.D.
Carrie A. Ganong, M.D.

A. In the history note symptoms of hyperkalemia such as anorexia, nausea, vomiting, and weakness. Identify predisposing factors such as renal disease, metabolic acidosis (diabetic ketoacidosis, aspirin intoxication), acute hemolysis, and acute rhabdomyolysis. Suspect excessive IV administration of potassium in patients receiving IV fluids.

B. In the physical examination note vital signs and assess the circulatory status (skin color, capillary refill). Suspect congenital adrenal hyperplasia in baby girls with ambiguous genitalia. Addison disease is associated with a characteristic slate-gray skin color. Note the signs of diabetic ketoacidosis (dehydration, Kussmaul respirations, acetone breath).

C. ECG findings in hyperkalemia include peaked T waves, which may progress to widening of the QRS complex, decreased P wave amplitude, and increased P-R interval. Serum potassium concentrations above 8 mEq/L may produce bradycardia, arrhythmias, and cardiac arrest.

D. Since potassium is the major intracellular cation, any significant cellular damage (acute hemolysis or rhabdomyolysis) may elevate serum potassium levels. Consider the possibility that hemolysis occurring during blood sampling is responsible for a false elevation of serum potassium. Metabolic acidosis elevates serum potassium as a result of displacement of potassium ions from within the cells by hydrogen ions.

E. When serum potassium levels are above 7 mEq/L and ECG changes are present, administer sodium bicarbonate 1 to 2 mEq/kg IV over 10 to 15 minutes as an isotonic (1:6 dilution) solution; calcium gluconate 50 to 100 mg/kg by IV drip over 5 to 10 minutes, with a maximal single dose of 1 g; and/or 25% glucose solution 2 ml/kg with regular insulin 0.1 U/kg IV over 10 to 15 minutes. Treat less urgent situations with 5% or 10% glucose in isotonic saline, 20 ml/kg over an hour, and consider furosemide (Lasix). When adrenal disorders are suspected, give hydrocortisone (Solu-Cortef) 75 to 100 mg/m² IV stat and the same dosage orally on a daily basis divided into four doses (see p 128). At the same time, give fludrocortisone (Florinef) 0.1 mg orally as a single daily dose (see p 128). In addition, lower serum potassium with a potassium-binding resin, sodium polystyrene sulfonate (Kayexalate) 1 g/kg by rectum as an enema. Serum potassium may be expected to decrease by 0.5 to 2 mEq/L with each enema. This may be repeated two or three times per day. In life-threatening situations consider peritoneal dialysis and/or hemodialysis as well as adrenal steroids.

TABLE 1 Severity of Illness in Hyperkalemia

Mild	Moderate	Severe	Very Severe
Serum K⁺ = 5.5–6 mEq/L and Asymptomatic	Serum K⁺ >6–7 mEq/L and Anorexia or weakness	Serum K⁺ >7–8 mEq/L or Prolonged P-R interval or Wide QRS or Persistent vomiting	Serum K⁺ >8 mEq/L or Absent P waves and sinusoidal pattern or Bradycardia, arrythmia, or cardiac arrest

F. Defects in mineralocorticoid secretion or action may result in excessive sodium excretion and potassium retention. Causes of a deficiency of mineralocorticoid (desoxycorticosterone and/or aldosterone) include deficiencies in the enzymes 20,22 desmolase, 3-β-ol-dehydrogenase, 21-hydroxylase, and 18-hydroxylase (see p 128). A defect in 20,22 desmolase results in the accumulation of cholesterol in the adrenal gland (lipoid hyperplasia), which is usually fatal in early infancy. Defects in 3-β-ol-dehydrogenase and 21-hydroxylase produce adrenal hyperplasia due to adrenocorticotropic hormone (ACTH) secretion, since cortisol synthesis is also compromised when either of these enzymes is defective. A defect in the 11-hydroxylase enzyme decreases aldosterone production but does not result in hyperkalemia because desoxycorticosterone has significant mineralocorticoid effect. Adrenal failure (Addison disease) caused by adrenal injury or autoantibodies manifests as mineralocorticoid and glucocorticoid deficiencies. Additional causes of hyperkalemia include end-organ unresponsiveness to aldosterone and adrenocortical hypoplasia congenita, a rare embryologic deficiency of the mature adrenal cortex.

References

Donaldson MDC, Thomas PH, Love JG, et al. Presentation, acute illness, and learning difficulties in salt wasting 21-hydroxylase deficiency. Arch Dis Child 1994; 70:214.

Einaudi S, Lala R, Corrias A, et al. Auxological and biochemical parameters in assessing treatment of infants and toddlers with congenital adrenal hyperplasia due to 21-hydroxylase deficiency. J Pediatr Endocrinol 1993; 6:173.

Feld LG, Kaskel FJ, Schoeneman MJ. Approach to fluid and electrolyte therapy in pediatrics. Adv Pediatr 1988; 35:497.

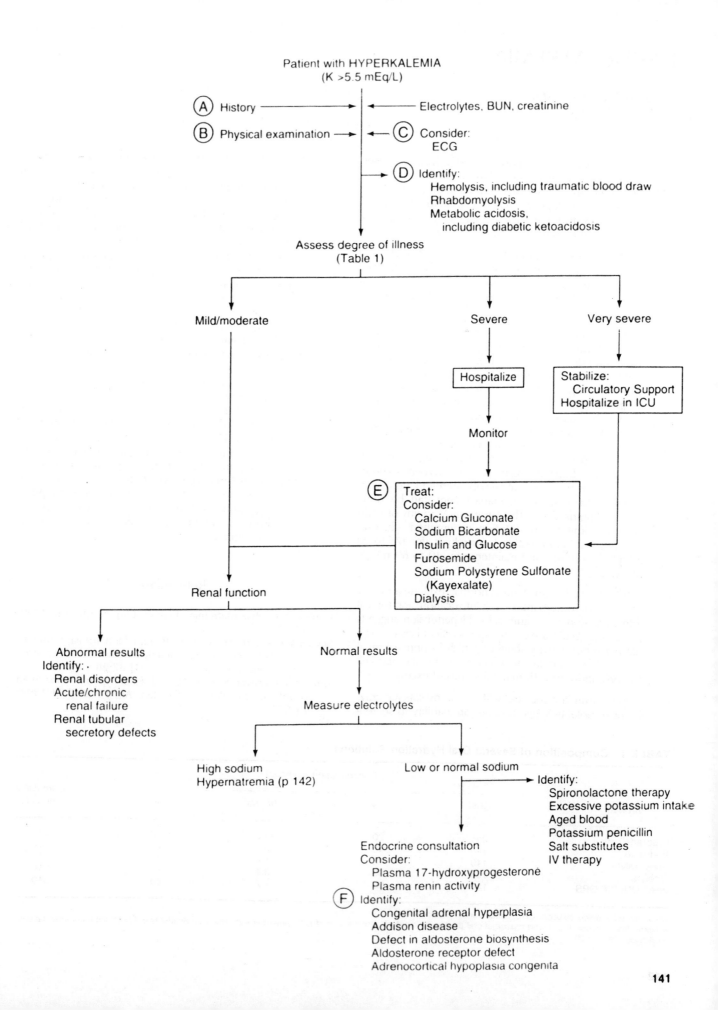

Patient with HYPERKALEMIA
(K >5.5 mEq/L)

(A) History ———→ ←——— Electrolytes, BUN, creatinine

(B) Physical examination ——→ ←— (C) Consider:
ECG

→ (D) Identify:
Hemolysis, including traumatic blood draw
Rhabdomyolysis
Metabolic acidosis,
including diabetic ketoacidosis

Assess degree of illness
(Table 1)

Mild/moderate   Severe   Very severe

Hospitalize   Stabilize:
Circulatory Support
Hospitalize in ICU

Monitor

(E) Treat:
Consider:
Calcium Gluconate
Sodium Bicarbonate
Insulin and Glucose
Furosemide
Sodium Polystyrene Sulfonate
(Kayexalate)
Dialysis

Renal function

Abnormal results   Normal results
Identify:
Renal disorders
Acute/chronic
renal failure
Renal tubular
secretory defects

Measure electrolytes

High sodium   Low or normal sodium
Hypernatremia (p 142)   → Identify:
Spironolactone therapy
Excessive potassium intake
Aged blood
Potassium penicillin
Salt substitutes
IV therapy

Endocrine consultation
Consider:
Plasma 17-hydroxyprogesterone
Plasma renin activity
(F) Identify:
Congenital adrenal hyperplasia
Addison disease
Defect in aldosterone biosynthesis
Aldosterone receptor defect
Adrenocortical hypoplasia congenita

HYPERNATREMIA

Carrie A. Ganong, M.D.
Michael S. Kappy, M.D., Ph.D.

A. In the history note any polyuria and polydipsia suggestive of diabetes insipidus. Identify children receiving steroid therapy or excessive sodium in oral or IV fluids. Rule out water deprivation and adipsia. Identify predisposing CNS disorders such as head injuries (surgery or trauma) and meningitis.

B. In the physical examination assess vital signs and hydration status. Note alterations in mental status and abnormal neurologic signs. Recognize cushingoid features (moon face, purplish striae, short stature, central adiposity).

C. Suspect hypertonic dehydration when patients with gastroenteritis have been managed at home with high-sodium fluids, such as boiled skim milk, and in infants and toddlers refusing fluids. Treat hypernatremic dehydration by replacing the fluid deficits and lowering the serum sodium at 0.5 to 1 mEq/L of sodium per hour. This can be accomplished by administering a two-thirds-normal IV solution. This contains small amounts of free water to correct fluid deficits without rapidly lowering serum sodium. When dehydration is not significant, administer the fluid with maintenance fluids over 48 hours as one-quarter-normal saline with 40 mEq/L potassium chloride. In some cases management can be done with oral fluids alone. The American Academy of Pediatrics Committee on Nutrition recommends glucose-electrolyte solutions (Table 1) for rehydration (75 to 90 mEq/L of sodium) and maintenance (40 to 60 mEq/L of sodium).

D. When the hydration status is normal, exclude a history of excessive sodium intake (salt intoxication) and topical administration of sodium salts. Hypertension suggests primary renal disease or a mineralocorticoid excess. The plasma renin activity should be high in primary renal disease (renovascular disorders or juxtaglomerular cell tumors) and low with mineralocorticoid excess.

E. Hypernatremia associated with low urine specific gravity or osmolality suggests either an inability to secrete antidiuretic hormone (ADH) (central diabetes insipidus) or an impairment of end-organ responsiveness to the hormone (nephrogenic diabetes insipidus). A trial of ADH distinguishes a primary deficiency from end-organ unresponsiveness. Patients with central diabetes insipidus respond within 20 to 30 minutes to a trial of 0.1 U/kg of aqueous pitressin (maximum 5 U) given IM by decreasing urine output and increasing urine specific gravity. Patients with nephrogenic diabetes insipidus fail to respond to pitressin. Causes of central diabetes insipidus include tumor of the hypothalamus or pituitary, histiocytosis X, trauma, toxins, and infections of the CNS. A sudden appearance of central diabetes insipidus in a patient with underlying CNS pathology is a poor prognostic sign frequently associated with brain death. A familial form of central diabetes insipidus due to an inherited decrease in the number of cells in the supraoptic or paraventricular nuclei in the hypothalamus is a rare cause of diabetes insipidus. Outpatients with central diabetes insipidus are best treated with intranasal 1-deamino-[8-D-arginine] vasopressin (DDAVP), a short-acting (8 to 12 hour) analogue of ADH, at 5 to 30 μg/day. Nephrogenic diabetes insipidus is an unusual condition that may be related to the failure of the distal tubular cells to generate cyclic adenosine monophosphate in response to ADH. End-organ unresponsiveness may also occur when serum concentrations of potassium or calcium are low.

References

Conley SB. Hypernatremia. Pediatr Clin North Am 1990; 37:365.

Snyder J. Use and misuse of oral therapy for diarrhea: Comparison of U.S. practices with American Academy of Pediatrics recommendations. Pediatrics 1991; 87:28.

Yercen N, Çaglayan S, Yücel N, et al. Fatal hypernatremia in an infant due to salting of the skin. Am J Dis Child 1993; 147:716.

TABLE 1   Composition of Several Oral Hydration Solutions

Product	Concentration (mmol/L)					Osmolality (mmol/L)
	CHO	Na	CHO-Na	K		
Gatorade	255	20	13.0	3		330
Pedialyte	140	45	3.1	20		250
Rehydralyte	140	75	1.9	20		310
Ricelyte	168	50	3.4	25		210
WHO/UNICEF ORS	111	90	1.2	20		310

ORS, oral rehydration solution; CHO, carbohydrate; Na, sodium.
Adapted from Snyder J. Use and misuse of oral therapy for diarrhea: Comparison of U.S. practices with American Academy of Pediatrics recommendations. Pediatrics 1991; 87:28.

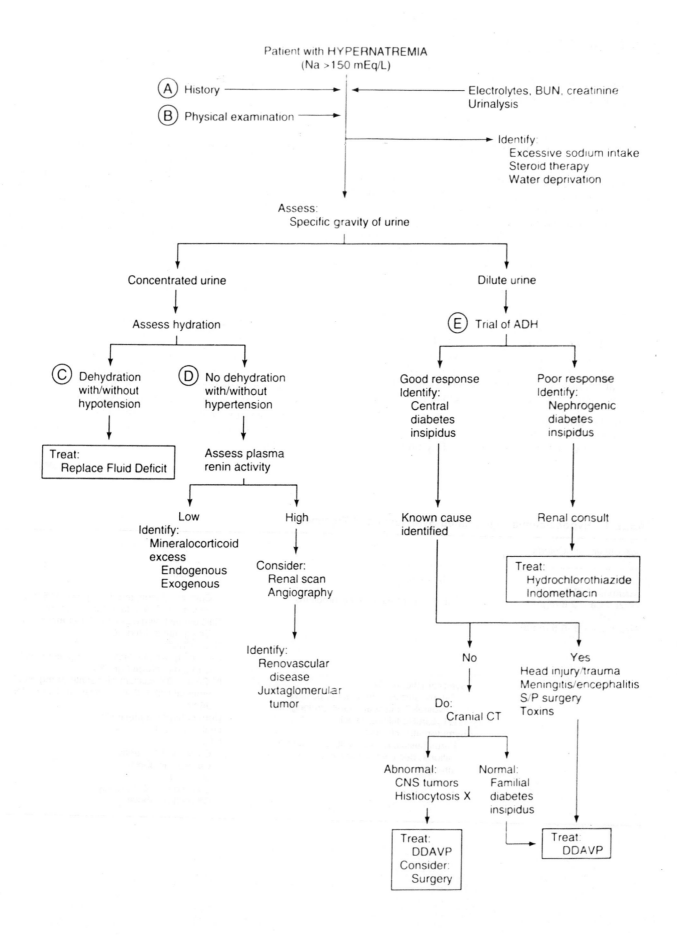

Patient with HYPERNATREMIA
(Na >150 mEq/L)

(A) History ⟶

(B) Physical examination ⟶

← Electrolytes, BUN, creatinine
Urinalysis

→ Identify:
Excessive sodium intake
Steroid therapy
Water deprivation

Assess:
Specific gravity of urine

Concentrated urine

Assess hydration

(C) Dehydration
with/without
hypotension

(D) No dehydration
with/without
hypertension

Treat:
Replace Fluid Deficit

Assess plasma
renin activity

Low
Identify:
Mineralocorticoid
excess
Endogenous
Exogenous

High

Consider:
Renal scan
Angiography

Identify:
Renovascular
disease
Juxtaglomerular
tumor

Dilute urine

(E) Trial of ADH

Good response
Identify:
Central
diabetes
insipidus

Poor response
Identify:
Nephrogenic
diabetes
insipidus

Known cause
identified

Renal consult

Treat:
Hydrochlorothiazide
Indomethacin

No

Do:
Cranial CT

Abnormal:
CNS tumors
Histiocytosis X

Normal:
Familial
diabetes
insipidus

Treat:
DDAVP
Consider:
Surgery

Yes
Head injury/trauma
Meningitis/encephalitis
S/P surgery
Toxins

Treat:
DDAVP

143

HYPOCALCEMIA

Carrie A. Ganong, M.D.
Michael S. Kappy, M.D., Ph.D.

DEFINITION

A normal serum calcium (Ca) level is 8.9 to 10.1 mg/dl or ionized Ca of 4.5 to 5.1 mg/dl. Levels in normal newborns are slightly lower. Premature newborns may have levels as low as 7 mg/dl. **Hypocalcemia** is serum Ca below 8 to 8.5 mg/dl in older children and below 7.5 mg/dl in neonates. Total protein or albumin is necessary to interpret total (but not ionized) Ca levels because 50% to 60% of Ca is protein bound. It may be asymptomatic.

A. In the history note symptoms such as lethargy, poor feeding, vomiting, diarrhea, photophobia, and tetany. Identify predisposing factors such as thyroid surgery (inadvertent removal of parathyroid glands), renal or liver disease, nutritional deficiency of Ca or vitamin D, and chronic use of medications (phenytoin, steroids) that interfere with normal vitamin D metabolism. Note any family history of hypocalcemia.

B. In the physical examination check for rickets since vitamin D deficiency may accompany hypocalcemia. Cystinosis, an inherited disorder of cystine catabolism, results in abnormal storage of cystine in the cornea, kidney, white blood cells, thyroid, and liver. An eye examination or white blood cell count may be diagnostic. DiGeorge syndrome, the most common cause of decreased or absent parathyroid tissue at birth, is often accompanied by aortic coarctation and decreased or absent thymic tissue. Careful cardiovascular examination, including blood pressures of all four extremities and the characteristic murmur of aortic coarctation, may be diagnostic. A chest film may document absent or greatly diminished thymic tissue in the neonate. Note absence of lymphoid tissue, adenoids, and tonsils.

C. In asymptomatic hypocalcemia begin oral therapy with vitamin D, calcitriol, and Ca (Table 1).

D. Treat acute symptomatic hypocalcemia with 10% calcium gluconate IV (Table 1). Monitor heart rate to identify arrhythmias caused by too-rapid infusion of Ca. Treat coexisting magnesium (Mg) deficiencies with magnesium chloride, citrate, or lactate (elemental Mg 24 to 48 mg/kg/day in divided doses; maximum 1 g/day).

(Continued on page 146)

TABLE 1 Hypocalcemia: Age-related Symptoms and Treatment

Age-dependent Criteria	Symptoms	Treatment

Neonate:
  Serum Ca <7.5 mg/dl
  Ionized Ca <2.8 mg/dl
Older child:
  Serum Ca <8–8.5 mg/dl
	Asymptomatic
	or
	Irritability, diarrhea, feeding problems
		Oral calcium
		Neonate:
		  Calcium gluconate 5 ml/kg/day (115 mg elemental Ca/kg/day) divided q4–6h
		  Calcium lactate/gluconate 75 mg elemental Ca/kg/day divided q6–8h
		Older Child:
		  Calcium gluconate/lactate 50 mg elemental Ca/kg/day divided q6–8h

	Symptomatic, acute:
	  Tetany, seizures, headache, positive Chvostek/Trousseau signs, prolonged QT, cardiac failure, shock
	Symptomatic, chronic:
	  Paresthesias, rickets, soft-tissue calcifications, decreased muscle tone or strength
		IV Ca as 10% calcium gluconate (9 mg/ml elemental Ca) 1–2 ml/kg over 10–15 min for 96 hr
		Correct hypomagnesemia
		Oral vitamin D
		Infant:
		  Calcitriol 0.1 μg/day
		  Ca (PO) as above
		Older child:
		  Calcitriol 0.1–0.3 μg/day
		  Ca (PO) as above

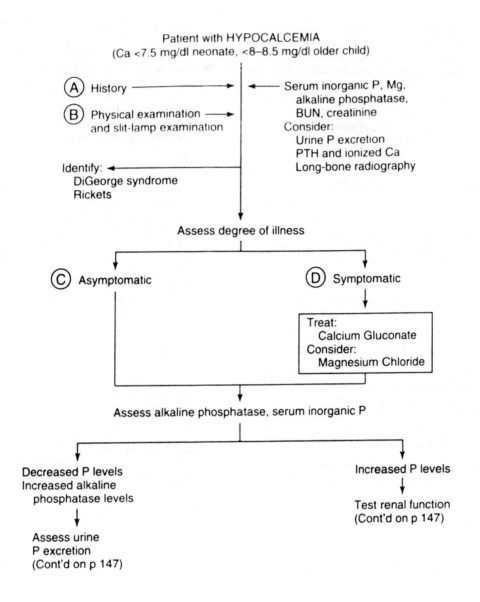

Patient with HYPOCALCEMIA
(Ca <7.5 mg/dl neonate, <8–8.5 mg/dl older child)

(A) History

(B) Physical examination
and slit-lamp examination

Serum inorganic P, Mg,
alkaline phosphatase,
BUN, creatinine
Consider:
Urine P excretion
PTH and ionized Ca
Long-bone radiography

Identify:
DiGeorge syndrome
Rickets

Assess degree of illness

(C) Asymptomatic

(D) Symptomatic

Treat:
Calcium Gluconate
Consider:
Magnesium Chloride

Assess alkaline phosphatase, serum inorganic P

Decreased P levels
Increased alkaline
phosphatase levels

Assess urine
P excretion
(Cont'd on p 147)

Increased P levels

Test renal function
(Cont'd on p 147)

E. If urinary phosphorus (P) is low or normal, consider nutritional deficiency of Ca and P (especially common in premature infants) or vitamin D. Nutritional deficiencies may be due to excessive loss through malabsorption (GI or liver disease). Abnormalities in vitamin D metabolism decrease formation of active vitamin D $-1,25(OH)_2D$. These conditions are not usually accompanied by severe hypocalcemia since elevated secretion of parathyroid hormone (PTH) tends to keep serum Ca from falling. Hypocalcemia may occur if the PTH effect is inadequate, particularly when serum vitamin D concentrations are very low.

F. In patients with high urinary P excretion suspect renal tubular disease such as Fanconi syndrome, cystinosis, Lowe syndrome, renal tubular acidosis, or X-linked dominant familial hypophosphatemic rickets. In these conditions hypophosphatemia is more common; however, hypocalcemia also may occur.

G. Decreased parathyroid tissue or diminished PTH secretion results in a low level of immunoreactive PTH (IPTH). Causes of decreased tissue include DiGeorge syndrome and removal during thyroid surgery. Decreased secretion may be related to autoimmune parathyroid insufficiency alone or as part of autoimmune polyglandular syndrome (APS) type I. APS type I most commonly includes persistent mucocutaneous candidiasis, hypoparathyroidism, and Addison disease. Other endocrinopathies are less commonly associated. Mg deficiency may also cause hypoparathyroidism.

H. Increased PTH secretion results from end organ unresponsiveness to PTH. In pseudohypoparathyroidism types Ia, Ib, II, and III, unresponsiveness is related to defects at or beyond the PTH receptors in bone and kidney. Type Ia (Albright hereditary osteodystrophy) is most easily recognized clinically; patients have round faces, short stature, mental retardation, and short fourth metacarpals. Patients with pseudopseudohypoparathyroidism have the same clinical features but normal laboratory values. Other causes of unresponsiveness to PTH are hypomagnesemia, hypernatremia, hypokalemia, and infection.

I. Renal parenchymal disease reduces P excretion. Elevated serum P levels lower serum Ca by forming insoluble calcium phosphate salts that are deposited in various tissues, including the kidney. The low serum Ca may be partially corrected by increased PTH secretion. Another cause of hypocalcemia is the relative inability of an abnormal kidney to convert vitamin D_3 to $1,25(OH)_2D$. The rate-limiting enzyme is deficient in the failing kidney and may result in $1,25(OH)_2D$ deficiency and hypocalcemia despite secondary hyperparathyroidism.

References

Gertner JM. Disorders of calcium and phosphorus homeostasis. Pediatr Clin North Am 1990; 37:1441.

Pollard AJ, Predergast M, Al-Hammouri F, et al. Different subtypes of pseudohypoparathyroidism in the same family with an unusual psychiatric presentation of the index case. Arch Dis Child 1994; 70:99.

Riley WJ. Autoimmune polyglandular syndromes. Horm Res 1992; 38(Suppl 2):9.

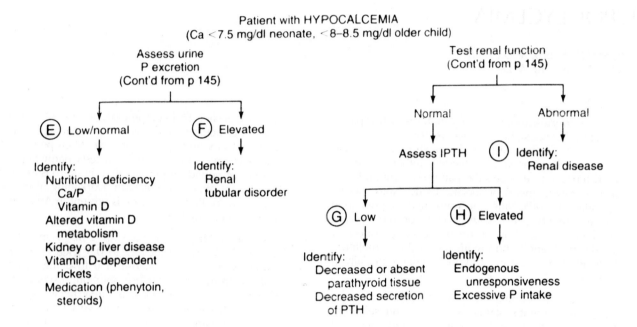

Patient with HYPOCALCEMIA
(Ca <7.5 mg/dl neonate, <8–8.5 mg/dl older child)

Assess urine
P excretion
(Cont'd from p 145)

Ⓔ Low/normal

Identify:
  Nutritional deficiency
    Ca/P
    Vitamin D
  Altered vitamin D
    metabolism
  Kidney or liver disease
  Vitamin D-dependent
    rickets
  Medication (phenytoin,
    steroids)

Ⓕ Elevated

Identify:
  Renal
    tubular disorder

Test renal function
(Cont'd from p 145)

Normal

Abnormal

Assess IPTH

Ⓘ Identify:
  Renal disease

Ⓖ Low

Identify:
  Decreased or absent
    parathyroid tissue
  Decreased secretion
    of PTH

Ⓗ Elevated

Identify:
  Endogenous
    unresponsiveness
  Excessive P intake

HYPOGLYCEMIA

Michael S. Kappy, M.D., Ph.D.
Carrie A. Ganong, M.D.

A. In the history ask about signs or symptoms such as pallor, sweating, dizziness, tachycardia, tremor, altered mental status, and seizures. Signs in the newborn are nonspecific, including apnea, poor feeding, lethargy, and low body temperature. Assess the pattern of signs and their relationship to meals or specific foods. Note specific episodes of febrile illness accompanied by poor food intake. Identify precipitating factors or predisposing conditions, e.g., drug or toxin ingestion (especially aspirin or ethanol) and insulin use (diabetes mellitus). Note any family history of hypoglycemia, especially in newborns.

B. In the physical examination assess vital signs and neurologic status (mental status, weakness, and seizures). Note pallor, tachycardia, tachypnea, and increased sweating. Consider large size for gestational age as a possible sign of hyperinsulinism (infant of diabetic mother or other). Low birth weight and premature infants are susceptible to hypoglycemia, primarily due to a deficiency of substrates and of enzymes for glycogen breakdown and gluconeogenesis, which are at full activity only at term. Consider galactosemia, liver failure, glycogen storage disease, or α_1-antitrypsin deficiency when jaundice or hepatomegaly is present. Cataracts suggest galactosemia. Congenital adrenal hyperplasia in a girl causes ambiguous genitalia. Micropenis in the hypoglycemic newborn boy suggests panhypopituitarism since gonadotropin secretion in utero is necessary for normal phallic size at birth. Darkening of the skin, especially in skinfold creases, is present in Addison disease in older children.

C. Treat acute hypoglycemia with 2 to 3 ml of 10% glucose/kg body weight (0.2 to 0.3 g/kg) IV, followed by an IV infusion of glucose of 6 to 8 mg/kg/minute *initially* using 10% glucose solution. Except in endogenous insulin excess, it is rarely necessary to use rates of glucose administration above 10 mg/kg/minute but be prepared to do so if necessary to maintain normoglycemia. Consider a dose of glucagon 0.03 mg/kg SC or IM, to a maximum of 1 mg. Prolonged difficulty in maintaining normal blood glucose levels may be alleviated by giving hydrocortisone 75 to 100 mg/m² IV followed by the same daily dose in three to four divided *oral* doses if necessary after blood studies have been obtained and until a diagnosis is made.

(Continued on page 150)

TABLE 1 Degree of Illness in Hypoglycemia

Mild	Moderate	Severe	Very Severe
Blood glucose 40–45 mg/dl and Asymptomatic	Blood glucose 30–40 mg/dl or Signs and symptoms such as pallor, tachycardia, tachypnea, sweating, weakness	Blood glucose 20–30 mg/dl or Seizures or Altered mental state	Blood glucose <20 mg/dl or Coma, shock, status seizures

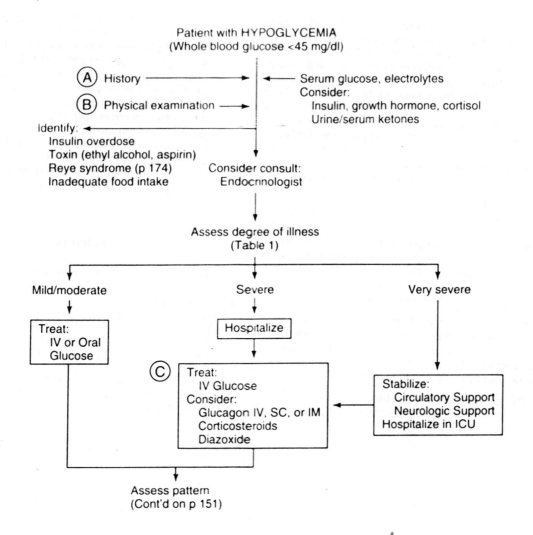

Patient with HYPOGLYCEMIA
(Whole blood glucose <45 mg/dl)

(A) History ⟶ ⟵ Serum glucose, electrolytes
Consider:
(B) Physical examination ⟶ Insulin, growth hormone, cortisol
  Urine/serum ketones

Identify: ⟵
  Insulin overdose
  Toxin (ethyl alcohol, aspirin)
  Reye syndrome (p 174) Consider consult:
  Inadequate food intake Endocrinologist

Assess degree of illness
(Table 1)

Mild/moderate   Severe   Very severe

Treat: Hospitalize
  IV or Oral
  Glucose

(C) Treat: Stabilize:
     IV Glucose   Circulatory Support
   Consider: Neurologic Support
     Glucagon IV, SC, or IM ⟵ Hospitalize in ICU
     Corticosteroids
     Diazoxide

Assess pattern
(Cont'd on p 151)

D. Exaggerated or morbid fasting (ketotic) hypoglycemia is the most common form of hypoglycemia in childhood. It usually occurs when the child is 1 to 5 years of age during periods of reduced food intake (e.g., during acute febrile illnesses). When glucose production is inadequate, the breakdown of fat stores for energy results in production and excretion of ketones in the urine. Ketonuria usually precedes hypoglycemia; therefore, the parents can test the child's urine for ketones at home, especially during an illness, and help prevent hypoglycemia by giving frequent small feedings of carbohydrate-rich foods if ketonuria is present.

E. The diagnosis of hyperinsulinism depends on documenting an inappropriately high serum insulin concentration for the glucose concentration (insulin-to-glucose ratio > 0.25) during hypoglycemia. In addition, serum ketones are absent, although urine ketones may be weakly positive. Consider diazoxide therapy 10 to 25 mg/kg/day PO in three divided doses prior to surgical intervention (subtotal pancreatectomy).

F. The adrenocorticotropic hormone (ACTH) test assesses adrenal cortex function. Low serum cortisol before and after stimulation suggests primary adrenal insufficiency; high cortisol after stimulation suggests that the patient has deficient pituitary secretion of ACTH.

G. In the fasting state normal blood glucose levels are maintained initially by the breakdown of glycogen and subsequently by the synthesis of glucose from muscle protein (gluconeogenesis). There are at least six major types of glycogen storage disease and many subtypes. Many cause hepatomegaly and failure to thrive. Disorders of gluconeogenesis (e.g., fructose-1,6-bisphosphatase deficiency, galactosemia, fructose intolerance) are associated with absent, defective, or blocked enzymes. Inborn errors of glycogen breakdown, gluconeogenesis, and amino acid metabolism are frequently associated with positive urinary and serum ketones, whereas errors of fatty acid use are not. Urinary organic acid and serum amino acid determination may help in the diagnosis of these rare causes of hypoglycemia.

References

Cornblath M, Schwartz R, Aynsley-Green A, et al. Hypoglycemia in infancy: The need for a rational definition. Pediatrics 1990; 85:834.

Kappy MS. Carbohydrate metabolism and hypoglycemia. In: Kappy MS, Blizzard RM, Migeon CJ, eds. The diagnosis and treatment of endocrine disorders in childhood and adolescence. 4th ed. Springfield, IL: Charles C. Thomas, 1994:919.

Worden FP, Freidenberg G, Pescovitz OH. The diagnosis and management of neonatal hyperinsulinism. Endocrinologist 1994; 4:196.

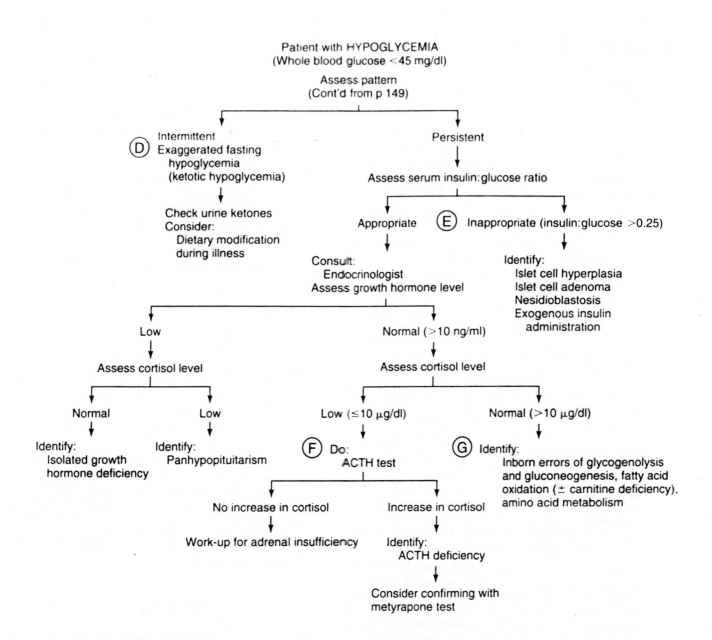

Patient with HYPOGLYCEMIA
(Whole blood glucose <45 mg/dl)

Assess pattern
(Cont'd from p 149)

(D) Intermittent
Exaggerated fasting
hypoglycemia
(ketotic hypoglycemia)

Check urine ketones
Consider:
Dietary modification
during illness

Persistent

Assess serum insulin:glucose ratio

Appropriate

(E) Inappropriate (insulin:glucose >0.25)

Consult:
Endocrinologist
Assess growth hormone level

Identify:
Islet cell hyperplasia
Islet cell adenoma
Nesidioblastosis
Exogenous insulin
administration

Low

Normal (>10 ng/ml)

Assess cortisol level

Assess cortisol level

Normal

Low

Low (≤10 μg/dl)

Normal (>10 μg/dl)

Identify:
Isolated growth
hormone deficiency

Identify:
Panhypopituitarism

(F) Do:
ACTH test

(G) Identify:
Inborn errors of glycogenolysis
and gluconeogenesis, fatty acid
oxidation (± carnitine deficiency),
amino acid metabolism

No increase in cortisol

Increase in cortisol

Work-up for adrenal insufficiency

Identify:
ACTH deficiency

Consider confirming with
metyrapone test

HYPOKALEMIA

Michael S. Kappy, M.D., Ph.D.
Carrie A. Ganong, M.D.

A. In the history note any weakness, lethargy, and vomiting. Identify predisposing factors and conditions such as diuretic therapy, steroid (glucocorticoid) therapy, persistent vomiting (pyloric stenosis), and renal disorders.

B. In the physical examination note vital signs, especially blood pressure. Moon face, purplish striae, and central adiposity suggest Cushing syndrome due to endogenous or exogenous glucocorticoid excess.

C. ECG findings of hypokalemia include flattened T waves, depressed ST segments, and a prominent U wave.

D. Diabetic ketoacidosis may lead to hypokalemia through loss of potassium in the urine as a result of osmotic diuresis and during therapy if bicarbonate is given. An inadequate potassium concentration in IV fluids may also lead to hypokalemia in the hospitalized patient.

E. Plasma renin activity is suppressed by primary mineralocorticoid excess (adrenal hyperactivity). Obtain a 24-hour urine collection and test for aldosterone (serum aldosterone concentrations fluctuate widely during the day). Clinical conditions characterized by suppressed renin activity without an elevation in daily aldosterone production include an inborn error of metabolism within the adrenal gland, such as 11-hydroxylase deficiency, where another mineralocorticoid (desoxycorticosterone) accumulates. This condition and Cushing syndrome result in increased mineralocorticoid activity, which produces hypokalemia.

F. Clinical signs of adrenal excess (Cushing syndrome) have various causes. One is bilateral adrenal hyperplasia caused by inappropriate secretion of adrenocorticotropic hormone (ACTH) by the pituitary; this is Cushing disease. Possible treatments of Cushing disease include pituitary irradiation, transsphenoidal hypophysectomy, the use of an antipituitary drug (cyproheptadine), and alternatively, drugs that are toxic to the adrenal gland. Other causes of Cushing syndrome include ingestion of pharmacologic doses of glucocorticoids, ectopic production of ACTH by tumors such as pheochromocytoma, neuroblastoma, pancreatic tumors, and Wilms tumors, and tumors of the adrenal gland (carcinoma or adenoma). Consider total adrenalectomy when Cushing syndrome is caused by an adrenal carcinoma or adenoma or when more conservative treatments for other conditions are ineffective.

G. Congenital adrenal hyperplasia due to deficiency of either 11-hydroxylase or 17-hydroxylase differs from that due to 21-hydroxylase deficiency in that mineralocorticoid synthesis is not impaired in the former conditions. Treat with glucocorticoid replacement alone. Boys and girls with 17-hydroxylase deficiency require testosterone or estrogen, respectively, during and after puberty because the 17-hydroxylase enzyme is necessary for the synthesis of androgen and estrogen in the gonads as well as the adrenal glands.

H. Plasma renin activity is high in certain renal disorders. A defect in chloride resorption (Bartter syndrome) results in a hypokalemic metabolic alkalosis associated with normal serum sodium and normal blood pressure despite the high renin. Elevated plasma renin activity, hypokalemia, and hypertension characterize renal vascular disease and tumors of the juxtaglomerular cells. The work-up for these disorders includes renal scan and digital subtraction angiography.

I. Treat Bartter syndrome with a sodium-wasting, potassium-sparing diuretic such as spironolactone and the supplemental use of potassium and magnesium as their chloride salts. This regimen blocks endogenous aldosterone action and restores electrolyte balances in potassium, magnesium, and chloride. Success has also been reported with the use of a prostaglandin synthesis inhibitor, indomethacin.

References

Melby JC. Diagnosis and treatment of primary aldosteronism and isolated hypoaldosteronism. In: De Groot LJ, Besser M, Burger HG, et al, eds. Endocrinology. Philadelphia: Saunders, 1989:1705.

Migeon CJ, Donohoue P. Adrenal disorders. In: Kappy MS, Blizzard RM, Migeon CJ, eds. The diagnosis and treatment of endocrine disorders in childhood and adolescence. 4th ed. Springfield, IL: Charles C. Thomas, 1994:717.

Odell G. Ectopic ACTH secretion. Endocrinol Metab Clin North Am 1991; 20:371.

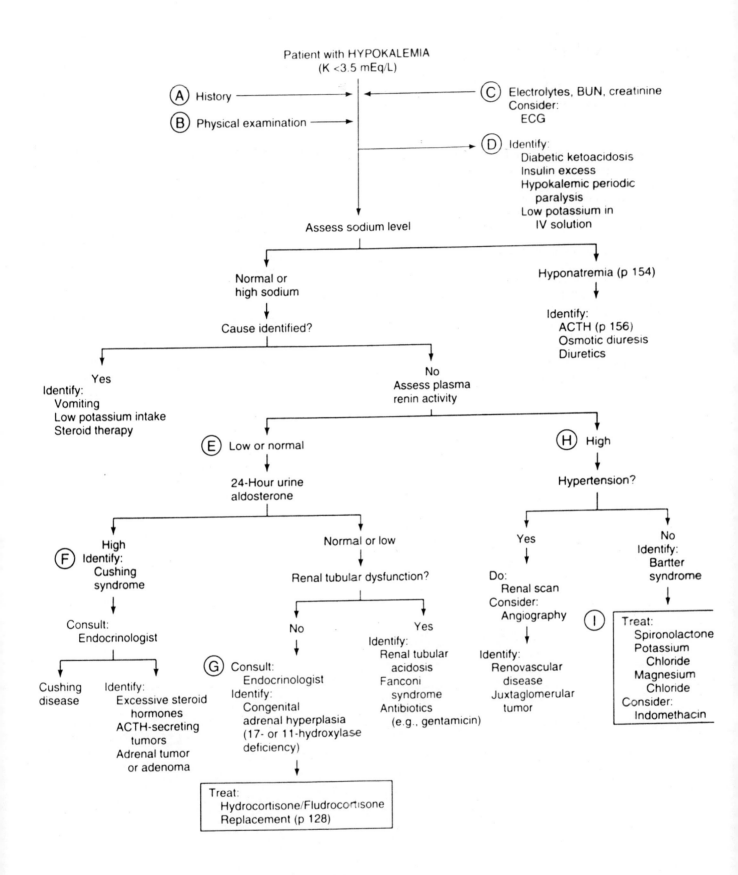

Patient with HYPOKALEMIA
(K <3.5 mEq/L)

(A) History

(B) Physical examination

(C) Electrolytes, BUN, creatinine
Consider:
ECG

(D) Identify:
Diabetic ketoacidosis
Insulin excess
Hypokalemic periodic
paralysis
Low potassium in
IV solution

Assess sodium level

Normal or
high sodium

Hyponatremia (p 154)

Identify:
ACTH (p 156)
Osmotic diuresis
Diuretics

Cause identified?

Yes
Identify:
Vomiting
Low potassium intake
Steroid therapy

No
Assess plasma
renin activity

(E) Low or normal

(H) High

24-Hour urine
aldosterone

Hypertension?

High
(F) Identify:
Cushing
syndrome

Normal or low

Yes

No
Identify:
Bartter
syndrome

Consult:
Endocrinologist

Renal tubular dysfunction?

Do:
Renal scan
Consider:
Angiography

(I) Treat:
Spironolactone
Potassium
Chloride
Magnesium
Chloride
Consider:
Indomethacin

Cushing
disease

Identify:
Excessive steroid
hormones
ACTH-secreting
tumors
Adrenal tumor
or adenoma

No

Yes
Identify:
Renal tubular
acidosis
Fanconi
syndrome
Antibiotics
(e.g., gentamicin)

Identify:
Renovascular
disease
Juxtaglomerular
tumor

(G) Consult:
Endocrinologist
Identify:
Congenital
adrenal hyperplasia
(17- or 11-hydroxylase
deficiency)

Treat:
Hydrocortisone/Fludrocortisone
Replacement (p 128)

HYPONATREMIA

Carrie A. Ganong, M.D.
Michael S. Kappy, M.D., Ph.D.

A. In the history identify predisposing factors such as diabetes mellitus, cystic fibrosis, CNS disorders or trauma, chemotherapy, malignancies, gastroenteritis, excessive water intake, diuretics, renal disease, exposure to heavy metals, pneumonia, and liver disease with ascites.

B. In the physical examination assess vital signs, circulatory status, and hydration status. Note signs of circulatory overload such as congestive heart failure with pulmonary edema, gallop, and hepatomegaly. Note signs of CNS disorder (altered mental status, abnormal or focal neurologic signs), respiratory distress (pneumonia, cystic fibrosis), liver disease (ascites, hepatomegaly, jaundice, portal hypertension), and renal disease. Suspect the syndrome of inappropriate antidiuretic hormone secretion (SIADH) in well-hydrated patients and cerebral salt wasting (CSW) in hypotensive patients with associated CNS pathology.

C. Identify patients whose plasma osmolality is increased by substances other than sodium. In hyperglycemia total body sodium may not be decreased, since movement of water from intracellular to vascular space causes an osmotic dilution of sodium. In hyperlipidemia the sodium measurement is falsely low, since the volume of lipid reduces the volume of serum in the centrifuged specimen of blood.

D. A low urinary sodium suggests insufficient sodium intake or excessive nonrenal sodium loss. Excessive sodium may be lost in sweat (cystic fibrosis) or from the GI tract (vomiting or diarrhea). Prolonged administration of clear fluids of low sodium content may produce hyponatremia.

(Continued on page 156)

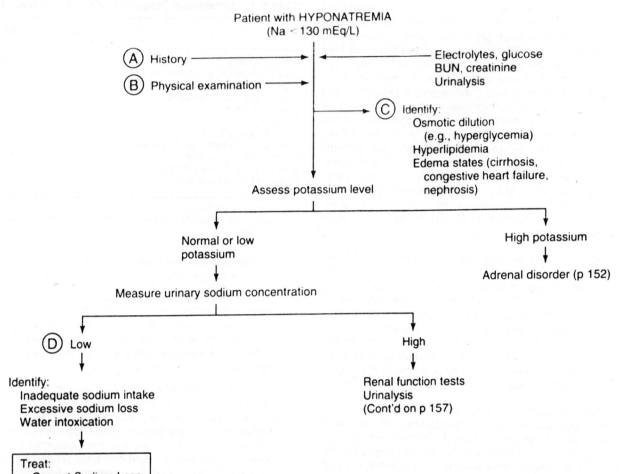

Patient with HYPONATREMIA
(Na < 130 mEq/L)

(A) History ——————→

(B) Physical examination ——→

←—————— Electrolytes, glucose
BUN, creatinine
Urinalysis

→ (C) Identify:
Osmotic dilution
(e.g., hyperglycemia)
Hyperlipidemia
Edema states (cirrhosis,
congestive heart failure,
nephrosis)

Assess potassium level

Normal or low
potassium

High potassium

Adrenal disorder (p 152)

Measure urinary sodium concentration

(D) Low

Identify:
Inadequate sodium intake
Excessive sodium loss
Water intoxication

Treat:
Correct Sodium Loss
Correct Fluid Deficit

High

Renal function tests
Urinalysis
(Cont'd on p 157)

E. When the urine osmolality exceeds the plasma osmolality, suspect SIADH. The hypothalamus produces ADH without physiologic cause. Patients with SIADH usually do not appear dehydrated, and they have a concentrated urine in the face of hyponatremia and lowered plasma osmolality. Consider CNS disorders such as head injury, meningitis, encephalitis, and brain tumor. Bronchopneumonia and chronic liver disease with ascites may stimulate appropriate secretion of ADH because of reduced blood flow to the atria and baroreceptor activation. Manage patients with SIADH by restricting the intake of free water. Consider replacing only insensible loss plus urine output. When SIADH results in severe hyponatremia (<120 mEq/L), consider using a hypertonic saline infusion and furosemide (Lasix) to increase serum sodium quickly.

F. Diuretics (thiazides and furosemide) inhibit renal tubular reabsorption of sodium and potassium. An important exception is spironolactone, which inhibits aldosterone action on the tubule, resulting in a selective loss of sodium with retention of potassium. Osmotic diuresis (hyperglycemia, mannitol, glycerol) also results in excessive urinary losses of sodium and potassium. In hyponatremia secondary to osmotic diuresis or diuretic therapy, the urine osmolality remains less than or equal to that of the serum.

G. Atrial natriuretic hormone (ANH) and brain natriuretic hormone (BNH) have been isolated from the organs of animals and humans. They are potent counterregulatory hormones for the renin-angiotensin-aldosterone system (blocking plasma renin activity, basal aldosterone, and angiotensin II–stimulated aldosterone release). Both produce sodium diuresis by increasing the glomerular filtration rate and by decreasing the proximal renal tubular resorption of sodium through interference with the generation of renin, angiotensin, aldosterone, as well as the peripheral action of aldosterone on the renal tubules. Furthermore, they are potent natriuretics causing excretion of large volumes of urine with a high salt concentration. This may be particularly important in congestive heart failure. It has become increasingly apparent that hyponatremia after head trauma or CNS surgery may not be due to SIADH (Table 1). Some patients excrete large volumes of high-salt urine, called cerebral salt wasting. Whether this is due to an inappropriate secretion of a natriuretic hormone has yet to be proved; however, preliminary evidence suggests that it is. A distinction between CSW and SIADH may be made primarily on the excessive urinary volume in the former. It is particularly important to differentiate be-

TABLE 1 Differential Diagnosis of CSW and SIADH

	CSW	SIADH
Plasma volume*	↓	↑
Clinical evidence of volume depletion*	+	−
Plasma sodium concentration	↓	↓
Urine sodium concentration	↑↑	Variable
Urine flow rate*	↑↑	↓ generally
Net sodium loss*	+++	+/−
Plasma renin activity	↓	↓
Plasma aldosterone concentration*	↓	↑
Plasma ADH concentration*	↓	↑
Serum uric acid concentration*	NL	↓
Plasma ANH concentration	↑	↑

*Main distinguishing features.
From Ganong CA, Kappy MS. Cerebral salt wasting in children. Am J Dis Child 1993; 147:167.

tween these two, since the treatment of SIADH is mainly fluid restriction, which can be fatal in CSW.

H. The treatment of CSW is to replace urine volume, using 0.9% or 3% saline for some or all of the urine loss. Urine volume is excessive, as is urine salt concentration, which is above 200 mEq/L in most cases. The occasional individual has benefited from continued oral supplementation with sodium chloride.

I. In Fanconi syndrome multiple transport functions of the tubule are disturbed, including impaired tubular reabsorption of glucose, amino acids, phosphate, bicarbonate, and electrolytes. These disorders may be secondary to tubular injury from exogenous toxic agents (heavy metals, outdated tetracyclines) or from toxic products of metabolic disorders such as cystinosis, tyrosinosis, and fructose intolerance. In chronic renal insufficiency urinary sodium excretion is high because the kidney fails to reabsorb normal amounts of sodium. In Bartter syndrome a primary disorder of chloride transport, the loss of potassium and chloride may be accompanied by hyponatremia during periods of low sodium intake.

References

Ganong CA, Kappy MS. Cerebral salt wasting in children. Am J Dis Child 1993; 147:167.

Gerigk M, Bald M, Rascher W. Clinical settings and vasopressin function in hyponatraemic children. Eur J Pediatr 1993; 152:301.

Gruskin AB, Sarnaik A. Hyponatremia: Pathophysiology and treatment, a pediatric perspective. Pediatr Nephrol 1992; 6:280.

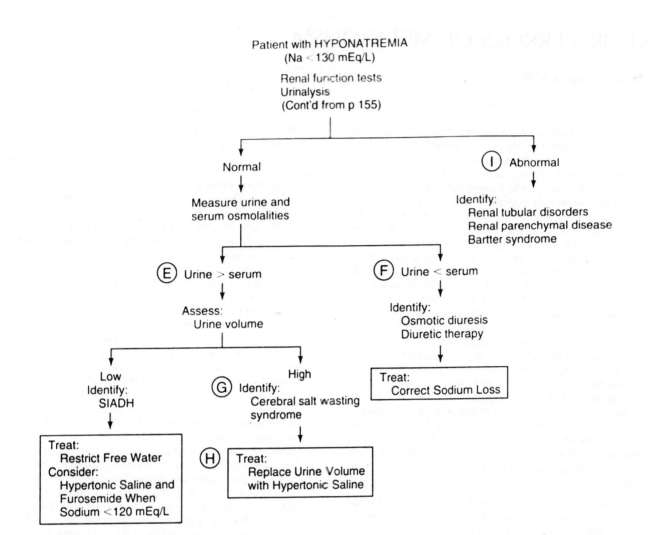

Patient with HYPONATREMIA
(Na < 130 mEq/L)

Renal function tests
Urinalysis
(Cont'd from p 155)

Normal

Measure urine and
serum osmolalities

(I) Abnormal

Identify:
    Renal tubular disorders
    Renal parenchymal disease
    Bartter syndrome

(E) Urine > serum

Assess:
Urine volume

(F) Urine < serum

Identify:
    Osmotic diuresis
    Diuretic therapy

Low
Identify:
    SIADH

High
(G) Identify:
    Cerebral salt wasting
    syndrome

Treat:
    Correct Sodium Loss

Treat:
    Restrict Free Water
Consider:
    Hypertonic Saline and
    Furosemide When
    Sodium <120 mEq/L

(H) Treat:
    Replace Urine Volume
    with Hypertonic Saline

INBORN ERRORS OF METABOLISM

Carol L. Greene, M.D.

In infants and children inborn errors of metabolism (IEM) manifest as nonspecific findings of altered mental status and/or acidosis that are often initially mistaken for poisoning, infection, or trauma. In some cases diagnosis of IEM is missed when an infection or trauma triggers deterioration although the apparent cause only partially explains the presentation. Laboratory findings may be mistakenly attributed to dehydration or asphyxia. Metabolic disease, like poisoning, should always be considered when the alteration in the mental status or acid-base status is not consistent with other aspects of the patient's clinical status. Although each IEM is rare, typically affecting fewer than 1 in 5000 to 1 in 100,000 children in the general population, collectively these disorders in the general population are more common than generally appreciated because there are many of them. More importantly, IEM are common in children who are in coma or require admission to control acidosis or hypoglycemia. Acute presentation of IEM may occur at any age from infancy to adulthood in a previously healthy individual with a negative family history. Individuals with IEM presenting after the neonatal period often have relatively mild biochemical defects with residual enzyme activity and may respond well to both acute and chronic treatment. Failure to consider IEM in acutely ill infants and children may delay appropriate treatment. Early suspicion and diagnosis provide the best chance for a good outcome.

A. Certain clinical histories raise the suspicion of IEM, but normal personal and family histories do not exclude it. Ask about a family history of consanguinity, mental retardation, seizures, sudden death (especially neonatal death or sudden infant death syndrome [SIDS]), recurrent emesis, or growth disturbance. The child's medical history may reveal previous episodes, e.g., admissions for "dehydration." History of growth disturbance, especially failure to thrive or microcephaly, and developmental problems increase suspicion. Feeding history is important; in the young child the first symptoms of IEM may appear with change in diet. Important changes include introduction of galactose (switch from soy to cow milk base); fructose (addition of juices or fruits or switch to certain soy formulas); higher protein (switch from breast milk to most formulas, or addition of foods); or increased fasting (longer sleep periods or intercurrent illness). Rashes, hair loss, and unusual odors may be clues.

B. On physical examination acute IEM often includes either altered mental status out of proportion to physiologic findings or physical findings that do not explain the lab findings (e.g., normal perfusion with acidosis in a vomiting child). Either hypertonia in a newborn or persistent hypotonia after age 1 or 2 years is typical of some IEM. Acute hypertonia in a previously normal child is typical of hyperammonemia and organic acidemias. Ataxia and movement disorders strongly suggest IEM. Tachypnea and apnea may be present in acidosis or hyperammonemia. Hepatomegaly and jaundice are common in some disorders. Macrocephaly with or without excess subdural fluid, rashes, hair changes, and cataracts may suggest specific disorders.

C. Laboratory findings are variable. They may include acidosis, alkalosis, hypoglycemia, hyperammonemia, and altered liver function. Collect metabolic samples at the time of presentation because management will alter study results (IV glucose affects urine ketones and organic acids). Consult the metabolic laboratory when the samples for amino and organic acids must be done stat. If IEM is unlikely, samples can be held frozen and sent later if an alternative diagnosis is not made and/or the patient's symptoms become more consistent with IEM. Hyperammonemia is often missed until all other attempts at diagnosis fail. Special handling is required for accurate blood ammonia, but the sample may be drawn with a tourniquet in emergencies. (Mishandling tends to increase the level, so normal ammonia always rules out hyperammonemia.) IEM (especially organic acidemia) can cause anemia, neutropenia, and thrombocytopenia. When an IEM such as galactosemia, fructose intolerance, tyrosinemia, or mitochondrial disease causes renal tubular acidosis, the acidosis may be associated with a normal anion gap. After the first weeks of life, catabolism causes ketogenesis, so finding no urine ketones in a child who has fasted suggests IEM. However, the presence of urine ketones does not exclude IEM, as patients with hypoketotic disorders (diseases of fatty acid oxidation) do make some ketones in response to fasting. When urine ketones are elevated in a nonfasting state, suspect a cross-reaction between organic metabolites and the reagent on the test strip. Consider measuring serum lactate and pyruvate and carnitine. An extremely high lactate in a patient with good peripheral perfusion and normal blood pressure suggests primary lactic acidosis. Very low carnitine levels may indicate a disorder of carnitine transport or be a secondary effect of other metabolic disorders. However, abnormal results must be interpreted with caution because normal values in an acutely ill child are not known.

D. Documentation of sepsis (especially with gram-negative enteric organisms) does not exclude IEM, as galactosemia and other disorders can predispose to sepsis. Respiratory syncitial virus or enterovirus may precipitate a metabolic crisis. A history of abuse, neglect, or nonaccidental trauma may accompany IEM since patients with IEM may have feeding difficulties or irritability, and parenting may be difficult. Documenting a specific nonmetabolic condition that explains all the child's symptoms and signs makes IEM less likely.

E. Special laboratory studies may be performed most rapidly after discussion with the appropriate consultant and laboratory. Laboratory diagnosis of certain IEM can

(Continued on page 160)

Patient with Suspected INBORN ERROR OF METABOLISM

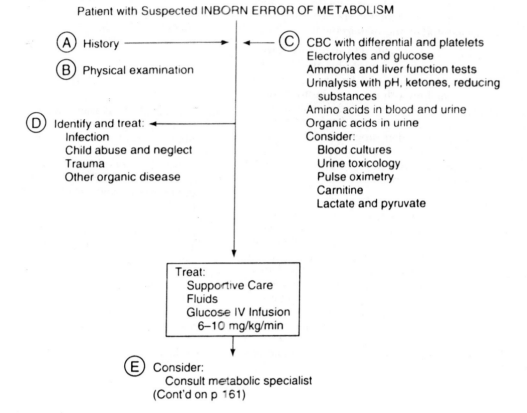

(A) History

(B) Physical examination

(C) CBC with differential and platelets
Electrolytes and glucose
Ammonia and liver function tests
Urinalysis with pH, ketones, reducing
   substances
Amino acids in blood and urine
Organic acids in urine
Consider:
   Blood cultures
   Urine toxicology
   Pulse oximetry
   Carnitine
   Lactate and pyruvate

(D) Identify and treat:
Infection
Child abuse and neglect
Trauma
Other organic disease

Treat:
   Supportive Care
   Fluids
   Glucose IV Infusion
   6–10 mg/kg/min

(E) Consider:
   Consult metabolic specialist
(Cont'd on p 161)

sometimes be made within hours. Discuss the patient with a metabolic consultant for specific suggestions about diagnostic studies and management.

F. Remember that children with IEM may have several types of clinical and biochemical abnormalities. The diagnosis of IEM is complicated by the variability in presentation of children with the same disorder and by the similarity of presentation of disorders in different categories. For example, both the fatty acid disorder medium chain acyl-CoA dehydrogenase (MCADD) and the amino acid disorder maple syrup urine disease (MSUD) may present with Reye syndrome. MCADD may also cause SIDS or apnea in babies.

G. In most patients with IEM high IV glucose infusions are required to stop catabolism, and only rare patients with severe primary lactic acidemia will become worse with IV glucose. Since protein cannot be withheld indefinitely, it must be resumed cautiously when the infant is stable. Elevated ammonia needs rapid treatment regardless of the cause. Treat with arginine and with sodium benzoate and sodium phenylacetate for pharmacologic dialysis. Lactulose and oral neomycin are not sufficient therapy for metabolic hyperammonemia. Treatment is available for specific conditions such as vitamin B_{12} for some types of methylmalonic acidemia.

H. Consider dialysis when mental status, severe acidosis, or hyperammonemia does not respond to other therapies.

References

Arens R, Gozal D, Williams JC, et al. Recurrent apparent life-threatening events during infancy: A manifestation of inborn errors of metabolism. J Pediatr 1993; 123:415.

Goodman SI, Greene CL. Metabolic disorders of the newborn. Pediatr Rev 1994; 15:359.

Greene CL, Blitzer MG, Shapira E. Inborn errors of metabolism and Reye syndrome: Differential diagnosis. J Pediatr 1988; 113:156.

Greene CL, Goodman SI. Inborn errors of metabolism. In: Hay WW, Groothuis JR, Hayward AR, Levin MJ, eds. Pediatric diagnosis and treatment. 12th ed. Norwalk, CT: Appleton & Lange, 1995:926.

Rowe PC, Valle D, Brusilow SW. Inborn errors of metabolism in children referred with Reye's syndrome: A changing pattern. JAMA 1988; 260:3167.

Surtees R, Leonard JV. Acute metabolic encephalopathy: A review of causes, mechanisms and treatment. J Inherit Metab Dis 1989; 12(Suppl):42.

Waber L. Inborn errors of metabolism. Pediatr Ann 1990; 19:105, 107.

Patient with Suspected INBORN ERROR OF METABOLISM

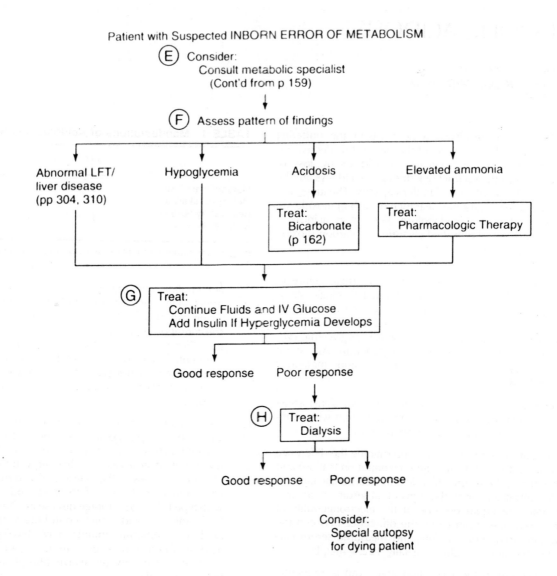

METABOLIC ACIDOSIS

Carrie A. Ganong, M.D.
Michael S. Kappy, M.D., Ph.D.

Metabolic acidosis results in a decrease in the buffering capacity (sodium bicarbonate) of the blood; this decrease is produced either by an increase in acid or by loss of bicarbonate from the GI tract or kidneys. The kidneys are the major site of the regulation of buffer capacity. The lungs also alter pH by determining the clearance of carbon dioxide, an end product of normal metabolism. Respiratory acidosis is associated with the diminished clearance of carbon dioxide from the lungs (Table 1).

A. In the history note any vomiting, diarrhea, failure to thrive, polyuria, fever, and altered neurologic status (seizures). Identify predisposing factors such as renal disease, diabetes mellitus, diarrhea and vomiting, hypothermia, toxin ingestion, known hypoglycemic syndrome, and inborn errors of metabolism. Ask about family history of neonatal death and metabolic disorders.

B. In the physical examination note the vital signs; assess the circulatory status. Note signs consistent with respiratory distress, sepsis, and CNS disorder.

C. Calculate the anion gap by determining the difference between the serum sodium concentration (cation) and the sum of the serum chloride and bicarbonate (anions) concentration. Since the sums of all serum anions and cations are equal because of the electroneutrality of the body, the anion gap is the difference between the unmeasured serum anions and measured serum cations. The normal value is usually 12 ± 4 mEq/L.

D. An increase in the calculated anion gap is frequently seen with increased acid production by the body, such as in inborn errors of metabolism or diabetic ketoacidosis, or with the ingestion of acid-producing toxins such as methanol and ethylene glycol. Aspirin intoxication is associated with a variable anion gap due to the

TABLE 1 Manifestations of Acidosis and Alkalosis

	pH	P_{CO_2}	HCO_3
Metabolic acidosis	↓	↓	↓
Metabolic alkalosis	↑	↑	↑
Respiratory acidosis	↓	↑	↑
Respiratory alkalosis	↑	↓	↓

P_{CO_2}, carbon dioxide partial pressure; HCO_3, bicarbonate radical.

accumulation of organic acids secondary to aspirin's effect on intermediary metabolism. A normal calculated anion gap may be present in the early stages of any of the conditions that traditionally have an increased anion gap; therefore, the anion gap alone is unreliable for the differential diagnosis of metabolic acidosis. Periodic reassessment of the patient's electrolyte status allows the recalculation of the anion gap if the diagnosis proves elusive.

E. Hypoglycemia, positive urinary ketones, and an elevated anion gap suggest a disorder of glycogenolysis or gluconeogenesis. Excessive ketone production is due to the use of fat stores to provide energy in the absence of glucose in excess of the liver's ability to metabolize the breakdown products of fatty acid oxidation. Patients with type I glycogen storage disease also produce excess lactic and uric acid, which contribute to the metabolic acidosis. Premature infants may develop metabolic acidosis when they receive an acid load that exceeds their renal capacity (excessive phosphate or protein from cow's milk).

F. Normal anion gaps are generally seen when both sodium and bicarbonate are lost from the body, as with diarrhea or through the kidney in proximal renal tubular acidosis type II.

(Continued on page 164)

METABOLIC ACIDOSIS Suspected

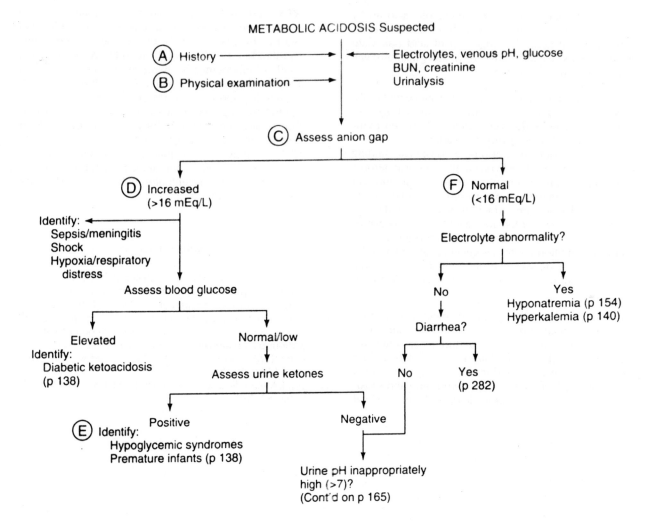

Ⓐ History ———————→ ←——— Electrolytes, venous pH, glucose
                                    BUN, creatinine
Ⓑ Physical examination ———→   Urinalysis

Ⓒ Assess anion gap

Ⓓ Increased   Ⓕ Normal
   (>16 mEq/L)   (<16 mEq/L)

Identify: ←   Electrolyte abnormality?
   Sepsis/meningitis
   Shock   No   Yes
   Hypoxia/respiratory   Hyponatremia (p 154)
      distress   Hyperkalemia (p 140)
   Assess blood glucose   Diarrhea?

Elevated   Normal/low   No   Yes
Identify: (p 282)
   Diabetic ketoacidosis   Assess urine ketones
   (p 138)

          Positive   Negative
Ⓔ Identify:
   Hypoglycemic syndromes
   Premature infants (p 138)
                                  Urine pH inappropriately
                                  high (>7)?
                                  (Cont'd on p 165)

G. Ingestion of toxins may cause a metabolic acidosis by producing any of a number of acids. Ethanol increases lactic acid and ketoacids. Ingestion of acid (salicylate intoxication, which also causes respiratory alkalosis) will also increase the anion gap.

H. Inborn errors of metabolism that can produce metabolic acidosis include deficiencies in pyruvate dehydrogenase enzyme complex and enzyme defects between pyruvate and phosphoenol-pyruvate, leading to lactic acidosis. Lactic acidosis may also be a nonspecific finding related to long periods of hypoxia, producing anaerobic tissue metabolism. Other causes are errors in amino acid oxidation (e.g., maple syrup urine disease) and disorders of fatty acid oxidation, which may be secondary to carnitine deficiency or the absence of specific enzymes crucial to β-oxidation of fatty acids. In these latter two groups of conditions, ketosis is generally absent and the qualitative and quantitative determination of organic acids in the urine may be an invaluable guide to the diagnosis.

I. Abnormal renal function produces metabolic acidosis because of impaired acid excretion and/or inability to retain sodium bicarbonate. Renal tubular disorders result in acidosis due to the failure to reabsorb sodium bicarbonate or excrete acid in normal amounts. Renal tubular disorders include Fanconi syndrome and proximal and distal renal tubular acidosis (RTA). In proximal RTA there is low threshold for the reabsorption of bicarbonate; patients can acidify the urine only when plasma bicarbonate falls below the lowered renal threshold (approximately 15 mEq/L). While the exact mode of inheritance is unknown, it appears to have a genetic component. In distal RTA the kidney is unable to excrete an acid urine at any plasma bicarbonate concentration. Impaired distal tubular hydrogen ion excretion results in excessive urinary loss of both potassium and phosphorus, leading to hypokalemic acidosis. Distal RTA also may result in mild to moderate antidiuretic hormone unresponsiveness at the renal tubule; the consequent polyuria accentuates both hypokalemia and hypophosphatemia.

References

Fitzgerald MJ, Goto M, Myers TF, Zeller WP. Early metabolic effects of sepsis in the preterm infant: Lactic acidosis and increased glucose requirement. J Pediatr 1992; 121:951.

Glaser B, Hirsch HJ, Landau H. Persistent hyperinsulinemic hypoglycemia of infancy: Long-term octreotide treatment without pancreatectomy. J Pediatr 1993; 123:637.

Halperin ML. Metabolic aspects of metabolic acidosis. Clin Invest Med 1993; 16:294.

Walter JH. Metabolic acidosis in newborn infants. Arch Dis Child 1992; 67:767.

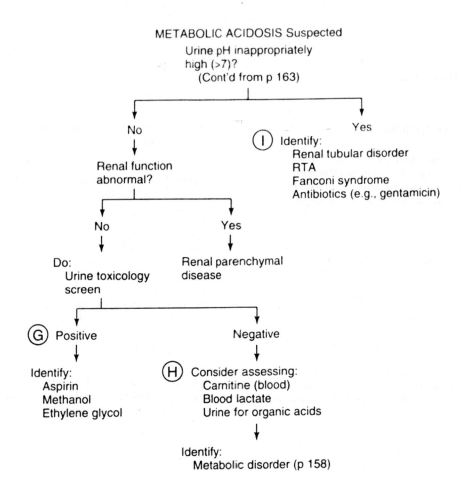

METABOLIC ACIDOSIS Suspected
Urine pH inappropriately
high (>7)?
(Cont'd from p 163)

No

Renal function
abnormal?

No

Do:
  Urine toxicology
  screen

(G) Positive

Identify:
  Aspirin
  Methanol
  Ethylene glycol

Negative

(H) Consider assessing:
  Carnitine (blood)
  Blood lactate
  Urine for organic acids

Identify:
  Metabolic disorder (p 158)

Yes

Renal parenchymal
disease

Yes

(I) Identify:
  Renal tubular disorder
  RTA
  Fanconi syndrome
  Antibiotics (e.g., gentamicin)

OBESITY

Carrie A. Ganong, M.D.
Michael S. Kappy, M.D., Ph.D.

DEFINITION

Obesity is present when the child's weight is at least 20% above the ideal weight for height. This may be estimated from a standard growth chart or the use of a life insurance company table. Most obesity in children is exogenous, and the children are tall for their age and family; they may also have advanced puberty.

A. A family history of obesity and/or excessive food intake and diminished activity is often diagnostic of exogenous obesity in childhood. Pattern of weight gain may identify specific periods that were stressful to the child and that may have provoked overeating. In addition, a history of CNS surgery, especially for tumors or lesions in the hypothalamic region, may identify the youngster who is obese because of damage to the satiety center in the hypothalamus. This is particularly evident in children who have been operated on for craniopharyngioma. A history of pharmacologic steroid ingestion should also be obtained, especially in children with asthma or those who must be immunosuppressed in the treatment of a chronic illness.

B. In the physical examination note the distribution of adipose tissue in the adolescent, specifically the characteristic buffalo hump and centripetal distribution compatible with Cushing syndrome. Younger children show this same pattern with exogenous obesity. The young child with Cushing syndrome is short for age and family and usually has a slow rate of growth. Hypogonadism may also identify other syndromes, for example, Prader-Willi syndrome, which also includes short stature, hypotonia, and mental retardation. A karyotype may reveal a defect in chromosome 15. In Laurence-Moon-Biedl syndrome obesity and hypogonadism are associated with mental retardation, polydactyly, and retinitis pigmentosa.

C. One of the discriminators in the evaluation of the obese child is the height and growth rate, since endocrine causes of obesity in children of normal height and normal growth rate are quite rare.

(Continued on page 168)

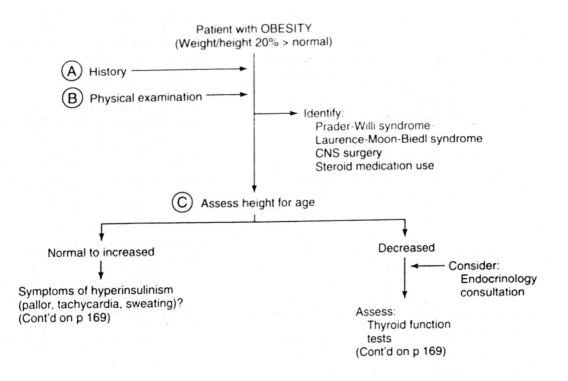

Patient with OBESITY
(Weight/height 20% > normal)

(A) History

(B) Physical examination

Identify:
Prader-Willi syndrome
Laurence-Moon-Biedl syndrome
CNS surgery
Steroid medication use

(C) Assess height for age

Normal to increased

Symptoms of hyperinsulinism
(pallor, tachycardia, sweating)?
(Cont'd on p 169)

Decreased

Consider:
Endocrinology
consultation

Assess:
Thyroid function
tests
(Cont'd on p 169)

D. Children who are obese because of hyperinsulinism usually have readily identifiable symptoms of hypoglycemia. In older children these are primarily catechol-mediated; they consist of pallor, tachycardia, sweating, and nervousness. Occasionally more severe symptoms such as lethargy and seizures occur. In the newborn the signs and symptoms of hypoglycemia are less distinct and may include only poor feeding, lethargy, and staring spells.

E. To screen for hyperinsulinism, assess the fasting insulin-to-glucose ratio. In most cases this should be 1:10 to 1:5, and an insulin-to-glucose ratio greater than 1:4 suggests hyperinsulinism. In the newborn period this is usually seen in infants of diabetic mothers who have secondary islet cell hyperplasia and in newborns with nesidioblastosis. In the older child islet cell adenomas become more common than hyperplasia or nesidioblastosis and require surgical intervention.

F. Exogenous obesity is probably the most common differential diagnosis in this section. Strongly determined by cultural-familial factors, it is not an endocrine problem. Although obesity is considered incurable by many physicians, a weight-loss program, preferably a structured one with behavior modification, may be effective. This should include a healthful exercise regimen in addition to normalization of the child's quantitative and qualitative food intake. Elevated fasting insulin-to-glucose ratios reflect the peripheral insulin resistance commonly seen in type II diabetes mellitus. The appearance of this early prediabetic insulin resistance may be an additional motivation for the family and the child in a weight-loss program.

G. Polycystic ovary syndrome (PCO) is secondary to increased androgen production by the ovary. Hirsutism, obesity, infertility, disturbances of the menstrual cycle, and multiple ovarian cysts seen on ultrasound are common. Acanthosis nigricans and type II diabetes mellitus often are part of PCO. Frequently there is a clear family history in a mother or siblings.

H. Primary hypothyroidism is associated with growth retardation more commonly than true obesity; however, the weight-to-height ratio is generally increased in these patients. Characteristically, a low thyroxine (T_4) or free T_4 combined with an elevation of thyroid-stimulating hormone (TSH) is found.

I. A low free T_4 and free thyroxine index (FTI) combined with a normal TSH suggests either secondary (pituitary) or tertiary (hypothalamic) hypothyroidism. In this case perform additional endocrine testing to assess total pituitary function, specifically growth hormone (GH) secretion, since GH deficiency may also produce short stature with a characteristically chubby appearance. Normal thyroid function studies should be noted, but the short, chubby child with a slow growth rate should still be evaluated for GH deficiency.

J. Children whose obesity is caused by hypothyroidism, GH deficiency, or cortisol excess (Cushing) characteristically have a delay in skeletal maturation (bone age), whereas children with exogenous obesity have advanced skeletal maturation. Cushing syndrome in children is much less common than supposed. In the adolescent it is manifested by a characteristic centripetal distribution of fat coupled with purple striae (although these may be present in simple obesity as well), occasional hypertension, hirsutism, and muscle wasting. Diagnosis may be helped by 24 hour urinary 17-hydroxycorticosteroids assessment of the patient's diurnal variation in plasma cortisol levels and the results of a dexamethasone suppression test. Urinary-free cortisol determinations before and after dexamethasone may also be diagnostic.

References

Bandini LG, Dietz WH. Myths about childhood obesity. Pediatr Ann 1992; 21:647.

Shulman DI. Literature reviews: Pathophysiology of hirsutism in the adolescent female. Adolesc Pediatr Gynecol 1993; 6:105.

Williams CL, Bollella M, Carter BJ. Treatment of childhood obesity in pediatric practice. Ann N Y Acad Sci 1993; 699:207.

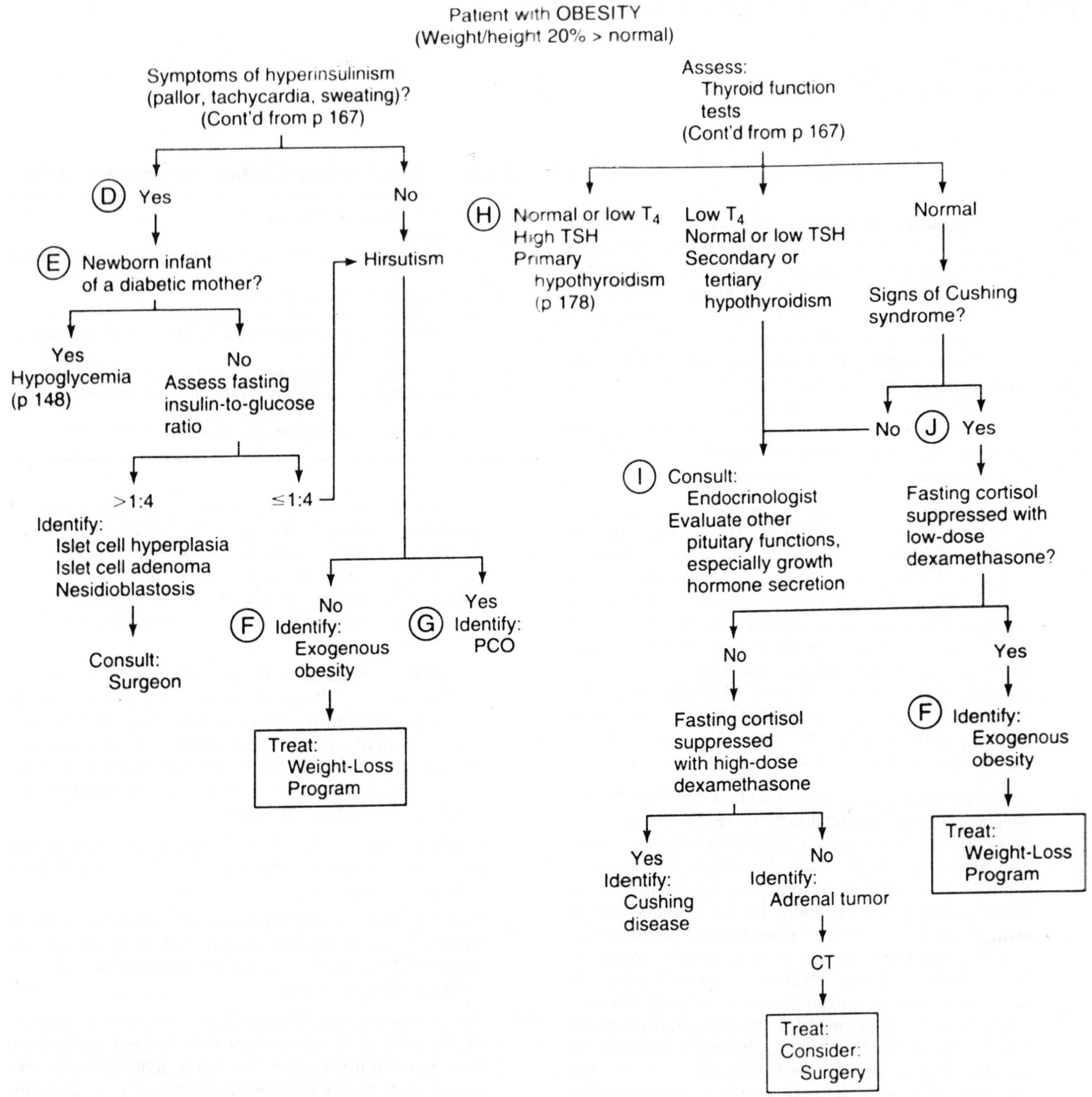

Patient with OBESITY
(Weight/height 20% > normal)

Symptoms of hyperinsulinism
(pallor, tachycardia, sweating)?
(Cont'd from p 167)

(D) Yes → No

(E) Newborn infant
of a diabetic mother? → Hirsutism

Yes
Hypoglycemia
(p 148)

No
Assess fasting
insulin-to-glucose
ratio

>1:4 → ≤1:4

Identify:
Islet cell hyperplasia
Islet cell adenoma
Nesidioblastosis

↓

Consult:
Surgeon

(F) No
Identify:
Exogenous
obesity

↓

Treat:
Weight-Loss
Program

(G) Yes
Identify:
PCO

Assess:
Thyroid function
tests
(Cont'd from p 167)

(H) Normal or low T$_4$
High TSH
Primary
hypothyroidism
(p 178)

Low T$_4$
Normal or low TSH
Secondary or
tertiary
hypothyroidism

Normal

↓

Signs of Cushing
syndrome?

No (J) Yes

(I) Consult:
Endocrinologist
Evaluate other
pituitary functions,
especially growth
hormone secretion

Fasting cortisol
suppressed with
low-dose
dexamethasone?

No → Yes

Fasting cortisol
suppressed
with high-dose
dexamethasone

(F) Identify:
Exogenous
obesity

↓

Treat:
Weight-Loss
Program

Yes
Identify:
Cushing
disease

No
Identify:
Adrenal tumor

↓

CT

↓

Treat:
Consider:
Surgery

PRECOCIOUS PUBERTY IN BOYS

Carrie A. Ganong, M.D.
Michael S. Kappy, M.D., Ph.D.

DEFINITIONS

Precocious puberty in boys is early *isosexual* pubertal development, or virilization. **True or central precocity** (gonadotropin-releasing hormone [GnRH] dependent) is early sexual development resulting from premature activation of the hypothalamopituitary axis. Virilization resulting from autonomous testicular or adrenal hyperfunction is generally called pseudo or **peripheral** (GnRH-independent) **precocity. Premature adrenarche,** the development of pubic hair and apocrine body odor (rarely accompanied by acne or axillary hair), is associated with normal or slightly increased plasma androgen concentrations and normal growth velocity. It is a benign, self-limited variant of normal development.

A. In the history note the age of onset of sexual development and recent increase in growth velocity. Identify predisposing CNS conditions such as head trauma, tumor, and meningitis. Obtain a family history of early male development that may be compatible with familial Leydig cell hyperplasia (testotoxicosis) and note parental heights. The normal mean onset of pubertal development (range in parentheses) in boys is as follows: testicular and penile enlargement, 11¾ years (9½ to 14 years); pubic hair, 12½ years (10¾ to 14 years); peak height growth velocity, 13¾ years (11¾ to 16 years); axillary hair, 14 years (12 to 16 years).

B. In the physical examination carefully plot height and weight and note parental heights. Assess the genitalia (testicular volume and stretched penile length) and note any acne and pubic hair. In peripheral precocity testosterone and/or other androgens are secreted without gonadotropin stimulation. Thus, the penis may be enlarged and pubic hair may be present, but the testes remain prepubertal in size (<4 cc volume using the Prader beads), unless a tumor is present (rare). In testotoxicosis or in congenital adrenal hyperplasia with adrenal rest tissue in the testes, the testes may be above 4 cc in volume, but they are usually smaller than normal for the degree of observed virilization. In central precocity early gonadotropin secretion stimulates the testes to grow and to produce testosterone prior to the normal pubertal age. Thus, penile enlargement is accompanied by appropriate testicular enlargement. Signs of androgen excess with moon face, central adiposity, and striae suggest Cushing syndrome.

C. Consider GnRH testing (measure serum luteinizing hormone [LH] concentration 30 minutes after a subcutaneous dose of GnRH [Factrel]) to determine the maturity of the hypothalamopituitary axis and whether precocity is GnRH-dependent (central) or GnRH-independent (peripheral).

D. A low plasma testosterone concentration in the presence of LH levels below 10 IU/L suggests abnormal secretion of other androgens, most commonly from the adrenal glands. Measure either the urinary excretion products of adrenal androgens (17-ketosteroids) or the hormones (androstenedione, dehydroepiandrosterone) and 17-hydroxyprogesterone (17-OHP) directly in the blood. If necessary, remeasure these hormones after adrenocorticotropic hormone (ACTH) testing if basal results are equivocal.

E. In patients with congenital adrenal hyperplasia (CAH) or Cushing disease, dexamethasone will suppress endogenous production of cortisol by inhibiting ACTH secretion. In patients whose virilization results from autonomously functioning adrenal tissue (adrenal tumor or an ectopic ACTH-secreting tumor), dexamethasone will not suppress cortisol secretion.

F. CAH accounts for 70% to 80% of boys with peripheral precocity. An elevated plasma (17-OHP) concentration suggests this diagnosis.

G. Familial Leydig cell hyperplasia (testotoxicosis) has been treated successfully with a combination of an antiandrogen (spironolactone) and an inhibitor of estrogen formation (testolactone).

H. The prevalence of CNS pathology decreases as the age of the patient at onset increases. Recent success in treating central precocity has been achieved with the use of agonists of GnRH given intranasally or subcutaneously as a daily regimen or with the use of a depot form of the agonist given monthly intramuscularly or subcutaneously (Table 1).

TABLE 1　Drug Therapy for Male Precocious Puberty

Central (GnRH-Dependent) Precocity
  GnRH agonist
    Leuprorelin (Lupron Depot-PED) 0.15–0.3 mg/kg/dose q4wk IM or SC
    Histrelin (Suprelin) 10 µg/kg qd SC
    Nafarelin (Synarel) 800–1600 µg b.i.d.-q.i.d. intranasally
Peripheral (GnRH-Independent) Precocity, McCune-Albright syndrome, or Testotoxicosis
  Ketoconazole 15–35 mg/kg/day divided into 2–3 doses PO
  Spironolactone 2–6 mg/kg/day divided into 2 doses PO
                                and
  Testolactone 20–40 mg/kg/day divided into 4 doses PO

References

Laue L, Jones J, Barnes KM, et al. Treatment of familial male precocious puberty with spironolactone, testolactone, and deslorelin. J Clin Endocrinol Metab 1993; 76:151.

Lee PA. Pubertal neuroendocrine maturation. Early differentiation and stages of development. Adolesc Pediatr Gynecol 1988; 1:3.

Rosenfield RL. Selection of children with precocious puberty for treatment with gonadotropin releasing hormone analogs. J Pediatr 1994; 124:989.

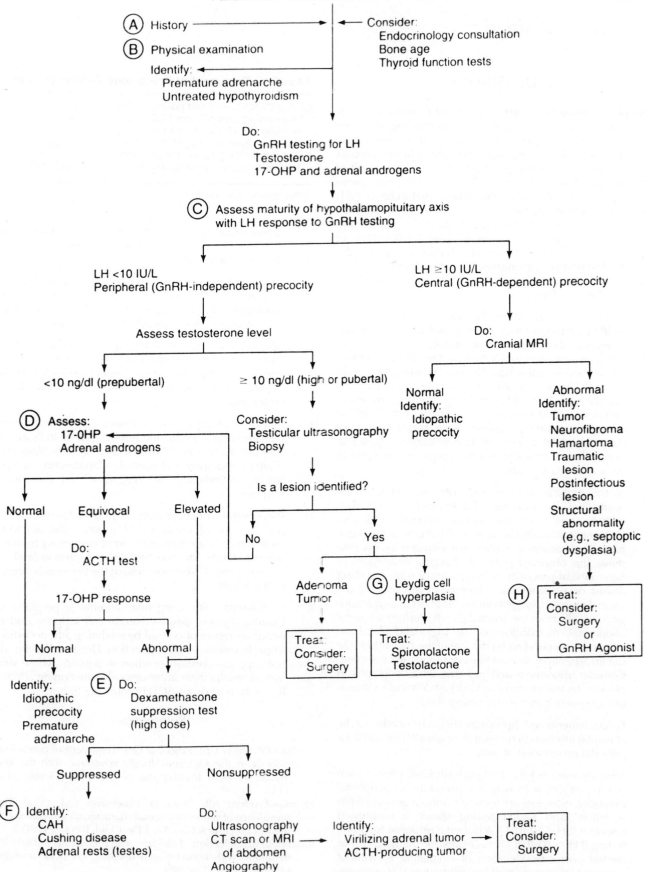

Patient with PRECOCIOUS PUBERTY (BOY)

(A) History — Consider:
    Endocrinology consultation
    Bone age
    Thyroid function tests

(B) Physical examination

Identify:
    Premature adrenarche
    Untreated hypothyroidism

Do:
    GnRH testing for LH
    Testosterone
    17-OHP and adrenal androgens

(C) Assess maturity of hypothalamopituitary axis
    with LH response to GnRH testing

LH <10 IU/L
Peripheral (GnRH-independent) precocity

LH ≥10 IU/L
Central (GnRH-dependent) precocity

Assess testosterone level

Do:
    Cranial MRI

<10 ng/dl (prepubertal)

≥ 10 ng/dl (high or pubertal)

Normal
Identify:
    Idiopathic
    precocity

Abnormal
Identify:
    Tumor
    Neurofibroma
    Hamartoma
    Traumatic
    lesion
    Postinfectious
    lesion
    Structural
    abnormality
    (e.g., septoptic
    dysplasia)

(D) Assess:
    17-OHP
    Adrenal androgens

Consider:
    Testicular ultrasonography
    Biopsy

Normal   Equivocal   Elevated

Is a lesion identified?

Do:
    ACTH test

No   Yes

17-OHP response

(H) Treat:
    Consider:
    Surgery
    or
    GnRH Agonist

Normal   Abnormal

Adenoma
Tumor

(G) Leydig cell
    hyperplasia

Identify:
    Idiopathic
    precocity
    Premature
    adrenarche

(E) Do:
    Dexamethasone
    suppression test
    (high dose)

Treat:
Consider:
Surgery

Treat:
Spironolactone
Testolactone

Suppressed   Nonsuppressed

(F) Identify:
    CAH
    Cushing disease
    Adrenal rests (testes)

Do:
    Ultrasonography
    CT scan or MRI
    of abdomen
    Angiography

Identify:
    Virilizing adrenal tumor
    ACTH-producing tumor

Treat:
Consider:
Surgery

PRECOCIOUS PUBERTY IN GIRLS

Michael S. Kappy, M.D., Ph.D.

DEFINITIONS

Precocious puberty in girls is isosexual pubertal development. True, or central (gonadotropin-releasing hormone [GnRH]-dependent) precocity, is a result of premature activation of the hypothalamopituitary axis, whereas pseudo, or peripheral (GnRH-independent) precocity, is a result of estrogen secretion autonomously by the ovaries or occasionally by the adrenal glands. **Premature thelarche** is early breast development in the absence of other signs of puberty. It is an innocent, nonpathologic finding and is not accompanied by rapid growth, advanced skeletal maturation, or pubertal plasma concentrations of estradiol or the gonadotropins. **Premature adrenarche** is early development of pubic hair without other signs of virilization. It is also a nonpathologic finding.

A. In the history ask about the age of onset of signs of puberty and recent increase in growth velocity. The age in years of normal mean onset of pubertal development (range in parentheses) is as follows: breast development, 11¼ (8 to 15); pubic hair, 12 (9 to 15); menarche, 13¾ (10½ to 16); peak height velocity, 12½ (9½ to 15); and axillary hair, 13¼ (11½ to 14½). Identify any exogenous source of hormones (e.g., birth control pills or estrogen-containing creams). Note family history of early pubertal development. Recent studies suggest that normal breast development may begin in some girls as early as 6 years of age.

B. In the physical examination note signs of CNS abnormalities. Rough-bordered café-au-lait spots or skeletal abnormalities suggest McCune-Albright syndrome. Document any adrenal aspects of puberty (acne, pubic hair). Their absence implies that estrogen excess produces the observed pubertal changes. Virilization, or heterosexual precocity without signs of estrogen effect (breast development or lightening of the color of the vaginal mucosa), suggests an excess of circulating androgens, usually from the adrenal glands. Perform a careful abdominal, rectoabdominal, or vaginoabdominal examination (depending on the age of the patient) to rule out an adrenal or ovarian mass or uterine enlargement. Consider abdominal and/or pelvic ultrasonography in place of rectoabdominal or vaginoabdominal examinations, especially in the very young child.

C. Follow patients with premature thelarche or adrenarche at regular intervals to monitor their growth rate and their pubertal progression, if any.

D. Measure estradiol (E_2) and perform GnRH testing (see p 170) in girls with isosexual precocity. In peripheral precocity, estrogens are secreted without gonadotropin secretion, and GnRH testing shows a suppressed response (LH < 10 IU/L). A pubertal response to GnRH testing (LH > 10 IU/L) is necessary for the diagnosis of central precocity. Elevation of circulating E_2 without concomitant elevation of gonadotropins (LH) suggests autonomous secretion of estrogens by a functional ovarian cyst, ovarian tumor, McCune-Albright syndrome, or adrenal tumor.

E. Recent studies have shown benefit in the treatment of central precocity from the use of a GnRH agonist given intranasally or SC daily, or from a depot form of the agonist given once a month IM or SC (Table 1).

F. Abnormal virilization in girls (pubic, axillary or facial hair, acne, clitoromegaly) warrants measurement of circulating androgens (testosterone, androstenedione, dehydroepiandrosterone [DHEA]) and 17-hydroxyprogesterone.

G. In a virilized girl who has elevated plasma testosterone concentrations, pelvic ultrasonography is indicated to rule out ovarian neoplasms such as arrhenoblastomas. If ultrasonography is abnormal, a laparoscopy or laparotomy is indicated for diagnostic and therapeutic purposes.

H. Prepubertal concentrations of plasma testosterone in the absence of elevated LH suggests the abnormal secretion of other androgens, most commonly from the adrenal glands. Measure the urinary excretion products of androgens (17-ketosteroids) or the hormones directly in the blood.

I. In patients with congenital adrenal hyperplasia or Cushing disease, dexamethasone will suppress endogenous secretion of cortisol by inhibiting adrenocorticotropic hormone (ACTH) secretion. Dexamethasone will not suppress cortisol secretion in patients whose virilization results from autonomously functioning adrenal tissue (tumor) or an ACTH-producing tumor.

TABLE 1 Treatment of Precocious Puberty in Girls

Central GnRH-dependent precocity: GnRH agonist
  leuprorelin (Lupron Depot-PED) 7.5–15 mg q4wk IM or SC
  Histrelin (Suprelin) 10 µg/kg qd SC
  Nafarelin (Synarel) 800–1600 µg b.i.d.-t.i.d. intranasally
Peripheral GnRH independent precocity
  Testolactone 20–40 mg/kg/day divided into 4 doses PO

GnRH, gonadotropin-releasing hormone.

References

Feuillan PP, Foster CM, Pescovitz OH. Treatment of precocious puberty in the McCune-Albright syndrome with the aromatase inhibitor testolactone. N Engl J Med 1986; 315: 1115.

Herman-Giddens ME, Slora EJ, Hasemeier CM, et al. The prevalence of secondary sexual characteristics in young girls seen in office practice. Am J Dis Child 1993; 147:455.

Rosenfield RL. Selection of children with precocious puberty for treatment with gonadotropin releasing hormone analogs. J Pediatr 1994; 124:989.

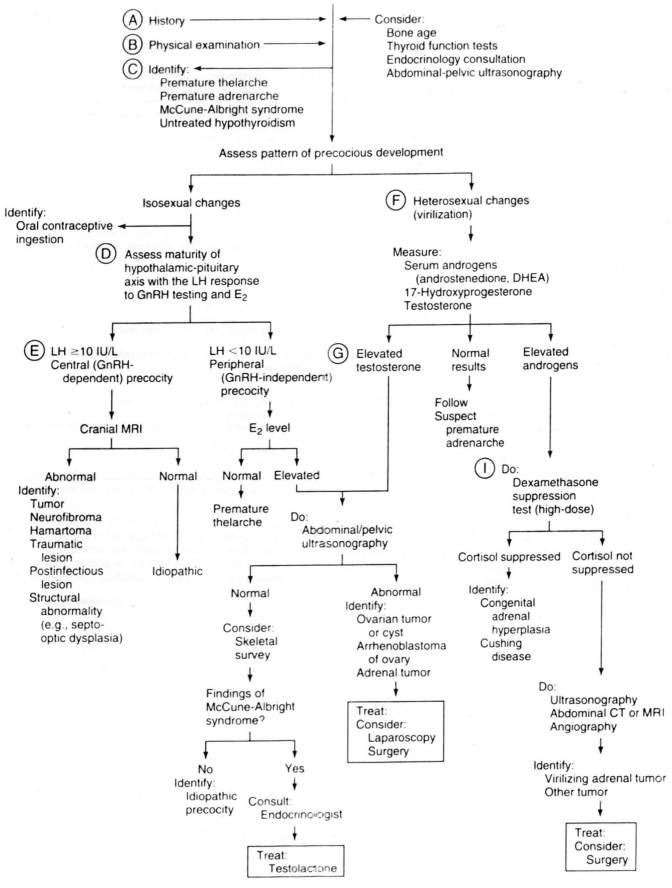

Patient with PRECOCIOUS PUBERTY (GIRL)

(A) History

(B) Physical examination

Consider:
  Bone age
  Thyroid function tests
  Endocrinology consultation
  Abdominal-pelvic ultrasonography

(C) Identify:
  Premature thelarche
  Premature adrenarche
  McCune-Albright syndrome
  Untreated hypothyroidism

Assess pattern of precocious development

Isosexual changes

Identify:
Oral contraceptive
  ingestion

(D) Assess maturity of
hypothalamic-pituitary
axis with the LH response
to GnRH testing and E_2

(E) LH ≥10 IU/L
Central (GnRH-
dependent) precocity

Cranial MRI

Abnormal
Identify:
  Tumor
  Neurofibroma
  Hamartoma
  Traumatic
    lesion
  Postinfectious
    lesion
  Structural
    abnormality
    (e.g., septo-
    optic dysplasia)

Normal

Idiopathic

LH <10 IU/L
Peripheral
(GnRH-independent)
precocity

E_2 level

Normal

Premature
thelarche

Elevated

Do:
Abdominal/pelvic
ultrasonography

Normal

Consider:
Skeletal
survey

Findings of
McCune-Albright
syndrome?

No
Identify:
  Idiopathic
  precocity

Yes

Consult:
Endocrinologist

Treat:
Testolactone

Abnormal
Identify:
  Ovarian tumor
  or cyst
  Arrhenoblastoma
  of ovary
  Adrenal tumor

Treat:
Consider:
  Laparoscopy
  Surgery

(F) Heterosexual changes
(virilization)

Measure:
  Serum androgens
  (androstenedione, DHEA)
  17-Hydroxyprogesterone
  Testosterone

(G) Elevated
testosterone

Normal
results

Follow
Suspect
premature
adrenarche

Elevated
androgens

(I) Do:
Dexamethasone
suppression
test (high-dose)

Cortisol suppressed

Identify:
  Congenital
  adrenal
  hyperplasia
  Cushing
  disease

Cortisol not
suppressed

Do:
  Ultrasonography
  Abdominal CT or MRI
  Angiography

Identify:
  Virilizing adrenal tumor
  Other tumor

Treat:
Consider:
  Surgery

173

REYE-LIKE SYNDROME

Stephen Berman, M.D.

Reye syndrome, a hepatic encephalopathy, is most likely related to altered mitochondrial metabolism. Viral illness, especially varicella and influenza, and ingestion of salicylates predispose to this syndrome. The Centers for Disease Control and Prevention (CDC) case definition is an alteration in mental status without CSF pleocytosis, evidence of hepatopathy by liver biopsy or a threefold or greater rise in AST, ALT, or serum ammonia and no reasonable explanation for cerebral or hepatic abnormalities. Nonspecific associated findings are hypoglycemia, hypophosphatemia, hyperuricemia, and metabolic acidosis. Most cases in children older than 2 years of age manifest as intractable vomiting, confusion, or irritability.

A. Some inborn errors of metabolism can cause a Reye-like syndrome of hepatic encephalopathy. Clinical features suggestive of metabolic disorder are unusual urine odor (isovaleric acidemia), age less than 2 years, recurrent Reye-like syndrome episodes, sibling history of Reye-like syndrome, abnormal growth and development, and a history of a recent dietary change. The work-up of Reye-like syndrome should include urine and plasma amino acids, urine organic acids, lactate and pyruvate, blood and urine carnitine, ammonia, blood glucose, pH, and electrolytes. Metabolic disorders that can present with a Reye-like syndrome can be classified according to metabolic acidosis, hypoglycemia, and elevated ammonia (Table 1). Specific therapy is available for deficiency of ornithine transcarbamylase (OTC), biotinidase, and carnitine and for some cases of methylmalonic acidemia and propionic or glutaric aciduria.

B. Reye-like syndrome is associated with acute or chronic liver failure. Causes include viral hepatitis, organic phosphate ingestion, mushroom poisoning, drugs (sedatives, tranquilizers, analgesics), malignancy, cirrhosis, congestive heart failure, and shock.

TABLE 1 Metabolic Disorders that Present with Reye-like Syndrome

Metabolic Acidosis with Hypoglycemia and Elevated Ammonia
Pyruvate carboxylase
Methylmalonic acidemia
Propionic acidemia
3-OH-3 methylglutaric aciduria
Carnitine deficiency
2-methyl-3-OH-butyric aciduria
Glutaric acidemia II
β-Ketothiolase deficiency
Isovaleric acidemia
Medium-chain acyl CoA dehydrogenase deficiency

Metabolic Acidosis with Hypoglycemia and Normal Ammonia
Maple syrup urine disease
Glycogen storage I, III
Biotinidase deficiency
Glutaric acidemia I
Fructose 1-6-diphosphatase
Hereditary fructose intolerance

Metabolic Acidosis without Hypoglycemia
Periodic hyperlysinemia

Elevated Ammonia with neither Metabolic Acidosis nor Hyperglycemia
Ornithine transcarbamylase deficiency
CPS deficiency
Transient hyperammonemia of newborn
Lysinuric protein intolerance
Hyperammonemia, hyperornithinemia, homocitrullinuria syndrome
ASA Tyase deficiency
Citrullinemia

CPS, carbamyl phosphate synthetase; ASA, argininosuccinate.

C. Stage the patient according to the following criteria: stage 1, vomiting and lethargy but response to commands; stage 2, disorientation, confusion, or combativeness with purposeful motor responses and no abnormal posturing; stage 3, comatose (unresponsive to

(Continued on page 176)

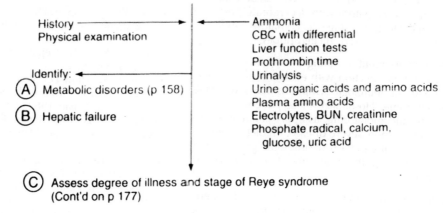

Patient with REYE-LIKE SYNDROME

History ——————————→ ←——— Ammonia
Physical examination   CBC with differential
                                        Liver function tests
                                        Prothrombin time
Identify: ◄————————————   Urinalysis
Ⓐ Metabolic disorders (p 158)   Urine organic acids and amino acids
                                        Plasma amino acids
Ⓑ Hepatic failure   Electrolytes, BUN, creatinine
                                        Phosphate radical, calcium,
                                            glucose, uric acid

Ⓒ Assess degree of illness and stage of Reye syndrome
   (Cont'd on p 177)

commands), periodic irregular breathing pattern, decorticate posturing, and doll's eyes (oculocephalic) reflexes; stage 4, comatose with decerebrate posturing and disconjugate gaze; stage 5, comatose, areflexia, flaccid paralysis, and fixed, dilated pupils.

D. Patients with frequent vomiting after varicella or an upper respiratory infection with evidence of liver dysfunction without neurologic symptoms may have stage 1 Reye syndrome. Hospitalize these patients for supportive care and monitoring, as approximately 5% to 10% progress to more severe disease. Predictors of progression are initial elevation of ammonia greater than 100 µg/dl and a prothrombin time 3 seconds longer than the control.

E. Oral lactulose treatment reduces high levels of ammonia that contribute to the encephalopathy. It acidifies the intestinal lumen, which facilitates the conversion of intestinal ammonia to ammonium ion that is excreted in the stool. Complications of treatment are osmotic diarrhea and electrolyte disturbances.

F. It is essential to monitor and manage increased intracranial pressure to maintain adequate cerebral perfusion. See page 100 for management guidelines.

References

Arrowsmith JB, Kennedy DL, Kuritsky JN, et al. National patterns of aspirin use and Reye syndrome reporting, United States, 1980 to 1985. Pediatrics 1987; 79:858.

Fraser CL, Arieff AI. Hepatic encephalopathy. N Engl J Med 1985; 313:865.

Frewen TC, Swedlow DB, Watcha M, et al. Outcome in severe Reye syndrome with early pentobarbital coma and hypothermia. J Pediatr 1982; 100:663.

Greene CL, Blitzer MG, Shapira E. Inborn errors of metabolism and Reye syndrome: Differential diagnosis. J Pediatr 1988; 113:156.

Heubi JE, Daugherty CC, Partin JS, et al. Grade I Reye's syndrome: Outcome and predictors of progression to deeper coma grades. N Engl J Med 1984; 311:1539.

Lichtenstein PK, Heubin JE, Daugherty CC, et al. Grade I Reye's syndrome — a frequent case of vomiting and liver dysfunction after varicella and upper respiratory-tract infection. N Engl J Med 1983; 309:133.

Rowe PC, Valle D, Brusilow SW. Inborn errors of metabolism in children referred with Reye's syndrome. JAMA 1988; 260:3167.

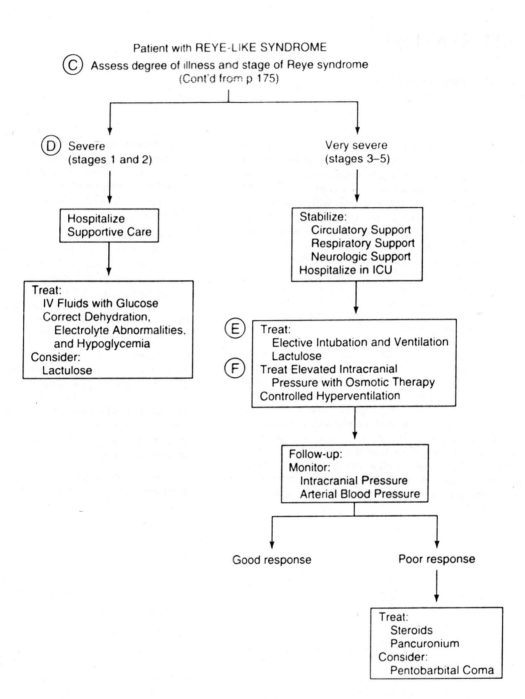

Patient with REYE-LIKE SYNDROME
Ⓒ Assess degree of illness and stage of Reye syndrome
(Cont'd from p 175)

Ⓓ Severe
(stages 1 and 2)

Very severe
(stages 3–5)

Hospitalize
Supportive Care

Stabilize:
  Circulatory Support
  Respiratory Support
  Neurologic Support
Hospitalize in ICU

Treat:
  IV Fluids with Glucose
  Correct Dehydration,
    Electrolyte Abnormalities,
    and Hypoglycemia
Consider:
  Lactulose

Ⓔ Treat:
  Elective Intubation and Ventilation
  Lactulose
Ⓕ Treat Elevated Intracranial
    Pressure with Osmotic Therapy
Controlled Hyperventilation

Follow-up:
Monitor:
  Intracranial Pressure
  Arterial Blood Pressure

Good response

Poor response

Treat:
  Steroids
  Pancuronium
Consider:
  Pentobarbital Coma

SHORT STATURE

Michael S. Kappy, M.D., Ph.D.
Carrie A. Ganong, M.D.

A. In the history ask about the heights of parents and siblings (familial short stature) and whether the mother had delayed menarche or father delayed puberty (late bloomer), usually associated with continued growth after high school (constitutional delay with short stature as an adolescent). Obtain an appropriate nutritional and psychosocial database. Identify predisposing conditions such as congenital infections, smallness for gestational age (SGA) at birth (primordial short stature), congenital syndromes, chronic illness involving major organ systems, especially the GI tract, cardiac, pulmonary, and/or renal systems, malnutrition, and medications, especially pharmacologic doses of glucocorticoids, e.g., in asthma.

B. In the physical examination accurately document the height, preferably using a stadiometer or a ruler attached to the wall so that the child is reliably vertical. The metal bar attached to the scale in most physicians' offices is not accurate or reproducible enough for evaluation and monitoring of a child with short stature. Calculate the weight to height ratio using a graph or by comparing the weight age with the height age (the ages for which the patient's measurements are the 50th percentile). Weight for height is usually normal in endocrine and metabolic disorders and reduced in malnutrition. Note any congenital abnormalities and/or dysmorphic appearance and assess the GI, cardiac, pulmonary, and renal systems. Note any goiter. Evaluate pubertal development and assess it according to age (see pp 170, 172). Assess dentition and state of nutrition.

C. Consider Turner syndrome in girls, recognizing that 60% of such patients do not have marked stigmata of the syndrome (webbed neck, wide-spaced nipples, wide carrying angle to the arms, etc.), especially girls with Turner mosaicism. After 9 to 10 years of age a random measurement of serum FSH and LH may signal ovarian failure (common in Turner syndrome); however, a karyotype is the definitive test.

D. Document the child's rate of growth over the longest period for which measurements are available. The lower limit of growth is approximately 4 cm/year for children 5 to 10 years old. The normal growth rate increases with age. Most standard pediatric texts have normal growth rate curves for comparison. A short child with a normal growth rate for age is unlikely to have significant illness or an endocrinopathy.

E. The bone age (single anteroposterior view of the left hand and wrist) is useful in correlating the degree of

(Continued on page 180)

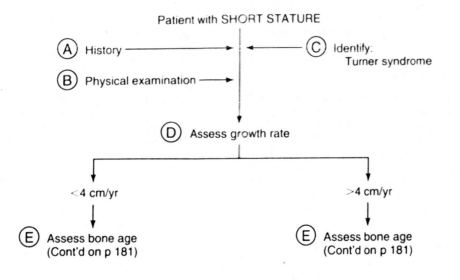

Patient with SHORT STATURE

(A) History ⟶
(B) Physical examination ⟶
(C) Identify:
    Turner syndrome

(D) Assess growth rate

<4 cm/yr
  (E) Assess bone age
  (Cont'd on p 181)

>4 cm/yr
  (E) Assess bone age
  (Cont'd on p 181)

physical maturation with chronologic age. It is usually delayed for chronologic age but normal for height age in constitutional delay of puberty. Other causes of delayed bone age include emotional deprivation, chronic illness, malnutrition, growth hormone (GH) deficiency, and thyroid hormone deficiency.

F. Rule out thyroid and/or GH deficiency in children with a significantly delayed bone age who are growing at a rate abnormal for age (> 2 standard deviations less than the mean for age). In primary hypothyroidism a low free T_4 or total T_4 is associated with elevated levels of thyroid stimulating hormone (TSH). Total or free T_4 may be normal in compensated hypothyroidism, but TSH is elevated. These children most likely have a thyroid disorder and should be treated with L-thyroxine 75 to 100 $\mu g/m^2$/day PO.

G. Children with familial short stature have a normal physical examination, normal (usually low-normal) growth rate for age, and bone age appropriate for chronologic age. Patients with primordial short stature were often SGA at birth or may have, in addition, a congenital syndrome (e.g., Russell-Silver syndrome).

H. In constitutional delay the child's tempo of physical maturation is slower than that of peers. The bone age is delayed for chronologic age but normal for height age. Pubertal maturation is appropriate for bone age. The ultimate height of these children is usually normal for their families since the pubertal growth spurt is not diminished but only delayed. In some boys for whom this delay causes undue psychological stress, a short course of low-dose, long-acting testosterone may be used. Testosterone depot 50 to 100 mg IM monthly for 4 to 6 months stimulates growth without unduly advancing the bone age. Although ultimate height is not increased by this treatment, the earlier growth spurt and appearance of secondary sexual characteristics make it a useful treatment option.

I. Rule out GH deficiency in children with normal thyroid function, delayed bone age, and an abnormal growth rate (usually < 4 cm/year).

J. Documentation of the extent of endogenous GH secretion is difficult. The standard provocative tests may yield normal results in children who are not growing well and who have low serum insulin-like growth factor-I (IGF-I) concentrations. Many of these children also respond well to a trial of GH therapy. Although such a trial has been advocated as a means of assessing or defining endogenous GH deficiency, many short normal children grow faster while on GH therapy. A concomitant increase in skeletal maturation also occurs, and therefore it is debatable whether this therapy actually adds inches to the child's ultimate height. Studies to answer this question are in progress. Treatment of GH deficiency in children is recombinant human growth hormone 0.3 mg/kg/week divided into 6 doses given subcutaneously.

K. A low T_4 not accompanied by an elevated TSH suggests thyroxine binding globulin deficiency, secondary (pituitary) disorders, or tertiary (hypothalamic) disorders. Refer patients with suspected pituitary or hypothalamic disorders for further evaluation.

References

Donaldson DL, Pan F, Hollowell JG, et al. Reliability of stimulated and spontaneous growth hormone (GH) levels for identifying the child with low GH secretion. J Clin Endocrinol Metab 1991; 72:647.

Frasier SD, Lippe BM. The rational use of growth hormone during childhood. J Clin Endocrinol Metab 1990; 71:269.

Moore KC, Donaldson DL, Ideus PL, et al. Clinical diagnoses of children with extremely short stature and their response to growth hormone. J Pediatr 1993; 122:687.

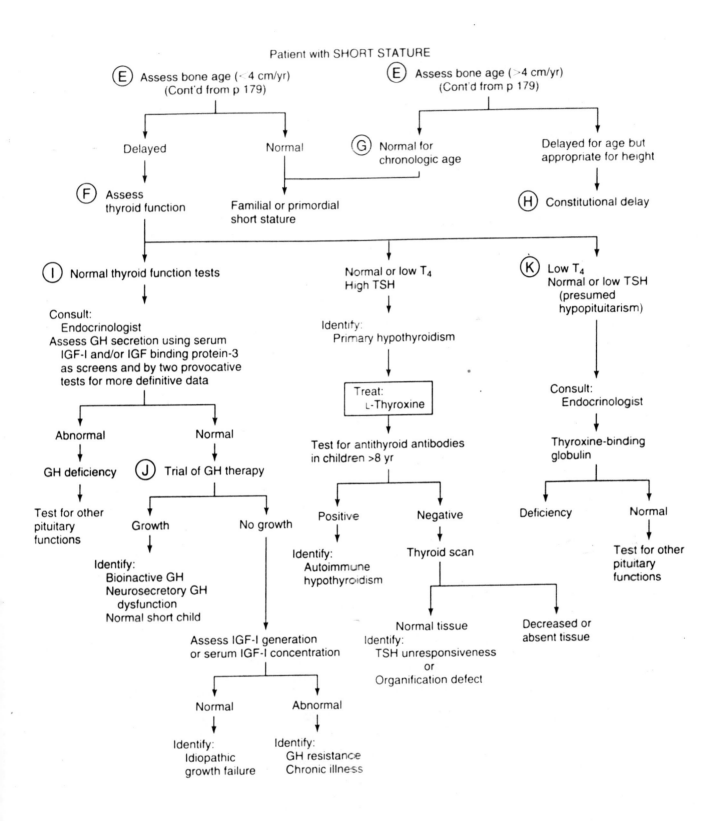

Patient with SHORT STATURE

Ⓔ Assess bone age (<4 cm/yr)
(Cont'd from p 179)

Ⓔ Assess bone age (>4 cm/yr)
(Cont'd from p 179)

Delayed

Normal

Ⓖ Normal for
chronologic age

Delayed for age but
appropriate for height

Ⓕ Assess
thyroid function

Familial or primordial
short stature

Ⓗ Constitutional delay

Ⓘ Normal thyroid function tests

Normal or low T_4
High TSH

Ⓚ Low T_4
Normal or low TSH
(presumed
hypopituitarism)

Consult:
Endocrinologist
Assess GH secretion using serum
IGF-I and/or IGF binding protein-3
as screens and by two provocative
tests for more definitive data

Identify:
Primary hypothyroidism

Consult:
Endocrinologist

Treat:
L-Thyroxine

Thyroxine-binding
globulin

Abnormal

Normal

Test for antithyroid antibodies
in children >8 yr

GH deficiency

Ⓙ Trial of GH therapy

Deficiency

Normal

Test for other
pituitary
functions

Growth

No growth

Positive

Negative

Identify:
Autoimmune
hypothyroidism

Thyroid scan

Test for other
pituitary
functions

Identify:
Bioinactive GH
Neurosecretory GH
dysfunction
Normal short child

Assess IGF-I generation
or serum IGF-I concentration

Normal tissue
Identify:
TSH unresponsiveness
or
Organification defect

Decreased or
absent tissue

Normal

Abnormal

Identify:
Idiopathic
growth failure

Identify:
GH resistance
Chronic illness

FEBRILE DISORDERS AND OTHER NONSPECIFIC PRESENTATIONS

ACUTE FEVER IN INFANTS LESS THAN 3 MONTHS OF AGE

Stephen Berman, M.D.

DEFINITIONS

Fever in early infancy is documentation of a rectal temperature of 38° C or more in an infant 1 to 12 weeks of age. **Fever without source** is an acute febrile illness in which a probable cause cannot be identified with a careful history and physical examination. **Serious bacterial infections (SBI)** include bacterial meningitis, bacteremia, bacterial pneumonia, urinary tract infections, bacterial enteritis, cellulitis, and bone and joint infections.

EPIDEMIOLOGY

Febrile illness during the first 3 months of life, though uncommon, is frequently serious. During the first 2 months of life 60% of febrile illnesses occur during the second month and 40% during the first month. Only 5% of febrile illnesses occur within the first 2 weeks of age. During the first 3 months of life bacterial infections account for approximately 20% of febrile illnesses, about half of these being serious. Among infants with fever without a source about 2.2% have bacteremia, 2.7% a urinary tract infection (UTI), 1.1% bacterial enteritis, and 1% bacterial meningitis. Viral infections can be identified in 40% of febrile illnesses occurring in young infants.

RISK FACTORS

Age: Bacteremia is more than twice as frequent in the first month of life (7.4%) as in the second month (3.1%). **Temperature:** For infants 4 to 8 weeks of age the frequency of SBI is 3.2% when the temperature is 38° to 38.9° C, 5.2% when 39° to 39.9° C, and 26% when over 40° C. **Prematurity:** The frequency of late onset group B *Streptococcus* (GBS) infection is higher in premature infants than full term infants.

ETIOLOGY

Bacterial pathogens responsible for meningitis and bacteremia are GBS, *Streptococcus pneumoniae*, *Escherichia coli*, *Haemophilus influenzae*, *Staphylococcus aureus*, group A streptococcus, enterococcus, *Listeria monocytogenes*, *Salmonella*, and *Shigella*. During the first month the most common pathogens are GBS and gram-negative enteric organisms; during the second month, *S. pneumoniae* and *H. influenzae*. Late-onset GBS infection can occur from 1 week to beyond 3 months of age. Serious GBS infections include sepsis (46%), meningitis (37%), UTI (7%), bone and joint infection (6%), pneumonia (4%), and cellulitis (4%). The most common viral pathogens are enteroviruses, which peak between July and September, and herpes simplex.

A. In the history ask about the following: onset, pattern, and degree of fever. Perinatal risk factors: prematurity, maternal fever, primary herpes infection, premature rupture of membranes, prolonged nursery stay with antibiotic treatment. Alterations in the mental status and normal level of activity: playfulness, irritability, feeding and sleeping patterns, responsiveness, seizures. Respiratory symptoms: cough, congestion, coryza, fast or difficult breathing, chest indrawing (retractions). Gastrointestinal symptoms: vomiting, diarrhea, abdominal distention, blood in stools.

B. On physical examination look, listen, and feel for findings that suggest the following: Meningitis: full fontanelle, too weak to feed, difficult to arouse, extremely irritable. It is difficult to evaluate infants who have not developed a social smile (4 to 6 weeks) or the ability to play or make eye contact. An infant smile is a useful negative predictor of meningitis. Perfusion: color and warmth of the extremities and capillary refill time (> 2 seconds is abnormal). Acute otitis media: tympanic membrane with decreased mobility, red/yellow color, bulging contour. Pneumonia: tachypnea, retractions, grunting, crackles. Soft-tissue cellulitis or abscess (especially omphalitis): swelling, erythema, induration, warmth of tissue. Bone or joint infection: painful swelling with limitation of motion. Enteroviral infection: rash, erythematous exanthem, hand, foot, and mouth lesions. *Neisseria meningitidis* bacteremia: petechiae, purpura.

C. The bacterial infections identified on physical examination and screening laboratory studies are acute otitis media (10%), pneumonia (7%), impetigo (4%), adenitis (2%), cellulitis (1%), omphalitis (1%), bacterial enteritis (bloody diarrhea) (1%), and septic arthritis/osteomyelitis (1%). The risk of an associated bacteremia is above 50% in infants with cellulitis, adenitis, or omphalitis. An associated bacteremia occurs in 10% to 30% of cases with bacterial enteritis and pneumonia. Some 10% of patients with UTI have bacteremia. Fewer than 5% of patients with acute otitis media have bacteremia or meningitis.

D. An infant older than 4 weeks whose degree of illness is assessed as mild or moderate can be managed as an outpatient. If blood and urine cultures have been obtained, there are two reasonable options: (1) treat with IM ceftriaxone or (2) observe closely and follow up without antibiotic therapy. Follow-up should be daily until culture results are available. Infants with pathogens isolated from blood should have a lumbar puncture and be admitted to the hospital for parenteral antibiotic therapy. Infants with pathogens isolated from urine can be treated with outpatient oral antibiotics if they are afebrile and appear well; if not, admission for parenteral antibiotics is appropriate.

(Continued on page 186)

Infant Under 3 Months of Age with ACUTE FEVER WITHOUT A SOURCE

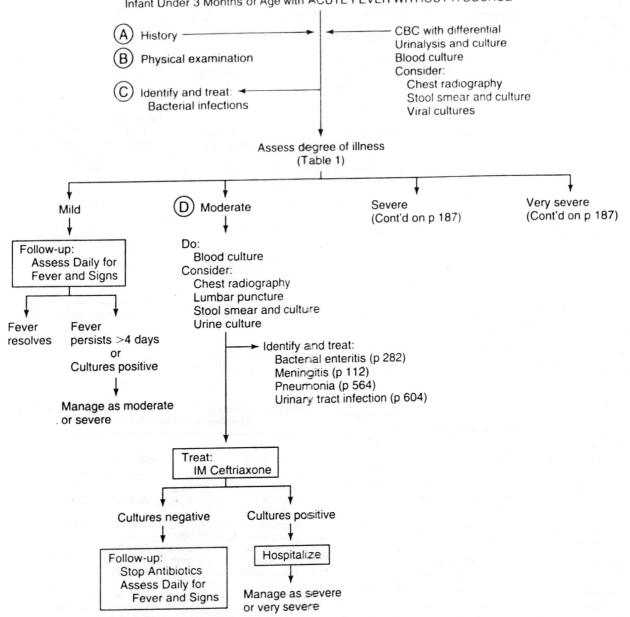

(A) History

(B) Physical examination

(C) Identify and treat:
Bacterial infections

CBC with differential
Urinalysis and culture
Blood culture
Consider:
Chest radiography
Stool smear and culture
Viral cultures

Assess degree of illness
(Table 1)

Mild

(D) Moderate

Severe
(Cont'd on p 187)

Very severe
(Cont'd on p 187)

Follow-up:
Assess Daily for
Fever and Signs

Fever
resolves

Fever
persists >4 days
or
Cultures positive

Manage as moderate
or severe

Do:
Blood culture
Consider:
Chest radiography
Lumbar puncture
Stool smear and culture
Urine culture

Identify and treat:
Bacterial enteritis (p 282)
Meningitis (p 112)
Pneumonia (p 564)
Urinary tract infection (p 604)

Treat:
IM Ceftriaxone

Cultures negative

Cultures positive

Follow-up:
Stop Antibiotics
Assess Daily for
Fever and Signs

Hospitalize

Manage as severe
or very severe

TABLE 1 Degree of Illness

Mild/Moderate	Severe	Very Severe
A. All infants age ≥ 4 weeks with temp. < 38.9° C without cardiopulmonary disease or a complicated nursery stay **and** B. Have reliable caretaker	A. Infants age < 4 weeks* **or** Infants with temp. > 38.9° C **or** Infants having cardiopulmonary disease or a complicated nursery stay regardless of degree of fever **or** B. Lack of a reliable caretaker **or**	
and Mental status: smiles and not irritable, alerts quickly, feeds well **and** No signs of dehydration and good peripheral perfusion: pink warm extremities **and** No signs of respiratory distress **and** Absolute band count < 1500/L, WBC 5000–15,000 **and** When diarrhea is present, < 5 WBC/high-power field in stool and no blood in stool	Mental status: irritable but consolable, poor eye contact (lethargic), feeds poorly **or** Signs of dehydration or poor perfusion: mottled, cool extremities **or** Respiratory rate > 60, retractions, grunting **or** Absolute band count ≥ 1500/L, WBC < 5000 or > 15,000 **or** When diarrhea is present, ≥ 5 WBC high-power field in stool or blood in stools	Mental status: irritable and not consolable, unresponsive, too weak to feed, or seizures **or** Shock, pale with thready pulse **or** Apnea, cyanosis, respiratory failure

*All febrile infants less than 4 weeks of age should be hospitalized and treated pending culture results because of the lack of data correlating clinical assessment with outcome.
Estimation of clinical usefulness of assessment criteria to identify cases with SBIs.
Sensitivity (proportion of SBI cases that will be classified as severe or very severe), 97% to 99%.
Positive predictive value (proportion of cases classified as severe or very severe with an SBI), 11.5% (range 5.9% to 24%).
Negative predictive value (proportion of cases classified as mild/moderate with no SBI), 97.3% (range 94.6% to 100%).

E. Perform a lumbar puncture as part of a work-up to diagnose meningitis in infants who are admitted, regardless of appearance. CSF pleocytosis is present when the total white blood cell count is above 10/ml. Most cases of meningitis are viral. Enteroviral meningitis occurs in 10% to 30% of febrile infants. Herpes simplex infection also produces an abnormal spinal fluid. The overall frequency of meningitis may be 10% to 14% of infants with temperatures higher than 38.9° C. Consider obtaining herpes cultures on nasal, rectal, and conjunctival swabs and rapid herpes diagnostic tests (PCR) on CSF.

F. Treat admitted patients with intravenous antibiotics (Table 2) pending culture results at 48 hours. In the first 2 weeks of age use ampicillin and gentamicin; from 2 to 8 weeks of age use ampicillin and cefotaxime or ceftriaxone. Ampicillin is recommended to cover Listeria and enterococcus. Substitute nafcillin or another semisynthetic penicillin for ampicillin if an infection with S. aureus is suspected because of bullous skin lesions or a nursery outbreak. Enterococcus infections often require IV treatment with both ampicillin and gentamicin for 10 days. IV antibiotics for Group B streptococcus and S. pneumoniae bacteremia can be continued for 7 to 10 days. Consider acyclovir therapy when herpes simplex infection is suspected because of skin lesions or seizures and in any infant assessed as very severe. Ceftriaxone should be used with caution in infants with hyperbilirubinemia.

References

Baraff LJ, Bass JW, Fleisher GR, et al. Practice guideline for the management of infants and children 0 to 36 months of age with fever without source. Pediatrics 1993; 92:1.

TABLE 2 Therapy for Presumed Bacteremia or Herpes Simplex in Early Infancy

Antibiotic	Dose	Product Availability
Inpatient		
Acyclovir (Zovirax)	10 mg/kg/dose q8h	500 mg
Ampicillin sodium	50 mg/kg/dose IV q6h	0.25, 0.5, 1, 2, 4 g
Cefotaxime (Claforan)	50 mg/kg/dose IV q8h (bacteremia), q6h (meningitis)	0.5, 1, 2 g
Ceftriaxone (Rocephin)		0.25, 0.5, 1 g
Gentamicin	75 mg/kg/dose IV q24h (bacteremia), 50 mg/kg/dose IV q12h (meningitis)	20, 80 mg
Nafcillin	2.5 mg/kg/dose IV q8h (neonates q12h)	250 mg
Outpatient Ceftriaxone (Rocephin)	25–50 mg/kg/dose IV q6h 50–75 mg/kg/dose IM q24h	0.25, 0.5, 1 g

Baskin M, O'Rourke E, Fleisher G. Outpatient treatment of febrile infants 28 to 89 days of age with intramuscular administration of ceftriaxone. J Pediatr 1992; 120:22.

Bonadio WA. Keeping febrile young infants out of the hospital. Contemp Pediatr 1994; 11:73.

Bonadio WA, Romine K, Gyuro J. Relationship of fever magnitude to rate of serous bacterial infections in neonates. J Pediatr 1990; 116:733.

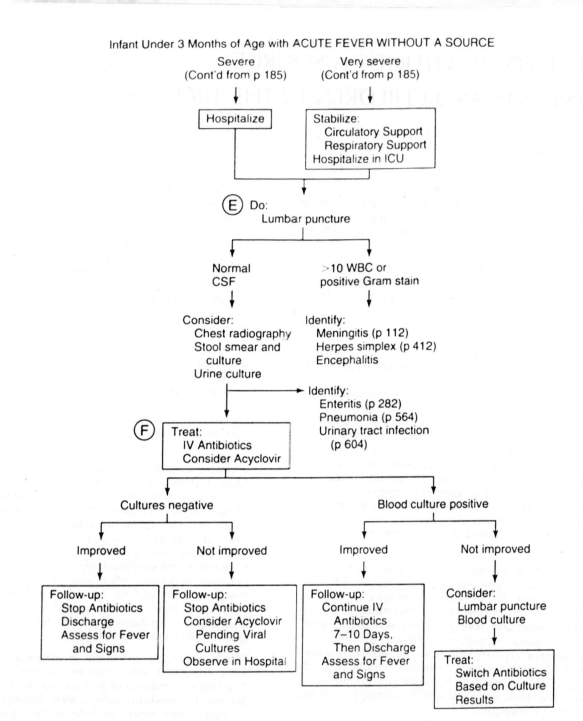

Bonadio WA, Smith D, Melzer M, et al. Reliability of observation variables in distinguishing infectious outcome of febrile young infants. Pediatr Infect Dis J 1993; 12:111.

Bonadio WA, Webster H, Wolfe A, et al. Correlating infectious outcome with clinical parameters of 1130 consecutive febrile infants aged 0–8 weeks. Pediatr Emerg Care 1993; 9:84.

Bramson RT, Meyer TL, Silbiger ML, et al. The futility of the chest radiograph in the febrile infant without respiratory symptoms. Pediatrics 1993; 92:524.

Crain EF, Gershel SC. Which febrile infants younger than 2 weeks of age are likely to have sepsis? A pilot study. Pediatr Infect Dis J 1988; 7:561.

DeAngelis C, Joffe A, Wilson M, et al. Iatrogenic risks and financial costs of hospitalizing febrile infants. Am J Dis Child 1983; 137:1146.

Hoberman A, Chao H-P, Keller DM, et al. Prevalence of urinary tract infection in febrile infants. J Pediatr 1993; 123:17.

Jaskiewicz JA, McCarthy CA, Richardson AC, et al. Febrile infants at low risk for serious bacterial infection: An appraisal of the rochester criteria and implications for management. Pediatrics 1994; 94:390.

McCarthy J, Powell K, Jaskiewicz J, et al. Outpatient management of selected infants younger than 2 months of age evaluated for possible sepsis. Pediatr Infect Dis J 1990; 9:385.

McCarthy PL. The febrile infant (commentary). Pediatrics 1994; 94:397.

Yagupsky P, Menegus MA, Powell KR. The changing spectrum of Group B streptococcal disease in infants: An 11-year experience in a tertiary care hospital. Pediatr Infect Dis J 1991; 10:801.

ACUTE FEVER WITHOUT A SOURCE IN INFANTS AND CHILDREN IN THE TROPICS

Stephen Berman, M.D.

The approach to the evaluation of a child who has recently visited or lives in a tropical developing country should be broadened to consider malaria, typhoid fever, rickettsial infections, and arthropod-borne viral and bacterial infections.

A. In the history ask about the following: onset, pattern, and degree of the fever. Relapsing fever suggests dengue fever, borreliosis, or brucellosis. Risk factors: travel within the past 12 months to an area with endemic malaria, use of chemoprophylaxis and other precautions (mosquito repellents, netting, and protective clothes) during travel to malarious areas, exposure to field rodents or rats, ingestion of unpasteurized milk products, underlying conditions such as severe malnutrition; cardiopulmonary, gastrointestinal, renal disease; sickle cell disease; and other conditions and therapy that compromise immunity, especially HIV infection. Alterations in the mental status and normal level of activity: playfulness, weakness, irritability, feeding and sleeping patterns, responsiveness, seizures. Respiratory symptoms: cough, congestion, coryza, sore throat, earache, fast or difficult breathing, chest indrawing (retractions). GI symptoms: nausea, vomiting, diarrhea, abdominal pain, blood in stools. Renal symptoms: dark urine, decreased urinary frequency, flank pain, lower abdominal pain.

B. On physical examination look, listen, and feel for findings that suggest multiorgan involvement. CNS: too weak to feed, difficult to arouse, unresponsive, seizures or coma with decerebrate or decorticate posturing. Dehydration and poor perfusion: skin turgor, tears, moist mucous membranes, color and warmth of the extremities, capillary refill time (>2 seconds is abnormal). Respiratory system: tachypnea, retractions, grunting, crackles. GI system: hepatomegaly, splenomegaly, jaundice. Musculoskeletal system: arthralgias, arthritis, weakness, myalgias.

C. All children suspected of having malaria require thick and thin smears of peripheral blood. Serial samples at 6 to 12 hour intervals for 48 hours may be necessary. The thick smear provides a screening test, and the thin smear is better for species identification. Low-grade parasitemia related to partial immunity or treatment can result in a negative smear. Even patients with cerebral malaria can have a negative smear at presentation. Therefore, when the clinical history and presentation suggest malaria, treatment should be initiated regardless of the identification of parasites on the smears. In Nigeria 67% of infants less than 12 months of age with acute fever without a source have malaria.

D. Dengue fever is a febrile episode often associated with a rash caused by an arbovirus, usually acquired by the daytime bite of the *Aedes aegypti* mosquito. The episode may also be associated with severe headache, arthralgias, and myalgias. It may progress to hemorrhage or shock. It is endemic to the Caribbean, South Pacific, Asia, Mexico, Latin America, and Africa.

E. Always consider bacteremia in a febrile child who appears moderately or severely ill. Severely malnourished children and those with a condition that impairs immunity are at high risk for bacteremia. The frequency of bacteremia in children with acute fever without a source living in Nigeria varied from 18.5% during the first year of life to 7% in 4 and 5 year old children. The height of the fever does not correlate with the risk of bacteremia, and combined infections with malaria are common. In Nigeria 86% of children with bacteremia have concurrent malaria. Severely malnourished children have high rates of coagulase-negative and coagulase-positive staphylococcal bacteremia as well as gram-negative enteric infections.

F. Febrile agglutinins are useful in diagnosing typhoid fever. Compared with culture results, titers of at least 1 : 40 have a sensitivity of 89% and specificity of 89%. The negative predictive value is 99%. Therefore, while a negative titer almost excludes typhoid fever, only about 50% of cases with a positive titer have typhoid fever.

(Continued on page 190)

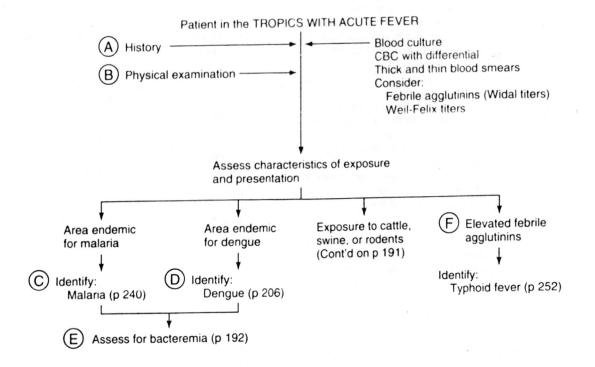

Patient in the TROPICS WITH ACUTE FEVER

(A) History ⟶ ← — Blood culture
CBC with differential
Thick and thin blood smears
Consider:
    Febrile agglutinins (Widal titers)
    Weil-Felix titers

(B) Physical examination ⟶

Assess characteristics of exposure
and presentation

| Area endemic for malaria | Area endemic for dengue | Exposure to cattle, swine, or rodents (Cont'd on p 191) | (F) Elevated febrile agglutinins |

(C) Identify:
Malaria (p 240)

(D) Identify:
Dengue (p 206)

Identify:
Typhoid fever (p 252)

(E) Assess for bacteremia (p 192)

G. Scrub typhus *(Rickettsia tsutsugamushi)*, usually acquired in a rural setting by a mite bite from an infected field rodent, begins with fever and hepatosplenomegaly. Pneumonia and meningitis can develop. Murine typhus *(Rickettsia typhi)*, an urban disease that fleas carry from infected rats, causes a skin rash and hepatomegaly. Diagnosis is suggested by a rise in the Weil-Felix agglutinins. A Weil-Felix titer of at least 1:320 for both *Proteus* OX-K and OX-19 antigens will identify about half of these infections. Since leptospirosis and other infections can cross-react with these antigens, confirmation by specific immunologic tests is needed. Treatment of typhus is with chloramphenicol or doxycycline. In Thailand about 9% of cases with acute fever without a source presenting to a rural hospital have a typhus infection.

H. Leptospirosis, a spirochetal infection transmitted from cattle, swine, or rodents, is a biphasic fever and can involve the CNS (headache, focal signs, meningitis), kidney (hematuria, renal failure), liver (jaundice, hepatomegaly, cholecystitis), and eyes (conjunctivitis), and it can cause a variety of rashes (petechiae, ecchymoses, erythema nodosum, vasculitis). Diagnostic tests include leptospiral agglutinins. Treatment is IV aqueous penicillin G 150,000/U/kg/day in 4 to 6 divided doses for 7 to 10 days. Doxycycline is an alternative for mild cases.

I. Borreliosis, or relapsing fever, a spirochetal infection transmitted by lice and ticks from infected rodents or humans, causes fever, rash, headache, and myalgia associated with hepatosplenomegaly. The initial febrile episode, which lasts 3 to 6 days, is followed by a week without fever and a relapse. Weil-Felix titers may be elevated. Spirochetes may be visible on thick smears or buffy-coat preparations. Treat with penicillin, erythromycin, or choramphenicol. Patients should be monitored closely for a Jarisch-Herxheimer reaction after the initial dose.

J. Brucellosis, an infection with *Brucella* (gram-negative coccobacilli) transmitted from direct contact with infected animals or ingestion of infected unpasteurized milk products causes fever, malaise, myalgias, and arthralgias. Diagnosis is made with blood cultures. Consider treatment with TMP-SMX plus rifampin for children or tetracycline (doxycycline) for older patients. Aminoglycosides may be added in more severe cases.

K. Other arbovirus infections include sandfly fever virus, equine encephalitis, Mayaro virus, Ross river virus, yellow fever, West Nile virus, Colorado tick fever, and tick-borne encephalitis.

References

Akpede GO, Abiodun PO, Sykes RM. Acute fevers of unknown origin in young children in the tropics. J Pediatr 1993; 122:79.

Christie CDC, Heinkens GT, Galden MHN. Coagulase-negative staphylococcal bacteremia in severely malnourished Jamaican children. Pediatr Infect Dis J 1992; 11:1030.

Khuri-Bulos NA, Doud AF, Azab SM. Treatment of childhood brucellosis: Results of a prospective trial on 113 children. Pediatr Infect Dis J 1993; 12:377.

Silpapojakul K, Chupupakarn S, Yuthasompob S, et al. Scrub and murine typhus in children with obscure fever in the tropics. Pediatr Infect Dis J 1991; 10:200.

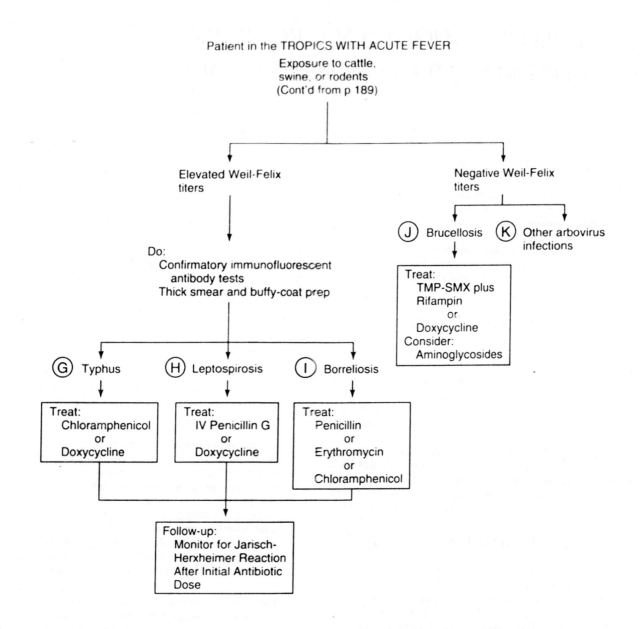

Patient in the TROPICS WITH ACUTE FEVER
Exposure to cattle,
swine, or rodents
(Cont'd from p 189)

Elevated Weil-Felix titers

Negative Weil-Felix titers

(J) Brucellosis   (K) Other arbovirus infections

Treat:
    TMP-SMX plus
    Rifampin
        or
    Doxycycline
Consider:
    Aminoglycosides

Do:
    Confirmatory immunofluorescent
    antibody tests
    Thick smear and buffy-coat prep

(G) Typhus   (H) Leptospirosis   (I) Borreliosis

Treat:
    Chloramphenicol
        or
    Doxycycline

Treat:
    IV Penicillin G
        or
    Doxycycline

Treat:
    Penicillin
        or
    Erythromycin
        or
    Chloramphenicol

Follow-up:
    Monitor for Jarisch-
    Herxheimer Reaction
    After Initial Antibiotic
    Dose

ACUTE FEVER WITHOUT A SOURCE IN INFANTS AND CHILDREN 3 TO 36 MONTHS OF AGE

Stephen Berman, M.D.

DEFINITIONS

Fever is documentation of a rectal temperature of at least 38° C (100.4° F) in an infant or child 3 to 36 months of age. **Fever without source** is an acute febrile illness in which no probable cause can be identified with a careful history and physical examination. **Serious bacterial infections** (SBI) include bacterial meningitis, bacteremia, bacterial pneumonia, urinary tract infections, bacterial enteritis, cellulitis, and bone and joint infections.

COMPLICATIONS OF BACTEREMIA

Complications of occult bacteremia include delayed-onset meningitis, periorbital or buccal cellulitis, pneumonia, epiglottitis, septic arthritis, osteomyelitis, and pericarditis. Untreated bacteremic children have a higher risk of persistent bacteremia (21%) and meningitis (7%) than treated children (persistent bacteremia 4% and meningitis 4.5%). Delayed-onset meningitis is more likely with *Neisseria meningitidis* (30% to 56%) and *Haemophilus influenzae* type B (27%) than with *Streptococcus pneumoniae* (6%). The overall probabilities of delayed-onset meningitis in a child who has fever without a source and does not receive antibiotic treatment are 0.21% for *S. pneumoniae* and 0.06% for *H. influenzae*.

EPIDEMIOLOGY

Fever in early childhood (3 to 24 months) is common, accounting for 26% of sick visits to pediatricians and 55% of sick visits to hospital pediatric clinics. Approximately 25% of febrile sick visits are associated with temperatures of 39° C (102° F) or higher. The clinician cannot identify a focus of bacterial or viral infection (excluding a mild upper respiratory tract infection) in 15% to 30% of these cases. The incidence of occult bacteremia in patients without obvious focus of infection varies with age and degree of fever.

RISK FACTORS

Rates are higher in 6 to 24 month old patients (4% to 11%) than in 2 to 5 month old (1% to 2%) and older patients (3%). The risk of occult bacteremia with a temperature below 39° C is 0.3%; with temperature 39° C to 40.4° C (104.7° F), 4%; with temperature 40.5° C, (104.9° F) to 41° C (105.8° F), 13%, and with temperature over 41° C, 23%.

ETIOLOGY

Occult bacteremia is usually caused by *S. pneumoniae* (85%), *H. influenzae* type B (10%) (uncommon in immunized populations), or *N. meningitidis* (3%). Less frequently *Salmonella, Staphylococcus aureus*, gram-negative enteric organisms, *Streptococcus pyogenes*, and *Neisseria gonorrhoeae* cause occult bacteremia. Causes of bacterial enteritis include *Salmonella, Campylobacter, Shigella, Yersinia*, and invasive or toxigenic strains of *Escherichia coli*.

A. In the history ask about the onset, pattern, and degree of the fever. Evaluate the family's ability to care for the child at home and their access to transportation and a telephone. Risk factors include immunization status, current medications, allergies, underlying conditions such as cardiopulmonary, GI, or renal disease, sickle cell disease, central venous catheter and other indwelling lines, and conditions and therapy that compromise immunity, especially HIV infection. Assess alterations in the mental status and normal level of activity: playfulness, irritability, feeding and sleeping patterns, responsiveness, and seizures. Note any respiratory symptoms: cough, congestion, coryza, sore throat, earache, fast or difficult breathing, or chest indrawing (retractions). Check for GI symptoms: vomiting, diarrhea, abdominal distention, abdominal pain, or blood in stools. Assess renal symptoms: pain with urination (dysuria), urinary frequency, flank pain, or lower abdominal pain.

B. On physical examination look, listen, and feel for findings that suggest the following: Meningitis: full fontanelle, too weak to feed, difficult to arouse, unresponsive, extreme or paradoxic irritability, nuchal rigidity, Brudzinski and Kernig signs. An infant smile is a useful negative predictor of meningitis. Dehydration and poor perfusion: skin turgor, tears, moist mucous membranes, color and warmth of the extremities and capillary refill time (>2 seconds is abnormal). Acute otitis media: tympanic membrane with decreased mobility, red or yellow color, bulging contour. Pneumonia: tachypnea, retractions, grunting, crackles. Adenitis, soft-tissue cellulitis or abscess: swelling, erythema, induration, warmth of tissue. Bone or joint infection: painful swelling with limitation of motion. Enteroviral infection: rash; erythematous exanthem; hand, foot,

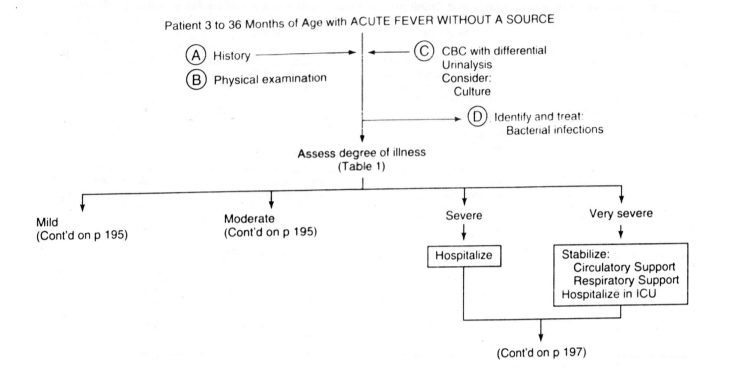

Patient 3 to 36 Months of Age with ACUTE FEVER WITHOUT A SOURCE

(A) History

(B) Physical examination

(C) CBC with differential
Urinalysis
Consider:
Culture

(D) Identify and treat:
Bacterial infections

Assess degree of illness
(Table 1)

Mild
(Cont'd on p 195)

Moderate
(Cont'd on p 195)

Severe

Very severe

Hospitalize

Stabilize:
Circulatory Support
Respiratory Support
Hospitalize in ICU

(Cont'd on p 197)

and mouth lesions. *N. meningitidis* bacteremia: pete-chiae, purpura.

C. Obtain a specimen from a catheter for a urinalysis and urine culture. Approximately 7% of boys 6 months or younger and 8% of girls younger than 1 year with fever without a source have a urinary tract infection (UTI). A leukocyte count of at least $10/mm^3$ and Gram stain of urine sediment are the most accurate screens for UTI. Since the sensitivity of a urinalysis or urine reagent strip test to identify an infection is only 80%, a culture should

always be done. A bacterial colony count of at least 50,000/ml appears to correlate best with a clinical infection.

D. Bacterial infections identified or suspected on history and physical examination are acute otitis media, pneumonia, impetigo, adenitis, sinusitis, cellulitis, bacterial enteritis (bloody diarrhea), and septic arthritis or osteomyelitis. Since approximately 13% of patients with acute otitis media also have bacteremia, these patients should be assessed independently of acute otitis.

TABLE 1   Degree of Illness in Infants and Children 3 to 6 Months of Age with Acute Fever without a Source

Mild	Moderate	Severe	Very Severe
All previously well infants and children with temperature <38.9° C	All infants and children with chronic illness regardless of temperature and all patients with temperature >38.9° C	All infants and children with a condition that compromises immunity	All infants and children with petechiae, purpura
and	or		
Who have a reliable caretaker	Who lack a reliable caretaker		
	or	or	or
and			
Mental status: smiles, playful, not irritable, alerts quickly, feeds well, cries strongly but is easily consoled by a caregiver	Mental status: brief smiles, irritable with crying and sobbing, still responsive to the caregiver and consolable, less playful and active than baseline	Mental status: irritable and not easily consolable, poor eye contact (lethargic), feeds poorly	Mental status: unresponsive, too weak to feed, seizures, or signs of meningeal irritation
and	or	or	
No signs of dehydration	Signs of mild or moderate dehydration	Signs of severe dehydration	
and	and	or	or
Good peripheral perfusion: pink, warm extremities	Good peripheral perfusion: pink, warm extremities	Poor perfusion: mottled, cool extremities	Shock, pale, with thready pulse
and	and	or	or
No signs of respiratory distress	No signs of respiratory distress	Respiratory rate >60, retractions, grunting	Apnea, cyanosis, respiratory failure

Estimation of clinical usefulness of assessment criteria to identify cases with serious bacterial infections:
Sensitivity (proportion of SBI cases that will be classified as severe or very severe), 44% to 74%.
Positive predictive value (proportion of cases classified as severe or very severe that will have a SBI), 33%.
Negative predictive value (proportion of cases classified as mild or moderate who will not have an SBI), 75%.

E. The CBC with differential can be used to screen moderately ill patients for occult bacteremia. Abnormal findings include an absolute band count greater than 500 and a WBC above 15,000 or below 5000. The risk of occult bacteremia is low in moderately ill patients with normal CBC. The risk of occult bacteremia or another occult bacterial focus of infection is 28% in patients who appear moderately ill with an abnormal CBC. The rate of bacteremia in patients with a WBC above 15,000 is 13%, compared with 2.6% in patients with a WBC between 5000 and 15,000.

F. Perform a lumbar puncture to diagnose meningitis in infants and children who are severely or very severely ill. Consider it in selected moderately ill patients who will be treated as outpatients. CSF pleocytosis is present when the total WBC is above 10/mm³. The most sensitive indicator of bacterial meningitis is the CSF Gram stain. The likelihood of isolating a bacterial pathogen from CSF is 1% or less when the Gram stain is negative and the cell count and chemistries are normal. Most meningitis is viral. Do not routinely obtain chest radiographs of children who have no signs of respiratory illness, as the likelihood of identifying an infiltrate is less than 1%. Obtain stool cultures when diarrhea with signs of invasive bacterial disease such as blood or five or more WBCs/high-power field are present. Consider empiric antibiotic treatment pending confirmation by stool culture.

G. Treat moderately ill patients without a source of infection with oral amoxicillin, IM ceftriaxone, or IM procaine penicillin. While studies suggest that parenteral, antibiotics are more effective than oral antibiotics in preventing delayed onset meningitis in bacteremic infants and children, the difference is attributed to infections with H. influenzae. Since immunization with H. influenzae type B vaccine has greatly reduced the frequency of these infections, oral antibiotics may adequately treat sensitive S. pneumoniae infections.

H. When a bacterial pathogen is isolated from the blood culture in a febrile patient managed as an outpatient, reassess the clinical status. All patients who remain febrile or who would continue to be assessed as moderately or severely ill should have a lumbar puncture and repeat blood culture and be admitted for IV antibiotics. Because of the increased risk of continuing invasive disease, consider doing a repeat blood culture and lumbar puncture and admitting children who are afebrile and appear well but who have N. meningitidis or H. influenzae isolated from blood. Treat afebrile patients assessed as mild in whom sensitive S. pneumoniae has been isolated with a second day of IM ceftriaxone and 10 days of oral therapy with amoxicillin or penicillin. Admit children with resistant or relatively resistant strains of S. pneumoniae for appropriate parenteral therapy. When only a urine culture is positive and the

(Continued on page 196)

Patient 3 to 36 Months of Age with ACUTE FEVER WITHOUT A SOURCE

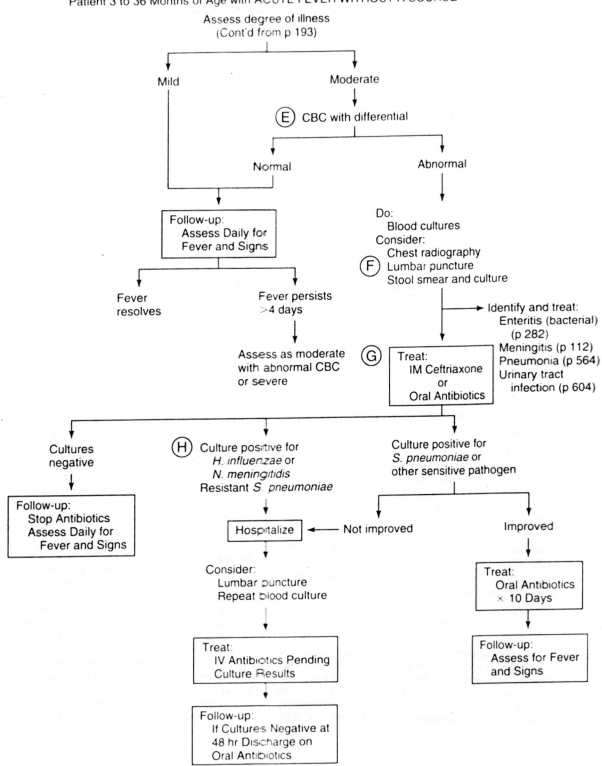

Assess degree of illness
(Cont'd from p 193)

Mild

Moderate

(E) CBC with differential

Normal

Abnormal

Follow-up:
  Assess Daily for
  Fever and Signs

Do:
  Blood cultures
Consider:
  Chest radiography
(F) Lumbar puncture
  Stool smear and culture

Fever
resolves

Fever persists
>4 days

Identify and treat:
  Enteritis (bacterial)
    (p 282)
  Meningitis (p 112)
  Pneumonia (p 564)
  Urinary tract
    infection (p 604)

Assess as moderate
with abnormal CBC
or severe

(G) Treat:
    IM Ceftriaxone
      or
    Oral Antibiotics

Cultures
negative

(H) Culture positive for
  H. influenzae or
  N. meningitidis
  Resistant S. pneumoniae

Culture positive for
S. pneumoniae or
other sensitive pathogen

Follow-up:
  Stop Antibiotics
  Assess Daily for
  Fever and Signs

Hospitalize ◄── Not improved

Improved

Consider:
  Lumbar puncture
  Repeat blood culture

Treat:
  Oral Antibiotics
  × 10 Days

Treat:
  IV Antibiotics Pending
  Culture Results

Follow-up:
  Assess for Fever
  and Signs

Follow-up:
  If Cultures Negative at
  48 hr Discharge on
  Oral Antibiotics

195

TABLE 2 Outpatient and Inpatient Antibiotics for the Treatment of Moderately to Severely Ill Children with Bacteremia

Antibiotic	Dose	Product Availability
Outpatient Antibiotics		
Erythromycin/sulfisoxazole (Pediazole)	10 mg E/kg/dose q.i.d.	Liquid: 200 mg (E) + 600 mg (S)/5 ml
Amoxicillin/clavulanate (Augmentin)	10–15 mg/kg/dose t.i.d.	Liquid: 125, 250 mg/5 ml
		Chewable: 125, 250 mg
		Tabs: 250, 500 mg
Amoxicillin	20–25 mg/kg/dose t.i.d.	Liquid: 125, 250 mg/5 ml
		Chewable: 125, 250 mg
		Caps: 250, 500 mg
Intramuscular Antibiotics		
Ceftriaxone (Rocephin)	50 mg/kg/dose q12–24h	Vials: 0.25, 0.5, 1 g
Penicillin G procaine	25,000 U/kg/dose q12–24h	Tubex: 600,000, 900,000, 1.2 million U
Initial Intravenous Antibiotics		
Cefotaxime (Claforan)	50–75 mg/kg/dose q6–8h	Vials: 0.5, 1, 2 g
Cefuroxime (Kefurox, Zinacef)	25–50 mg/kg/dose q8h	Vials: 0.75, 2.5 g
Ceftriaxone (Rocephin)	75 mg/kg/dose q24h	Vials: 0.25, 0.5, 1 g
Clindamycin (Cleocin)	8–13 mg/kg/dose q8h	Vials: 2, 4, 6 ml (150 mg/ml)
Ampicillin sodium	50–75 mg/kg/dose q6h	Vials: 0.25, 0.5, 1, 2, 4 g
Vancomycin (Vancocin)	10–15 mg/kg/dose q8h	Vials: 500, 1000 mg
		Caps: 125, 250 mg

TMP-SMX, trimethoprim-sulfamethoxazole; T, trimethoprim component; E, erythromycin component in Pediazole; S, sulfisoxazole component in Pediazole.

patient is assessed as improved (well or mild illness), continue outpatient treatment with oral antibiotics. If the patient does not improve, consider admission for parenteral therapy.

I. Treat admitted patients assessed as severely ill with an IV cephalosporin antibiotic (Table 2) pending culture results at 48 hours. Treat patients assessed as very severe with vancomycin and a cephalosporin such as cefotaxime to provide additional coverage for *S. aureus* and resistant *S. pneumoniae*. Clindamycin should be considered if anaerobes or *S. aureus* is suspected. In a hospitalized child with a suspected nosocomial bacteremia, add an aminoglycoside to cover *Enterobacter* and other gram-negative enterics that are resistant to third-generation cephalosporins.

References

Baraff LJ, Bass JW, Fleisher GR, et al. Practice guideline for the management of infants and children 0 to 36 months of age with fever without source. Pediatrics 1993; 92:1.

Baraff LJ, Oslund S, Prather M. Effect of antibiotic therapy and etiologic microorganism on the risk of bacterial meningitis in children with occult bacteremia. Pediatrics 1993; 92:140.

Baron MA, Fink HD, Cicchetti DV. Blood cultures in private pediatric practice: An 11 year experience. Pediatr Infect Dis J 1989; 8:2.

Fleisher GR, Rosenberg N, Vinci R, et al. Intramuscular versus oral antibiotic therapy for the prevention of meningitis and other bacterial sequelae in young febrile children at risk for occult bacteremia. J Pediatr 1994; 124:504.

Forman PM, Murphy TV. Reevaluation of the ambulatory pediatric patient whose blood culture is positive for *Haemophilus influenzae* type b. J Pediatr 1991; 118:503.

Haberman A, Wald ER, Reynolds EA, et al. Pyuria and bacteriuria in urine specimens obtained by catheter from young children with fever. J Pediatr 1994; 124:513.

Harper MB, Bachur R, Fleisher GR. Effect of antibiotic therapy on the outcome of outpatients with unsuspected bacteremia. Pediatr Infect Dis J 1995; 14:760.

Kramer MS, Lane DA, Mills EL. Should blood cultures be obtained in the evaluation of young febrile children without evident focus of bacterial infection? A decision analysis of diagnostic management strategies. Pediatrics 1989; 84:18.

Long S. Antibiotic therapy in febrile children: "Best-laid schemes . . ." J Pediatr 1994; 124:585.

Woods ER, Merola JL, Bithoney WG, et al. Bacteremia in an ambulatory setting: Improved outcome in children treated with antibiotics. Am J Dis Child 1990; 144:1195.

Patient 3 to 36 Months of Age with ACUTE FEVER WITHOUT A SOURCE

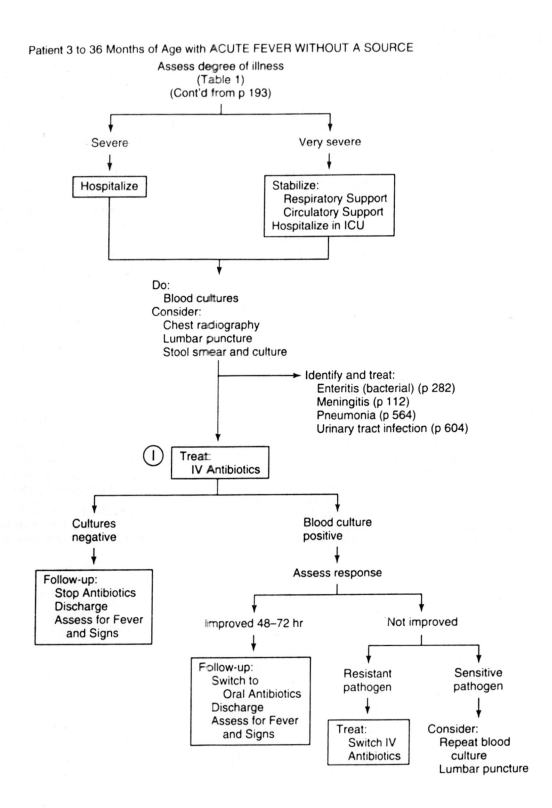

CHEST PAIN

Stephen Berman, M.D.

Chest pain, a common complaint among children, has many causes: idiopathic (21%), musculoskeletal (15%), cough (10%), costochondritis (8%), psychogenic (9%), asthma (7%), trauma (5%), pneumonia (4%), sickle cell crisis (2%), and other miscellaneous conditions (1%).

A.   In the history ask about onset, duration, location, and severity of pain. Pain that awakens the patient is likely caused by organic illness. Note associated symptoms such as fever, vomiting, cough, and migraine headache. Note the effect of the pain on daily activities and school attendance. Note possible precipitating factors, especially trauma, exercise, weight lifting, foreign body ingestion, caustic ingestion, acute respiratory infection, and underlying illness or conditions, especially Kawasaki disease or congenital heart disease. Obtain a family history of cardiac disease, peptic ulcer disease, and rheumatoid disease. Assess the psychosocial situation (see p 8) and identify sources of stress and anxiety. If appropriate, ask about cigarette smoking and use of birth control pills.

B.   Perform a complete physical examination and note signs of respiratory distress, reactive airway disease, cardiac disease, arthritis, and abdominal masses. Palpate each rib cartilage with only one finger; two or more fingers may splint the affected cartilage and not reproduce the pain. Costochondritis causes tenderness over the costochondral or costosternal junctions. Anterior chest wall syndromes cause chest wall pain that is exacerbated by trunk or shoulder movements.

C.   Cardiac causes of chest pain include ischemia, infarction, arrhythmias, mitral valve prolapse, pulmonic or aortic stenosis, pericarditis or pericardial defects, pulmonary hypertension, and dissecting aortic aneurysm. Risk factors for cardiac disease include a family history of early myocardial infarction or hypercholesterolemia, a history of Kawasaki disease, hypertension, or congenital disease. Findings that suggest cardiac disease are heart murmurs, increased intensity of the second heart sound, clicks, gallop rhythm, friction rub, hypertension, and decreased femoral pulses. Findings on chest radiography and ECG may suggest cardiac disease. Pericarditis and myocarditis related to an infection or vasculitis will present with cardiomegaly and ST-T wave changes. Aortic stenosis and idiopathic hypertrophic subaortic stenosis cause a systolic heart murmur and left-ventricular hypertrophy. Primary pulmonary hypertension and pulmonary stenosis produce right-ventricular hypertrophy. Coronary artery disease related to Kawasaki disease, hypercholesterolemia, aberrant left coronary artery, and lesions associated with decreased coronary artery blood flow such as severe aortic stenosis or idiopathic hypertrophic subaortic stenosis produce ischemic ST-T wave changes. Arrhythmias such as atrioventricular block, sick sinus syndrome, and supraventricular tachycardia are associated with ECG findings of abnormal conduction patterns.

D.   Pulmonary diseases produce pain of muscle strain (related to cough), pleural irritation or pleurisy, diaphragmatic irritation (pneumonia, bronchitis), asthma, a

(Continued on page 200)

Patient with CHEST PAIN

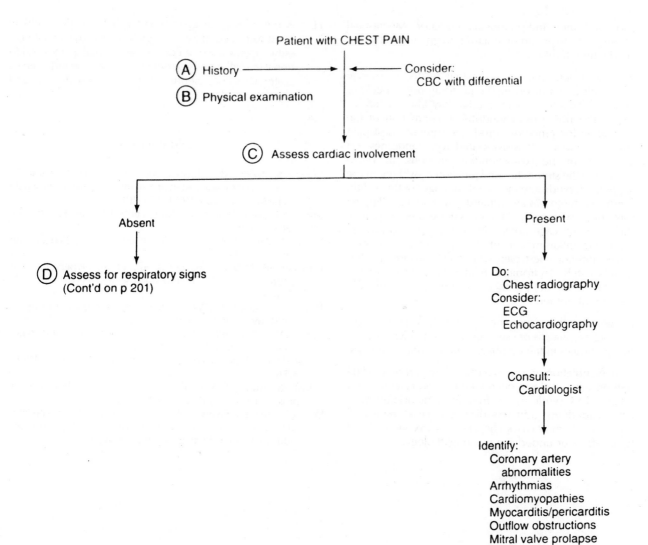

(A) History ⟶ ← Consider:
CBC with differential

(B) Physical examination

(C) Assess cardiac involvement

Absent

Present

(D) Assess for respiratory signs
(Cont'd on p 201)

Do:
Chest radiography
Consider:
ECG
Echocardiography

Consult:
Cardiologist

Identify:
Coronary artery
abnormalities
Arrhythmias
Cardiomyopathies
Myocarditis/pericarditis
Outflow obstructions
Mitral valve prolapse

thoracic tumor, and pulmonary infarction. Mediastinal causes include pneumomediastinum, mediastinitis, or a mediastinal tumor.

E.   Musculoskeletal pain is most often related to muscle strain or trauma involving the pectoral, upper back, or shoulder muscles. Direct trauma may also fracture or bruise the ribs. Costochondritis, inflammation of the costochondral junctures, produces anterior chest pain that may radiate. It is associated with tenderness on palpation of the costochondral junctions. In Tietze syndrome the sternochondral junction is swollen. In the slipping rib syndrome the costal cartilages of the eighth, ninth, and tenth ribs are irritated and produce a slipping movement with pain. The pain is duplicated by pulling the lower rib cage anteriorly. In the xyphoid process syndrome inflammation of the xyphoid process produces anterior chest pain with chest movement. Precordial catch syndrome is related to irritation of the parietal pleura that produces a stabbing pain along the left sternal border.

F.   GI disorders that cause chest pain include peptic ulcer disease, esophagitis or esophageal spasm, odynophagia, foreign bodies in the esophagus, and caustic ingestions.

G.   Hyperventilation produces reduction in carbon dioxide tension with alkalosis, decreased ionized calcium, and tetany. This syndrome is frequently associated with light-headedness, giddiness, dizziness, paresthesias, and chest pain. In most cases a high level of anxiety is related to life stress or underlying psychopathology.

H.   A breast mass or gynecomastia in the male results in chest pain secondary to a high level of anxiety related to either appearance or concern about malignancy. Additional miscellaneous causes of chest pain include herpes zoster infection, nephrolithiasis, thoracic tumor, and cigarette smoking.

References

Berezin S, Medow MS, Glassman M, et al. Use of the intraesophageal acid perfusion test in provoking nonspecific chest pain in children. J Pediatr 1989; 115:709.

Brown RT. Costochondritis in adolescents. J Adolesc Health Care 1981; 1:198.

Brown RT. Recurrent chest pain in adolescents. Pediatr Ann 1991; 20:194.

Herman SP, Stickler GB, Lucas AR, et al. Hyperventilation syndrome in children and adolescents. Pediatrics 1981; 67:183.

Pantell RH, Goodman BW Jr. Adolescent chest pain: A prospective study. Pediatrics 1983; 71:881.

Perry LW. Pinpointing the cause of pediatric chest pain. Contemp Pediatr 1985; February:71.

Selbst SM. Evaluation of chest pain in children. Pediatr Rev 1986; 8:56.

Selbst SM, Ruddy RM, Clark BJ, et al. Pediatric chest pain: A prospective study. Pediatrics 1988; 82:319.

Wiens L, Sabath R, Ewing L, et al. Chest pain in otherwise healthy children and adolescents is frequently caused by exercise-induced asthma. Pediatrics 1992; 90:350.

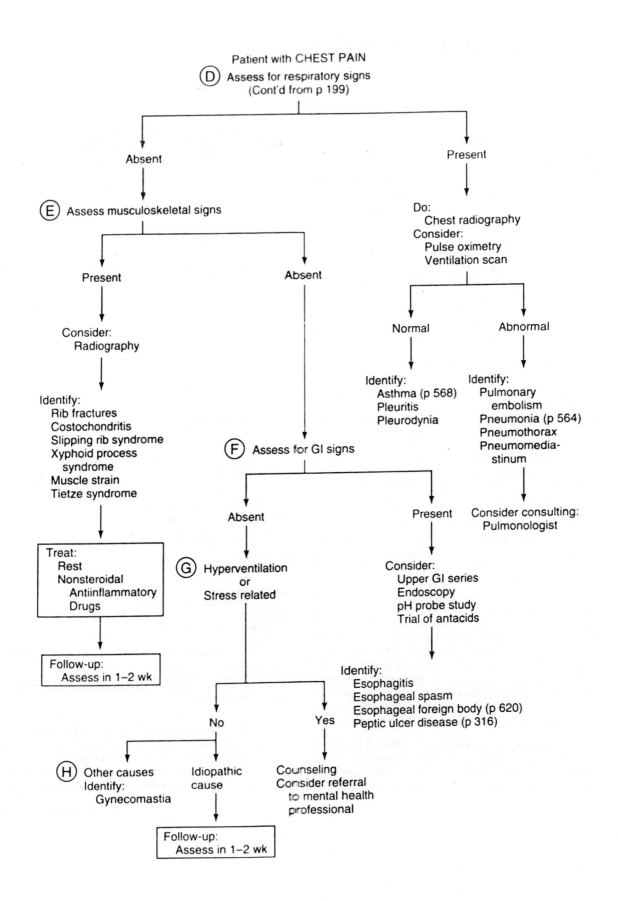

Patient with CHEST PAIN
(D) Assess for respiratory signs
(Cont'd from p 199)

Absent

(E) Assess musculoskeletal signs

Present

Consider:
    Radiography

Identify:
    Rib fractures
    Costochondritis
    Slipping rib syndrome
    Xyphoid process
        syndrome
    Muscle strain
    Tietze syndrome

Treat:
    Rest
    Nonsteroidal
        Antiinflammatory
        Drugs

Follow-up:
    Assess in 1–2 wk

Absent

(F) Assess for GI signs

Absent

(G) Hyperventilation
    or
    Stress related

No

(H) Other causes
    Identify:
        Gynecomastia

Idiopathic
cause

Follow-up:
    Assess in 1–2 wk

Yes

Counseling
Consider referral
to mental health
professional

Present

Consider:
    Upper GI series
    Endoscopy
    pH probe study
    Trial of antacids

Identify:
    Esophagitis
    Esophageal spasm
    Esophageal foreign body (p 620)
    Peptic ulcer disease (p 316)

Present

Do:
    Chest radiography
Consider:
    Pulse oximetry
    Ventilation scan

Normal

Identify:
    Asthma (p 568)
    Pleuritis
    Pleurodynia

Abnormal

Identify:
    Pulmonary
        embolism
    Pneumonia (p 564)
    Pneumothorax
    Pneumomedia-
        stinum

Consider consulting:
    Pulmonologist

CRYING/ACUTE, EXCESSIVE

Steven R. Poole, M.D.

DEFINITION

Acute, excessive crying manifests in infants with the sudden onset of crying or fussiness without fever, for which there is no cause that is obvious to the parents. The differential diagnosis includes a variety of harmless causes and a number of serious ones (Table 1).

A. In the history ask about previous episodes, recent immunization, medications, constipation, emesis, diarrhea, blood in the stool, fever, trauma, overstimulation, changes in diet, possible ingestion, the child's location at the onset, and any suspicions the parents may have. The parents' suspicions are correct fewer than half of the times when they have a strong suspicion. The consolability and time of onset do not appear to correlate with the severity of the cause. History will reveal helpful clues 20% of the time but will also uncover symptoms that may be unrelated to the correct diagnosis 20% of the time. Therefore, carefully corroborate clues in the history with appropriate physical examination or testing.

B. Physical examination alone will identify a cause approximately 40% of the time. The physical examination must be meticulous and should include (1) assessment of the level of toxicity, (2) complete inspection of every bit of the surface of the infant's body, (3) careful palpation of the body for subtle signs of tenderness, (4) otoscopy, (5) eversion of the eyelids, (6) fluorescein staining of the corneas, (7) complete observation of the oropharynx (consider using a laryngoscope), (8) careful abdominal examination, (9) rectal examination with hematest of the stool, (10) auscultation of the heart, (11) retinal examination, and (12) careful neurologic and developmental assessment. A bruise, bite, or hair tourniquet may be hiding under clothing. Fractures may present without visible swelling and may be diagnosable only on careful palpation and observation. Corneal abrasion most often causes only crying, without tearing, blepharospasm, or conjunctival redness. Pharyngeal foreign bodies may not be visible without a laryngoscope. Retinal hemorrhages may be the only physical sign of shaking injury or head trauma.

C. When the diagnosis is apparent on physical examination, treat accordingly, keeping in mind that 5% of patients have two causes of fussiness. Follow-up contact should be maintained until crying has ceased. When

TABLE 1 Diagnoses in 56 Infants with an Episode of Unexplained Excessive Crying

Diagnosis	No. With Diagnosis
Idiopathic	10
Colic	6
Infectious causes	
Otitis media*	10
Viral illness with anorexia, dehydration*	2
Urinary tract infection*	1
Mild prodrome of gastroenteritis	1
Herpangina*	1
Herpes stomatitis*	1
Trauma	
Corneal abrasion*	3
Foreign body in eye*	1
Foreign body in oropharynx*	1
Tibial fracture*	1
Clavicular fracture*	1
Brown recluse spider bite*	1
Hair tourniquet syndrome (toe)*	1
Gastrointestinal tract	
Constipation	3
Intussusception*	1
Gastroesophageal reflux and esophagitis*	1
Central nervous system	
Subdural hematoma*	1
Encephalitis*	1
Pseudotumor cerebri*	1
Drug reaction/overdose	
DTP† reaction*	1
Inadvertent pseudoephedrine overdose*	1
Behavioral	
Night terrors	1
Overstimulation	1
Cardiovascular	
Supraventricular tachycardia*	2
Metabolic	
Glutaric aciduria, type I*	1
Total	56

* Conditions considered serious.
† Diphtheria-tetanus-pertussis vaccine.
From Poole SR. The infant with acute, unexplained crying. Pediatrics 1991; 88:450, with permission.

you suspect a particular diagnosis but are not certain, keep in mind that the differential includes many serious conditions. Therefore, it is dangerous to jump to a diagnosis based only on suspicion. A brief period of observation may be necessary to confirm the suspicion.

(Continued on page 204)

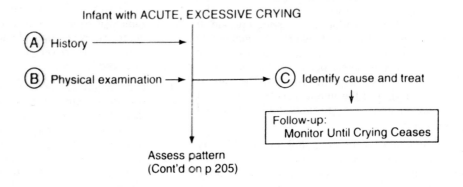

Infant with ACUTE, EXCESSIVE CRYING

(A) History

(B) Physical examination ➔ (C) Identify cause and treat

Follow-up:
    Monitor Until Crying Ceases

Assess pattern
(Cont'd on p 205)

D. Many infants have ceased crying by the time they are seen by the physician and the crying does not recur. This syndrome is called idiopathic acute crying episode. It must include the following elements: (1) unalarming history, (2) normal physical examination, (3) cessation of crying prior to seeing the physician, (4) lack of signs of toxicity, and (5) no subsequent episodes. The parents can be reassured, and the infants can be followed at home. However, if the crying resumes, the infant should be reexamined.

E. The cause may not be apparent after the initial history and physical examination of as many as one in three infants with this type of episode. Infants who continue to cry and have no apparent diagnosis on initial examination often have a serious cause requiring specific treatment. Screening tests are of limited value; only urinalysis and urine culture have been shown to be effective. A period of observation lasting 1 to 2 hours with repeated observation and examination (including all of the special examinations described earlier) will often uncover clues to the diagnosis. For many infants crying is the first symptom of an illness that will manifest other more helpful signs or symptoms in a matter of hours (i.e., gastroenteritis, viral exanthems, enanthems, infectious illnesses, intussusception, encephalitis).

F. Some infants cease crying during the observation. The infant should be observed for a time since many serious causes have temporary asymptomatic periods.

G. For infants who continue to cry or fuss and for whom the diagnosis is still in question, consider additional studies that are both invasive and expensive. Follow clues or instincts in selecting from this list: (1) skeletal x-rays, (2) lumbar puncture, (3) barium enema, (4) CT scan of the head, (5) electrolytes and pH, (6) toxicology, (7) ECG or ECHO, (8) pulse oximetry, and (9) foreign body radiologic series. It is unwise to discharge an infant with acute, excessive, unexplained crying prior to making a diagnosis. Therefore, many of these infants must be observed longer.

H. Colic includes all of the following: (1) recurrent spells of excessive crying or fussiness, (2) occurrence at predictable times more than 3 days a week, (3) duration of 3 or more hours a day, (4) beginning in the first 3 weeks of life and resolving by 3 to 4 months of age, (5) an infant who is developing and growing normally, (6) without other concerning symptoms, and (7) with a normal physical examination when seen by the physician. Without each of the seven elements described above, the diagnosis should not be made. Therefore, it is difficult to make the diagnosis with complete confidence on the first night of colic, and follow-up is needed to confirm it.

I. Soothing techniques include rhythmic motion such as rocking and stroller or car rides; monotonous noise from a radio, tape, or clock; a pacifier; and warm water bottle next to the abdomen. Being carried in a sack may help. Parents may need support for leaving the infant with a babysitter for an evening out. The effectiveness of formula changes is unclear. Pharmacologic therapy should be discouraged.

Reference

Poole SR. The infant with acute, unexplained, excessive crying. Pediatrics 1991; 88:450.

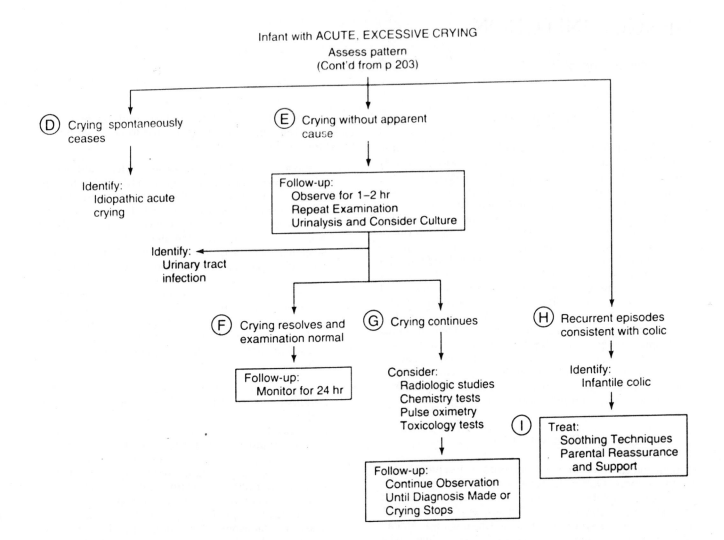

Infant with ACUTE, EXCESSIVE CRYING
Assess pattern
(Cont'd from p 203)

D Crying spontaneously
   ceases

Identify:
   Idiopathic acute
   crying

E Crying without apparent
   cause

Follow-up:
   Observe for 1–2 hr
   Repeat Examination
   Urinalysis and Consider Culture

Identify:
   Urinary tract
   infection

F Crying resolves and
   examination normal

Follow-up:
   Monitor for 24 hr

G Crying continues

Consider:
   Radiologic studies
   Chemistry tests
   Pulse oximetry
   Toxicology tests

Follow-up:
   Continue Observation
   Until Diagnosis Made or
   Crying Stops

H Recurrent episodes
   consistent with colic

Identify:
   Infantile colic

I Treat:
   Soothing Techniques
   Parental Reassurance
   and Support

DENGUE INFECTION

Stephen Berman, M.D.

DEFINITIONS

Dengue fever is a mild, self-limited febrile episode often associated with a rash. It is caused by an arbovirus, usually acquired by the daytime bite of the *Aedes aegypti* mosquito. Dengue fever begins with fever, respiratory symptoms (sore throat, coryza, and cough), and headache. Back pain, myalgias, arthralgias, conjunctivitis, and nausea with vomiting may also occur. A transient macular rash usually develops within 48 hours. The initial fever resolves within approximately 1 week, and a few days later a generalized morbilliform or maculopapular rash develops. Fever often returns with the rash. **Dengue hemorrhagic fever** is progression of dengue fever to dehydration with hemoconcentration, thrombocytopenia, or coagulation abnormalities, including disseminated intravascular coagulation (DIC). **Dengue shock syndrome** is progression of hemorrhagic fever (in about 20% to 30% of cases) to severe hypovolemia and shock. Fatality rates vary from 12% to 44%. Complications include encephalopathy (40%), liver dysfunction or failure (20% to 30%), pneumonia (18%), and pulmonary hemorrhage (3%).

EPIDEMIOLOGY

Dengue infections occur worldwide but are most prevalent in Southeast Asia. Outbreaks have occurred in the Western Hemisphere, notably in Central and South America. In Thailand large outbreaks of hemorrhagic fever occur every 1 to 2 years. Similar syndromes include Chikungunya (Africa), West Nile fever, and O'nyong-nyong fever. Denguelike illnesses without a rash include Colorado tick fever, sandfly fever, Ross River fever, and Rift Valley fever.

PATHOPHYSIOLOGY

The pathogenesis of the infection involves activation of the complement system with release of chemical mediators that markedly increase capillary leak and produce DIC. The capillary leak predisposes to pulmonary edema, pleural effusion, and ascites as well as intravascular compromise and hemoconcentration. Bleeding (epistaxis, purpura, petechiae, GI hemorrhage, menorrhagia) is related to DIC with thrombocytopenia and liver damage.

A. In the history ask about the onset, pattern, and degree of the fever and evaluate the family's ability to care for the child at home and their access to transportation and a telephone. Risk factors include recent travel to an area with endemic dengue fever, such as Southeast Asia. Assess alterations in the mental status and normal level of activity: playfulness, weakness, irritability, feeding and sleeping patterns, responsiveness, and seizures. Note any respiratory symptoms: cough, congestion, coryza, sore throat, earache, fast or difficult breathing, chest indrawing (retractions). Assess GI symptoms (nausea, vomiting, diarrhea, abdominal pain, blood in stools, and jaundice) and renal symptoms (dark urine, decreased urinary frequency, flank pain, lower abdominal pain).

B. On physical examination look, listen, and feel for findings that suggest progression to hemorrhagic fever and shock syndrome. These include CNS involvement: too weak to feed, difficult to arouse, unresponsive, seizures, irritability, coma with decerebrate or decorticate posturing. Also look for dehydration and poor perfusion: skin turgor, tears, moist mucous membranes, color and warmth of the extremities and capillary refill time (>2 seconds is abnormal), low blood pressure, narrowing of the pulse pressure to 20 mm Hg or less. Assess any tachypnea, retractions, grunting, crackles, hepatomegaly, splenomegaly, jaundice, arthralgias, arthritis, weakness, myalgias, petechiae, purpura, hemoptysis, bloody vomitus, and bloody stools.

C. Leukopenia and neutropenia are characteristic findings. In dengue hemorrhagic fever and dengue shock syndrome the most common laboratory findings are hemoconcentration (an increase of at least 20% in the hematocrit), thrombocytopenia, increase in prothrombin time, and abnormalities in fibrinogen and other coagulation factors. Liver function may be impaired. Virus isolation and serologic tests are confirmatory.

(Continued on page 208)

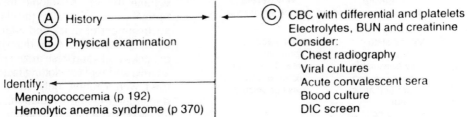

Patient with DENGUE INFECTION

(A) History ⟶ ← (C) CBC with differential and platelets
Electrolytes, BUN and creatinine
(B) Physical examination
Consider:
    Chest radiography
    Viral cultures
Identify: ←
    Acute convalescent sera
  Meningococcemia (p 192)
    Blood culture
  Hemolytic anemia syndrome (p 370)
    DIC screen
  Bleeding disorders (p 364)
    Liver function tests

Assess pattern of infection, degree of illness
(Table 1)

(Cont'd on p 209)

TABLE 1 Degree of Illness in Dengue Infection

Moderate (dengue fever)	Severe (hemorrhagic fever)	Very Severe (shock syndrome)
Mental status: headache, malaise, irritable but consolable	Mental status: irritible but easily consolable, poor eye contact (lethargic), feeds poorly	Mental status: unresponsive or too weak to feed or extreme weakness or seizures
and	or	or
No signs of dehydration and good peripheral perfusion with pink arm extremities	Signs of moderate dehydration with hemoconcentration, good peripheral perfusion	Signs of severe dehydration with shock, poor peripheral perfusion with cold, mottled extremities, capillary refill > 2 seconds, low BP
and	or	or
No signs of respiratory distress or pulmonary edema	Signs of respiratory distress (pneumonia or pulmonary edema)	Signs of severe respiratory distress (pneumonia, pulmonary edema, or congestive heart failure) with respiratory rate > 60, retractions, grunting, cyanosis, or respiratory failure
and	or	or
No signs of severe anemia or bleeding	Signs of severe anemia or bleeding (petechiae, purpura, GI hemorrhage, hematuria)	Life-threatening anemia, bleeding associated with DIC
and	and	or
No signs of metabolic or end organ failure	No signs of metabolic or end organ failure	Metabolic disorder including hypoglycemia, metabolic acidosis, or liver or renal failure

D. Hospitalize patients with very severe cases in an intensive care unit. Manage shock with a sufficient volume (IV) of an isotonic fluid (Ringer's lactate or normal saline) to stabilize the circulation. See page 120 for treatment of shock and additional use of vasopressors and monitoring. Consider whole-blood transfusions or packed cells and fresh frozen plasma to correct severe anemia and replace clotting factors. Heparin should be used with caution only when DIC persists despite stabilization of the circulation, correction of acidosis, and good oxygenation. Systemic steroids do not appear to affect outcome.

References

Feigin RD, Cherry JD. Dengue and dengue hemorrhagic fever. In: Feigin RD, Cherry JD, eds. Textbook of pediatric infectious diseases, volume II. Philadelphia: Saunders, 1987: 1510.

Halstead SB. Selective primary health care: Strategies for control of disease in the developing world. XI. Dengue. Rev Infect Dis 1984; 6:251.

Maneekarn N, Morita K, Tanaka M, et al. Applications of polymerase chain reaction for identification of dengue viruses isolated from patient sera. Microbiol Immunol 1993; 37:41.

Sangkawibha N, Rojansuphot S, Ahandrik S, et al. Risk factors in dengue shock syndrome: A prospective epidemiologic study in Rayong, Thailand. Am J Epidemiol 1984; 120:653.

Tassniyom S, Vasanawathana S, Chirawatkul A, et al. Failure of high-dose methylprednisolone in established dengue shock syndrome: A placebo-controlled, double-blind study. Pediatrics 1993; 92:111.

Technical guides for diagnosis, treatment, surveillance, prevention and control of dengue haemorrhagic fever for the South-East Asian and Western Pacific Regions. Manila: World Health Organization, 1980.

Patient with DENGUE INFECTION
Assess pattern of infection, degree of illness
(Table 1)
(Cont'd from p 207)

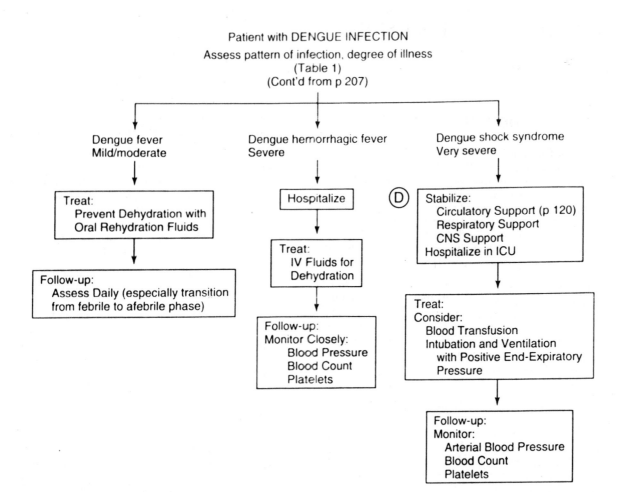

Dengue fever
Mild/moderate

Treat:
   Prevent Dehydration with
   Oral Rehydration Fluids

Follow-up:
   Assess Daily (especially transition
   from febrile to afebrile phase)

Dengue hemorrhagic fever
Severe

Hospitalize

Treat:
   IV Fluids for
   Dehydration

Follow-up:
Monitor Closely:
   Blood Pressure
   Blood Count
   Platelets

Dengue shock syndrome
Very severe

Ⓓ Stabilize:
   Circulatory Support (p 120)
   Respiratory Support
   CNS Support
Hospitalize in ICU

Treat:
Consider:
   Blood Transfusion
   Intubation and Ventilation
     with Positive End-Expiratory
     Pressure

Follow-up:
Monitor:
   Arterial Blood Pressure
   Blood Count
   Platelets

FEVER, RED EYES, RED SKIN

Stephen Berman, M.D.

DEFINITION

Erythema multiforme is a complex of symptoms of the skin and mucous membranes. It has two forms, minor and major. The minor form, not associated with systemic signs, is characterized by lesions with concentric zones of color change and a central dusky area (target or iris lesions). These lesions usually persist for 1 to 3 weeks. The major form, associated with systemic signs and sloughing of the skin and mucous membranes, is called Stevens-Johnson syndrome (SJS) and toxic epidermal necrolysis (TEN).

A. In the history ask about the onset of fever, rash, conjunctivitis, photophobia, and other associated symptoms such as sore throat; mouth lesions; coryza; cough; swelling of hands, feet, or joints; diarrhea; abdominal pain; and current and past medications. Ask about the distribution of the rash. Note any allergies. Note the temporal relationship of the onset of different symptoms and their duration.

B. On physical examination note whether the conjunctivitis is purulent or hyperemic. Characterize the type of rash (morbilliform, maculopapular, erythrodermal), as well as its distribution, and note any bullae, blisters, ulcerations, or impetiginous lesions. Press on the lateral edge of a blister; extension and enlargement constitute a positive Nikolsky sign. Look for mouth lesions (fissuring and crusting of lips, Koplik spots on the buccal mucosa, strawberry tongue, oropharyngeal lesions or injection). Characterizing the rash and conjunctivitis is helpful diagnostically. A purulent conjunctivitis and a diffuse erythroderma with bullae, tender skin, and a positive Nikolsky sign suggest SJS or staphylococcal scalded skin syndrome (SSSS). Conjunctival hyperemia with an erythroderma suggests toxic shock syndrome, Kawasaki disease, scarlet fever syndromes, or leptospirosis. A morbilliform rash with Koplik spots suggests measles. Other conditions with a morbilliform rash are rubella, infectious mononucleosis, drug eruptions, and Kawasaki disease. Erythema multiforme is characterized by iris and target lesions.

C. Measles is associated with a 3 or 4 day prodrome of cough, coryza, fever, and conjunctivitis. The rash, which starts on the head and face, moves downward to involve the trunk and extremities. Lesions on the face, neck, and upper trunk become confluent. Koplik spots are usually present on the buccal mucosa. The rash resolves in approximately 1 week (see p 244).

D. SJS and TEN present with bullous lesions, a positive Nikolsky sign, and mucous membrane involvement. Unlike SSSS, they are often preceded by erythema multiforme with iris and target lesions and evolve over 3 to 5 days rather than a few hours. SJS is associated with epidermal necrosis and subepidermal blister formation. Agents most frequently associated with SJS and TEN are herpes simplex, *Mycoplasma pneumoniae, Streptococcus pyogenes,* Epstein-Barr virus, and tuberculosis. The most commonly associated drugs are sulfonamides, barbiturates, dilantin, salicylate, and penicillin. The use of steroids in SJS is controversial.

E. Suspect Kawasaki disease (mucocutaneous lymph node syndrome) when an erythematous rash and conjunctival hyperemia are associated with fever for more than 5 days, mouth lesions (fissuring and crusting of the lips, strawberry tongue, or oropharyngeal injection), alterations of the hands and/or feet (erythema, edema, and induration followed by desquamation), and lymphadenopathy (see p 232).

F. Rubella is not usually associated with a prodrome. A red macular rash starts on the face and progresses downward, becoming generalized within 24 to 48 hours. Lesions are usually discrete rather than confluent; clearing is noted on the face and trunk by day 3 or 4. Mild conjunctivitis may be present.

(Continued on page 212)

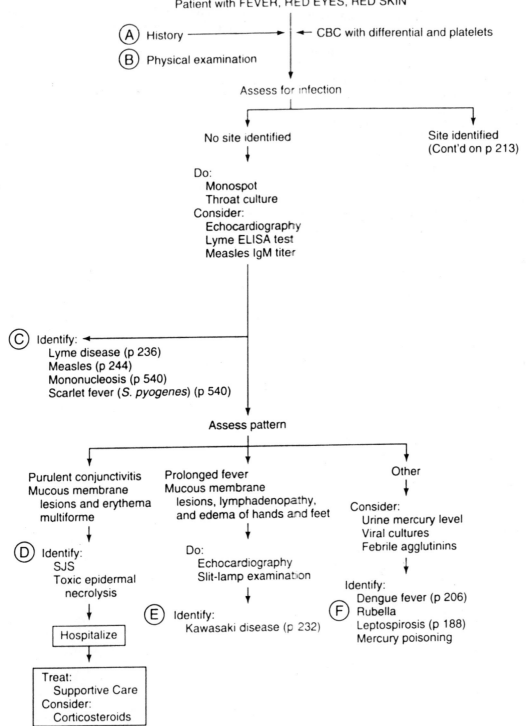

Patient with FEVER, RED EYES, RED SKIN

(A) History ⟶ ← CBC with differential and platelets

(B) Physical examination

Assess for infection

No site identified

Site identified
(Cont'd on p 213)

Do:
    Monospot
    Throat culture
Consider:
    Echocardiography
    Lyme ELISA test
    Measles IgM titer

(C) Identify: ◄
    Lyme disease (p 236)
    Measles (p 244)
    Mononucleosis (p 540)
    Scarlet fever (*S. pyogenes*) (p 540)

Assess pattern

Purulent conjunctivitis
Mucous membrane
  lesions and erythema
  multiforme

Prolonged fever
Mucous membrane
  lesions, lymphadenopathy,
  and edema of hands and feet

Other

Consider:
    Urine mercury level
    Viral cultures
    Febrile agglutinins

(D) Identify:
    SJS
    Toxic epidermal
      necrolysis

Do:
    Echocardiography
    Slit-lamp examination

Identify:
    Dengue fever (p 206)
(F) Rubella
    Leptospirosis (p 188)
    Mercury poisoning

Hospitalize

(E) Identify:
    Kawasaki disease (p 232)

Treat:
    Supportive Care
Consider:
    Corticosteroids

G. Oral erythromycin estolate or ethyl succinate, cephalosporins, dicloxacillin, and clindamycin are comparable for treating superficial *Staphylococcus aureus* infections.

H. Toxic shock syndrome is caused by a staphylococcal phage-related toxin. It can be caused by skin and wound infections, tampon use, vaginal infections, nasal packing, childbirth and abortion infections, and postinfluenza bacterial respiratory tract infections (tracheitis, pneumonia). Suspect toxic shock syndrome when erythroderma is associated with fever, altered mental status, diarrhea, hypotension, disseminated intravascular coagulation, and renal failure. Hospitalize these patients, stabilize their circulation, and begin IV antistaphylococcal antibiotic coverage.

I. Suspect SSSS when lateral pressure on the edge of the blister enlarges and extends the blister (Nikolsky sign) or bullous impetigo is present. The rash may be local or general such as in Ritter disease of the newborn. A toxin associated with *S. aureus* of the phage group II causes separation of the granular layer of the stratum corneum of the skin (intraepidermal blisters). Hospitalize and treat patients with antistaphylococcal antibiotics.

References

Ben-Amitai D, Ashkenazi S. Common bacterial skin infections in childhood. Pediatr Ann 1993; 22:225.

Cohen B. The many faces of erythema multiforme. Contemp Pediatr 1994; 11:19.

Rasmussen JE. Impetigo: Changing bacteria, changing therapies. Contemp Pediatr 1992; 9:14.

Roujeau JC, Stern RS. Severe adverse cutaneous reactions to drugs. N Engl J Med 1994; 10:1272.

Weston WL, Lane AT. Color textbook of pediatric dermatology. St. Louis: Mosby, 1991.

Yagupsky P. Bacterial aspects of skin and soft tissue infections. Pediatr Ann 1993; 22:217.

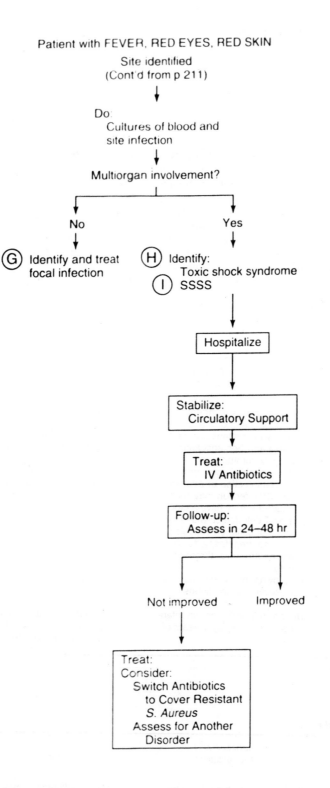

Patient with FEVER, RED EYES, RED SKIN
Site identified
(Cont'd from p 211)

Do:
    Cultures of blood and
    site infection

Multiorgan involvement?

No

Yes

(G) Identify and treat
    focal infection

(H) Identify:
    Toxic shock syndrome
(I) SSSS

Hospitalize

Stabilize:
    Circulatory Support

Treat:
    IV Antibiotics

Follow-up:
    Assess in 24–48 hr

Not improved

Improved

Treat:
Consider:
    Switch Antibiotics
       to Cover Resistant
       S. Aureus
    Assess for Another
       Disorder

FREQUENT INFECTIONS

Stephen Berman, M.D.

DEFINITIONS

Frequent invasive bacterial infections consist of two invasive bacterial infections such as meningitis, bone or joint infections, or bacteremia within 2 years. **Serious bacterial infections (SBI)** include bacterial meningitis, bacteremia, bacterial pneumonia, urinary tract infections (UTI), bacterial enteritis, cellulitis, and bone and joint infections. **Immunodeficiency disorders** are defects in the T-lymphocyte system (T cells and lymphokines), B-lymphocyte system (B cells and immunoglobulins), neutrophil function, or complement system. They can be primary or secondary related to infection, drugs, malnutrition, or protein loss.

EPIDEMIOLOGY

The incidence of asymptomatic IgA deficiency is 20:10,000, and the incidences of other primary immunodeficiency diseases are about 1:10,000. The risk of a primary immunodeficiency depends on the mode of inheritance (X-linked or autosomal recessive) and the carrier status of a family. Carrier identification and antenatal diagnosis are available for many disorders when a primary immunodeficiency has been identified in a family.

A. In the history ask about the following: types of infection and the pathogens isolated. Document the onset

TABLE 1 B-Cell Disorders

Disorder	Genetics and Presentation	Defect	Treatment
Bruton agammaglobulinemia	X-linked recessive inheritance; prenatal diagnosis available	Arrest in differentiation of pre-B cells	Monthly IVIG
Immunoglobulin deficiency with high IgM	Unknown inheritance; neutropenia and hepatosplenomegaly common	Isotype switching from IgM to IgG, IgA, and IgE	Monthly IVIG
Common variable immunodeficiency or late-onset hypogammaglobulinemia	Unknown inheritance; congenital infection or postnatal EBV infection may have occurred; may have associated T-cell defect; may have signs of collagen vascular disease, hepatosplenomegaly, neutropenia, thrombocytopenia	B cells do not differentiate into plasma cells	Consider IVIG
Selective immunoglobulin deficiencies/IgA, IgG subclass, and IgM	Unknown inheritance; may have autoimmune conditions	Unclear	Consider IVIG for patients with marked deficiencies and severe infections
Transient hypogammaglobulinemia of infancy	Unknown inheritance; spontaneous recovery by 4 years of age	Delayed maturation; response of B cells to T cell–dependent stimulation depressed	Treat with IVIG only for severe infections

IVIG, intravenous immunoglobulin.

TABLE 2 T-Cell Disorders

Disorder	Genetics and Presentation	Defect	Treatment
Purine-nucleoside phosphorylase deficiency	AR inheritance; prenatal diagnosis available; may present with autoimmune hemolytic anemia	Enzyme deficiency causes increase in deoxyguanosine triphosphate, which kills dividing T cells	Consider BMT, irradiated red cell transfusions to replace enzyme
Thymic hypoplasia (DiGeorge syndrome)	Intrinsic genetic factors, extrinsic factors (diabetes, alcoholism, isotretinoin exposure); no prenatal diagnosis, abnormal facial features, neonatal tetany	Malformations of cardiac outflow tract, absent or hypoplastic thymus, parathyroid glands	Consider graft with fetal thymus or thymic epithelial cells or BMT

AR, autosomal recessive; BMT, bone marrow transplantation.

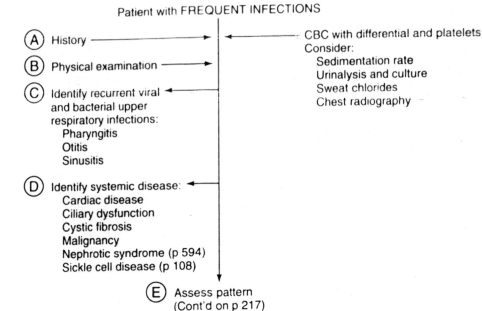

Patient with FREQUENT INFECTIONS

(A) History ⟶

(B) Physical examination ⟶

(C) Identify recurrent viral
and bacterial upper
respiratory infections:
    Pharyngitis
    Otitis
    Sinusitis

(D) Identify systemic disease:
    Cardiac disease
    Ciliary dysfunction
    Cystic fibrosis
    Malignancy
    Nephrotic syndrome (p 594)
    Sickle cell disease (p 108)

(E) Assess pattern
    (Cont'd on p 217)

CBC with differential and platelets
Consider:
    Sedimentation rate
    Urinalysis and culture
    Sweat chlorides
    Chest radiography

severity, response to therapy, and pattern of infections. Onset of infections soon after birth suggests defects in cell-mediated immunity, neutrophil function, or complement, because maternal antibody protects infants with B-cell disorders for 3 to 6 months. Family history: early unexplained infant deaths, other family members with frequent severe infections or known immunodeficiency diseases, especially HIV infection and malignancies. Risk factors: immunization status and adverse reactions to vaccines, current medications, allergies, underlying conditions such as collagen vascular, cardiopulmonary, GI, and renal disease, sickle cell disease, central venous catheter and other indwelling lines, conditions and/or therapies that compromise immunity, especially HIV infection. CNS symptoms, including alterations in the mental status and normal level of activity: playfulness, irritability, feeding and sleeping patterns, schoolwork, responsiveness, and seizure activity. Respiratory symptoms: cough, recurrent sore throats and ear infections, pneumonia episodes, and periods of fast or difficult breathing with chest indrawing (retractions). GI symptoms: chronic diarrhea, weight loss, malnutrition, failure to thrive. Renal symptoms: pain with urination (dysuria), urinary frequency, flank pain, lower abdominal pain, nephrosis, glomerulonephritis. Dermatology symptoms: chronic *Candida* infection (involvement of skin, nails, and mucous membranes), rashes, eczema, impetigo.

B. On physical examination look, listen, and feel for findings that suggest a current infection or sequelae of past infections. Note lymphoid tissue (lymph nodes and tonsils); assess growth and development. Note petechiae (Wiskott-Aldrich syndrome), telangiectasia, and neurologic findings (ataxia telangiectasia syndrome), scarring from adenitis (chronic granulomatous disease), hepatosplenomegaly (HIV and immune disorders), and partial albinism (Chediak-Higashi syndrome).

C. Children under 6 years of age may have 6 to 12 viral infections/year. These episodes of upper respiratory infections and diarrhea are usually mild and self-limited. Children who attend nursery school or day care centers are most likely to have frequent viral infections.

D. A systemic disorder or malignancy may cause frequent infections because of neutropenia, impaired mucociliary clearance (cystic fibrosis, atopy, ciliary dysfunction), or abnormal vascular perfusion (diabetes, nephrosis, congestive heart failure, infarction). Metabolic disorders and systemic diseases that predispose to frequent infection include diabetes mellitus, cystic fibrosis, severe malnutrition, allergic disorders (allergic rhinitis, eczema, reactive airway disease), CNS disorders (recurrent aspiration), and gastroesophageal reflux. Therapy with a corticosteroid or other immunosuppressive for renal disease, rheumatoid arthritis, or reactive airway disease alters immune defenses and may result in frequent infections.

E. Most patients fall into one of the following four patterns: pattern 1 (consider anatomic/structural defects and B-cell defects), SBIs involving one system only such as recurrent meningitis, pneumonia, or osteomyelitis; pattern 2, (consider B-cell defects, Tables 1 and 3), multiple SBIs in different systems, especially respiratory (sinopulmonary disease) and GI tracts; pattern 3 (consider T-cell defects, Tables 2 and 3), severe infections with opportunistic and/or intracellular pathogens, including viruses (cytomegalovirus, Epstein-Barr virus, respiratory syncytial virus), fungi, protozoa (pneumocystis), and intracellular bacteria (tuberculosis); and pattern 4 (neutrophil function defects), recurrent abscesses, soft-tissue, and skin infections. These groups are not mutually exclusive, and combined immunodeficiency disorders with defects in both antibody and cell-mediated immunity will cause infections that fit several groups.

F. Suspect a defect in nonimmunologic defenses when two or more SBIs occur in the same anatomic site without infections in other sites. Nonimmunologic defects that allow frequent infections include anatomic alterations (ureteral stenosis, vesicoureteral reflux, eustachian tube dysfunction, tracheoesophageal fistula, skull defects or fractures, sinus tracts), impaired barriers (eczema, burns), and foreign bodies (catheters, heart valves).

G. Neutrophil disorders can cause quantitative as well as qualitative alterations resulting from intrinsic or extrinsic factors. Quantitative alterations include problems with bone marrow production (congenital and cyclic neutropenia, reticular dysgenesis), storage (bone marrow necrosis), migration or sequestration (hypersplenism, burns, trauma), and destruction (antineutrophil antibodies, infection, inflammation). Qualitative alterations

TABLE 3 Combination B- and T-Cell Disorders

Disorder	Genetics and Presentation	Defect	Treatment
Severe combined immuno-deficiency (SCID)	X-linked and AR inheritance; prenatal diagnosis, carrier detection available for some forms	Adenosine deaminase deficiency in 50% of cases with AR SCID; other forms have varying T- and B-cell abnormalities	BMT; consider enzyme replacement
Ataxia-telangiectasia syndrome	AR inheritance; carrier state detection possible; findings include elevated serum α-fetoprotein, cerebellar ataxia, telangiectasias (2–8 years of age), high incidence of malignancy	Inability to repair DNA damage, interference with rearrangement of T- and B-cell genes	Supportive care, antibiotics for specific infections
Wiskott-Aldrich syndrome	X-linked recessive; prenatal and carrier detection available; eczema, thrombocytopenia, bloody diarrhea, cerebral hemorrhage	Expression of a cell surface sialophorin	BMT; consider IVIG, prednisone, splenectomy
Chronic mucocutaneous candidiasis	Unknown genetics; skin, nail, mucous membrane involvement; association with endocrinopathies, signs of autoimmune disorders	Unknown	Ketoconazole

AR, autosomal recessive; BMT, bone marrow transplantation; IVIG, intravenous immuno globulin.

TABLE 4 Neutrophil Function Disorders

Disorder	Genetics and Presentation	Defect	Treatment
Chronic granulomatous disease	X-linked or AR inheritance; prenatal diagnosis available	Respiratory burst O$_2$ production	γ-Interferon, BMT; gene therapy being studied
Leukocyte adhesion disorder	AR inheritance; prenatal diagnosis available; neutrophilia	Adhesion	BMT; gene therapy being studied
Chediak-Higashi syndrome	AR inheritance; prenatal diagnosis available, partial albinism, giant granules in neutrophils, melanocytes	Transport of granules including melanins and neurotransmitters	Vitamin C
Actin dysfunction	AR inheritance; prenatal diagnosis available	Granule transportation causing altered chemotaxis and phagocytosis	No treatment
Reticular dysgenesis	AR inheritance; no prenatal diagnosis; neutropenia	Uncertain	BMT
Congenital and cyclic neutropenias	AR inheritance; no prenatal diagnosis	Uncertain	Granulocyte-monocyte colony stimulating factor in trials
Isoimmune neutropenia	Unknown inheritance; no prenatal diagnosis	Auto antineutrophil antibodies	Intravenous immunoglobulin
Hyper-IgE (Job's) syndrome	Unknown inheritance; no prenatal diagnosis; severe eczema, elevated IgE	Chemotaxis, T-cell function	Trials of γ-interferon, H$_2$ antagonists, vitamins C, E under way
Juvenile periodontitis	Unknown inheritance; no prenatal diagnosis	Surface of glycoprotein that causes isolated periodontitis	No treatment

AR, autosomal recessive; BMT, bone marrow transplantation.

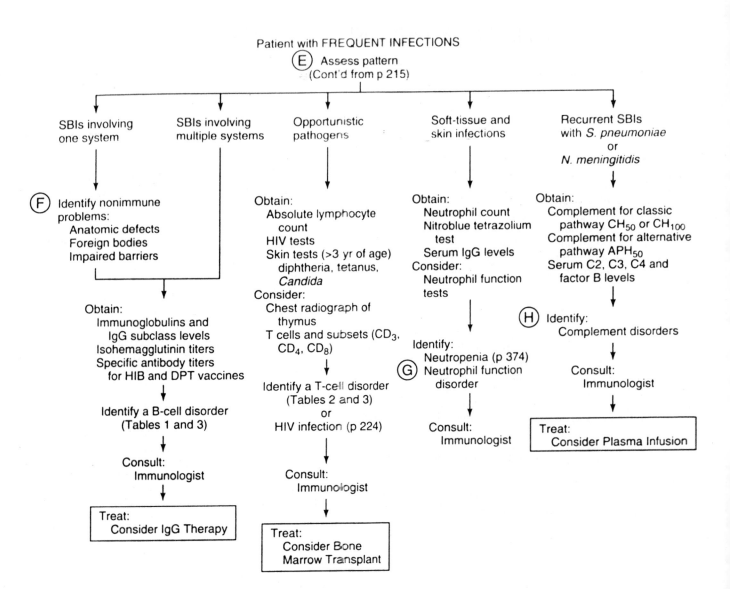

Patient with FREQUENT INFECTIONS

(E) Assess pattern
(Cont'd from p 215)

SBIs involving one system

(F) Identify nonimmune problems:
Anatomic defects
Foreign bodies
Impaired barriers

SBIs involving multiple systems

Obtain:
Immunoglobulins and IgG subclass levels
Isohemagglutinin titers
Specific antibody titers for HIB and DPT vaccines

Identify a B-cell disorder (Tables 1 and 3)

Consult:
Immunologist

Treat:
Consider IgG Therapy

Opportunistic pathogens

Obtain:
Absolute lymphocyte count
HIV tests
Skin tests (>3 yr of age) diphtheria, tetanus, Candida
Consider:
Chest radiograph of thymus
T cells and subsets (CD_3, CD_4, CD_8)

Identify a T-cell disorder (Tables 2 and 3)
or
HIV infection (p 224)

Consult:
Immunologist

Treat:
Consider Bone Marrow Transplant

Soft-tissue and skin infections

Obtain:
Neutrophil count
Nitroblue tetrazolium test
Serum IgG levels
Consider:
Neutrophil function tests

Identify:
Neutropenia (p 374)
(G) Neutrophil function disorder

Consult:
Immunologist

Recurrent SBIs with *S. pneumoniae* or *N. meningitidis*

Obtain:
Complement for classic pathway CH_{50} or CH_{100}
Complement for alternative pathway APH_{50}
Serum C2, C3, C4 and factor B levels

(H) Identify:
Complement disorders

Consult:
Immunologist

Treat:
Consider Plasma Infusion

---

include problems with adhesion (leukocyte adhesion disorder), migration/chemotaxis (lazy leukocyte syndrome; hyper-IgE, or Job's, syndrome; actin dysfunction; and systemic conditions such as diabetes mellitus and collagen vascular disorders), phagocytosis (actin dysfunction, opsonin deficiency caused by hypogammaglobulinemia or complement deficiency, asplenium, Wiskott-Aldrich syndrome), bactericidal activity and cytotoxicity (enzyme defects), and respiratory burst activities (chronic granulomatous disease). Patients with chronic granulomatous disease do not respond to phagocytosis with chemoluminescence (emission of energy as light). Specific tests are available to evaluate both quantitative and qualitative alterations. Neutrophil disorders are summarized in Table 4.

H. Disorders of complement have various clinical manifestations. Patients may be asymptomatic or have signs of immune disease (systemic lupus erythematosus, angioedema, urticaria), failure to thrive, chronic diarrhea, seborrheic dermatitis, or recurrent severe infection with *S. aureus*, *Neisseria meningitidis*, or gram-negative enteric bacteria. Specific additional complement studies other than C3 and total hemolytic levels are functional levels of C1 to C9b, C1 Inh, assays of complement split-products C3a, C4a, C5a, and

complement activation. The roles of plasma infusions and steroids remain unclear.

References

Ambrosino DM, Siber GR, Chilmonczyk BA, et al. Immunodeficiency characterized by impaired antibody responses to polysaccharides. N Engl J Med 1987; 316:790.

Herrod HG, Blaiss MS, Valenski WR, Gross S. Cell-mediated status of children with recurrent infection. J Pediatr 1995; 126:530.

Hong R. Recurrent infections. Pediatr Rev 1989; 11:180.

Lyall EG, Eden OB, Dixon R, et al. Assessment of a clinical scoring system for the detection of immunodeficiency in children with recurrent infections. Pediatr Infect Dis J 1991; 10:673.

Rosen FS, Cooper MD, Wedgwood JP. The primary immunodeficiencies. N Eng J Med 1995; 333:431.

Shackelford PG, Polmar SH, Mayus JL, et al. Spectrum of IgG2 subclass deficiency in children with recurrent infections. Prospective study. J Pediatr 1986; 108:647.

Shyur S-D, Hill HR. Immunodeficiency in the 1990's. Pediatr Infect Dis J 1991; 10:595.

Yang KD, Hill HR. Assessment of neutrophil function disorders. Practical and preventive interventions. Pediatr Infect Dis J 1994; 13:906.

GROWTH DEFICIENCY/FAILURE TO THRIVE

Janet A. Weston, M.D.

DEFINITION

Growth deficiency in infancy is present when the weight age is disproportionately low compared with the height and head circumference ages. Infants should regain their birth weight by the 2 week visit and have a steady weight gain. During infancy failure to gain weight over 2 months indicates growth failure. In longstanding growth failure weight drops first, followed by length, and finally head circumference for age. In severe cases all three parameters may drop below the third percentile. Severe growth failure can result in marasmus or kwashiorkor.

A. Obtain a detailed medical history. Note predisposing conditions such as intrauterine growth retardation, perinatal stress, prematurity, and chronic disease. Note the frequency of intercurrent acute illnesses such as acute otitis media, vomiting, diarrhea, respiratory infection, or urinary infection. Obtain a detailed history of diet and feeding. Determine family composition; assess employment and financial status, degree of social isolation, and level of family stress. Determine the infant's immunization history, missed appointment rate, and accessibility of medical care. Assess the mother-child interaction and level of family functioning.

B. Do a complete physical examination. Determine the median ages for the patient's height (height age), weight (weight age), and head circumference (head circumference age). On physical examination note signs of neglect or abuse such as bruises, burns, dirty appearance, severe diaper rash, impetigo, flat occiput, or bald spot. Assess the infant's developmental status with a full Denver Developmental Standardized Test. Note any dysmorphic features or signs of CNS, pulmonary, or cardiac disease.

C. A 3 day diet history calorie count is important in investigating growth deficiency. If the caloric counts are adequate for growth (110 cal/kg/day up to 6 months of age, 105 cal/kg/day for 6 to 12 months of age, 100 cal/kg/day for 12 to 24 months of age), consider a systemic disorder causing growth deficiency and evaluate caloric loss or altered metabolic stress. If the parent does not bring in a 3 day diet history, if the diet history is incomplete, or if it shows inadequate caloric intake for growth, investigate nonorganic growth deficiency. Unusual feeding patterns recorded on the diet history also point at nonorganic growth deficiency.

D. If the family does not understand the child's nutritional needs, the child may not grow. Fear of cholesterol and other health beliefs may result in an inadequate diet. Overuse of juice and inadequate intake of formula or breast milk may result in poor growth. Prolonged breast-feeding without sufficient additional foods may not provide adequate nutrition. Nutritional counseling to institute a diet providing enough calories is needed.

(Continued on page 220)

Patient with GROWTH DEFICIENCY OR FAILURE TO THRIVE*

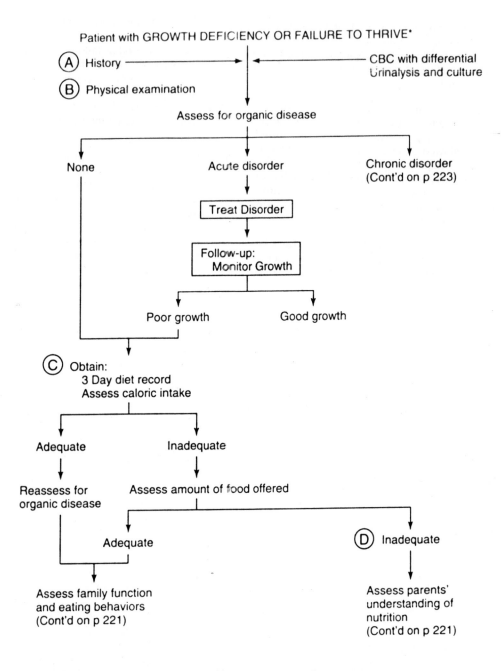

(A) History ——————→ ←—— CBC with differential
                                    Urinalysis and culture

(B) Physical examination

Assess for organic disease

None   Acute disorder   Chronic disorder
                                       (Cont'd on p 223)

Treat Disorder

Follow-up:
Monitor Growth

Poor growth   Good growth

(C) Obtain:
3 Day diet record
Assess caloric intake

Adequate   Inadequate

Reassess for   Assess amount of food offered
organic disease

Adequate   (D) Inadequate

Assess family function   Assess parents'
and eating behaviors   understanding of
(Cont'd on p 221)   nutrition
                                (Cont'd on p 221)

*Failure to thrive has become a legal term indicating neglect or abuse.
It should not be used as a diagnosis when neglect or abuse is not evident.

E. If there is evidence of lack of food in the home, dilution of formula, or use of large amounts of juice, tea, or water in the diet, refer the family for supplemental foods and nutritional counseling. If eligible, refer the family for financial assistance.

F. Poor eating behavior may be caused by diet deficiencies, such as iron, zinc, and vitamins, that depress appetite. More frequently poor eating behavior is learned. Children are allowed to graze, eating small amounts frequently, which depresses appetite. Inconsistent meals or disrupted meals also promote poor eating behavior. Day care can often provide a more structured environment and better feeding for the child. Nutritional counseling should be a part of this treatment.

G. Poor feeding may be related to family dysfunction. Children who are abused, neglected, or exposed to poorly controlled mental illness should be referred to social services. If nonaccidental trauma is suspected, obtain a skeletal bone series to identify fracture. (These cases may be defined as failure to thrive. Often parents have a history of being abused or have poor parenting skills.) Disposition options to be considered include home placement with support services, close medical follow-up visits, temporary foster placement while a parent receives therapy, and long-term foster placement.

H. High-calorie diets to promote regrowth and frequent monitoring of growth are essential. Growth is monitored in g/day and mm/day (0 to 3 months of age, 20 to 30 g/day; 3 to 6 months of age, 15 to 20 g/day; 6 to 9 months of age, 10 to 15 g/day; 9 to 12 months of age, 6 to 11 g/day; 12 to 18 months of age, 5 to 8 g/day; 18 to 24 months of age, 3 to 7 g/day). Length growth is harder to assess but should be 0.2 to 0.4 mm/day in most children.

(Continued on page 222)

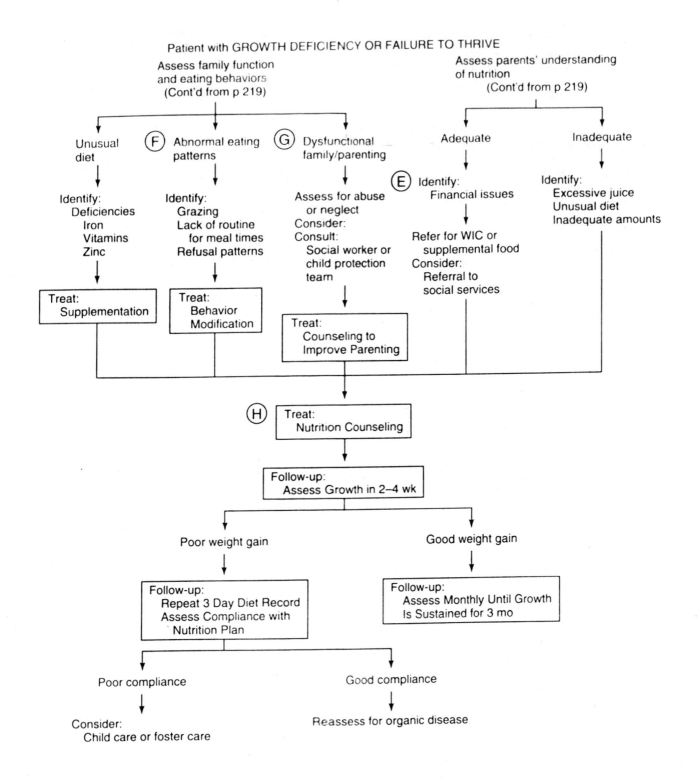

Patient with GROWTH DEFICIENCY OR FAILURE TO THRIVE

Assess family function
and eating behaviors
(Cont'd from p 219)

Assess parents' understanding
of nutrition
(Cont'd from p 219)

Unusual
diet

(F) Abnormal eating
patterns

(G) Dysfunctional
family/parenting

Adequate

Inadequate

Identify:
Deficiencies
Iron
Vitamins
Zinc

Identify:
Grazing
Lack of routine
for meal times
Refusal patterns

Assess for abuse
or neglect
Consider:
Consult:
Social worker or
child protection
team

(E) Identify:
Financial issues

Identify:
Excessive juice
Unusual diet
Inadequate amounts

Refer for WIC or
supplemental food
Consider:
Referral to
social services

Treat:
Supplementation

Treat:
Behavior
Modification

Treat:
Counseling to
Improve Parenting

(H) Treat:
Nutrition Counseling

Follow-up:
Assess Growth in 2–4 wk

Poor weight gain

Good weight gain

Follow-up:
Repeat 3 Day Diet Record
Assess Compliance with
Nutrition Plan

Follow-up:
Assess Monthly Until Growth
Is Sustained for 3 mo

Poor compliance

Good compliance

Consider:
Child care or foster care

Reassess for organic disease

I. When poor weight gain is associated with vomiting or rumination, consider gastroesophageal reflux, pyloric stenosis, duodenal stenosis or atresia, vascular rings, metabolic disease, renal disease, adrenal disease, or CNS disease (mass lesion, hydrocephalus, cerebral atrophy, subdural hematoma, infection).

J. When poor weight gain is associated with diarrhea or malabsorption, consider viral, bacterial, or parasitic enteritis, cystic fibrosis, celiac disease, milk protein intolerance, disaccharidase deficiencies, pancreatic insufficiency, short bowel syndrome, and inflammatory bowel disease. Diarrhea may also be seen with grazing.

K. Suspect a hypermetabolic state when adequate caloric intake does not result in weight gain. Possible causes include hyperthyroidism, diabetes mellitus, adrenal disorders, chronic infection, malignancy, inflammatory bowel disease, collagen vascular disease, and diencephalic syndrome.

L. Laboratory studies are helpful in identifying causes of organic growth deficiency only after a thorough history and complete physical examination have been performed. Order lab studies to confirm suspected diagnoses and not in a shotgun attempt to define possible causes.

References

Chatoor I, Egan J. Nonorganic failure to thrive and dwarfism due to food refusal: A separation disorder. J Am Assoc Child Psychiatry 1983; 22:294.

Chatoor I, Schaefer S, Dickson K, Egan J. Nonorganic failure to thrive: A developmental perspective. Pediatr Ann 1984; 13:829.

Fomon SJ. Infant nutrition. St. Louis: Mosby, 1993.

Frank DA, Zeisel SH. Failure to thrive. Pediatr Clin North Am 1988; 35:1187.

Pugliese MT, Wayman-Dawn M, Moses N, Lifshitz F. Parental health beliefs as a cause of non organic failure to thrive. Pediatrics 1987; 80:175.

Sills RH. Failure to thrive: The role of clinical and laboratory evaluation. Am J Dis Child 1978; 132:967.

Smith MM, Lifshitz F. Excess fruit juice consumption in failure to thrive. Pediatrics 1994; 93:438.

Weston JA, Colloton M. A legacy of violence in nonorganic failure to thrive. Child Abuse Negl 1993; 17:709.

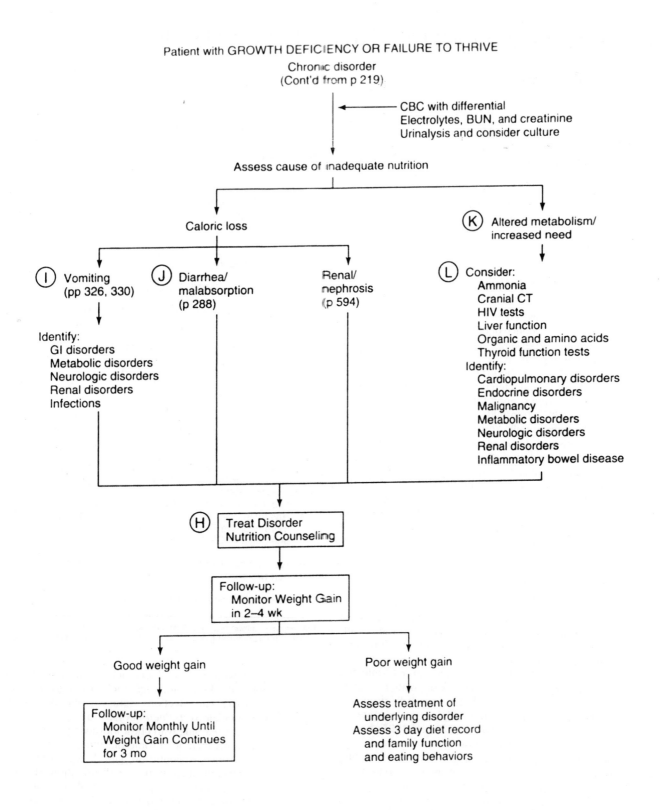

Patient with GROWTH DEFICIENCY OR FAILURE TO THRIVE
Chronic disorder
(Cont'd from p 219)

CBC with differential
Electrolytes, BUN, and creatinine
Urinalysis and consider culture

Assess cause of inadequate nutrition

Caloric loss

Ⓚ Altered metabolism/
increased need

Ⓘ Vomiting
(pp 326, 330)

Ⓙ Diarrhea/
malabsorption
(p 288)

Renal/
nephrosis
(p 594)

Ⓛ Consider:
Ammonia
Cranial CT
HIV tests
Liver function
Organic and amino acids
Thyroid function tests
Identify:
Cardiopulmonary disorders
Endocrine disorders
Malignancy
Metabolic disorders
Neurologic disorders
Renal disorders
Inflammatory bowel disease

Identify:
GI disorders
Metabolic disorders
Neurologic disorders
Renal disorders
Infections

Ⓗ Treat Disorder
Nutrition Counseling

Follow-up:
Monitor Weight Gain
in 2–4 wk

Good weight gain

Poor weight gain

Follow-up:
Monitor Monthly Until
Weight Gain Continues
for 3 mo

Assess treatment of
underlying disorder
Assess 3 day diet record
and family function
and eating behaviors

HUMAN IMMUNODEFICIENCY VIRUS INFECTION

Stephen Berman, M.D.

DEFINITION

HIV is a cytopathic human retrovirus that destroys CD_4 T helper lymphocytes and other cells, including macrophages that have CD_4 receptors. Table 1 shows the 1994 Centers for Disease Control and Prevention (CDC) diagnostic classification for infants born to HIV-infected mothers and children younger than 13 years of age. Table 2 shows the CDC definition of AIDS.

EPIDEMIOLOGY

In the United States children and adolescents account for 2% of AIDS cases. The incidence of HIV infection varies with risk factors for specific, especially minority, populations. As HIV infection is acquired more frequently from heterosexual intercourse, adolescents become more vulnerable. The average age at first sexual intercourse is 16 years, and one in four high school students report four or more sexual partners by twelfth grade. HIV is transmitted by blood, semen, cervical secretions, and human milk. Young children are infected by maternal transmission. In developed countries transmission by contaminated blood products is now rare. Intrauterine or intrapartum transmission, the most frequent cause of HIV-infected children, is increasing proportionately with the number of HIV-infected women of childbearing age. Older children and adolescents can also be infected through IV drug use. The risk of infection after a needlestick exposure to HIV-infected blood is about 0.3%. Among infected children the prognosis is worst for infants who develop AIDS during their first year of life and those who have *Pneumocystis carinii* pneumonia (PCP), progressive neurologic disease, or severe failure to thrive with wasting.

A. In the history ask about the types of infections suffered and the pathogens isolated. Document the onset, severity, response to therapy, pattern of infections, and current episodes of fevers and sweating. Relevant risk factors and family history include an HIV-infected parent or a parent from a high-risk population such as Haitians, Africans, those with a history of IV drug use, male homosexual activity, or multiple sexual partners; a history of transfusion between 1978 and 1985; hemophilia or other coagulation disorder and transfusion of blood products or clotting factor concentrates during the same period; and history of sexual or parenteral exposure to HIV. In addition, note immunization status and adverse reactions to vaccines, current medications (zidovudine [AZT], zalcitabine [DDC], didanosine [DDI], TMP-SMX); allergies; underlying conditions such as cardiopulmonary, GI, or renal disease; malignancies; and situations that further predispose to bacterial infection (indwelling catheters). CNS signs include developmental delay or deterioration of developmental milestones and motor skills, vision disturbances, seizures, recent alterations in the mental status and normal level of activity (playfulness, irritability, feeding and

TABLE 1 Diagnosis of HIV Infection in Children

HIV Infected

I. A child < 18 mo of age who is known to be HIV seropositive or born to an HIV-infected mother

    and

A. Has positive results on two separate determinations (excluding cord blood) from one or more of the following HIV detection tests:

    1. HIV culture
    2. HIV polymerase chain reaction
    3. HIV antigen

    or

B. Meets criteria for AIDS diagnosis based on the 1987 AIDS surveillance case definition.

II. A child ≥ 18 mo of age born to an HIV-infected mother or any child infected by blood, blood products, or other known modes of transmission (e.g., sexual contact) who

A. Is HIV-antibody positive by repeatedly reactive enzyme immunoassay (EIA) and confirmatory test (e.g., Western blot or immunofluorescence assay [IFA])

    or

B. Meets any of the criteria in I. above

Perinatally Exposed (prefix E)

I. A child who does not meet the criteria above who

A. Is HIV seropositive by EIA and confirmatory test (e.g., Western blot or IFA) and is < 18 mo of age at the time of test

    or

B. Has unknown antibody status but was born to a mother known to be infected with HIV

Seroreverter (SR)

I. A child who is born to an HIV-infected mother and who

A. Has been documented as HIV-antibody negative (i.e., two or more negative EIA tests performed at 6–18 mo of age or one negative EIA test after 18 mo of age)

    and

B. Has had no other laboratory evidence of infection (has not had two positive viral detection tests, if performed)

    and

C. Has not had an AIDS-defining condition

EIA, enzyme immunoassay; IFA, immunofluorescence assay.
Adapted from Diagnosing HIV infection in children. MMWR 1994; 43(RR-12):3.

sleeping patterns, social interactions with peers, and school work). Respiratory signs include cough, recurrent sore throats, ear infections, sinusitis, pneumonia episodes (especially with *Pneumocystis*), and periods of fast or difficult breathing with chest indrawing (retractions). GI symptoms include chronic diarrhea, weight loss or failure to thrive, malnutrition, jaundice, and hepatitis. Renal symptoms include pain with urination (dysuria), urinary frequency, flank pain, lower abdominal pain, dark or bloody urine, and edema. Ask about chronic candidal infection (thrush, vaginitis or involvement of other mucous membranes, skin, and nails), rashes, eczema, impetigo, and warts.

B. On physical examination look, listen, and feel for findings that suggest a current infection or HIV involvement of multiple organ systems. In the CNS these include microcephaly or signs of encephalopathy (too weak to feed, difficult to arouse, unresponsive, weak,

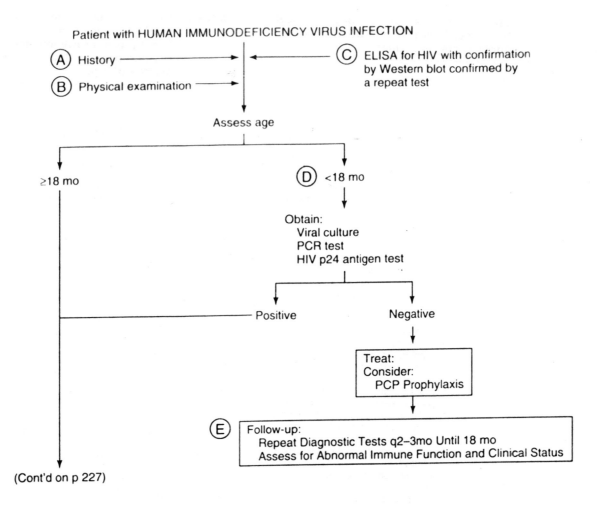

Patient with HUMAN IMMUNODEFICIENCY VIRUS INFECTION

(A) History

(B) Physical examination

(C) ELISA for HIV with confirmation by Western blot confirmed by a repeat test

Assess age

≥18 mo

(D) <18 mo

Obtain:
Viral culture
PCR test
HIV p24 antigen test

Positive

Negative

Treat:
Consider:
  PCP Prophylaxis

(E) Follow-up:
  Repeat Diagnostic Tests q2–3mo Until 18 mo
  Assess for Abnormal Immune Function and Clinical Status

(Cont'd on p 227)

disoriented, having seizures), personality change, developmental delay or loss of milestones, vision loss, ataxia, pseudobulbar palsy, myoclonus, increased tone, and spasticity. Check for dehydration and poor perfusion by assessing skin turgor, tears, moist mucous membranes, color and warmth of the extremities, and capillary refill time (> 2 seconds is abnormal). Look for retinitis, acute otitis media, salivary gland enlargement (parotitis), cervical adenopathy, tachypnea, retractions, grunting, wheezing, and crackles. Listen to the heart for gallop rhythm, murmurs, signs of congestive heart failure (tachypnea, tachycardia, lung crackles, hepatomegaly, and decreased peripheral pulses), and myocarditis. Identify any adenitis, soft-tissue cellulitis, or abscess (swelling, erythema, induration, warmth of tissue). Look for lymphadenopathy, splenomegaly, hepatomegaly, jaundice, failure to thrive, wasting, signs of nephropathy such as proteinuria, hematuria, and hypertension, and signs of bone or joint infection such as painful swelling with limitation of motion. Also look for an erythematous exanthem; hand, foot, and mouth lesions; *Candida* rashes; warts; vesicular lesions of herpes; petechiae; and purpura.

C. Enzyme-linked immunoabsorbent assay (ELISA) and Western blot detect antibody to HIV. Since the ELISA may be false-positive, it is necessary to confirm positives with a repeat ELISA and Western blot test. Polymerase

chain reaction (PCR) techniques to identify HIV DNA sequences, HIV p24 antigen assay, and HIV culture can also be used to diagnose HIV infection. Initially HIV-infected patients may have negative antibody tests. These patients can usually be diagnosed with cultures or antigen testing.

D. The transmission rate from infected mother to infant varies from 13% to 39%. The mechanism of transmission may be infection in utero, at delivery, or postpartum through breast feeding or contact with blood. Maternal risk factors for transmission include high viral concentrations identified by HIV p24 antigenemia, low peripheral CD_4 T lymphocyte counts, and advanced disease. Treatment of pregnant women who have mild disease with antepartum and intrapartum zidovudine followed by treatment of the newborn for 6 weeks reduces the risk of vertical transmission by about two thirds. The clinical course of HIV-infected neonates varies; the median age at onset of AIDS is 3.5 years, but 50% of infants with perinatal acquisition are symptomatic, and 5% to 15% develop AIDS within 6 months. Half of HIV-infected neonates survive to 8 years.

E. Diagnosis in infants is complicated by placental transfer of maternal antibodies against HIV, which may persist as long as 18 months. HIV infection can be proved in 95% of infections by 3 to 6 months of age using a

TABLE 2 CDC Surveillance Case Definition of AIDS: Diagnoses Indicative of AIDS in Children, Adolescents, and Adults

Age Group	Diagnoses
All ages	Candidiasis of the esophagus[a,b]
	Candidiasis of the trachea, bronchi, or lungs[a]
	Coccidioidomycosis, disseminated or extrapulmonary[c]
	Cryptococcosis, extrapulmonary[a]
	Cryptosporidiosis, chronic intestinal[a]
	Cytomegalovirus disease (other than liver, spleen, nodes) onset before 1 mo of age[a]
	Cytomegalovirus retinitis with loss of vision[a,b]
	Herpes simplex ulcer, chronic (>1 mo duration) or pneumonitis or esophagitis onset after 1 mo of age[a]
	HIV encephalopathy[c]
	Histoplasmosis, disseminated or extrapulmonary[c]
	Isoporiasis, chronic intestinal (>1 mo duration)[c]
	Kaposi sarcoma[a,b]
	Lymphoma, primary brain[a]
	Lymphoma (Burkitt, or immunoblastic sarcoma)[c]
	Mycobacterial infections: avium complex, *M. kansasii*[a] or *M. tuberculosis*[c]; other species or unidentified species, disseminated or extrapulmonary[b]
	Pneumocystis carinii pneumonia[a,b]
	Progressive multifocal leukoencephalopathy[a]
	Toxoplasmosis of brain, onset at 1 mo of age[a,b]
	Wasting syndrome due to HIV[c]
Children <13 yr	Lymphoid interstitial pneumonitis[a,b]
	Multiple or recurrent serious bacterial infections[c]
Adolescents ≥13 yr and adults	Cervical cancer, invasive[c]
	M. tuberculosis, pulmonary[c]
	Pneumonia, recurrent[c]
	Salmonella septicemia, recurrent[c]
	CD$_4$ T lymphocyte count <200 cells/mm^3 or a CD$_4$ percentage of <14[c]

[a]If indicator disease is diagnosed definitively (e.g., by biopsy or culture) and no other cause of immunodeficiency is present, laboratory documentation of HIV infection is not required.
[b]Presumptive diagnosis of indicator disease is accepted if laboratory evidence of HIV infection is present.
[c]Laboratory evidence of HIV infection is required.
Adapted from Centers for Disease Control and Prevention. 1993 revised classification system for HIV infection and expanded surveillance case definition for AIDS among adolescents and adults. MMWR. 1992; 41 (RR-17):19.

combination of viral culture, PCR, and HIV p24 antigen detection. HIV infection can also be diagnosed by the combination of HIV antibody, evidence of both cellular and humoral deficiency, and illnesses considered evidence of symptomatic infection, or by symptoms meeting the CDC case definition of AIDS. Follow seropositive infants with negative cultures and other diagnostic tests with ELISA and Western blot tests and CD$_4$ lymphocyte values every 3 months for the first year and then at 18 and 24 months. Consider prophylaxis with TMP-SMX for *Pneumocystis* (Table 3) during the first year, while the diagnosis is still uncertain. When HIV

TABLE 3 Recommendations for Initiation of *Pneumocystis carinii* Pneumonia Prophylaxis for HIV-infected or HIV-seropositive Children Less Than 12 Months of Age

Age	Prophylaxis
Birth to 6 wk	No prophylaxis
6 wk–4 mo	Everyone, including indeterminate infections
4–12 mo	Prophylaxis for documented infections
1–2 yr	Prophylaxis if CD$_4$ <750 mm^3 or <15% of total lymphocytes
2–6 yr	Prophylaxis if CD$_4$ <500 mm^3 or <15% of total lymphocytes
6–12 yr	Prophylaxis if CD$_4$ <200 mm^3 or <15% of total lymphocytes

Data from Presentation 1994 AIDS Clinical Trials Group Meeting.

antibody is negative by 18 months and other diagnostic tests (culture, PCR, and p24 antigen) are negative, the child is an uninfected seroreverter.

F. Laboratory findings associated with HIV infection include a decrease in the absolute number of T lymphocytes (often suggested by lymphopenia); a decrease in the number of CD$_4$ relative to the number of CD$_8$ cells (or total T lymphocytes), and HIV p24 antigenemia. These markers correlate with progression of disease in children less than in adults. Early in the disease B lymphocytes are usually normal in number and serum IgG is often very high.

G. While HIV infection is uniformly fatal, children should receive the best care available. Assess the child's state with respect to the CDC classification to determine the need for antiretroviral treatment, other therapy, and prophylaxis (Table 4).

H. Oral zidovudine is the first line of HIV therapy (Table 5). Treatment can improve laboratory findings of immune function and decrease antigenemia as well as stabilize or improve the clinical condition (especially neurodevelopmental status and failure to thrive) for long periods. Modify the dosage in children with progressive neurologic disease and preexisting anemia and neutropenia. Monitor patients for drug toxicity (anemia and neutropenia) by obtaining a CBC with differential and reticulocyte count every 2 to 4 weeks during the first 2 months of therapy, then less frequently. To determine whether worsening anemia or neutropenia is related to the drug or the disease, it may be helpful either to reduce the dose by 30% or to discontinue the drug. If the presumed toxic effect improves, try to maintain the child with a reduced dose. If the condition does not improve when the drug is discontinued, consider changing the drug and/or instituting corrective therapy (blood transfusions or erythropoietin). Follow the status of the disease with clinical assessments, including neurodevelopmental testing every 1 to 3 months and with laboratory tests of liver and kidney function (electrolytes, BUN, creatinine, liver enzymes) and lymphocyte subsets every 3 months depending on the progression of the disease.

I. Several general principles apply to immunization in these patients. HIV-infected children are likely to have

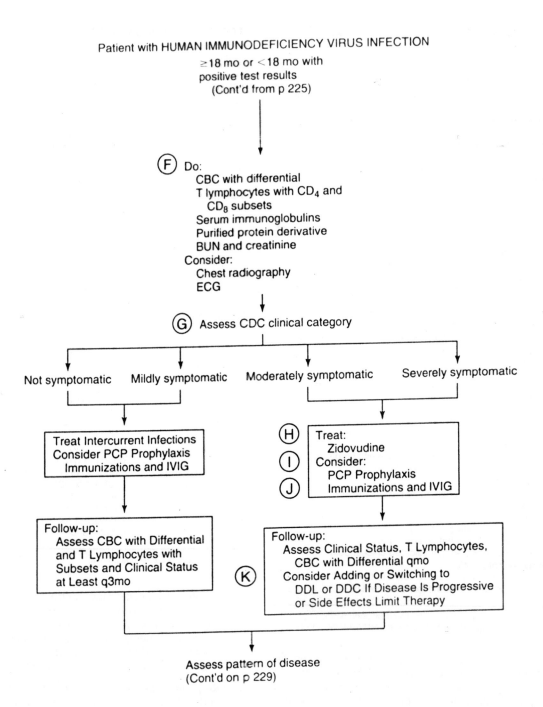

Patient with HUMAN IMMUNODEFICIENCY VIRUS INFECTION
≥18 mo or <18 mo with
positive test results
(Cont'd from p 225)

(F) Do:
CBC with differential
T lymphocytes with CD_4 and
CD_8 subsets
Serum immunoglobulins
Purified protein derivative
BUN and creatinine
Consider:
Chest radiography
ECG

(G) Assess CDC clinical category

Not symptomatic   Mildly symptomatic   Moderately symptomatic   Severely symptomatic

Treat Intercurrent Infections
Consider PCP Prophylaxis
Immunizations and IVIG

(H) (I) (J) Treat:
Zidovudine
Consider:
PCP Prophylaxis
Immunizations and IVIG

Follow-up:
Assess CBC with Differential
and T Lymphocytes with
Subsets and Clinical Status
at Least q3mo

(K) Follow-up:
Assess Clinical Status, T Lymphocytes,
CBC with Differential qmo
Consider Adding or Switching to
DDL or DDC If Disease Is Progressive
or Side Effects Limit Therapy

Assess pattern of disease
(Cont'd on p 229)

family members who are immunosuppressed. Live attenuated-virus vaccines, such as oral poliovirus vaccine, can cause serious harm to immunocompromised hosts; therefore, inactivated polio vaccine should be substituted. However, wild infections, i.e., with measles in patients with HIV, can be devastating; therefore, they should receive MMR vaccine. Patients are at increased risk for infections caused by *Haemophilus influenzae, Pneumococcus,* and influenza virus due to underlying immunodeficiency; give HIB (*H. influenzae* type B), Pneumovax (>2 years), and influenza vaccines. Unfortunately, these children may not respond to vaccines as well as normal children. Children exposed to measles and varicella should receive immunoglobin therapy.

J. HIV-infected children are susceptible to frequent and persistent invasive bacterial infections because of impaired B cell antibody immune function. In addition to treating episodes with IV antibiotics, try to prevent bacterial and viral infections with IV immunoglobulin (IVIG) in children who have any of the following indications: (1) hypogammaglobulinemia (IgG < 250 mg/ml), (2) recurrent serious bacterial infections, (3) failure to form antibodies to common antigens, (4) failure to develop antibodies to two doses of MMR vaccine who live where measles is prevalent.

K. Add or switch to DDI when 4 to 6 months of zidovudine has failed to halt progression of HIV disease (failure to thrive, neurologic deterioration, development of end

TABLE 4 Clinical Categories of Children with HIV infection

N: Not Symptomatic

Children who have no signs or symptoms considered to be the result of HIV infection or who have only one of the conditions listed in category A

A: Mildly Symptomatic

Children with two or more of the conditions listed below but none of the conditions listed in categories B and C

- Lymphadenopathy (≥ 0.5 cm at more than two sites; bilateral counts as one site)
- Hepatomegaly
- Splenomegaly
- Dermatitis
- Parotitis
- Recurrent or persistent upper respiratory infection, sinusitis, or otitis media

B: Moderately Symptomatic

Children who have symptomatic conditions other than those listed for category A or C that are attributed to HIV infection. Examples of conditions in clinical category B include but are not limited to the following:

- Anemia (< 8 g/dl), neutropenia ($< 1000/mm^3$), or thrombocytopenia ($< 100,000/mm^3$) persisting ≥ 30 days
- Bacterial meningitis, pneumonia, or sepsis (single episode)
- Candidiasis, oropharyngeal (thrush), persisting (> 2 mo) in children age > 6 mo
- Cardiomyopathy
- Cytomegalovirus infection with onset before age 1 mo
- Diarrhea, recurrent or chronic
- Hepatitis
- HSV stomatitis (more than two episodes within 1 yr)
- HSV bronchitis, pneumonitis, or esophagitis with onset before age 1 mo
- Herpes zoster (shingles) involving at least two distinct episodes or more than one dermatorme
- Leiomyosarcoma
- LIP or pulmonary lymphoid hyperplasia complex
- Nephropathy
- Nocardiosis
- Persistent fever (lasting > 1 mo)
- Toxoplasmosis, onset before age 1 mo
- Varicella, disseminated (complicated chickenpox)

C: Severely Symptomatic

Children who have any condition listed in the 1987 surveillance case definition for AIDS, with the exception of LIP

HSV, herpes simplex virus; LIP, lymphoid interstitial pneumonia.
Adapted from Diagnosing HIV infection in children. MMWR 1994; 43(RR-12):6.

TABLE 5 Therapies for HIV

Drug	Dosage	Product Availability
Intravenous gamma globulin	400 mg/kg q4wk to prevent bacterial infections 500–1000 mg/kg/day for 3–5 days for thrombocytopenia 600 mg/kg q4wk for bronchiectasis	Vials: 30, 60, 120 mg/ml
TMP-SMX	20 mg/kg/day IV for 14–21 days for PCP; 5 mg/kg TMP/dose b.i.d. 3 times a week for PCP prophylaxis	Injection: 16 mg TMP, 80 mg SMX Susp: 40 TMP/200 mg SMX/5 ml Tabs: 80 mg TMP/400 mg SMX
Pentamidine	4 mg/kg/day IV for 14–21 days for PCP	Injection: 300 mg
Methylprednisolone	0.5 mg/kg/dose q6h (max 40 mg) for 7–10 days	Injection: 40, 125, 500 mg, 1 g
Zidovudine (Retrovir)	0–6 wk of age: 2 mg/kg/dose PO q6h; 6 wk–13 yr: 180 mg/m²/dose PO q6h; > 13 yr: max 500 mg/day	Caps: 100 mg Liquid: 50 mg/5 ml
DDI (Videx)	90–135 mg/m²/dose PO q12h	Susp: 10 mg/ml
Ganciclovir (Cytovene)	5 mg/kg/dose IV q12h for 14–21 days, then 5 mg/kg qd (or 5 of 7 days/wk) for maintenance	Injection: 500 mg

PCP, Pneumocystis carinii pneumonia.

organ disease such as cardiomyopathy) or when the patient cannot tolerate zidovudine. Adverse reactions to DDI are pancreatitis in 5% of children and in 5% peripheral retinal depigmentation that is not associated with vision defects. Combination treatments with protease inhibitors are promising.

L. HIV-associated nephropathy, usually identified on biopsy as focal segmental glomerulosclerosis or diffuse mesangial hyperplasia, can progress to renal failure. Other causes of renal disease in HIV-infected patients include effects of nephrotoxic drugs, acute tubular necrosis, infections, and an infiltrative process (malignancy).

M. Hematologic abnormalities are common in HIV-infected children and must be followed closely. Anemia is almost universal and may require transfusions with irradiated CMV-negative buff coat-poor blood. Severe anemia resistant to therapy may require an evaluation to rule out a specific cause such as lymphoma, infection, or bone marrow infiltrative disorder. Any thrombocytopenia is usually due to platelet destruction. When thrombocytopenia becomes life threatening, treatment options in addition to antiviral agents include IV γ-globulin, corticosteroids, and splenectomy.

N. Respiratory disease is common in HIV-infected children and is the most common cause of death. Rapid onset and progression of respiratory distress suggests an acute infection and/or congestive heart failure. Infections with *Pneumocystis*, bacterial pathogens, common viral respiratory pathogens (respiratory syncytial virus, parainfluenza, influenza, and adenovirus) are most common. Tuberculosis, mycobacterium avium-intracellulare, cytomegalovirus (CMV), and while less frequent, other opportunistic agents must also be considered (Table 6). Acute distress can also arise from reactive airway disease. More slowly progressive disease is compatible with PCP, other opportunistic pathogens (*Mycobacterium avium*, fungi) and lymphocytic interstitial pneumonitis. This condition may be related to a lymphproliferative response to Epstein-Barr virus DNA in lung tissue.

(Continued on page 230)

Patient with HUMAN IMMUNODEFICIENCY VIRUS INFECTION
Assess pattern of disease
(Cont'd from p 227)

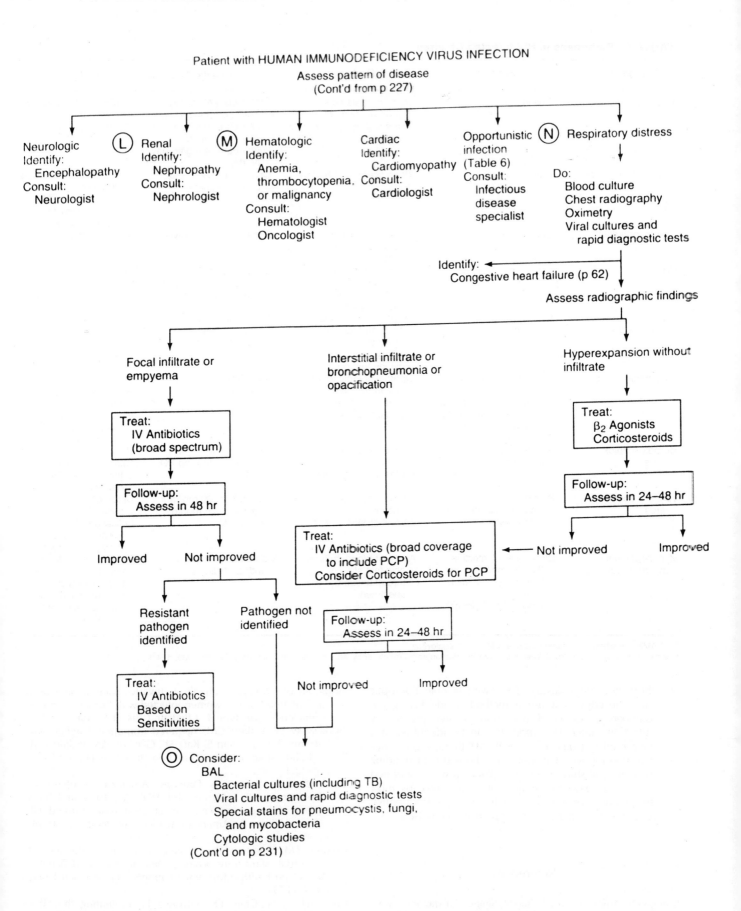

Neurologic
Identify:
  Encephalopathy
Consult:
  Neurologist

(L) Renal
Identify:
  Nephropathy
Consult:
  Nephrologist

(M) Hematologic
Identify:
  Anemia,
  thrombocytopenia,
  or malignancy
Consult:
  Hematologist
  Oncologist

Cardiac
Identify:
  Cardiomyopathy
Consult:
  Cardiologist

Opportunistic
infection
(Table 6)
Consult:
  Infectious
  disease
  specialist

(N) Respiratory distress

Do:
  Blood culture
  Chest radiography
  Oximetry
  Viral cultures and
    rapid diagnostic tests

Identify:
  Congestive heart failure (p 62)

Assess radiographic findings

Focal infiltrate or
empyema

Interstitial infiltrate or
bronchopneumonia or
opacification

Hyperexpansion without
infiltrate

Treat:
  IV Antibiotics
  (broad spectrum)

Treat:
  β_2 Agonists
  Corticosteroids

Follow-up:
  Assess in 48 hr

Follow-up:
  Assess in 24–48 hr

Improved   Not improved

Treat:
  IV Antibiotics (broad coverage
    to include PCP)
  Consider Corticosteroids for PCP

Not improved   Improved

Resistant
pathogen
identified

Pathogen not
identified

Follow-up:
  Assess in 24–48 hr

Treat:
  IV Antibiotics
  Based on
  Sensitivities

Not improved   Improved

(O) Consider:
  BAL
    Bacterial cultures (including TB)
    Viral cultures and rapid diagnostic tests
    Special stains for pneumocystis, fungi,
      and mycobacteria
    Cytologic studies
(Cont'd on p 231)

TABLE 6 Pathogens in HIV-infected Children

Organism	Syndrome	Diagnosis	Treatment	Comments
Pneumocystis carinii	Pneumonia	Pneumocysts seen on special stains of respiratory specimen or tissue	TMP-SMX (20 mg/kg TMP component/day IV, PO) or pentamidine isethionate Isethionate (4 mg/kg/day IV, IM)	Toxic effects of therapy common Treat 21 days
Toxoplasma gondii	Brain abscess	Brain scans and biopsy	Oral sulfadiazine and pyrimethamine	Toxic effects of therapy common Use folinic acid; lifelong therapy to prevent relapse
Cryptosporidium	Gastroenteritis	Stool examination (special procedure), biopsies	Consider paromomycin	Chronic infection
Candida	Thrush, esophagitis	Wet mount or Gram stain of lesions (thrush) Esophagoscopy and biopsy (esophagus)	Nystatin, clotrimazole, ketoconazole, fluconazole amphotericin B	Relapses common Consider maintenance therapy but be wary of resistance
Cryptococcus neoformans	Meningitis, fungemia, pneumonia	Cryptococcal antigen tests on blood, CSF Culture of blood, respiratory specimen, CSF India ink test on CSF	Amphotericin B Flucytosine can be used if tolerated	Chronic suppressive therapy with flucytosine required to prevent relapse
Cytomegalovirus	Chorioretinitis, pneumonitis, hepatitis, colitis, esophagitis, encephalitis, disseminated CMV (including adrenals) $CD_4 < 100/mm^3$	Ophthalmologic examination (retinitis), tissue biopsy, culture (urine, sputum, buffy coat)	Ganciclovir (investigational)	Relapses after therapy Suppressive regimen required Isolation of virus does not alone provide diagnosis
Herpes simplex virus	Stomatitis, perianal infection	Tzanck preparation, culture FA test or skin smear	Acyclovir (750 mg/m²/day IV, or 400 mg PO t.i.d.)	Recurrences frequent Chronic suppressive therapy may be needed
Varicella zoster virus	Primary varicella, local or disseminated zoster	Tzanck preparation, culture FA test or skin smear	Acyclovir (1500 mg/m²/day IV or 20 mg/kg PO q.i.d.)	Chronic or relapsing zoster lesions Indications for effectiveness of oral therapy not clear
Mycobacterium avium-intracellulare	Disseminated infection (blood, bone marrow, liver, spleen, GI tract, nodes) Usually <50 CD₄/mm³	Acid-fast blood culture, acid-fast stain or culture of tissue or fluid specimen	Combination therapy with 2–4 drugs	Drugs used include clarithromycin, rifabutin, clofazimine, ethambutal, amikacin, isoniazid, ethionamide

TMP-SMX, trimethoprim-sulfamethoxazole; CMV, cytomegalovirus.
Modified from Falloon J, Eddy J, Wiener L, Pizza PA. Human immunodeficiency virus infection in children. J Pediatr 1989; 114:1.

O. Bronchoalveolar lavage (BAL) with flexible fiberoptic bronchoscopy is a useful method of identifying the pathogens associated with unresponsive pulmonary infection. Since *Pneumocystis* can be identified in a lavage after 4 days of IV TMP-SMX therapy, presumptive therapy for PCP should not be withheld pending BAL. In one study pathogenic bacteria were identified in 57% of lavages, fungi in 42% (*C. albicans* most frequently), viruses in 29% (CMV most frequently), *Pneumocystis* in 22%, and mycobacteria in 14%.

References

Abadco DL, Amaro-Galvez R, Rao M, Steiner P. Experience with flexible fiberoptic bronchoscopy with bronchoalveolar lavage as a diagnostic tool in children with AIDS. Am J Dis Child 1992; 146:1056.

Andiman WA, Mezger J, Shapiro E. Invasive bacterial infections in children born to women infected with human immunodeficiency virus type 1. J Pediatr 1994; 124:846.

Borkowsky W, Wilfert CM. Acquired immunodeficiency syndrome. In: Krugman S, Katz SL, Gershon AA, Wilfert CM, eds. Infectious diseases of children. 9th ed. St. Louis: Mosby, 1992:1.

Committee on Infectious Diseases, American Academy of Pediatrics. HIV infection and AIDS. In: 1994 Red book report of the committee on infectious disease. 23rd ed. Elk Grove Village, IL: American Academy of Pediatrics, 1994: 254.

Conner EM, Sperling RS, Gelber R, et al. Reduction of maternal-infant transmission of human immunodeficiency virus type 1 with zidovudine treatment. N Engl J Med 1994; 331:1173.

Cunningham SJ, Crain EF, Bernstein LJ. Evaluating the HIV-infected child with pulmonary signs and symptoms. Pediatr Emerg Care 1991; 7:32.

Farley JJ, King JC Jr, Nair P, et al. Invasive pneumococcal disease

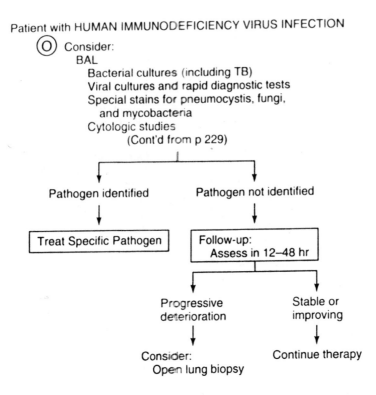

Patient with HUMAN IMMUNODEFICIENCY VIRUS INFECTION

Ⓞ Consider:
BAL
Bacterial cultures (including TB)
Viral cultures and rapid diagnostic tests
Special stains for pneumocystis, fungi,
and mycobacteria
Cytologic studies
(Cont'd from p 229)

Pathogen identified → Treat Specific Pathogen

Pathogen not identified → Follow-up:
Assess in 12–48 hr

Progressive deterioration → Consider:
Open lung biopsy

Stable or improving → Continue therapy

among infected and uninfected children of mothers with human immunodeficiency virus infection. J Pediatr 1994; 124:853.

Husson RN, Shirasaka T, Butler KM, et al. High-level resistance to zidovudine but not to zalcitabine or didanosine in human immunodeficiency virus from children receiving antiretroviral therapy. J Pediatr 1993; 123:9.

Mueller BU, Butler KM, Stocker VL, et al. Clinical and pharmacokinetic evaluation of long-term therapy with didanosine in children with HIV infection. Pediatrics 1994; 94:724.

The National Institutes of Health-University of California Expert Panel for Corticosteroids as Adjunctive Therapy for Pneumocystis Pneumonia. Consensus statement on the use of corticosteroids as adjunctive therapy for Pneumocystis pneumonia. N Engl J Med 1990; 323:1500.

Ogino MT, Dankner WM, Spector SA. Development and significance of zidovudine resistance in children infected with human immunodeficiency virus. J Pediatr 1993; 123:1.

Peckham C, Gibb D. Current concepts: Mother-to-child transmission of the human immunodeficiency virus. N Engl J Med 1995; 333:298.

Prober CG, Gershon AA. Medical management of newborns and infants born to human immunodeficiency virus-seropositive mothers. Pediatr Infect Dis J 1991; 10:684.

Spector SA, Gelber RD, McGrath N, et al. A controlled trial of intravenous immune globulin for the prevention of serious bacterial infections in children receiving zidovudine for advanced human immunodeficiency virus infection. N Engl J Med 1994; 331:1181.

Wilfert CM, Pizzo PA. A blueprint for care, treatment, and prevention of HIV/AIDS in children. Pediatr Infect Dis J 1994; 13:920.

Working Group on Antiretroviral Therapy: National Pediatric HIV Resource Center. Antiretroviral therapy and medical management of the human immunodeficiency virus infected child. Pediatr Infect Dis J 1993; 12:513.

KAWASAKI DISEASE

Stephen Berman, M.D.

DEFINITION

Kawasaki disease, a multisystem vasculitis, is characterized by fever for at least 5 days with four of the following five signs in the absence of a known disease or infection: (1) bilateral conjunctival hyperemia; (2) mouth lesions consisting of dry, fissured lips, injected pharynx, or a strawberry tongue; (3) changes of peripheral extremities such as edema, erythema, or induration of hands and feet and desquamation 10 to 20 days after onset of fever; (4) a nonvesicular erythematous rash (morbilliform, maculopapular, scarlatiniform, or erythema multiforme); and (5) lymphadenopathy, often cervical, with enlargement of a node to more than 1.5 cm in diameter. Patients with fever and fewer than four of these features can be diagnosed with Kawasaki disease when coronary artery disease is detected. Additional findings that may present within 3 weeks include arthritis or arthralgia, diarrhea, abdominal pain, hepatitis, obstructive jaundice, acute hydrops of the gallbladder, aseptic meningitis, urethritis, and cardiac disease. The median age for onset of Kawasaki disease is 2 years, most patients being younger than 5 years. Infants less than 6 months of age who have Kawasaki disease may fail to meet the case definition. These patients appear to be at increased risk for severe disease and coronary artery aneurysm. An association with carpet cleaning has been described.

A. Laboratory evaluation may show leukocytosis, thrombocytosis (approximately 1 to 2 weeks after onset), high sedimentation rate, and sterile pyuria. Identify *Streptococcus pyogenes* pharyngitis. Uveitis is seen in 80% of cases on slit-lamp examination during the first week of illness.

B. Patients with very severe illness have unstable vital signs (shock), severe dehydration, myocarditis, constrictive pericarditis, or signs of congestive heart failure.

C. During the acute symptomatic phase of the illness (initial 14 days) treat with oral aspirin 80 to 100 mg/kg/day. Continue high-dose aspirin longer if fever or other signs of active inflammation persist or develop. Monitor serum salicylate levels (18 to 28 mg/dl) and follow for signs of toxicity such as vomiting, hyperpnea, lethargy, and liver function alterations. When acute signs resolve, lower aspirin to 3 to 5 mg/kg/day for 6 to 8 weeks for patients without coronary artery findings and indefinitely for patients with those findings. If the patient on aspirin develops varicella infection or influenza, switch to dipyrimadole, an alternative antiplatelet drug, to prevent Reye syndrome.

D. As early in the course of the illness as is feasible after the diagnosis is established, treat with IV gamma globulin 2 g/kg given during 10 to 12 hours as a single dose to prevent coronary artery lesions. Treatment is most effective when given during the first 10 days of the illness; treatment of symptomatic cases after the tenth day is controversial. Side effects include fever, chills, back pain, and headaches. Anaphylaxis is rare. Immunoglobulin preparations have been screened for hepatitis and human immunodeficiency viruses. Measles-mumps-rubella vaccine should not be given within 5 months of treatment.

E. Cardiac complications include pericardial effusion, myocarditis with arrhythmias or congestive heart failure, coronary artery aneurysms, late coronary artery occlusion with myocardial infarction, acute and chronic

(Continued on page 234)

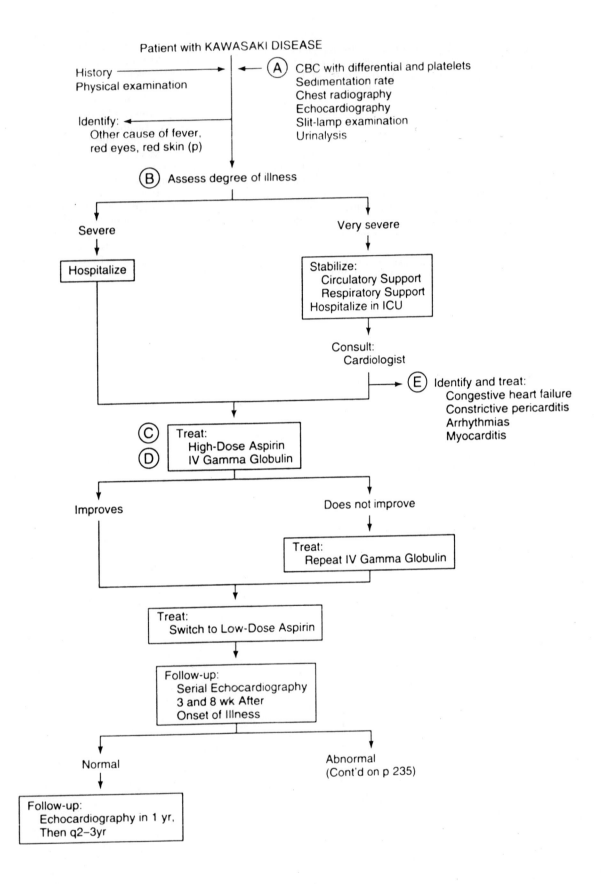

Patient with KAWASAKI DISEASE

History ——————————→ ←——— (A) CBC with differential and platelets
Physical examination   Sedimentation rate
                                  Chest radiography
                                  Echocardiography
Identify: ←————   Slit-lamp examination
    Other cause of fever,   Urinalysis
    red eyes, red skin (p)

(B) Assess degree of illness

Severe   Very severe

Hospitalize   Stabilize:
                                             Circulatory Support
                                             Respiratory Support
                                         Hospitalize in ICU

                                         Consult:
                                             Cardiologist

                                                 ——→ (E) Identify and treat:
                                                             Congestive heart failure
                                                             Constrictive pericarditis
                                                             Arrhythmias
(C) Treat: Myocarditis
(D)   High-Dose Aspirin
         IV Gamma Globulin

Improves   Does not improve

                                         Treat:
                                             Repeat IV Gamma Globulin

Treat:
    Switch to Low-Dose Aspirin

Follow-up:
    Serial Echocardiography
    3 and 8 wk After
    Onset of Illness

Normal   Abnormal
                                                  (Cont'd on p 235)

Follow-up:
    Echocardiography in 1 yr,
    Then q2–3yr

valvulitis, and aneurysms of the aorta and other noncoronary arteries. Patients who develop giant coronary aneurysms (≥ 8 mm) are at high risk for obstruction and myocardial ischemia. Deaths are most frequent between days 20 and 40 of the illness.

References

Akagi T, Rose V, Benson LN, et al. Outcome of coronary artery aneurysms after Kawasaki disease. J Pediatr 1992; 121:689.

Burns JC, Mason WH, Glode MP, et al. Clinical and epidemiologic characteristics of patients referred for evaluation of possible Kawasaki disease. J Pediatr 1991; 118:680.

Burns JC, Wiggins JW, Toews WH, et al. Clinical spectrum of Kawasaki disease in infants younger than 6 months of age. J Pediatr 1986; 109:759.

Kato H, Inoue O, Akagi T. Kawasaki disease: Cardiac problems and management. Pediatr Rev 1988; 9:209.

Melish ME. Kawasaki syndrome. In: Krugman S, Katz SL, Gershon AE, Wilfert C, eds. Infectious diseases of children. 9th ed. St. Louis: Mosby, 1992:211.

Newburger JW, Takahashi M, Beiser AS, et al. A single intravenous infusion of gamma globulin as compared with four infusions in the treatment of acute Kawasaki syndrome. N Engl J Med 1991; 324:1633.

Newburger JW, Takahashi M, Burns JC, et al. The treatment of Kawasaki syndrome with intravenous gamma globulin. N Engl J Med 1986; 315:341.

NIH Consensus Conference. Intravenous immunoglobulin: Prevention and treatment of disease. JAMA 1990; 264:3189.

Rosenfeld EA, Corydon KE, Shulman ST. Kawasaki disease in infants less than one year of age. J Pediatr 1995; 126:524.

Shulman ST, Bass JL, Bierman F, et al. Management of Kawasaki syndrome: A consensus statement prepared by North American participants of the Third International Kawasaki Disease Symposium, Tokyo, Japan, December, 1988. Pediatr Infect Dis J 1989; 8:663.

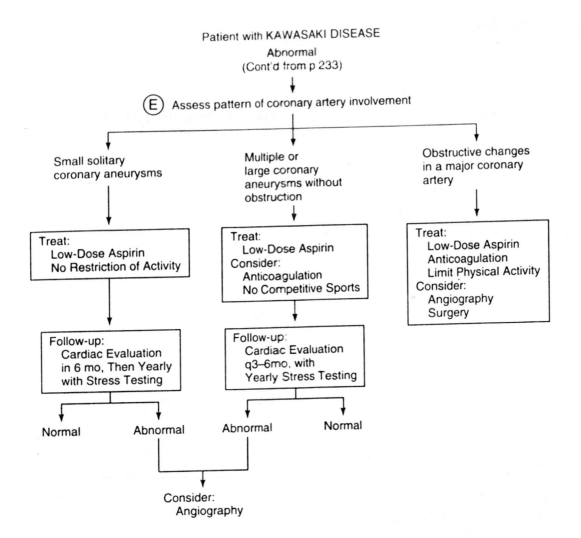

Patient with KAWASAKI DISEASE
Abnormal
(Cont'd from p 233)

(E) Assess pattern of coronary artery involvement

Small solitary coronary aneurysms

Treat:
  Low-Dose Aspirin
  No Restriction of Activity

Follow-up:
  Cardiac Evaluation in 6 mo, Then Yearly with Stress Testing

Normal   Abnormal

Multiple or large coronary aneurysms without obstruction

Treat:
  Low-Dose Aspirin
Consider:
  Anticoagulation
  No Competitive Sports

Follow-up:
  Cardiac Evaluation q3–6mo, with Yearly Stress Testing

Abnormal   Normal

Consider:
  Angiography

Obstructive changes in a major coronary artery

Treat:
  Low-Dose Aspirin
  Anticoagulation
  Limit Physical Activity
Consider:
  Angiography
  Surgery

LYME DISEASE

Stephen Berman, M.D.

DEFINITION

Lyme disease is a multisystem immune-mediated inflammatory disorder caused by infection with *Borrelia burgdorferi,* a spirochete. The disease is transmitted by the bite of a tick and has been confirmed on at least three continents.

A. In the history ask about exposure to ticks and tick bites and development of skin rashes and/or a flulike illness. Generalized symptoms of fever, malaise, fatigue, conjunctivitis, sore throat, arthralgias, nausea, vomiting, stiff neck, and headache often accompany the initial rash.

B. In the physical examination note skin lesions. The initial manifestation, usually developing 4 to 20 days after the tick bite, is erythema migrans (seen in 30% to 60% of cases). This skin lesion starts as an erythematous papule and expands to a large red lesion that may reach a diameter of 60 cm. The lesion may resemble cellulitis, the center may vesiculate or ulcerate, and secondary lesions may develop. The lesion is present for about 4 to 6 weeks but may recur during the following year. Additional signs may include lymphadenopathy, hepatomegaly (anicteric hepatitis), splenomegaly, and testicular swelling.

C. Assess the pattern of disease. Lyme disease has early and late stages. Early localized disease is limited to a skin lesion of erythema migrans with fever, headache, and myalgia. Early disseminated disease occurs when secondary erythema migrans lesions develop within several weeks and/or there is involvement of the nervous system (aseptic meningitis, facial nerve palsy, encephalitis) or heart (heart block or myocarditis). Late disease occurs months after the initial infection, usually as arthritis of the large joints such as knees and rarely with neurologic disease or keratitis. Without treatment the arthritis usually lasts several weeks but recurs. It can become recurrent or persistent and debilitating.

D. Treat early localized disease accompanied by erythema migrans, arthralgias, headaches, and other early manifestations with oral tetracycline (for children 8 years of age and older) or ampicillin (for younger children) for 10 days. Erythromycin can be used by patients allergic to penicillin (Table 1).

E. Treatment of early disease appears to prevent the manifestations of late disease. Follow-up should continue for 6 months. All symptoms and signs should resolve during this period, and patients should be asymptomatic. Advise patients to take appropriate precautions for preventing further tick bites such as protective clothing, use of insect repellents, and inspection for tick bites.

F. Treat patients with early disseminated disease having neurologic or cardiac complications with intravenous high-dose penicillin G or ceftriaxone for 10 to 14 days.

G. Cardiac manifestations usually develop 3 to 21 weeks after the bite and include arrhythmias, atrioventricular block, myocarditis, and left ventricular dysfunction. Carditis most often resolves within 6 weeks. Consider aspirin and/or prednisone for those with cardiac involvement who fail to respond to antibiotics. Efficacy data on the antiinflammatory agents are limited.

H. Neurologic abnormalities can be present initially but more often develop 4 to 6 weeks after the tick bite. The most frequent manifestations are meningitis, encephalitis, cranial nerve palsies (Bell's palsy), and peripheral radiculoneuropathies. Less common are transverse myelitis, Guillain-Barré syndrome, cerebellar ataxia, and pseudotumor cerebri. Neurologic abnormalities may progress in untreated cases over months or years

TABLE 1 Drugs Used in the Treatment of Lyme Disease

Drugs	Dosage	Product Availability
Antibiotics		
Amoxicillin	15 mg/kg/dose PO t.i.d.	Liquid: 125, 250 mg/5 ml Tabs: 250, 500 mg
Ceftriaxone	50–80 mg/kg/dose q24h IV or IM (max 2 g/day)	Vials: 0.25, 0.5, 1, 2 g
Doxycycline	2–5 mg/kg/day qd to b.i.d. (max 200 mg/day)	Tabs: 50, 100 mg Caps: 50, 100 mg Susp: 25, 50 mg/ 5 ml
Erythromycin ethyl succinate	10 mg/kg/dose PO q.i.d.	Susp: 200, 400 mg/5 ml Tabs: 200, 400 mg
Penicillin G sodium	50,000–75,000 U/kg/dose q6h IV (max 20 million U/day)	Vial: 5 million U
Antiinflammatory agents		
Aspirin	15 mg/kg/dose PO q.i.d.	Tabs: 65, 81, 325, 500, 650 mg
Prednisone	0.5–1 mg/kg/dose PO b.i.d. (max 40 mg/dose)	Liquid: 5 mg/5 ml Tabs: 2.5, 5, 10, 20, 50 mg

(Continued on page 238)

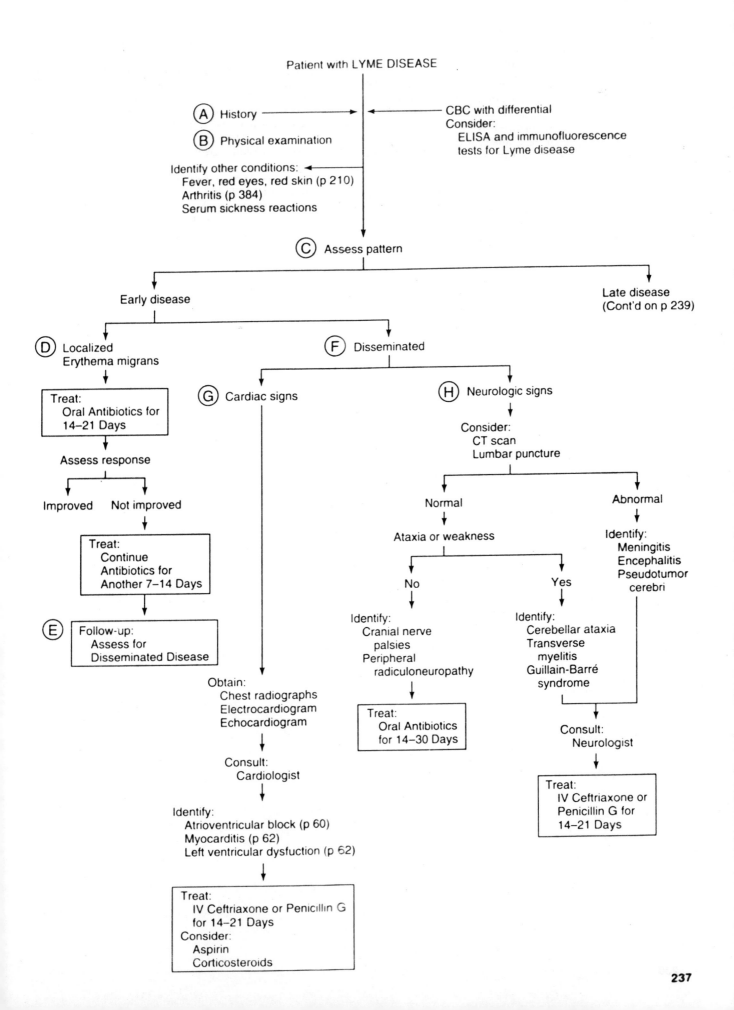

Patient with LYME DISEASE

Ⓐ History

Ⓑ Physical examination

CBC with differential
Consider:
   ELISA and immunofluorescence
   tests for Lyme disease

Identify other conditions:
   Fever, red eyes, red skin (p 210)
   Arthritis (p 384)
   Serum sickness reactions

Ⓒ Assess pattern

Early disease

Late disease
(Cont'd on p 239)

Ⓓ Localized
Erythema migrans

Treat:
   Oral Antibiotics for
   14–21 Days

Assess response

Improved   Not improved

Treat:
   Continue
   Antibiotics for
   Another 7–14 Days

Ⓔ Follow-up:
   Assess for
   Disseminated Disease

Ⓕ Disseminated

Ⓖ Cardiac signs

Ⓗ Neurologic signs

Consider:
   CT scan
   Lumbar puncture

Normal

Abnormal

Ataxia or weakness

Identify:
   Meningitis
   Encephalitis
   Pseudotumor
   cerebri

No   Yes

Identify:
   Cranial nerve
   palsies
   Peripheral
   radiculoneuropathy

Identify:
   Cerebellar ataxia
   Transverse
   myelitis
   Guillain-Barré
   syndrome

Treat:
   Oral Antibiotics
   for 14–30 Days

Consult:
   Neurologist

Treat:
   IV Ceftriaxone or
   Penicillin G for
   14–21 Days

Obtain:
   Chest radiographs
   Electrocardiogram
   Echocardiogram

Consult:
   Cardiologist

Identify:
   Atrioventricular block (p 60)
   Myocarditis (p 62)
   Left ventricular dysfuction (p 62)

Treat:
   IV Ceftriaxone or Penicillin G
   for 14–21 Days
Consider:
   Aspirin
   Corticosteroids

into chronic syndromes. Bell's palsy is common and can be treated with oral antibiotics.

I. Arthritis usually develops within 4 to 6 weeks of the tick bite. The pattern is variable and can be monoarticular, oligoarticular, and migratory or additive. The knee is most often involved, followed by the shoulder, elbow, temporomandibular joint, ankle, wrist, and hip. Joints are often quite hot and swollen but rarely red. Recurrent episodes are common.

References

Baltimore RS, Shapiro ED. Lyme disease. Pediatr Rev 1994; 15:167.

Christy C, Siegel DM. Lyme disease—what it is, what it isn't. Contemp Pediatr 1995; 12:64.

Eichenfield AH, Goldsmith DP, Benach JL, et al. Childhood Lyme arthritis: Experience in an endemic area. J Pediatr 1986; 109:753.

Feder HM Jr, Zalneraitis EL, Reik L Jr. Lyme disease: Acute focal meningoencephalitis in a child. Pediatrics 1988; 82:931.

Salazar JC, Gerber MA, Goff CW. Long-term outcome of Lyme disease in children given early treatment. J Pediatr 1993; 122:591.

Stechenberg BW. Lyme disease: The latest great imitator. Pediatr Infect Dis J 1988; 402.

Szer IS, Taylor E, Steere AC. The long-term course of Lyme arthritis in children. N Engl J Med 1991; 325:159.

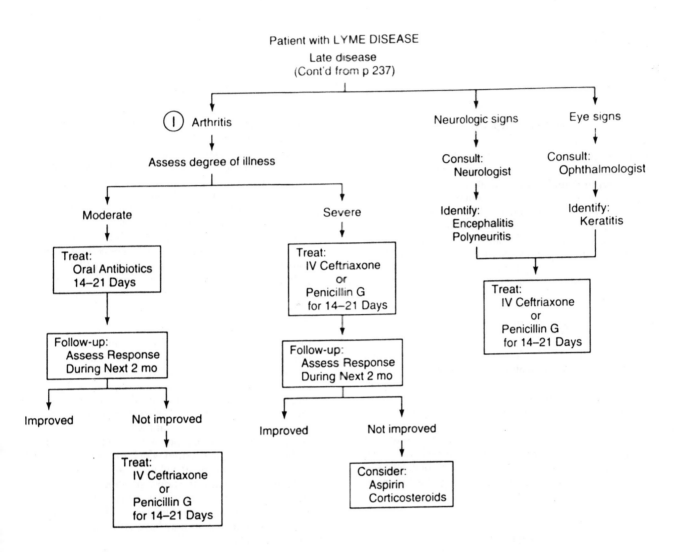

Patient with LYME DISEASE

Late disease
(Cont'd from p 237)

Ⓘ Arthritis

Assess degree of illness

Moderate

Treat:
Oral Antibiotics
14–21 Days

Follow-up:
Assess Response
During Next 2 mo

Improved   Not improved

Treat:
IV Ceftriaxone
or
Penicillin G
for 14–21 Days

Severe

Treat:
IV Ceftriaxone
or
Penicillin G
for 14–21 Days

Follow-up:
Assess Response
During Next 2 mo

Improved   Not improved

Consider:
Aspirin
Corticosteroids

Neurologic signs

Consult:
Neurologist

Identify:
Encephalitis
Polyneuritis

Eye signs

Consult:
Ophthalmologist

Identify:
Keratitis

Treat:
IV Ceftriaxone
or
Penicillin G
for 14–21 Days

MALARIA

Stephen Berman, M.D.

DEFINITIONS

Suspicion of malaria arises for a febrile child who has traveled in the past 12 months to an area where malaria is endemic. **Cerebral malaria** is parasitemia identified in the blood associated with signs of acute encephalopathy (coma and seizures), normal CSF, and no other identifiable cause (meningitis, viral encephalitis, metabolic abnormalities). After a seizure, unresponsiveness (coma) should last longer than 30 minutes (postictal period). Sludging of parasitized red blood cells in the CNS capillaries may contribute to the condition. Mortality varies from 15% to 50%.

EPIDEMIOLOGY

Worldwide there are 300 million cases of malaria each year and 1 million to 2 million deaths. Most deaths occur in children under 5 years of age. Malaria occurs predominantly in two settings: (1) areas in southeast Asia and Latin America, where transmission is seasonal or limited to specific focal areas, so that the general population does not have a high level of acquired immunity (children and adults are at high risk for severe disease); and (2) areas in Africa where the disease is widespread and endemic, leading to high levels of acquired immunity (young children at very high risk for severe disease).

ETIOLOGY

Malaria caused by *Plasmodium vivax, Plasmodium malariae,* and *Plasmodium ovale* usually results in mild or moderate disease. *Plasmodium falciparum* often results in life-threatening disease and severe anemia. The emergence of multidrug-resistant *P. falciparum* is a global problem.

A. In the history ask about the onset, pattern, and degree of fever. Evaluate the family's ability to care for the child at home and their access to transportation and a telephone. Establish any risk factors (travel in the past 12 months to an area with endemic malaria; use of chemoprophylaxis and other precautions, including mosquito repellents, netting, and protective clothes during travel to malarious areas; underlying conditions such as cardiopulmonary, GI or renal disease, sickle cell disease, and conditions and/or therapy that compromise immunity, especially HIV infection). Note any alterations in mental status and normal level of activity, including playfulness, weakness, irritability, feeding and sleeping patterns, responsiveness, and seizures. Evaluate respiratory symptoms (cough, congestion, coryza, sore throat, earache, fast or difficult breathing, chest indrawing [retractions]), GI symptoms (nausea, vomiting, diarrhea, abdominal pain, blood in stools), and renal symptoms (dark urine, decreased urinary frequency, flank pain, lower abdominal pain).

B. On physical examination look, listen, and feel for findings that can be caused by malaria. CNS signs include being irritable, too weak to feed, difficult to arouse, unresponsive, seizures, and coma with decerebrate or decorticate posturing. Also look for dehydration and poor perfusion: skin turgor, tears, moist mucous membranes, color and warmth of the extremities, and capillary refill time (>2 seconds is abnormal). In the cardiovascular system watch for tachycardia and signs of congestive heart failure. The respiratory signs include tachypnea, retractions, grunting, and crackles. The hematopoetic system may reveal severe anemia with hepatomegaly, splenomegaly, and jaundice. The musculoskeletal system may have arthralgias, myalgias, arthritis, and weakness.

C. All children suspected of having malaria require thick and thin smears of peripheral blood. Serial samples at 6 to 12 hour intervals for 48 hours may be necessary. The thick smear provides a screening test and the thin smear is better for species identification. Low-grade parasitemia related to partial immunity or treatment can result in a negative smear. Even patients with cerebral malaria can be smear negative at presentation. Therefore, when the clinical history and presentation suggest malaria, begin treatment regardless of parasites on the smears.

(Continued on page 242)

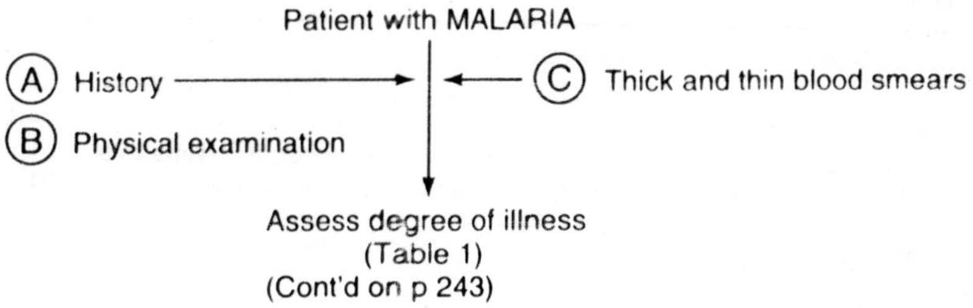

Patient with MALARIA

(A) History ──────────→ | ←── (C) Thick and thin blood smears

(B) Physical examination

Assess degree of illness
(Table 1)
(Cont'd on p 243)

TABLE 1 Degree of Illness in Malaria

Moderate	Severe	Very Severe
Headache, malaise, irritable but consolable	Irritable and not easily consolable, poor eye contact (lethargic), feeds poorly	Unresponsive, too weak to feed or extreme weakness, or seizures
and	or	or
No signs of dehydration and good peripheral perfusion with pink warm extremities	Signs of mild or moderate dehydration, good peripheral perfusion	Signs of severe dehydration with shock, poor peripheral perfusion with cold, mottled extremities, capillary refill > 2 seconds, low BP
and	or	or
No signs of respiratory distress or pulmonary edema	No signs of respiratory distress or pulmonary edema	Signs of respiratory distress or pulmonary edema with respiratory rate > 60, retractions, grunting, cyanosis, or respiratory failure
and	or	or
No signs of severe anemia or bleeding	Pallor but no signs of severe anemia or bleeding	Severe normocytic anemia, hemoglobinuria, or bleeding associated with disseminated intravascular coagulation
and	and	or
No signs of metabolic or end organ failure	No signs of metabolic or end organ failure	Metabolic disorder, including hypoglycemia, metabolic acidosis, or renal failure
and	or	or
Parasitemia < 2%.	Parasitemia > 2% and < 5%	Parasitemia ≥ 5%

TABLE 2 Treatment of P. Falciparum Malaria

Drug of Choice	Age/ Dosage*	Maximum/ Dose
Chloroquine-sensitive		
Chloroquine	10 mg base/kg, then 5 mg base/kg 6 hr later; 5 mg base/kg/dose at 24 and 48 hr	600 mg base
Chloroquine-resistant, uncomplicated		
Quinine sulfate	30 mg/kg/day salt in 3 doses for 3–7 days†	650 mg salt
plus Pyrimethamine/ sulfadoxine (Fansidar)	< 1 yr: ¼ tablet once 1–3 yr: ½ tablet once 4–8 yr: 1 tablet once 9–14 yr: 2 tablets once > 14 yr: 3 tablets once	3 tablets once
or Quinine as above plus tetracycline	5 mg/kg/dose 4 times a day for 7 days	250 mg
or Mefloquine hydro chloride (Lariam)‡	15 mg/kg once	1250 mg
Chloroquine-resistant, severe and complicated		
Quinidine gluconate	10 mg/kg loading dose IV over 1–2 hr, then 0.02 mg/kg/ min continuous infusion until oral therapy can be given	600 mg load

*All drugs are oral except quinidine gluconate.
†Seven days is recommended for infections acquired in Thailand.
‡Safety of mefloquine in children < 15 kg has not been established.
From McCaslin RI, Pikis A, Rodriquez WJ, Pedia Plasmodium falciparium malaria: A 10-year-experiment from Washington, D.C. Pediatr Infect Dis J 1994; 13:709.

D. Treat all forms of malaria except for chloroquine-resistant P. falciparum with oral or nasogastric chloroqine phosphate. Patients with P. ovale or P. vivax should have a 12 to 14 day follow-up course of primaquine phosphate to prevent relapses. Indications for exchange transfusion vary according to the quality of intensive care facilities and availability and safety of blood products. The theoretic benefits of an exchange transfusion are reduction in parasitemia, correction of anemia, improved oxygenation, and enhanced capillary blood flow. The relative benefit of whole blood versus component exchange and the minimum exchange volume has not been well documented. The CDC recommends exchange transfusion with component therapy when children have signs of very severe illness with more than 10% parasitemia. The exchange should be continued until the level has dropped below 5%. It is not necessary to repeat the loading dose of IV quinidine.

E. Chloroquine-resistant strains of P. falciparum are common throughout many regions. In Africa these strains are usually still treatable with quinine; however, as in southeast Asia and the Amazon basin, many strains are resistant to pyrimethamine (Fansidar) and require therapy with quinine plus tetracycline or mefloquine alone. Alternative drugs not available in the United States and undergoing clinical trials are halofantrine and qinghao derivatives.

F. Treat very severely ill patients with IV quinidine as outlined in Table 2. Children must be monitored in an intensive care unit for ECG changes (QT interval), arrhythmias, cinchonism (tinnitus, nausea, headache, and visual changes), and hypoglycemia. Discontinue IV quinidine as soon as the child has improved and switch to oral or nasogastric quinine to complete a 3 day course. Assume that all malarial infections are caused by resistant strains unless proved otherwise. Treat children who may have acquired malaria in southeast Asia (Thailand) and east Africa for 7 days because of multiple resistant strains.

G. Treat children with severe and very severe illness with antibiotics for possible bacteremia pending the results of blood and CSF cultures. In Nigeria 86% of children with bacteremia may have concurrent malaria.

H. Recommendations for malaria prophylaxis vary by the region visited and the age of the traveler. If resistant

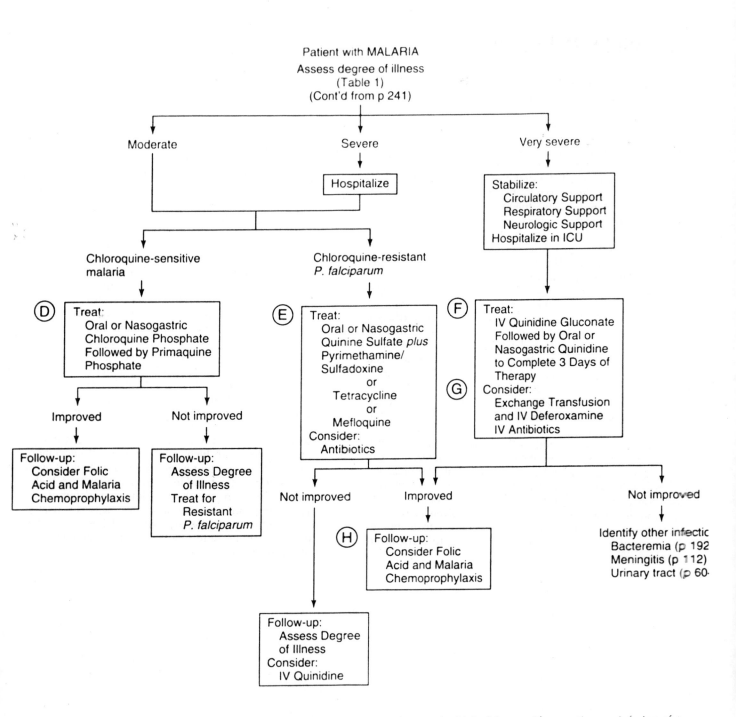

Patient with MALARIA

Assess degree of illness
(Table 1)
(Cont'd from p 241)

Moderate

Severe → Hospitalize

Very severe → Stabilize:
Circulatory Support
Respiratory Support
Neurologic Support
Hospitalize in ICU

Chloroquine-sensitive malaria

Chloroquine-resistant *P. falciparum*

(D) Treat:
Oral or Nasogastric
Chloroquine Phosphate
Followed by Primaquine
Phosphate

Improved → Follow-up:
Consider Folic
Acid and Malaria
Chemoprophylaxis

Not improved → Follow-up:
Assess Degree
of Illness
Treat for
Resistant
P. falciparum

(E) Treat:
Oral or Nasogastric
Quinine Sulfate *plus*
Pyrimethamine/
Sulfadoxine
or
Tetracycline
or
Mefloquine
Consider:
Antibiotics

(F) Treat:
IV Quinidine Gluconate
Followed by Oral or
Nasogastric Quinidine
to Complete 3 Days of
Therapy
(G) Consider:
Exchange Transfusion
and IV Deferoxamine
IV Antibiotics

Not improved

Improved → (H) Follow-up:
Consider Folic
Acid and Malaria
Chemoprophylaxis

Not improved → Identify other infectic
Bacteremia (p 192
Meningitis (p 112)
Urinary tract (p 60·

Follow-up:
Assess Degree
of Illness
Consider:
IV Quinidine

P. falciparum is not a concern, prophylaxis should be weekly chloroquine phosphate. Mefloquine is recommended for prophylaxis in children over 15 kg traveling to areas with resistant *P. falciparum* such as Africa. Since recommendations change frequently, consult the CDC hotline (404-332-4555) for advice.

References

Emanuel B, Aronson N, Shulman S. Malaria in children in Chicago. Pediatrics 1993; 92:83.

McCaslin RI, Pikis A, Rodriguez WJ. Pediatric *Plasmodium falciparum* malaria: A 10-year experience from Washington, D.C. Pediatr Infect Dis J 1994; 13:709.

Miller KD, Greenberg AE, Campbell CC. Treatment of severe malaria in the United States with a continuous infusion of quinidine gluconate and exchange transfusion. N Engl J Med 1989; 321:65.

Moran JS, Bernard KW. The spread of chloroquine-resistant malaria in Africa. JAMA 1989; 262:245.

Steele RW, Baffoe-Bonnie B. Cerebral malaria in children. Pediatr Infect Dis J 1995; 14:281.

Taylor TE, Molyneux ME, Wirima JJ, et al. Blood glucose levels in Malawian children before and during the administration of intravenous quinine for severe falciparum malaria. N Engl J Med 1988; 319:1040.

World Health Organization, Division of Control of Tropical Diseases. Severe and complicated malaria. Trans R Soc Trop Med Hyg 1990; 84 (Suppl 2):1.

World Health Organization. Practical chemotherapy of malaria. Report of a WHO Scientific Group. Geneva: World Health Organization Technical Report Series, 1990.

MEASLES INFECTION

Stephen Berman, M.D.
Perla Santos Ocampo, M.D.

Measles (rubeola), a viral infection, remains a major cause of worldwide childhood mortality despite the availability of an effective vaccine. Following an incubation period of 10 to 12 days, the clinical syndrome begins with fever, cough, coryza, and conjunctivitis, followed on day 3 or 4 by a morbilliform or maculopapular erythematous rash. The rash is preceded for 1 to 2 days by the appearance of Koplik spots, small red irregular lesions with blue-white centers, on the buccal mucosa. The rash begins in the hairline and forehead, then moves downward to involve the face, neck, extremities, and trunk. It becomes confluent in the upper body and discrete on the lower body and can become brownish after 3 or 4 days because of capillary hemorrhages. It fades after 6 to 8 days. Desquamation may occur in areas of intense involvement. Associated physical findings include localized (cervical, postauricular, occipital) or generalized lymphadenopathy. Bloody diarrhea occurs in 10% of cases. Most children lose up to 20% of body weight regardless of diarrhea. In the marginally nourished child measles often results in marasmus or kwashiorkor. Measles can cause subacute sclerosing panencephalitis (SSPE), a neurodegenerative disease associated with persistent measles virus infection. Effective community measles immunization can reduce mortality by at least 30%. Current immunization strategies in developing countries are either to immunize as soon as possible after 9 months of age or to institute a two-dose schedule; the initial dose is given at 6 or 15 months of age and followed by a second 4 to 6 months later. Approximately 50% of children fail to seroconvert despite previous immunization.

A. Immunize contacts exposed within 72 hours with live virus vaccine. Immunoglobulin can be given between 72 hours and 6 days of exposure. It should be used for household contacts, especially infants, immunocompromised patients, and susceptible pregnant women. The recommended dose is 0.25 ml/kg IM for patients without underlying disorders and 0.50 ml/kg IM for patients with immunodeficiency disorders.

B. Treat all hospitalized children 6 months to 2 years of age with vitamin A. In addition, treat all patients regardless of age who (1) live in areas with a high prevalence of vitamin A deficiency; (2) have an immunodeficiency disorder; (3) have impaired intestinal absorption such as short bowel syndrome, cystic fibrosis, or biliary disease; or (4) have ophthalmologic signs of vitamin A deficiency such as Bitot spots or xerophthalmia. The dose is 100,000 U for infants and 200,000 U for children older than 12 months. To prevent corneal ulceration repeat the dose the next day and in 4 weeks for patients with ophthalmologic signs of vitamin A deficiency. Vitamin A deficiency is associated with high fatality rates and high rates of corneal ulceration. Vitamin A is important in maintaining epithelization of the respiratory tract and in the recovery process. It also plays a role in the body's immune defenses. In developing countries mortality from measles is related to the intensity of the exposure and host nutritional and immunologic status. Secondary cases in the household are at greater risk than index cases.

(Continued on page 246)

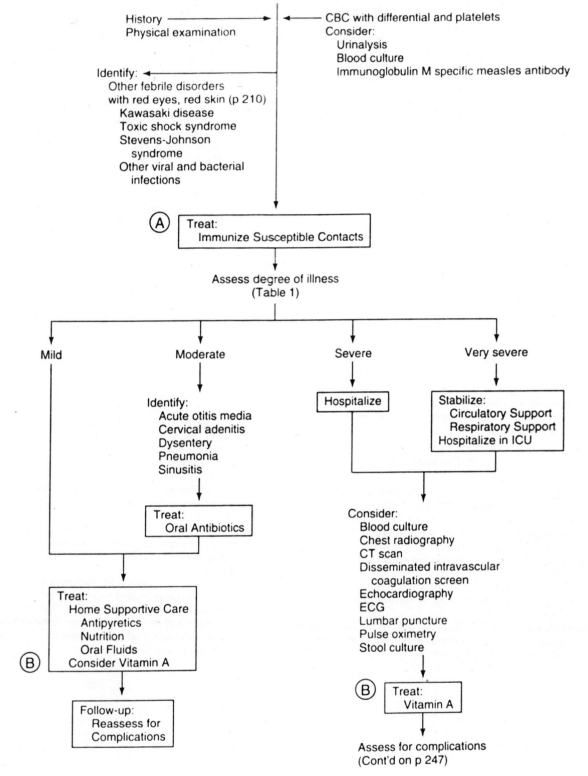

Patient with MEASLES INFECTION

History → ← CBC with differential and platelets
Physical examination
Consider:
　Urinalysis
　Blood culture
　Immunoglobulin M specific measles antibody

Identify: ←
　Other febrile disorders
　with red eyes, red skin (p 210)
　　Kawasaki disease
　　Toxic shock syndrome
　　Stevens-Johnson
　　　syndrome
　　Other viral and bacterial
　　　infections

Ⓐ Treat:
　Immunize Susceptible Contacts

Assess degree of illness
(Table 1)

Mild　　Moderate　　Severe　　Very severe

Moderate:
Identify:
　Acute otitis media
　Cervical adenitis
　Dysentery
　Pneumonia
　Sinusitis

Treat:
　Oral Antibiotics

Severe:
Hospitalize

Very severe:
Stabilize:
　Circulatory Support
　Respiratory Support
Hospitalize in ICU

Ⓑ Treat:
　Home Supportive Care
　　Antipyretics
　　Nutrition
　　Oral Fluids
　　Consider Vitamin A

Follow-up:
　Reassess for
　Complications

Consider:
　Blood culture
　Chest radiography
　CT scan
　Disseminated intravascular
　　coagulation screen
　Echocardiography
　ECG
　Lumbar puncture
　Pulse oximetry
　Stool culture

Ⓑ Treat:
　Vitamin A

Assess for complications
(Cont'd on p 247)

TABLE 1 Degree of Illness in Measles Infection

Mild	Moderate	Severe	Very Severe
Fever resolves within 4 days and rash within 8 days without signs of complication	Signs of secondary bacterial upper respiratory infection such as acute otitis media, sinusitis, or cervical adenitis	Respiratory distress with tachypnea, retractions or Oxygen desaturation or Stridor or Heart murmurs or ECG changes or Ophthalmologic signs of vitamin A deficiency or corneal ulcerations or Bloody diarrhea, jaundice, abdominal pain, or moderate to severe dehydration or Purpura (hemorrhagic measles) or Severe malnutrition, immunodeficiency disorders, cardiopulmonary disorders, or tuberculosis	Altered mental status with coma, seizures, or focal neurologic signs or Shock with poor peripheral perfusion or Impending upper airway obstruction; signs of respiratory failure or Signs of congestive heart failure or Acute abdominal pain with peritoneal signs

C. Measles alters the immune system and predisposes to the reactivation of tuberculosis. The tuberculin skin test is often negative because of the anergy. These alterations in immunity may also predispose to secondary bacterial pneumonia, especially infection with *Staphylococcus aureus*.

References

Aaby P, Bukh J, Hoff G. High measles mortality in infancy related to intensity of exposure. J Pediatr 1986; 109:40.

Aaby P, Pedersen IR, Knudsen K. Child mortality related to seroconversion or lack of seroconversion after measles vaccination. Pediatr Infect Dis 1989; 8:197.

Axton JHM. Measles: A protein losing enteropathy. BMJ 1975; 3:79.

Barclay AJG, Foster A, Sommer A. Vitamin A supplements and mortality related to measles: A randomized clinical trial. BMJ 1989; 294:294.

Brown DW, Ramsay ME, Richards AF, Miller R. Salivary diagnosis of measles: A study of notified cases in the United Kingdom, 1991–1993. BMJ 1994; 308:1015.

Butler JC, Havens PL, Sowell AL, et al. Measles severity and serum retinol (vitamin A) concentration among children in the United States. Pediatrics 1993; 91:1176.

Cohn ML, Robinson ED, Faerber M, et al. Measles vaccine failures: Lack of sustained measles-specific immunoglobulin G responses in revaccinated adolescents and young adults. Pediatr Infect Dis J 1994; 13:34.

Gindler JS, Atkinson WL, Markowitz LE, Hutchins SS. Epidemiology of measles in the United States in 1989 and 1990. Pediatr Infect Dis J 1992; 11:841.

Hussey GD, Klein M. A randomized, controlled trial of vitamin A in children with severe measles. N Engl J Med 1990; 323:160.

Johnson CE, Nalin DR, Chiu LW, et al. Measles vaccine immunogenicity in 6- versus 15-month-old infants born to mothers in the measles vaccine era. Pediatrics 1994; 93(6 Pt 1):939.

Kaplan LJ, Daum RS, Smaron M, McCarthy CA. Severe measles in immunocompromised patients. JAMA 1992; 267:1237.

Tamashiro VG, Perez HH, Griffin DE. Prospective study of the magnitude and duration of changes in tuberculin reactivity during uncomplicated and complicated measles. Pediatr Infect Dis 1989; 6:451.

Patient with MEASLES INFECTION

Assess for complications
(Cont'd from p 245)

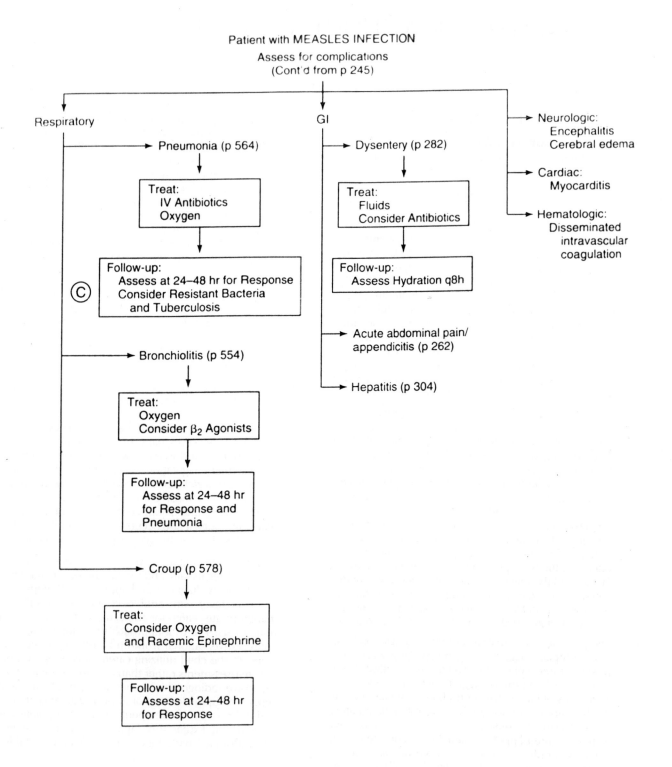

Respiratory

GI

Pneumonia (p 564)

Treat:
  IV Antibiotics
  Oxygen

Ⓒ Follow-up:
  Assess at 24–48 hr for Response
  Consider Resistant Bacteria
  and Tuberculosis

Bronchiolitis (p 554)

Treat:
  Oxygen
  Consider β₂ Agonists

Follow-up:
  Assess at 24–48 hr
  for Response and
  Pneumonia

Croup (p 578)

Treat:
  Consider Oxygen
  and Racemic Epinephrine

Follow-up:
  Assess at 24–48 hr
  for Response

Dysentery (p 282)

Treat:
  Fluids
  Consider Antibiotics

Follow-up:
  Assess Hydration q8h

Acute abdominal pain/
appendicitis (p 262)

Hepatitis (p 304)

Neurologic:
  Encephalitis
  Cerebral edema

Cardiac:
  Myocarditis

Hematologic:
  Disseminated
  intravascular
  coagulation

PROLONGED FEVER WITHOUT A SOURCE

Stephen Berman, M.D.

DEFINITION

Prolonged fever without a source is an unexplained fever that persists beyond 7 to 10 days. The fever may resolve, and the cause often remains unclear.

ETIOLOGY

Half of cases are infectious. The remainder are related to collagen vascular disease (15%), neoplasms (7%), inflammatory bowel disease (4%), and other causes (12%). Infections include viral syndromes (2% to 18%), upper respiratory infection (2% to 10%), lower respiratory infection (4% to 8%), urinary tract infection (3% to 4%), gastroenteritis (<2%), osteomyelitis (<2%), CNS infections (3% to 4%), tuberculosis (<3%), bacteremia (<2%), subacute bacterial endocarditis (<2%), mononucleosis (<2%), abscess (<1%), brucellosis (<1%), and malaria (<1%). Associated collagen vascular diseases are rheumatoid arthritis (10%), systemic lupus erythematosus (3%), and vasculitis (1%). Associated malignancies are leukemia, lymphoma, and neuroblastoma.

A. The characteristics of the fever (onset, duration, and pattern) and nonspecific symptoms such as anorexia, fatigue, chills, headache, and mild abdominal pain are rarely helpful in diagnosis. Ask about animal exposures: ticks (Lyme disease, relapsing fever), rats (plague, rat-bite fever, leptospirosis), hamsters (lymphocytic choriomeningitis virus), rabbits (tularemia), cattle, goats, dogs (brucellosis), birds (psittacosis), and cats (cat-scratch fever). Also note any history of pica, travel or foreign contacts, and drug exposure (salicylism). Specific symptoms referable to organ system dysfunction are often helpful. Note predisposing conditions such as risk factors for HIV infection (exposure to possibly contaminated blood transfusions, drug abuse, perinatal HIV transmission), sickle cell disease, malignancies, immune deficiency states, diabetes mellitus, and dysautonomia.

B. The presence of arthralgia, arthritis, myalgia, or localized limb pain suggests collagen vascular disease, neoplasms, or infections (osteomyelitis, septic arthritis). Significant heart murmurs suggest bacterial endocarditis. Note signs of GI involvement; abdominal pain, bloody stools, diarrhea, or weight loss suggests inflammatory bowel disease. Abdominal pain or mass may be present with a ruptured appendix. Jaundice is consistent with hepatitis; a rash may indicate collagen vascular disease, neoplasms, or infection. Pharyngitis, tonsillitis, or peritonsillar abscess can be caused by the usual bacteria or infectious mononucleosis, cytomegalovirus, tularemia, or leptospirosis. Respiratory distress may relate to an underlying neoplasm, collagen vascular disease, or infection. Meningeal or focal neurologic signs suggest encephalitis, meningitis, or neoplasm. While lymphadenopathy and hepatosplenomegaly are nonspecific findings that may be related to any of several infectious or noninfectious causes, consider malignancy.

C. The CBC with differential may help guide the work-up. Pancytopenia, unexplained neutropenia with thrombocytopenia, or lymphoblasts on the peripheral smear require a hematology/oncology consult and bone marrow test. Reactive lymphocytes on differential suggest mononucleosis or other viral infection. Severe neutropenia in a mildly to moderately ill patient is consistent with many infections. Leukocytosis and elevated sedimentation rate suggest infection and collagen vascular disease. Hemolytic anemia suggests collagen vascular disease or endocarditis. Nonhemolytic anemia suggests chronic illness or malignancy. Pyuria and bacteriuria suggest urinary tract infection; hematuria suggests endocarditis.

D. Children with prolonged fever without a source who live in or have traveled to tropical areas in developing countries are at risk for infections such as malaria (see p 240), dengue fever (see p 206), typhoid fever (see p 252), scrub and murine typhus (see p 188), borreliosis (see p 188), brucellosis (see p 188), and leptospirosis (see p 188).

E. Suspect Rocky Mountain spotted fever when fever is associated with an erythematous macular rash that begins on the wrists and ankles and spreads rapidly to the trunk. It can occur without the characteristic rash. It can progress to involve many organ systems (CNS, lungs, heart, kidney, and liver) as well as cause disseminated intravascular coagulation, shock, and death. The pathogen *Rickettsia rickettsi* is transmitted by the bite of ticks. The disease is most common in the south Atlantic, southeastern, and south-central areas of the United States, although it also occurs in the upper Rocky Mountain states. Treat with chloramphenicol or tetracycline.

F. Inappropriate antibiotics may alter typical signs of occult infections (especially abdominal abscess or osteomyelitis) and delay diagnosis and appropriate therapy. Resolution of fever with antibiotics may also result in an inappropriate search for an occult bacterial focus when none exists. The best approach to prolonged fever is a conservative, rational work-up based on the severity of illness in the child utilizing careful follow-up and periodic reassessments rather than the indiscriminate use of expensive radiographic studies and scans. With the exception of aspirin in cases of suspected juvenile rheumatoid arthritis, avoid therapeutic trials of antibiotics and other drugs. Exploratory laparotomy without signs of intraabdominal pathology is not indicated in children.

References

Chantada G, Casak S, Plata JD, et al. Children with fever of unknown origin in Argentina: An analysis of 113 cases. Pediatr Infect Dis J 1994; 13:260.

Hayani A, Mahoney DH, Fernback DJ. Role of bone marrow examination in the child with prolonged fever. J Pediatr 1990; 116:919.

Kleinman MB. The complaint of persistent fever. Pediatr Clin North Am 1982; 29:201.

Lohr JA, Hendley JO. Prolonged fever of unknown origin: A

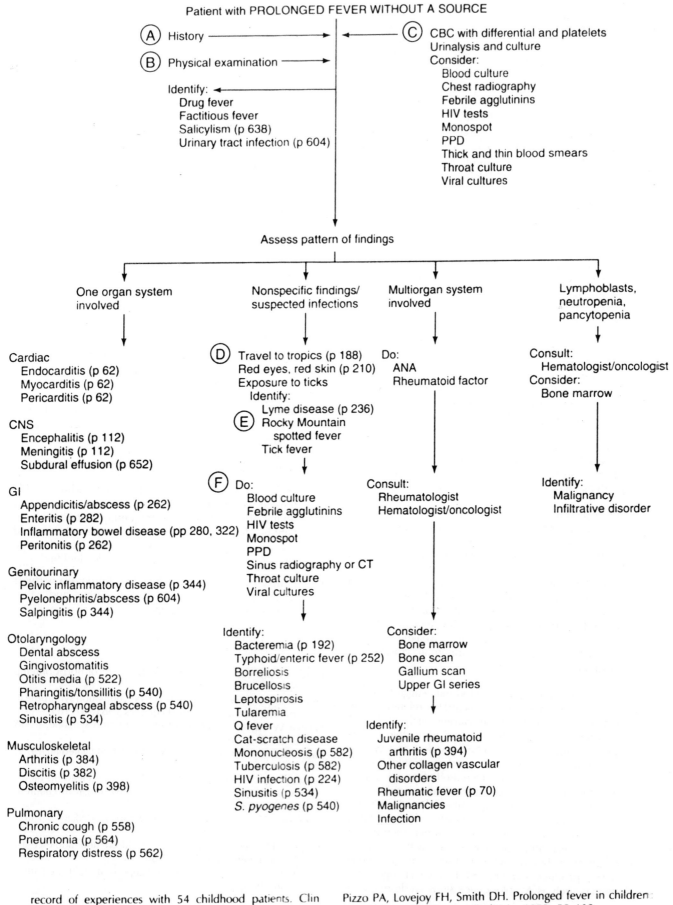

Patient with PROLONGED FEVER WITHOUT A SOURCE

Ⓐ History ⟶
Ⓒ CBC with differential and platelets
Urinalysis and culture
Consider:
    Blood culture
    Chest radiography
    Febrile agglutinins
    HIV tests
    Monospot
    PPD
    Thick and thin blood smears
    Throat culture
    Viral cultures

Ⓑ Physical examination ⟶

Identify:
    Drug fever
    Factitious fever
    Salicylism (p 638)
    Urinary tract infection (p 604)

Assess pattern of findings

One organ system involved

Cardiac
    Endocarditis (p 62)
    Myocarditis (p 62)
    Pericarditis (p 62)

CNS
    Encephalitis (p 112)
    Meningitis (p 112)
    Subdural effusion (p 652)

GI
    Appendicitis/abscess (p 262)
    Enteritis (p 282)
    Inflammatory bowel disease (pp 280, 322)
    Peritonitis (p 262)

Genitourinary
    Pelvic inflammatory disease (p 344)
    Pyelonephritis/abscess (p 604)
    Salpingitis (p 344)

Otolaryngology
    Dental abscess
    Gingivostomatitis
    Otitis media (p 522)
    Pharingitis/tonsillitis (p 540)
    Retropharyngeal abscess (p 540)
    Sinusitis (p 534)

Musculoskeletal
    Arthritis (p 384)
    Discitis (p 382)
    Osteomyelitis (p 398)

Pulmonary
    Chronic cough (p 558)
    Pneumonia (p 564)
    Respiratory distress (p 562)

Nonspecific findings/ suspected infections

Ⓓ Travel to tropics (p 188)
Red eyes, red skin (p 210)
Exposure to ticks
    Identify:
        Lyme disease (p 236)
Ⓔ   Rocky Mountain
            spotted fever
        Tick fever

Ⓕ Do:
    Blood culture
    Febrile agglutinins
    HIV tests
    Monospot
    PPD
    Sinus radiography or CT
    Throat culture
    Viral cultures

Identify:
    Bacteremia (p 192)
    Typhoid/enteric fever (p 252)
    Borreliosis
    Brucellosis
    Leptospirosis
    Tularemia
    Q fever
    Cat-scratch disease
    Mononucleosis (p 582)
    Tuberculosis (p 582)
    HIV infection (p 224)
    Sinusitis (p 534)
    S. pyogenes (p 540)

Multiorgan system involved

Do:
    ANA
    Rheumatoid factor

Consult:
    Rheumatologist
    Hematologist/oncologist

Consider:
    Bone marrow
    Bone scan
    Gallium scan
    Upper GI series

Identify:
    Juvenile rheumatoid
        arthritis (p 394)
    Other collagen vascular
        disorders
    Rheumatic fever (p 70)
    Malignancies
    Infection

Lymphoblasts, neutropenia, pancytopenia

Consult:
    Hematologist/oncologist
Consider:
    Bone marrow

Identify:
    Malignancy
    Infiltrative disorder

record of experiences with 54 childhood patients. Clin Pediatr 1977; 16:768.

McClung HJ. Prolonged fever of unknown origin in children. JAMA 1972; 124:544.

Pizzo PA, Lovejoy FH, Smith DH. Prolonged fever in children: Review of 100 cases. Pediatrics 1975; 55:468.

Van der Jagt EW. Fever of unknown origin. In: Hoekelman, ed. Primary pediatric care. St. Louis: Mosby, 1987:691.

SYNCOPE

Stephen Berman, M.D.

DEFINITIONS

Syncope is a transient loss of consciousness and muscle tone. **Near syncope** is a transient alteration in consciousness without a period of unconsciousness.

ETIOLOGY

The most frequent causes of syncope in patients attending an emergency room are vasovagal reaction (50%), orthostatic hypotension (20%), seizures (7.5%), migraine headache (5%), and head trauma (5%). The most frequent causes of near syncope are light-headedness (29%), seizure (18%), tension headache (12%), and migraine (6%). Approximately half of patients have a contributing condition such as dehydration, seizures, anemia, cardiac disease, or hypoglycemia.

A. The history should clarify predisposing conditions and any precipitating events such as prolonged or sudden standing, prolonged fasting, micturition, paroxysm of coughing, physical exercise, recent closed head trauma, or a sudden, strong emotion. Note history of cardiac or pulmonary diseases. Risk factors for cardiac disease include a family history of early myocardial infarction or hypercholesterolemia, a history of Kawasaki disease, hypertension, and congenital heart disease.

B. Perform a complete physical examination. Note signs of cardiac disease (see p 56), respiratory distress (see p 118), and neurologic disease (see p 448). Findings that suggest cardiac disease are heart murmurs, increased intensity of the second heart sound, clicks, gallop rhythm, friction rub, hypertension, and decreased femoral pulses. Signs of respiratory distress are tachypnea, retractions, decreased breath sounds, wheezing, rales, and cyanosis. Signs of CNS disease include altered mental status, focal neurologic signs, weakness, abnormal tone and reflexes, and abnormal growth and development.

C. Findings on chest x-ray and ECG may suggest cardiac disease. Pericarditis and myocarditis related to an infection or vasculitis cause cardiomegaly and ST-T wave changes. Aortic stenosis and idiopathic hypertrophic subaortic stenosis (IHSS) manifest as a systolic heart murmur and left-ventricular hypertrophy. Coarctation syndromes cause decreased femoral pulses and left-ventricular hypertrophy. Primary pulmonary hypertension and pulmonary stenosis produce right-ventricular hypertrophy. Coronary artery disease related to Kawasaki disease, hypercholesterolemia, aberrant left coronary artery, and lesions associated with decreased coronary artery blood flow, such as severe aortic stenosis or IHSS, produce ischemic ST-T wave changes. Arrhythmias such as AV block, sick sinus syndrome, and supraventricular tachycardia are associated with ECG findings of abnormal conduction patterns.

D. Seizure activity is suggested when a syncopal episode lasts longer than 2 minutes, is followed by confusion or impaired mental status (postictal state), or is associated with incontinence, muscle jerks, or cyanosis. Frequent recurrent episodes also suggest seizures.

E. Orthostatic syncope is associated with a fall in blood pressure upon standing. Rarely, syncope may follow micturition, when rapid bladder decompression produces postural hypotension and decreased cardiac return.

F. Vasovagal syncope is caused by a sudden decrease in peripheral vascular resistance. It is usually precipitated by sudden fear, anger, or another strong emotion.

G. Breath holding occurs in children under 6 years of age and is precipitated by crying, sudden pain, or fear. Loss of tone and consciousness is followed by stiffening and clonus. Cyanosis, if present, should precede any abnormal movements. No postictal or confusional state occurs. The prognosis is excellent; spells of breath holding usually are discontinued by 6 years of age. Treatment is reassuring the parents of the benign nature of the problem.

H. Hyperventilation produces reduction in carbon dioxide tension with alkalosis, decreased ionized calcium, and tetany. This syndrome is frequently associated with light-headedness, giddiness, dizziness, paresthesias, and chest pain. In most cases high anxiety related to life stress or underlying psychopathology is identified.

I. Paroxysmal coughing produced by *Bordetella pertussis* or asthma may decrease cardiac output and cause hypoxia resulting in syncope.

References

Hardy CE. Syncope and chest pain: To worry, or not? Contemp Pediatr 1994; 11:19.

Herman SP, Stickler GB, Lucas AR. Hyperventilation syndrome in children and adolescents. Pediatrics 1981; 67:183.

Kapoor WN, Peterson JR, Karpf M. Micturition syncope. JAMA 1985; 253:796.

Katz RM. Cough syncope in children with asthma. J Pediatr 1979; 77:48.

Lerman-Sagie T, Rechavia E, Strasberg B, et al. Head-up tilt for the evaluation of syncope of unknown origin in children. J Pediatr 1991; 118:676.

Lombroso CT, Lerman P. Breathholding spells. Pediatrics 1967; 39:563.

Pratt JL, Fleisher GR. Syncope in children and adolescents. Pediatr Emerg Care 1989; 5:80.

Woody RC, Kiel EA. Swallowing syncope in a child. Pediatrics 1986; 78:507.

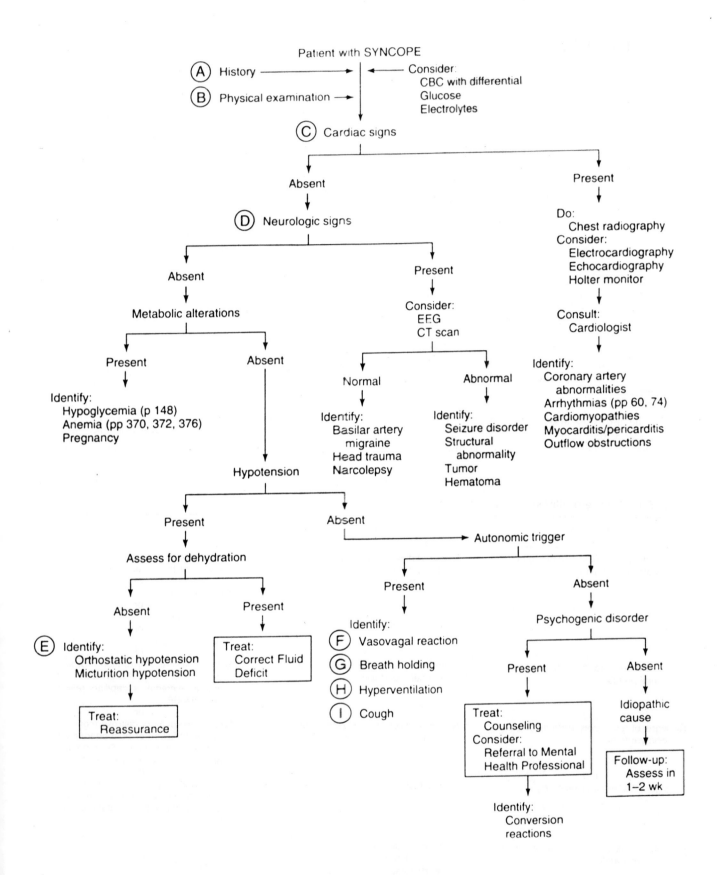

Patient with SYNCOPE

(A) History ⟶ ← Consider:
CBC with differential
(B) Physical examination ⟶ Glucose
Electrolytes

(C) Cardiac signs

Absent

(D) Neurologic signs

Absent

Metabolic alterations

Present

Identify:
Hypoglycemia (p 148)
Anemia (pp 370, 372, 376)
Pregnancy

Absent

Hypotension

Present

Assess for dehydration

Absent

(E) Identify:
Orthostatic hypotension
Micturition hypotension

Treat:
Reassurance

Present

Treat:
Correct Fluid
Deficit

Present

Consider:
EEG
CT scan

Normal

Identify:
Basilar artery
migraine
Head trauma
Narcolepsy

Abnormal

Identify:
Seizure disorder
Structural
abnormality
Tumor
Hematoma

Absent ⟶ Autonomic trigger

Present

Identify:
(F) Vasovagal reaction
(G) Breath holding
(H) Hyperventilation
(I) Cough

Absent

Psychogenic disorder

Present

Treat:
Counseling
Consider:
Referral to Mental
Health Professional

Identify:
Conversion
reactions

Absent

Idiopathic
cause

Follow-up:
Assess in
1–2 wk

Present

Do:
Chest radiography
Consider:
Electrocardiography
Echocardiography
Holter monitor

Consult:
Cardiologist

Identify:
Coronary artery
abnormalities
Arrhythmias (pp 60, 74)
Cardiomyopathies
Myocarditis/pericarditis
Outflow obstructions

TYPHOID FEVER

Perla Santos Ocampo, M.D.
Stephen Berman, M.D.

Typhoid fever, or enteric fever, an infection with *Salmonella typhi,* presents with fever, abdominal pain, headache, malaise, and listlessness. Diarrhea is variable. Fever can persist in untreated cases for 3 to 4 weeks. Erythematous maculopapular skin lesions about 2 to 3 mm in diameter may develop at the end of the first week of the illness. These lesions, called rose spots, may become hemorrhagic. Intestinal bleeding occurs in 4% to 7% of cases and perforation in about 2%. Additional complications include toxic encephalopathy, pneumonia, pyelonephritis, meningitis, cerebral vein thrombosis, pericarditis, arthritis, osteomyelitis, hepatitis, and cholecystitis. A similar syndrome can be caused by other *Salmonella* organisms: *S. paratyphi* A and B and *S. choleraesuis.* Immunization for typhoid fever may be recommended for travelers, especially in highly endemic areas. The IM Ty21₄ vaccine is found to be more practical and offers a better alternative than past vaccines due to better compliance and tolerance.

A. In the history ask about contact with *Salmonella* carriers or exposure to contaminated food or water. Note the onset of fever and associated symptoms.

B. Perform a complete physical examination. Assess mental status and note meningeal signs. Look for rose spots. Note signs of respiratory distress (tachypnea, retractions, rales) and cardiac abnormalities. Bradycardia is often present despite high fever. Carefully palpate the abdomen for hepatomegaly, splenomegaly, and localized tenderness. Note peritoneal signs that suggest perforation. Note swollen joints and tender swelling over bones.

C. Isolation of *S. typhi* is highest from blood, followed by isolation from stool and urine. Febrile agglutinins (Widal test) is positive in only 50% of cases and is not reliable in endemic areas where constant exposure is high. Serologic tests for specific H (flagella) and O (cell wall) antigens are available. Leukopenia, anemia, and abnormal liver function tests are common nonspecific findings.

D. Treatment regimens for sensitive organisms include chloramphenicol or IV ampicillin for 3 weeks or ceftriaxone for 5 to 10 days (Table 2). In very severe cases with circulatory instability, start therapy with dexamethasone

TABLE 1 Degree of Illness in Typhoid Fever

Moderate	Severe	Very Severe
Mental status: headache, malaise but consolable and alert	Mental status: headache, malaise, irritable and not easily consolable, poor eye contact (lethargic), feeds poorly	Mental status: unresponsive, disoriented, or too weak to feed or Meningeal signs or Extreme weakness or Seizures
and No or mild dehydration with good peripheral perfusion	or Signs of moderate dehydration, good peripheral perfusion	or Signs of severe dehydration with shock, poor peripheral perfusion with cold mottled extremities, capillary refill >2 sec, low BP
and No signs of respiratory distress or pulmonary edema	or No signs of respiratory distress or pulmonary edema	or Signs of respiratory distress (congestive heart failure or pulmonary edema) with respiratory rate >60, retractions, grunting, cyanosis, or respiratory failure
and No signs of anemia or bleeding	or No signs of severe anemia or bleeding	or Severe normocytic anemia, hemoglobinuria, or bleeding associated with disseminated intravascular coagulation
and Mild abdominal pain, diarrhea or constipation, or vomiting	or Moderate to severe abdominal pain, abnormal liver function tests, intestinal bleeding	or Peritoneal signs or Liver failure

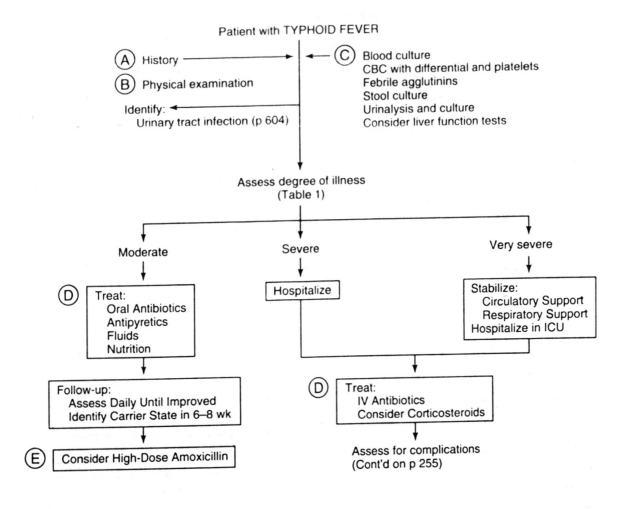

Patient with TYPHOID FEVER

(A) History
(B) Physical examination

Identify:
    Urinary tract infection (p 604)

(C) Blood culture
    CBC with differential and platelets
    Febrile agglutinins
    Stool culture
    Urinalysis and culture
    Consider liver function tests

Assess degree of illness
(Table 1)

Moderate | Severe | Very severe

(D) Treat:
    Oral Antibiotics
    Antipyretics
    Fluids
    Nutrition

Hospitalize

Stabilize:
    Circulatory Support
    Respiratory Support
Hospitalize in ICU

Follow-up:
    Assess Daily Until Improved
    Identify Carrier State in 6–8 wk

(D) Treat:
    IV Antibiotics
    Consider Corticosteroids

(E) Consider High-Dose Amoxicillin

Assess for complications
(Cont'd on p 255)

plus IV antibiotics and switch to oral chloramphenicol or IM ceftriaxone when the patient becomes stable. When resistant organisms are identified, base antibiotic treatment on the sensitivity pattern. If the organism is resistant to ampicillin, chloramphenicol, and cephalosporins, consider ciprofloxacin or furazolidone. TMP-SMX and amoxicillin are oral alternative therapies for moderate cases with sensitive organisms. If fever persists longer than 10 days, assess for complications and/or a resistant organism. Consider a bone marrow culture to identify a resistant organism. Relapse of fever, abdominal pain, and headache requiring a second course of antibiotics may occur in 15% of treated cases.

E. Approximately 3% of patients with typhoid fever become carriers. The best method of identifying carriers is with a hemagglutination test Vi (envelope) antigen titer 1:160 or higher. The eradication of the carrier state is difficult. The efficacy of high-dose amoxicillin is unclear.

TABLE 2   Drugs Used in the Treatment of Typhoid Fever

Drug	Dosage	Product Availability
Chloramphenicol	75–100 mg/kg/24 hr divided q6h until fever resolves, then 50 mg/kg/24 hr to complete 3 wk	Vial: 1 g
Ceftriaxone	100 mg/kg/24 hr IV divided q12h or 80 mg/kg IM qd	Vial: 0.25, 0.5, 1 g
Ampicillin	200 mg/kg/24 hr divided q6h IV	Vial: 125, 250, 500, 1000, 2000 mg
Amoxicillin	100 mg/kg/24 hr divided q.i.d. PO	Liquid: 125, 500 mg/5 ml
		Caps: 250, 500 mg
		Chewable: 125, 250 mg
TMP-SMX	5 mg (T) kg/dose b.i.d. or 0.5 ml/kg/dose b.i.d.	Liquid: 40 mg (T)/5 ml
		Tabs: 80, 160 mg
		T:S = 1:5
Dexamethasone	3 mg/kg IV, then 8 doses of 1 mg/kg q6h	Vials: 4, 10 mg/ml
Ciprofloxacin	5 mg/kg/24 hr IV q12h 20–30 mg/kg/24 hr PO divided q12h	Vial: 10 mg/ml (20 ml)
		Tabs: 250, 500, 750 mg
Furazolidone	7.5 mg/kg/24 hr PO divided q6h	Liquid: 50 mg/15 ml

T, trimethoprim component.

References

Casanueva VE, Cid X, Cavicchioli G, et al. Serum adenosine deaminase in the early diagnosis of typhoid fever. Pediatr Infect Dis J 1992; 11:828.

Constanza V, Hernandez H, Kay B, et al. Efficacy of bone marrow, blood, stool and duodenal contents cultures for bacteriologic confirmation of typhoid fever in children. Pediatr Infect Dis 1985; 4:496.

Dutta P, Rasaily R, Saha MR, et al. Ciprofloxacin for treatment of severe typhoid fever in children. Antimicrob Agents Chemother 1993; 37:1197.

Dutta P, Rasaily R, Saha MR, et al. Randomized clinical trial of furazolidone for typhoid fever in children. Scand J Gastroenterol 1993; 28:168.

Girgis NI, Kilpatrick ME, Farid Z, et al. Cefixime in the treatment of enteric fever in children. Drugs Exp Clin Res 1993; 19:47.

Girgis NI, Sultan Y, Hammad O, Farid Z. Comparison of the efficacy, safety and cost of cefixime, ceftriaxone and aztreonam in the treatment of multidrug-resistant Salmonella Typhi septicemia in children. Pediatr Infect Dis J 1995; 14:603.

Gupta A. Multidrug-resistant typhoid fever in children: Epidemiology and therapeutic approach. Pediatr Infect Dis J 1994; 13:134.

Kizilcan F, Tanyel FC, Buyukpamukcu N, Hicsonmez A. Complications of typhoid fever requiring laparotomy during childhood. J Pediatr Surg 1993; 28:1490.

Punjabi NH, Pulungsih P, Woodward TE. Treatment of severe typhoid fever in children with high dose dexamethasone. Pediatr Infect Dis J 1988; 7:598.

Rahman S, Barr W, Hilton E. Use of oral typhoid vaccine strain Ty21a in a New York state travel immunization facility. Am J Trop Med Hyg 1993; 48:823.

Rodriguez WJ. Typhoid Fever. In: Kaplan SL, ed. Current therapy in pediatric infectious disease. 3rd ed. St. Louis: Mosby, 1993:256.

Sharma A, Gathwala G. Clinical profile and outcome in enteric fever. Indian Pediatr 1993; 30:47.

Thisyakorn U, Mansuwan P, Taylor DN. Typhoid and paratyphoid fever in 192 hospitalized children in Thailand. Am J Dis Child 1987; 141:862.

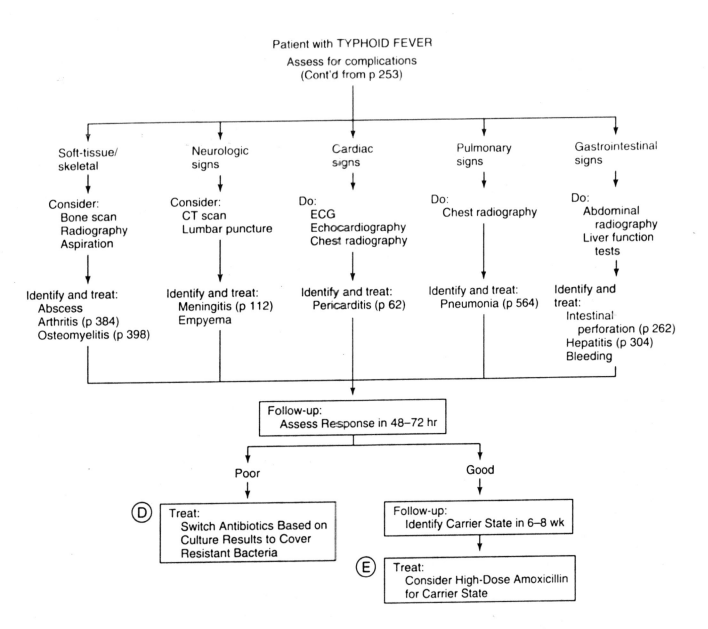

Patient with TYPHOID FEVER
Assess for complications
(Cont'd from p 253)

Soft-tissue/skeletal
↓
Consider:
  Bone scan
  Radiography
  Aspiration
↓
Identify and treat:
  Abscess
  Arthritis (p 384)
  Osteomyelitis (p 398)

Neurologic signs
↓
Consider:
  CT scan
  Lumbar puncture
↓
Identify and treat:
  Meningitis (p 112)
  Empyema

Cardiac signs
↓
Do:
  ECG
  Echocardiography
  Chest radiography
↓
Identify and treat:
  Pericarditis (p 62)

Pulmonary signs
↓
Do:
  Chest radiography
↓
Identify and treat:
  Pneumonia (p 564)

Gastrointestinal signs
↓
Do:
  Abdominal radiography
  Liver function tests
↓
Identify and treat:
  Intestinal perforation (p 262)
  Hepatitis (p 304)
  Bleeding

Follow-up:
Assess Response in 48–72 hr

Poor
↓
(D) Treat:
  Switch Antibiotics Based on Culture Results to Cover Resistant Bacteria

Good
↓
Follow-up:
  Identify Carrier State in 6–8 wk
↓
(E) Treat:
  Consider High-Dose Amoxicillin for Carrier State

GASTROENTEROLOGIC DISORDERS

Abdominal Mass
Abdominal Pain — Acute
Abdominal Pain — Persistent or Recurrent
Ascites
Bloody Stools
Constipation
Crohn Disease
Diarrhea — Acute
Diarrhea—Chronic
Gastroesophageal Reflux

Hematemesis
Hepatitis
Hepatomegaly
Jaundice After 6 Months of Age
Pancreatitis
Peptic Ulcer Disease
Splenomegaly
Ulcerative Colitis
Vomiting After Infancy
Vomiting During Infancy

ABDOMINAL MASS

Perla Santos Ocampo, M.D.
Stephen Berman, M.D.

The most common neoplasms that present with an abdominal mass are neuroblastoma and Wilms tumor. Abdominal masses in newborns are often benign.

A. In the history ask about the age of the child when the mass was detected and systemic manifestations such as fever, anorexia, weight loss, bleeding, pallor, ascites, vomiting, and diarrhea. Note the rate at which the mass grows; a slow-growing mass is usually benign.

B. In the physical examination carefully palpate the mass. Intraabdominal masses can generally be palpated either anteriorly (intraperitoneal) or posteriorly (retroperitoneal). If a posterior mass is huge, it can be palpated anteroposteriorly. Some intraperitoneal masses that are normal include the neonatal liver, intestines with gas and/or feces, a pregnant uterus, and a distended bladder. Soft cystic masses are usually benign; malignancy often presents as a hard mass. If a malignancy is suspected, palpate gently and briefly, and limit the number of examinations. Caution: undue palpation may disseminate tumor cells. Look for other masses in the body.

C. CBC with differential may suggest malignancy because of abnormal cells, anemia, neutropenia, or pancytopenia.

D. Fothergill test is done by increasing the intraabdominal pressure (e.g., Valsalva maneuver). If the mass becomes more prominent with this maneuver, it is in the abdominal wall.

(Continued on page 260)

TABLE 1   The International Neuroblastoma Staging System

Stage 1	Localized tumor confined to area of origin, complete gross excision, with or without microscopic residual disease; identifiable lymph nodes negative microscopically
Stage 2	Unilateral tumor with incomplete gross excision; identifiable lymph nodes negative microscopically
Stage 3	Unilateral tumor with complete or incomplete gross excision; positive ipsilateral regional lymph nodes; identifiable contralateral lymph nodes negative microscopically
Stage 4	Dissemination of tumor to distant lymph nodes, bone, bone marrow, liver, or other organs (except as defined in stage 4S)
Stage 4S	Localized primary tumor as defined for stage 1 or 2 with dissemination limited to liver, skin, or bone marrow

TABLE 2   Staging Classification for Wilms Tumor

Stage I	Tumor limited to kidney and completely excised
Stage II	Tumor extends beyond kidney but completely excised
Stage III	Residual nonhematogenous tumor confined to abdomen a. Lymph nodes involved b. Diffuse peritoneal contamination by tumor c. Peritoneal implants found d. Tumor beyond surgical margins (microscopic or gross) e. Unresectable tumor infiltrating into vital structures
Stage IV	Hematogenous metastases (e.g., lung, liver)
Stage V	Bilateral renal involvement at diagnosis

Patient with ABDOMINAL MASS

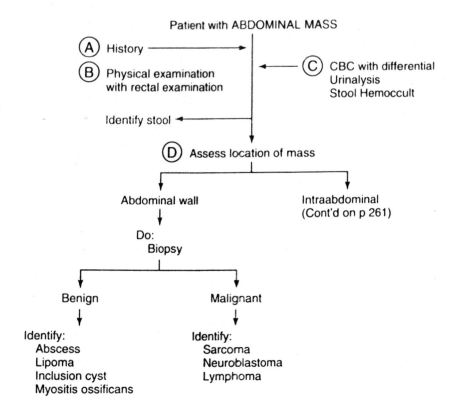

(A) History

(B) Physical examination
with rectal examination

(C) CBC with differential
Urinalysis
Stool Hemoccult

Identify stool

(D) Assess location of mass

Abdominal wall

Intraabdominal
(Cont'd on p 261)

Do:
Biopsy

Benign

Malignant

Identify:
Abscess
Lipoma
Inclusion cyst
Myositis ossificans

Identify:
Sarcoma
Neuroblastoma
Lymphoma

E. Lymphomas, mesenteric cysts, and tuberculous masses may be found in all quadrants of the abdomen. An ovarian tumor may be palpated anywhere in the lower half of the abdomen. Ovarian malignancies are usually unilateral. Masses in the lower left quadrant, other than stool, are more likely malignant than masses in the right lower quadrant.

F. Ultrasonography or IV pyelography will show whether the pathology is intrinsically renal or extrarenal. If the mass originates outside of the kidney, an MRI or CT scan will give its exact location and extent.

G. Neuroblastoma, a neural crest cell malignancy, is the most common malignancy in infancy and early childhood. Some 75% occur in children younger than 4 years of age. Additional clinical manifestations include systemic symptoms, signs of excessive catecholamine activity (episodes of sweating, headache, hypertension, flushing, pallor, or diarrhea), myoclonus and opsoclonus, or evidence of metastatic spread (subcutaneous nodules, skeletal involvement, liver, bone marrow, retroorbital space). Laboratory evidence of neuroblastoma includes elevation of serum norepinephrine and its metabolites in urine vanillylmandelic acid and homovanillic acid as well as elevated urinary cystathionine. Neuroblastoma is staged as shown in Table 1. Therapy usually includes surgery, radiotherapy, and chemotherapy.

Generally, the younger the patient, the higher the survival rate: under 1 year, 74%; 1 to 2 years, 26%; over 2 years, 12%.

H. Wilms tumor, or nephroblastoma, the most common malignancy of the genitourinary tract, has a peak incidence at 3 to 4 years. Additional clinical manifestations include microscopic hematuria (25%), hypertension (25%), congenital aniridia (1 in 70 children with Wilms tumor), congenital hemihypertrophy, and chromosome abnormalities. In 10% of tumors calcification is seen on radiographs. Wilms tumor metastasizes to the lungs, brain, bone, and bone marrow. The staging classification is shown in Table 2. Rarely, Wilms tumor can be bilateral. Cure rates of over 90% for stages I, II, and III are possible; stage IV has a cure rate of about 60%.

References

Brodeur AE, Brodeur GM. Abdominal masses in children: Neuroblastoma, Wilms tumor, and other considerations. Pediatr Rev 1991; 12:196.

Lanzkowsky P. Cancers in childhood. In: Hoekelman RA, Blatman S, Friedman SB, et al, eds: Primary pediatric care. St. Louis: Mosby, 1987:1165.

Tunnessen WW. A 10-year-old boy with hepatomegaly. Contemp Pediatr 1987; March:121.

Patient with ABDOMINAL MASS
Intraabdominal
(Cont'd from p 259)

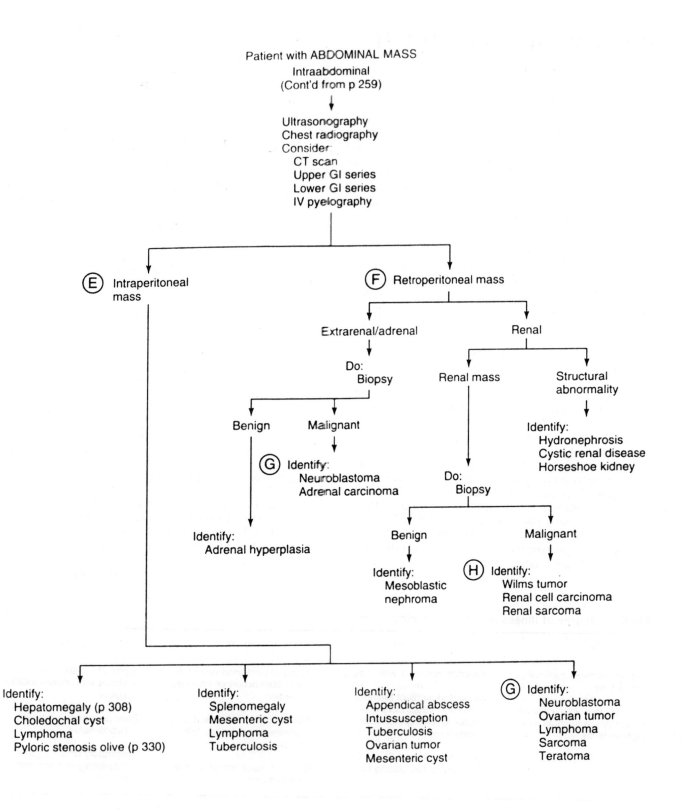

Ultrasonography
Chest radiography
Consider:
CT scan
Upper GI series
Lower GI series
IV pyelography

Ⓔ Intraperitoneal mass

Ⓕ Retroperitoneal mass

Extrarenal/adrenal

Do:
Biopsy

Benign

Malignant

Ⓖ Identify:
Neuroblastoma
Adrenal carcinoma

Identify:
Adrenal hyperplasia

Renal

Renal mass

Structural abnormality

Identify:
Hydronephrosis
Cystic renal disease
Horseshoe kidney

Do:
Biopsy

Benign

Identify:
Mesoblastic nephroma

Malignant

Ⓗ Identify:
Wilms tumor
Renal cell carcinoma
Renal sarcoma

Identify:
Hepatomegaly (p 308)
Choledochal cyst
Lymphoma
Pyloric stenosis olive (p 330)

Identify:
Splenomegaly
Mesenteric cyst
Lymphoma
Tuberculosis

Identify:
Appendical abscess
Intussusception
Tuberculosis
Ovarian tumor
Mesenteric cyst

Ⓖ Identify:
Neuroblastoma
Ovarian tumor
Lymphoma
Sarcoma
Teratoma

ABDOMINAL PAIN—ACUTE

Stephen Berman, M.D.

A. In the history determine the onset, frequency, severity, pattern, and location of the pain. Note associated symptoms of urinary tract involvement (dysuria, frequency) and any fever, vomiting, diarrhea, rectal bleeding, jaundice, weight loss, and arthritis. Identify precipitating factors and predisposing conditions, including constipation, trauma, medications, menses, spider bite, sickle cell disease, pregnancy, prior abdominal surgery, and inflammatory bowel disease.

B. In the physical examination assess the circulatory and hydration status. Note signs of peritoneal irritation such as ileopsoas rigidity (psoas sign), pain with external thigh rotation (obturator test), pain with jarring movements, difficulty or inability to walk or jump, hyperesthesia, and referred pain to the neck or shoulder. Signs of intestinal obstruction include abdominal distention, decreased bowel sounds, and persistent vomiting. Gently palpate the abdomen with the patient's legs slightly raised to relax the abdominal rectus muscles. Signs of peritonitis include rigidity of the abdominal muscles, rebound tenderness, decreased bowel sounds, abdominal distention, and shock. Locate the sites of maximal pain and radiation of pain. With epigastric pain, consider peptic ulcer disease, hiatal hernia, gastroesophageal reflux, esophagitis, and pancreatitis. Right upper quadrant pain suggests hepatitis, liver abscess or tumor, Fitz-Hugh-Curtis syndrome, cholecystitis, or cholangitis. When mild abdominal pain is diffuse, periumbilical, or left-sided, consider constipation, mesenteric adenitis, food poisoning, pharyngitis, muscle strain, gastroenteritis, and psychogenic pain.

C. Signs that suggest systemic disease or infection include jaundice (hepatitis); perianal lesions, weight loss, bloody stools (inflammatory bowel disease); bloody stools with antibiotic use (pseudomembranous colitis); bloody stools, hematuria, anemia, renal failure (hemolytic uremic syndrome); bloody diarrhea, fever, no vomiting (bacterial enteritis); palpable purpura, arthritis, hematuria (Henoch-Schönlein purpura); prolonged fever, conjunctivitis, mucosal lesions, rash (Kawasaki disease); tick bite, erythema chronicum migrans (Lyme disease); vaginal discharge (pelvic inflammatory disease); fever, weight loss, lymphadenopathy, hepatosplenomegaly (malignancy); anemia (sickle cell disease); cough, rales, decreased breath sounds (lower lobe pneumonia); sore throat, exudate, adenitis (*Streptococcus pyogenes* pharyngitis); and bruises, fractures, abdominal distention (nonaccidental trauma).

D. Ultrasonography is a cost-effective diagnostic technique to identify many causes of acute abdominal pain, including appendicitis, intussusception, gallbladder disorders, biliary tract disease, pelvic masses, and renal disorders. It often fails to identify pelvic inflammatory disease, hepatitis, and pancreatitis. A negative sonogram does not exclude appendicitis or abscess. The sensitivity of ultrasonography for appendicitis is 75%.

E. Suspect ulcer disease when recurrent abdominal pain is associated with nausea, vomiting, hematemesis, or melena. The pain in older children is often epigastric, is relieved by food or antacids, and awakens the patient from sleep.

(Continued on page 264)

TABLE 1 Degree of Illness in Acute Abdominal Pain

Mild	Moderate	Severe	Very Severe
Pain that interferes minimally with activity or Pain associated with a known benign cause such as viral gastroenteritis	Pain that interferes with activity or Associated signs of bacterial infection (respiratory distress, UTI, *Streptococcus pyogenes*) or A history of prior abdominal surgery or necrotizing enterocolitis	Signs of peritonitis or intestinal obstruction or intussusception or Alterations in mental status (delirium, confusion, lethargy) or Signs of moderate or severe dehydration	Signs of sepsis or septic shock with altered mental status or Poor peripheral perfusion, hypotension or Respiratory distress (adult respiratory distress syndrome)

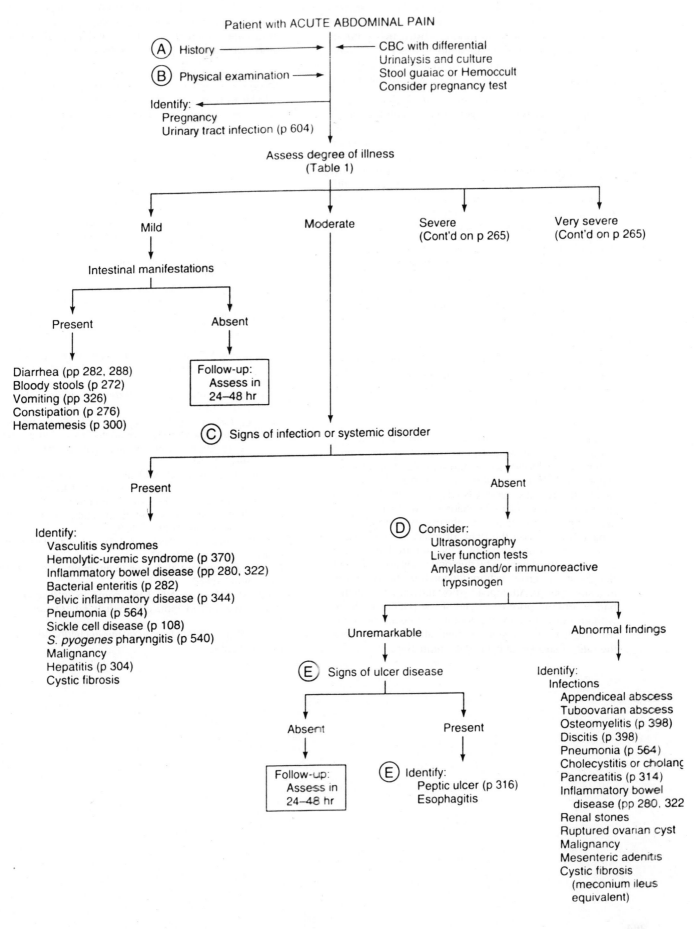

Patient with ACUTE ABDOMINAL PAIN

(A) History → ← CBC with differential
Urinalysis and culture
Stool guaiac or Hemoccult
Consider pregnancy test

(B) Physical examination →

Identify: ←
  Pregnancy
  Urinary tract infection (p 604)

Assess degree of illness
(Table 1)

Mild | **Moderate** | **Severe** (Cont'd on p 265) | **Very severe** (Cont'd on p 265)

Intestinal manifestations

Present

Diarrhea (pp 282, 288)
Bloody stools (p 272)
Vomiting (pp 326)
Constipation (p 276)
Hematemesis (p 300)

Absent

Follow-up:
Assess in
24–48 hr

(C) Signs of infection or systemic disorder

Present

Identify:
  Vasculitis syndromes
  Hemolytic-uremic syndrome (p 370)
  Inflammatory bowel disease (pp 280, 322)
  Bacterial enteritis (p 282)
  Pelvic inflammatory disease (p 344)
  Pneumonia (p 564)
  Sickle cell disease (p 108)
  S. pyogenes pharyngitis (p 540)
  Malignancy
  Hepatitis (p 304)
  Cystic fibrosis

Absent

(D) Consider:
  Ultrasonography
  Liver function tests
  Amylase and/or immunoreactive
    trypsinogen

Unremarkable

(E) Signs of ulcer disease

Absent

Follow-up:
Assess in
24–48 hr

Present

(E) Identify:
  Peptic ulcer (p 316)
  Esophagitis

Abnormal findings

Identify:
  Infections
    Appendiceal abscess
    Tuboovarian abscess
    Osteomyelitis (p 398)
    Discitis (p 398)
    Pneumonia (p 564)
    Cholecystitis or cholang
    Pancreatitis (p 314)
    Inflammatory bowel
      disease (pp 280, 322
    Renal stones
    Ruptured ovarian cyst
    Malignancy
    Mesenteric adenitis
    Cystic fibrosis
      (meconium ileus
      equivalent)

263

F. Abnormal radiographic findings include fecaliths (appendicitis), pneumatosis intestinalis (necrotizing enterocolitis), free air (perforation), obstructive patterns (mechanical and functional), air in an abscess, abdominal mass, and abdominal calcifications. Renal stones, pneumonia, or osteomyelitis may also be identified.

G. Suspect acute pancreatitis when acute abdominal pain radiates to the back or right upper quadrant and is associated with vomiting. Ascites, abdominal distention, and peritoneal signs may be present. Elevation of serum amylase or a radioimmune assay of pancreatic trypsinogen suggests pancreatitis. Ultrasonography may show inflammation or a pseudocyst. Causes of pancreatitis include acquired or congenital structural defects, trauma, metabolic disorders, infection, hemolytic uremia syndrome, and drug toxicity.

H. Appendicitis presents classically with fever, vomiting, point tenderness over McBurney's point, and signs of peritoneal irritation. The findings are variable, reflecting the location of the appendix (iliac, ascending, pelvic), the acuity of the inflammation, and following rupture, the size and site of the abscess. On rectal examination a tender right lower quadrant mass may be palpated. Diarrhea or pyuria may occur. Leukocytosis is common but nonspecific. The absence of fever and vomiting suggests an alternative diagnosis (negative predictive value, 0.97). Perforation is most likely if treatment is delayed more than 36 hours or if the patient is under 8 years of age.

I. Consider an intussusception when intermittent crampy abdominal pain is associated with vomiting, abdominal distention, or bloody stools and an epigastric sausage-shaped mass. Intussusception may cause an alteration in mental status that suggests CNS disease. Intussusception most commonly occurs in children 4 to 24 months of age. Plain abdominal radiography may be normal, show a paucity of gas on the right, or indicate small-bowel obstruction. Ultrasonography is the preferred method of confirming the diagnosis by demonstrating a sonolucent doughnut on cross-section (edematous head of the intussusception). Attempt a hydrostatic reduction with a barium enema prior to surgery if the patient is stable without signs of shock or perforation (free air, peritonitis). The use of analgesic premedication may increase the rate of successful hydrostatic reduction.

J. Nonaccidental abdominal trauma, suggested by a positive history or associated bruises or fractures, causes traumatic pancreatitis, intramural duodenal hematuria, and lacerations of the liver, spleen, or bladder.

K. Acute ovarian torsion has signs of an acute abdomen. When the right ovary is involved, the presentation is similar to that of acute appendicitis. It is diagnosed by ultrasonography. Early diagnosis and surgery are necessary to save the ovary and fallopian tube.

References

Brender JD, Marcuse EK, Koepsell TD, et al. Childhood appendicitis: Factors associated with perforation. Pediatrics 1985; 76:301.

Caty MG, Azizkhan RG. Acute surgical conditions of the abdomen. Pediatr Ann 1994; 23:192.

Goldberg PJ, Tunnessa WW. On being sore in the right lower quadrant. Contemp Pediatr 1991; September:51.

Hubert BC, Toyama WM. Analgesic premedication in the management of ileocolic intussusception. Pediatrics 1987; 79:432.

O'Shea JS, Bishop ME, Alario AJ, et al. Diagnosing appendicitis in children with acute abdominal pain. Pediatr Emerg Care 1988; 4:172.

Reif S, Sloven DG, Lebenthal E. Gallstones in children. Am J Dis Child 1991; 145:105.

Rothrock SG, Green SM, Harding M, et al. Plain abdominal radiography in the detection of acute medical and surgical disease in children: A retrospective analysis. Pediatr Emerg Care 1991; 7:281.

Seashore JH, Touloukian RJ. Midgut volvulus: An ever-present threat. Arch Pediatr Adolesc Med 1994; 148:43.

See CC, Glassman M, Berezin S, et al. Emergency ultrasound in the evaluation of acute-onset abdominal pain in children. Pediatr Emerg Care 1988; 4:169.

Stevenson RJ, Ziegler MM. Abdominal pain unrelated to trauma. Pediatr Rev 1993; 14:302.

Swischuk LE. Protuberant abdomen in an infant. Pediatr Emerg Care 1989; 5:117.

Tenenbein M, Wiseman NE. Early coma in intussusception: Endogenous opioid induced? Pediatr Emerg Care 1987; 3:22.

Weizman Z, Durie PR. Acute pancreatitis in childhood. J Pediatr 1988; 113:24.

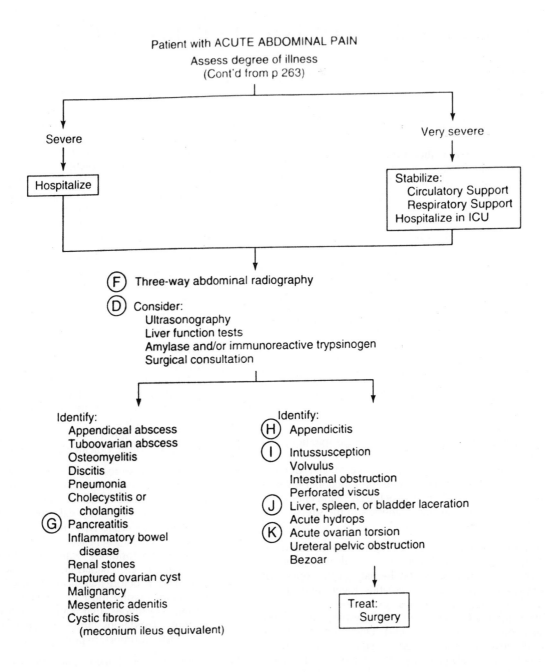

Patient with ACUTE ABDOMINAL PAIN
Assess degree of illness
(Cont'd from p 263)

Severe

Very severe

Hospitalize

Stabilize:
  Circulatory Support
  Respiratory Support
Hospitalize in ICU

(F) Three-way abdominal radiography
(D) Consider:
  Ultrasonography
  Liver function tests
  Amylase and/or immunoreactive trypsinogen
  Surgical consultation

Identify:
  Appendiceal abscess
  Tuboovarian abscess
  Osteomyelitis
  Discitis
  Pneumonia
  Cholecystitis or
    cholangitis
(G) Pancreatitis
  Inflammatory bowel
    disease
  Renal stones
  Ruptured ovarian cyst
  Malignancy
  Mesenteric adenitis
  Cystic fibrosis
    (meconium ileus equivalent)

Identify:
(H) Appendicitis
(I) Intussusception
  Volvulus
  Intestinal obstruction
  Perforated viscus
(J) Liver, spleen, or bladder laceration
  Acute hydrops
(K) Acute ovarian torsion
  Ureteral pelvic obstruction
  Bezoar

Treat:
Surgery

ABDOMINAL PAIN—PERSISTENT OR RECURRENT

Stephen Berman, M.D.

DEFINITION

Persistent or recurrent abdominal pain is usually acute episodes occurring at least monthly for a minimum of 3 months. It is most common in children 10 to 12 years of age (prevalence 10% to 15%).

ETIOLOGY

Causes fall into three groups: organic, dysfunctional, and psychogenic disorders. Multiple causes within each of these groups may be present in a patient. Often there are interactions between dysfunctional and organic disorders, personality and emotional characteristics, habits and lifestyle routines, and critical events and sources of stress.

A. In the history determine the onset, frequency, severity, pattern, and location of the pain. Note associated GI manifestations such as diarrhea and constipation as well as extraintestinal manifestations, including fever, rash, weight loss, arthritis, hematuria, frequency, and dysuria. Note any nonspecific autonomic symptoms such as headache, limb pains, nausea, pallor, perspiration, and vomiting. Identify precipitating factors or predisposing conditions such as medications, sickle cell disease, menses, and foods. Determine the functional level of impairment, the anxiety level of the child and family, the family history of functional illness, and the stress in the child's life.

B. In the physical examination note the site of the pain. With epigastric pain consider nonulcer dyspepsia, peptic ulcer disease, hiatal hernia, gastroesophageal reflux, esophagitis, and pancreatitis. Right upper quadrant pain suggests hepatitis, liver abscess or tumor, Fitz-Hugh-Curtis syndrome, cholecystitis, cholangitis, gallstones, or choledochal cyst. Document any point tenderness, peritoneal signs, rigidity of abdominal muscles, and rebound. Do a rectal examination for impaction or mass. Note signs of pneumonia and other extraintestinal manifestations such as arthritis, ascites, hepatosplenomegaly, jaundice, lymphadenopathy, and purpura.

C. A lack of concern about the effect of the recurrent abdominal pain on the patient's lifestyle suggests a psychogenic disorder. Such a patient often has low self-esteem, a withdrawn personality, and few if any good friends. There may be inappropriate fears and inability to cope with change. Academic performance is often low. Frequent absenteeism from school suggests a school phobia (see p 44). Note any crisis such as recent divorce, illness, or death in family or of friend; move; or fight with parents or friends. Counseling to reduce stress and minimize secondary gain may not be effective. In these cases refer the patient to a mental health professional.

D. Signs of an intestinal dysfunction include intermittent diarrhea and/or constipation, cramping, excessive flatus, mouth breathing, a history of infantile colic, and a family history of irritable bowel syndrome. Weight gain is normal. Colonic distention caused by intestinal spasm produces referred pain to periumbilical and hypogastric areas. Mechanisms that increase gas or liquid proximal to the spasm (lactase deficiency and certain foods) increase the distention and pain.

E. Suspect lactose intolerance when symptoms of cramping, bloating, flatus, or diarrhea develop about 2 hours after the ingestion of milk products. A positive family history is also suggestive. The frequency of lactose intolerance as the primary cause of recurrent abdominal pain is unclear.

F. Lactose intolerance is diagnosed with a lactose breath hydrogen test. A lactose load of 2 g/kg with a maximum of 50 g is given as a 20% solution in water. The hydrogen is measured in exhaled breath prior to the lactose ingestion and at 30 minute intervals for 3 hours. Hydrogen is produced when lactose is fermented by bacteria in the intestines. An increase greater than 20 ppm of hydrogen indicates lactose intolerance.

G. When a lactose-restricted diet is implemented, it is important to monitor intake to ensure adequate consumption of protein, calcium, and calories. Yogurt with active cultures contains β-galactosidase and can usually be tolerated. Certain types of cheese, such as cheddar, are also low in lactose. Lactase supplements, bacterial or yeast β-galactosidases, can be added to lactose-containing foods. Lactaid liquid can be added to milk several hours before ingestion, or capsules can be taken with food. Dosing must be individualized. Recognize organic conditions that cause constipation such as anatomic conditions (anterior displacement of anus), neurologic disorders, hypothyroidism, and drugs.

H. There are recognized guidelines for targeting the work-up for suspected organic disease. When bloody stools, weight loss, perianal lesions, fever, rash, arthritis, or elevated sedimentation rate is present, suspect inflammatory bowel disease and do an upper GI series, barium enema, and endoscopy. If you see persistent nausea, vomiting, hemepositive stools, epigastric or nocturnal pain, and/or positive family history, suspect peptic ulcer disease and work-up with endoscopy or upper GI series. When pain radiates to the back and there is concomitant vomiting and elevated amylase or trypsinogen, suspect recurrent pancreatitis and work-up with ultrasonography. Right upper quadrant pain that radiates to the right shoulder, jaundice, fatty food intolerance, hemolytic disorder may indicate hepatobiliary disease; work-up with ultrasonography and liver function tests. Suspect malignancy when weight loss, fever, lymphadenopathy, hepatospleno-

(Continued on page 268)

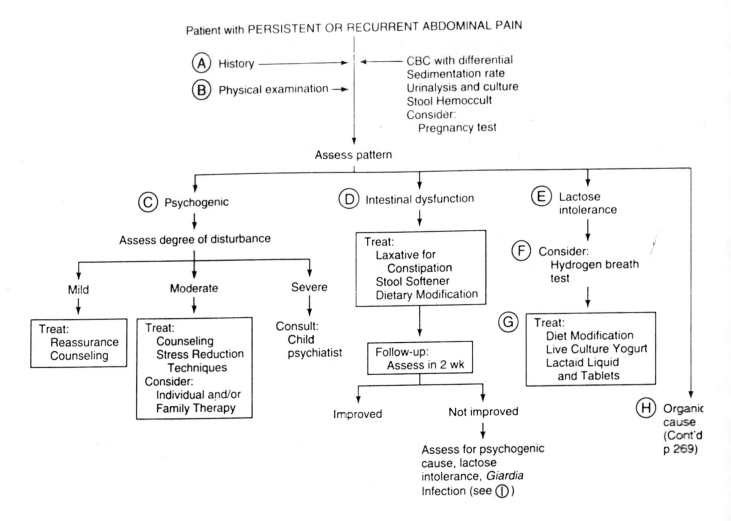

Patient with PERSISTENT OR RECURRENT ABDOMINAL PAIN

(A) History ———————→ ←—— CBC with differential
                                    Sedimentation rate
(B) Physical examination →   Urinalysis and culture
                                    Stool Hemoccult
                                    Consider:
                                        Pregnancy test

Assess pattern

(C) Psychogenic   (D) Intestinal dysfunction   (E) Lactose
                                                              intolerance

Assess degree of disturbance   Treat: (F) Consider:
                                    Laxative for   Hydrogen breath
                                      Constipation   test
Mild   Moderate   Severe   Stool Softener
                                    Dietary Modification
                                                         (G) Treat:
Treat: Treat: Consult: Diet Modification
  Reassurance Counseling   Child   Follow-up: Live Culture Yogurt
  Counseling   Stress Reduction psychiatist Assess in 2 wk   Lactaid Liquid
               Techniques   and Tablets
             Consider:
               Individual and/or   Improved   Not improved
               Family Therapy   (H) Organic
                                                                cause
                                         Assess for psychogenic   (Cont'd
                                         cause, lactose   p 269)
                                         intolerance, *Giardia*
                                         Infection (see (I))

megaly, or abdominal mass is seen, and work-up with ultrasonography, CT scan, biopsy, or bone marrow examination. Palpable purpura, hematuria, and/or arthritis may indicate Henoch-Schönlein purpura.

I. Diagnosis of *Giardia* is based on identification of either trophozoites or cysts on a smear of the stool or duodenal fluid. An enzyme immunoassay of *Giardia* antigens is also available. Testing three stools increases the sensitivity to about 95%. Treat with furazolidine (Furoxone), which is 80% effective, or metronidazole, which is 90% effective but not recommended for children because safety has not been established.

References

Chong SKF, Lou Q, Asnicar MA, et al. *Helicobacter pylori* infection in recurrent abdominal pain in childhood: Comparison of diagnostic tests and therapy. Pediatrics 1995; 96:211

Coleman WL, Levine MD. Recurrent abdominal pain: The cost of the aches and the aches of the cost. Pediatr Rev 1986; 8:143.

Davidson M. Recurrent abdominal pain: Look to dyskinesia as the culprit. Contemp Pediatr 1986; 3:16.

Feldman W, McGrath P, Hodgson C, et al. Am J Dis Child 1985; 139:1216.

Flotte TR. Dietl syndrome: Intermittent ureteropelvic junction obstruction as a cause of episodic abdominal pain. Pediatrics 1988; 82:792.

Gartner JC. Recurrent abdominal pain — who needs a work up? Contemp Pediatr 1989; September:62.

Glassman M, Spivak W, Miniberg D, et al. Chronic idiopathic intestinal pseudoobstruction: A commonly misdiagnosed disease in infants and children. Pediatrics 1989; 83:603.

Oberlander TF, Rappaport LA. Recurrent abdominal pain during childhood. Pediatr Rev 1993; 14:313.

Rings EHHM, Grand RJ, Buller HA. Lactose intolerance and lactase deficiency in children. Curr Opin Pediatr 1994; 6:562.

Silverberg M. Chronic abdominal pain in adolescents. Pediatr Ann 1991; 20:179.

Patient with PERSISTENT OR RECURRENT ABDOMINAL PAIN
Organic cause
(Cont'd from p 267)

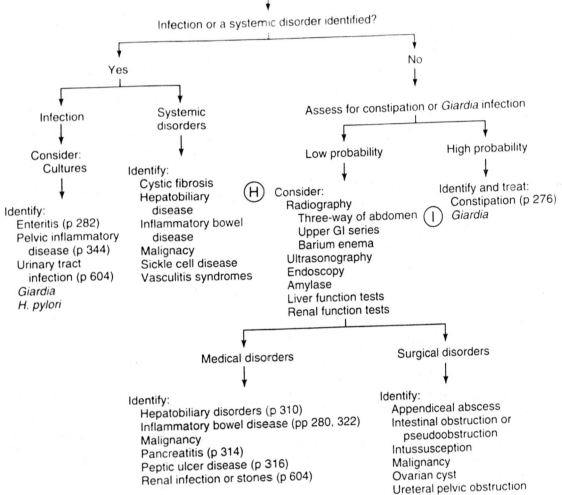

Infection or a systemic disorder identified?

Yes

Infection

Consider:
   Cultures

Identify:
   Enteritis (p 282)
   Pelvic inflammatory
     disease (p 344)
   Urinary tract
     infection (p 604)
   Giardia
   H. pylori

Systemic
disorders

Identify:
   Cystic fibrosis
   Hepatobiliary
     disease
   Inflammatory bowel
     disease
   Malignacy
   Sickle cell disease
   Vasculitis syndromes

No

Assess for constipation or *Giardia* infection

Low probability

(H) Consider:
   Radiography
     Three-way of abdomen
     Upper GI series
     Barium enema
   Ultrasonography
   Endoscopy
   Amylase
   Liver function tests
   Renal function tests

High probability

Identify and treat:
   Constipation (p 276)
(I) *Giardia*

Medical disorders

Identify:
   Hepatobiliary disorders (p 310)
   Inflammatory bowel disease (pp 280, 322)
   Malignancy
   Pancreatitis (p 314)
   Peptic ulcer disease (p 316)
   Renal infection or stones (p 604)

Surgical disorders

Identify:
   Appendiceal abscess
   Intestinal obstruction or
     pseudoobstruction
   Intussusception
   Malignancy
   Ovarian cyst
   Ureteral pelvic obstruction

ASCITES

Perla Santos Ocampo, M.D.

DEFINITION

Ascites is the accumulation of fluid in the peritoneal cavity. The ascites frequently is a component or a complication of hepatic cirrhosis, congestive heart failure, nephrosis, or carcinoma. In such disorders the fluid has the characteristic of a transudate (< 25 g/L of protein, specific gravity < 1.016, and white blood cell count $< 250/m^3$).

A. Shifting dullness to percussion is the most sensitive clinical sign of ascites.

B. Ascites can be confirmed by ultrasonography.

C. Diagnostic paracentesis should be part of the routine examination of the patient with no obvious cause of ascites. Examine the fluid for its gross appearance, specific gravity, protein content, total lipids, serum and fluid lactate, cell count, and differential. Gram stain, acid-fast stain, and culture are requested if an infection is suspected. Cytology and cell block can identify cells that may help determine the cause of the ascites.

D. Cloudy or turbid peritoneal fluid with a predominance of polymorphonuclear cells, a positive Gram stain, and a lactate level or pH less than that of the serum are characteristic of bacterial peritonitis. If most cells are lymphocytes, suspect tuberculosis and order an acid-fast bacilli (AFB) stain and culture. Since Gram stain and AFB stain are negative in a high proportion of cases, culture of the peritoneal fluid is mandatory.

E. Blood-stained or hemorrhagic peritoneal fluid is usually seen in patients with malignancy with peritoneal seeding. The red blood cell count is usually greater than 10,000/mm³ in 20% of cases. A cytology and cell block should always be requested when the peritoneal fluid is bloody. The differential diagnosis of hemorrhagic peritoneal fluid includes pancreatic ascites secondary to pancreatitis and pancreatic pseudocyst. An increase in amylase levels in the ascitic fluid supports the diagnosis of pancreatic involvement. Tuberculous peritonitis may sometimes manifest as bloody peritoneal fluid.

F. Chylous ascites refers to a turbid, milky, or creamy peritoneal fluid. On Sudan staining the fluid shows fat globules microscopically. This disorder results from a congenital or acquired intestinal lymph obstruction. Among the causes of acquired lymphatic obstruction are trauma, tumor, tuberculosis, nephrosis, and filariasis and previous surgery with trauma to the main lymphatic ducts.

G. A fluid that is turbid because of leukocytes or tumor cells may be confused with chylous fluid. Ether extraction of the chylous fluid will lead to clearing if the turbidity is a result of lipids. Chylous ascites may sometimes be seen in patients with nephrosis or malignancy.

References

Behrman RE, Speck WT. Peritoneum and allied structures. In: Behrman RE, Vaughan VC, eds. Textbook of pediatrics. Philadelphia: Saunders, 1983:986.

Friedman H, Kurtzberg J. Abdominal distention. In: Hoekelman RA, Blatman S, Friedman SB, et al, eds. Primary pediatric care. St. Louis: Mosby, 1987:840.

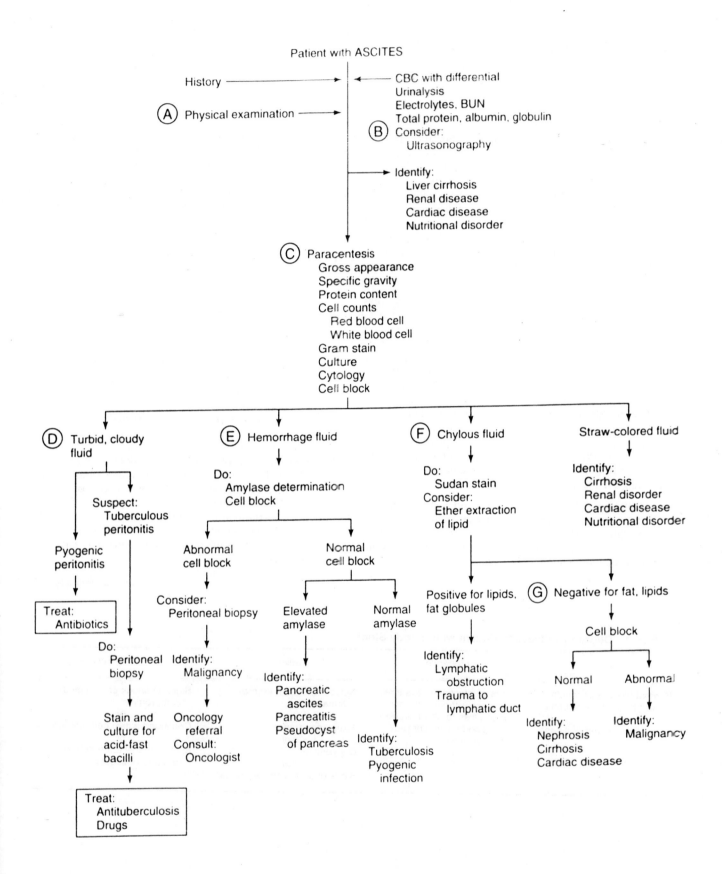

Patient with ASCITES

History

(A) Physical examination

(B) CBC with differential
Urinalysis
Electrolytes, BUN
Total protein, albumin, globulin
Consider:
   Ultrasonography

Identify:
   Liver cirrhosis
   Renal disease
   Cardiac disease
   Nutritional disorder

(C) Paracentesis
   Gross appearance
   Specific gravity
   Protein content
   Cell counts
      Red blood cell
      White blood cell
   Gram stain
   Culture
   Cytology
   Cell block

(D) Turbid, cloudy fluid

Suspect:
   Tuberculous peritonitis

Pyogenic peritonitis

Treat:
Antibiotics

Do:
   Peritoneal biopsy

Stain and culture for acid-fast bacilli

Treat:
Antituberculosis Drugs

(E) Hemorrhage fluid

Do:
   Amylase determination
   Cell block

Abnormal cell block

Consider:
   Peritoneal biopsy

Identify:
   Malignancy

Oncology referral
Consult:
   Oncologist

Normal cell block

Elevated amylase

Identify:
Pancreatic ascites
Pancreatitis
Pseudocyst of pancreas

Normal amylase

Identify:
   Tuberculosis
   Pyogenic infection

(F) Chylous fluid

Do:
   Sudan stain
Consider:
   Ether extraction of lipid

Positive for lipids, fat globules

Identify:
   Lymphatic obstruction
   Trauma to lymphatic duct

(G) Negative for fat, lipids

Cell block

Normal

Identify:
Nephrosis
Cirrhosis
Cardiac disease

Abnormal

Identify:
Malignancy

Straw-colored fluid

Identify:
Cirrhosis
Renal disorder
Cardiac disease
Nutritional disorder

BLOODY STOOLS

Stephen Berman, M.D.

Bloody stools can be bright red (hematochezia) or dark and tarry (melena). Hematochezia usually indicates lower intestinal bleeding; however, massive upper intestinal hemorrhage can produce bright red blood. Melena is associated with gastric or small bowel bleeding. The most common causes of lower intestinal bleeding by age are as follows: less than 2 months, allergic milk protein, necrotizing enterocolitis or volvulus with malrotation; 2 to 24 months, anal fissure, allergic (milk protein) colitis, or intussusception; 2 to 5 years, colonic polyp; more than 5 years, peptic ulcer disease and inflammatory bowel disease.

A. In the history determine the onset, type of bloody stools, and quantity of blood loss. Ask about associated GI symptoms such as diarrhea, vomiting, constipation, anorexia, abdominal pain, or distention. Note extraintestinal symptoms including fever, weight loss, delayed puberty, arthritis, purpura, rash, or jaundice. Exclude ingestion of substances that may be mistaken for melena or hematochezia, such as iron supplementation, bismuth, chocolate, grape juice, spinach, blueberries, food coloring, beets, Jell-O, and red antibiotics. Identify possible precipitating factors or predisposing conditions such as drug ingestions (maternal or child), current antibiotic use, constipation, bleeding disorders, or milk/soy protein intolerance.

B. Obtain a CBC with differential and platelet count to document any anemia. Consider hemolytic-uremic syndrome when thrombocytopenia and a microangiopathic hemolytic anemia are present. Obtain a coagulation screen when hemorrhagic disease of the newborn or other bleeding disorder is suspected. A low serum albumin is associated with a protein-losing enteropathy. An elevated sedimentation rate suggests infection, inflammatory bowel disease, or malignancy. In the newborn period the Apt-Downey or Kleihauer test distinguishes maternal blood from newborn blood. A positive nasogastric aspirate identifies bleeding proximal to the ligament of Treitz.

C. During infancy anal fissures are the most common cause of superficial blood on the stools. Fissures, usually caused by constipation, are also associated with infections of *Candida* and *Streptococcus pyogenes*. Suspect child abuse when a preschool child has anal fissures.

D. Nonspecific colitis related to milk/soy protein intolerance presents in infants under 6 months of age with loose bloody stools and is often associated with vomiting, abdominal pain, and distention. Rarely, it may occur in the newborn or in infants of breast-feeding mothers who drink large amounts of cow's milk. When it is suspected, change to a semielemental formula (Pregestimil, Alimentum, or Nutramigen). Bloody stools should resolve within 2 weeks. Consider a milk challenge in 2 months in a controlled setting to document recurrence of blood in stools. Anaphylaxis is a rare complication of challenge with cow's milk protein. Endoscopy reveals nonspecific findings of superficial aphthoid ulcerations with erythematous margins. Consider using a soy formula in older infants but remember that 30% to 40% of infants with cow's milk protein allergy also react to soy formula.

(Continued on page 274)

TABLE 1 Degree of Illness in Patient with Bloody Stools

Mild	Moderate	Severe	Very Severe
Minimal blood loss insufficient to produce anemia and No systemic signs of illness	Signs of infection or systemic disease without sufficient blood loss to affect circulating blood volume or produce anemia	Newborn, even if asymptomatic or Toxic appearance or Dehydration or Signs of significant blood loss	Signs of shock or circulatory compromise or Continued active hemorrhage or Acute surgical abdomen (peritonitis or acute obstruction)

Patient with BLOODY STOOLS

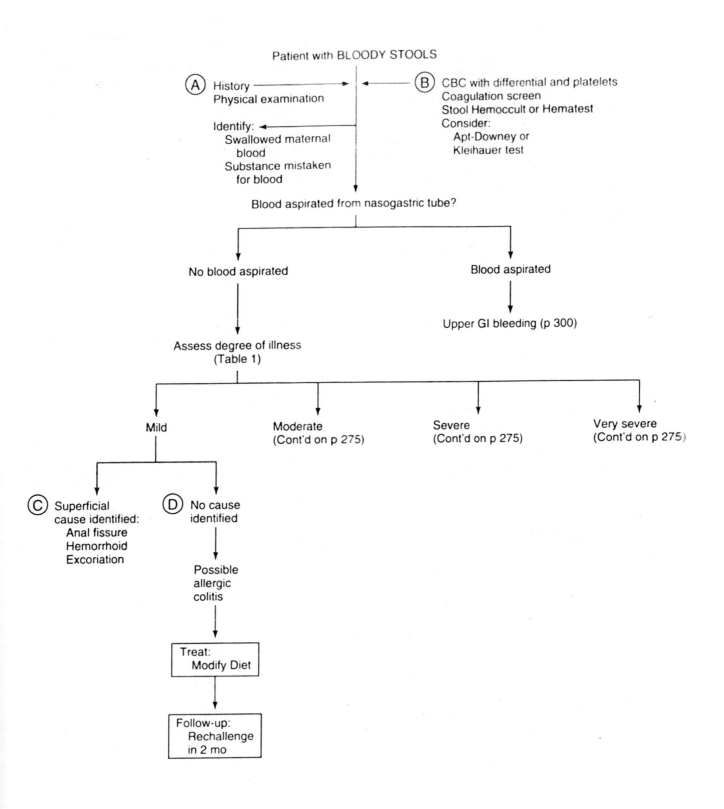

A. History — Physical examination

B. CBC with differential and platelets
Coagulation screen
Stool Hemoccult or Hematest
Consider:
   Apt-Downey or
   Kleihauer test

Identify:
   Swallowed maternal blood
   Substance mistaken for blood

Blood aspirated from nasogastric tube?

No blood aspirated

Blood aspirated

Upper GI bleeding (p 300)

Assess degree of illness (Table 1)

Mild

Moderate (Cont'd on p 275)

Severe (Cont'd on p 275)

Very severe (Cont'd on p 275)

C. Superficial cause identified:
   Anal fissure
   Hemorrhoid
   Excoriation

D. No cause identified

Possible allergic colitis

Treat:
   Modify Diet

Follow-up:
   Rechallenge in 2 mo

E. Pseudomembranous colitis or *Clostridium difficile*–induced antibiotic-associated colitis is toxin mediated. Diagnosis is made by an assay for the *C. difficile* toxin. The two exotoxins are toxin A, an enterotoxin, and toxin B, a cytotoxin. Initial therapy is with metronidazole or vancomycin. Options for persistent or recurrent disease include anion exchange resins to bind the toxins, *Lactobacillus*, other antibiotics, or IV γ-globulin therapy. Pseudomembranous colitis is frequently associated with penicillins, cephalosporins, and clindamycin. Causes of infectious enteritis include *Salmonella, Shigella, Campylobacter, Yersinia, Escherichia coli*, rotavirus, and *Entamoeba histolytica*.

F. Meckel diverticulum, usually within 100 cm of the ileocecal valve, contains gastric parietal cells that irritate adjacent intestinal mucosa. The usual presentation is painless bleeding. A sodium pertechnetate scan often is concentrated in the gastric tissue (sensitivity 85%, specificity 95%). Enteric duplication can also contain ectopic gastric tissue and cause bleeding.

G. Most polyps are the juvenile type and do not have malignant potential. Bleeding from a polyp can be differentiated from hemorrhoids by using a saline enema to soften the stool. Continued bleeding suggests a polyp. When a polyp is suspected, ultrasonography with a saline enema is an acceptable alternative to air contrast barium enema or endoscopy. In Peutz-Jeghers syndrome multiple polyps in the small and large bowel are associated with mucocutaneous pigmentation. Multiple large-bowel polyps associated with soft-tissue tumors or bony abnormalities suggest Gardner syndrome, which is associated with a high risk of malignancy.

H. Suspect a vascular malformation when aortic stenosis, Turner syndrome, or a mucocutaneous disorder (Rendu-Osler-Weber syndrome) is present. Endoscopy (sigmoidoscopy, colonoscopy) is the method most likely to diagnose a lesion. When the bleeding is extensive, arteriography may be necessary to identify the source.

I. Suspect intussusception when bloody stools are associated with intermittent abdominal pain, abdominal distention, or vomiting. Intussusception usually occurs during the first 2 years of life (61% of patients are 4 to 10 months of age). Ultrasonography confirms the diagnosis, and in 80% of cases a barium enema or manometric air insufflation results in hydrostatic reduction.

References

Berezin S, Schwarz SM, Glassman M, et al. Gastrointestinal milk intolerance of infancy. Am J Dis Child 1989; 143:361.

Dutro JA, Santanello SA, Unger F, et al. Rectal bleeding in a 4-month-old boy. JAMA 1986; 256:2239.

Lake AM. Practical proctoscopy for the office. Contemp Pediatr 1984:63.

Lake AM, Whitington PF, Hamilton SR. Dietary protein–induced colitis in breast-fed infants. J Pediatr 1982; 101:906.

Milov DE, Andres JM. Sorting out the causes of rectal bleeding. Contemp Pediatr 1988; October:80.

Nagita A, Amemoto K, Yoden A, et al. Ultrasonographic diagnosis of juvenile colonic polyps. J Pediatr 1994; 124:535.

Odze RD, Wershil BK, Leichtner AM, Antonioli DA. Allergic colitis in infants. J Pediatr 1995; 126:163.

Sampson H, Bernhisel-Broadbent J, Yang E, Scanlon SM. Safety of case in hydrolysate formula in children with milk allergy. J Pediatr 1991; 118:520.

Sibler G. Lower gastrointestinal bleeding. Pediatr Rev 1990; 12:85.

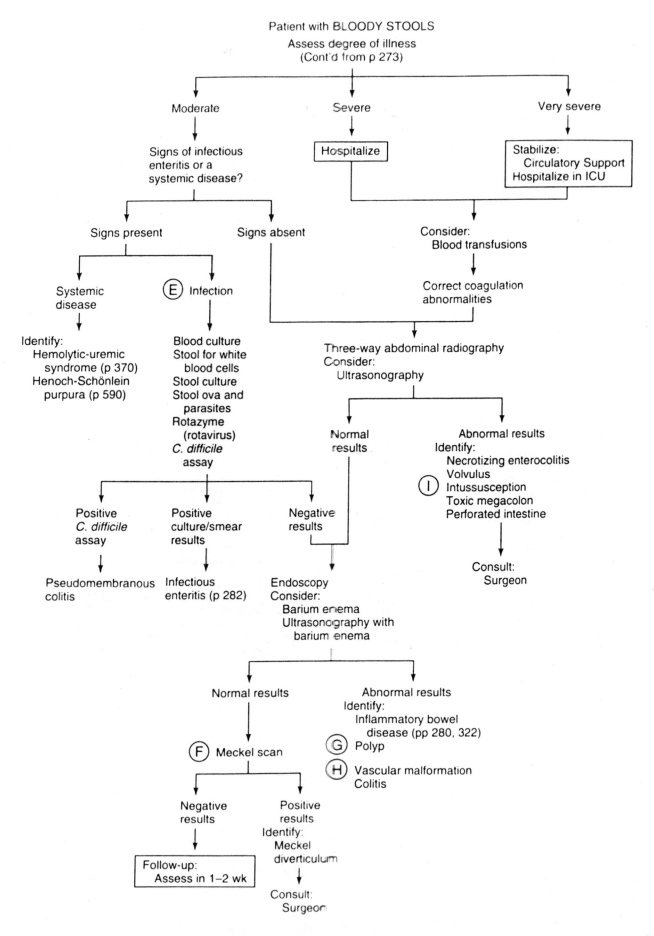

Patient with BLOODY STOOLS
Assess degree of illness
(Cont'd from p 273)

Moderate

Severe

Very severe

Signs of infectious
enteritis or a
systemic disease?

Hospitalize

Stabilize:
  Circulatory Support
  Hospitalize in ICU

Signs present

Signs absent

Consider:
  Blood transfusions

Systemic
disease

Ⓔ Infection

Correct coagulation
abnormalities

Identify:
  Hemolytic-uremic
    syndrome (p 370)
  Henoch-Schönlein
    purpura (p 590)

Blood culture
Stool for white
  blood cells
Stool culture
Stool ova and
  parasites
Rotazyme
  (rotavirus)
C. difficile
  assay

Three-way abdominal radiography
Consider:
  Ultrasonography

Normal
results

Abnormal results
Identify:
  Necrotizing enterocolitis
  Volvulus
Ⓘ Intussusception
  Toxic megacolon
  Perforated intestine

Positive
C. difficile
assay

Positive
culture/smear
results

Negative
results

Consult:
  Surgeon

Pseudomembranous
colitis

Infectious
enteritis (p 282)

Endoscopy
Consider:
  Barium enema
  Ultrasonography with
    barium enema

Normal results

Abnormal results
Identify:
  Inflammatory bowel
    disease (pp 280, 322)
Ⓖ Polyp

Ⓕ Meckel scan

Ⓗ Vascular malformation
  Colitis

Negative
results

Positive
results
Identify:
  Meckel
  diverticulum

Follow-up:
  Assess in 1–2 wk

Consult:
  Surgeon

275

CONSTIPATION

Stephen Berman, M.D.

DEFINITION

Constipation is the painful passage of stool, usually associated with crying in young children and infants, stool retention with voluntary withholding, or a stool frequency of fewer than three bowel movements a week.

A.   In the history ask about stool pattern, size, and consistency. Assess the diet. By 4 months infants usually have one or two bowel movements/day. When an infant is affected, ask whether the parents add honey to the feeds (botulism). Note patient and family history of Hirschsprung disease or other GI disorder, neurologic disorder, endocrine or metabolic disorder, and collagen vascular disease. Inquire about a toddler's toilet training. When appropriate, assess for sexual abuse. Ask about pain with defecation and blood on the stools (anal fissures). Note current medications that may cause constipation such as antacids, anticholinergics, bismuth, iron, and opiates. Ask older patients about psychologic disorders such as depression, anorexia, and sleep disturbances.

B.   In the physical examination perform a rectal examination and note any impaction and presence of stool in the vault. Note anatomic abnormalities such as anal stenosis, corrected imperforate anus, ectopic anus, and anteriorly displaced anus as well as acquired lesions such as anal fissures, perianal abscess, cellulitis, and dermatitis. Examine the patient for signs of neurologic disease, endocrine or metabolic disorders, GI disease, and collagen vascular disease.

C.   Neurologic causes of constipation include cerebral palsy, hypotonia (myotonic dystrophy and other myopathies), spinal cord lesions (spina bifida, meningomyelocele, sacral teratoma), spinal cord trauma, Down syndrome, and mental retardation. Chronic intestinal pseudoobstruction related to a myopathy or neuropathy can cause severe intractable constipation.

D.   Breast-feeding constipation can result in bowel movements as infrequent as every 5 to 7 days. Usually these patients are growing well and have soft normal stools and no abdominal distention. No therapy other than parental reassurance is needed. However, if the infant does not grow, the lactation problems must be assessed and treated. If lactation problems cannot be corrected, supplementation is indicated.

E.   A barium enema will identify approximately 80% of cases with Hirschsprung disease. Findings include documentation of a transition zone that separates a small distal colon from a dilated segment. Additional diagnostic methods are anorectal manometry and tissue biopsy. Most physicians rely on tissue biopsies that can be obtained with a suction biopsy instrument. The presence of ganglion cells excludes Hirschsprung disease, and the absence of ganglion cells is an indication for a surgical procedure to obtain full-thickness biopsies.

F.   Hirschsprung disease, occurring in 1:5000 live births, causes constipation in early infancy. The internal anal sphincter fails to relax with rectal distention because neural ganglia are absent from the distal intestine. The aganglionic segment often extends through the rectum and sigmoid. Delayed passage of meconium suggests Hirschsprung disease, but 60% of patients with this disorder pass meconium in the first 48 hours. Onset of constipation occurs in the newborn period or early infancy and is often associated with abdominal distention and other obstructive symptoms. Treatment of Hirschsprung disease is surgical placement of a diverting ostomy to prevent life-threatening complications of enterocolitis, sepsis, and perforation.

G.   During infancy consider diet modification when constipation is associated with normal growth. This may include supplemental water feedings or the addition of corn syrup to the formula. The addition of cereal, fruits, and vegetables after 3 to 5 months often improves the constipation.

(Continued on page 278)

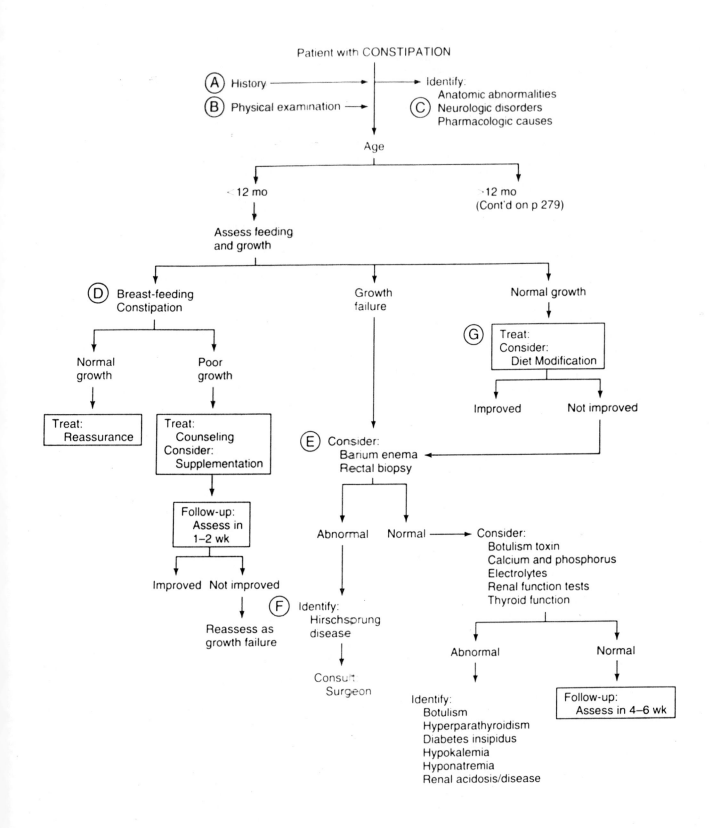

Patient with CONSTIPATION

(A) History ⟶ ⟶ Identify:
(B) Physical examination ⟶   Anatomic abnormalities
    (C) Neurologic disorders
    Pharmacologic causes

Age

<12 mo

>12 mo
(Cont'd on p 279)

Assess feeding
and growth

(D) Breast-feeding
Constipation

Growth
failure

Normal growth

(G) Treat:
Consider:
Diet Modification

Improved   Not improved

Normal
growth

Poor
growth

Treat:
Reassurance

Treat:
Counseling
Consider:
Supplementation

(E) Consider:
Barium enema
Rectal biopsy

Follow-up:
Assess in
1–2 wk

Abnormal   Normal ⟶ Consider:
    Botulism toxin
    Calcium and phosphorus
    Electrolytes
    Renal function tests
    Thyroid function

Improved   Not improved

Reassess as
growth failure

(F) Identify:
Hirschsprung
disease

Abnormal   Normal

Consult:
Surgeon

Identify:
    Botulism
    Hyperparathyroidism
    Diabetes insipidus
    Hypokalemia
    Hyponatremia
    Renal acidosis/disease

Follow-up:
Assess in 4–6 wk

H. Functional fecal retention and withholding not associated with medications or other disorders are the most common cause of constipation in the toddler and school-age child. Withholding may result from discomfort during defecation or problems with toilet training. When the stool is held too long in the rectum by the external sphincter, it dries out, becomes hard, and produces pain with passage. This reinforces withholding and retention. Eventually a very large mass may be passed and/or the child may develop encopresis (see p 36). Rectal examination usually reveals impacted stool in the ampulla.

I. Remove the impaction with two or three hyperphosphate enemas or give 1 oz/year of age/day (8 oz maximum) of mineral oil by mouth for 3 to 4 days. Treat the child with a stool softner such as mineral oil, magnesium salts (Milk of Magnesia), or lactulose for 3 months, until the diameter and tone of the bowel return to normal. Treat children who hold back because of pain or negativism with a laxative in addition to the stool softener. Recommend a diet that includes increased amounts of bran, fresh fruits and vegetables, and decreased milk products. Instruct the parents that the older child should also sit on the toilet three times a day, or the program will fail. Some children will not sit on the toilet unless offered incentives. The physcian's continued involvement is critical even if the child needs referral to a psychologist or psychiatrist.

References

Fitzgerald JF. Constipation in children. Pediatr Rev 1987; 8:299.

Gleghorn EE, Heyman MB, Rudolph CD. No-enema therapy for idiopathic constipation and encopresis. Clin Pediatr 1991; 30:669.

Loening-Baucke V. Constipation in children. Curr Opin Pediatr 1994; 5:556.

Nolan T, Debelle G, Oberklaid F, et al. Randomised trial of laxatives in treatment of childhood encopresis. Lancet 1991; 338:523.

Pettei MJ. Chronic constipation. Pediatr Ann 1987; 16:796.

Reisner SH, Silvan Y, Nitzan M, et al. Determination of anterior displacement of the anus in newborn infants and children. Pediatrics 1984; 73:216.

Rockney RM, McQuade WH, Days AL. The plain abdominal roentgenogram in the management of encopresis. Arch Pediatr Adolesc Med 1995; 149:623.

Rudolph C, Benaroch L. Hirschsprung disease. Pediatr Rev 1995; 16:5.

Sondheimer JM. Helping the child with chronic constipation. Contemp Pediatr 1985; March:12.

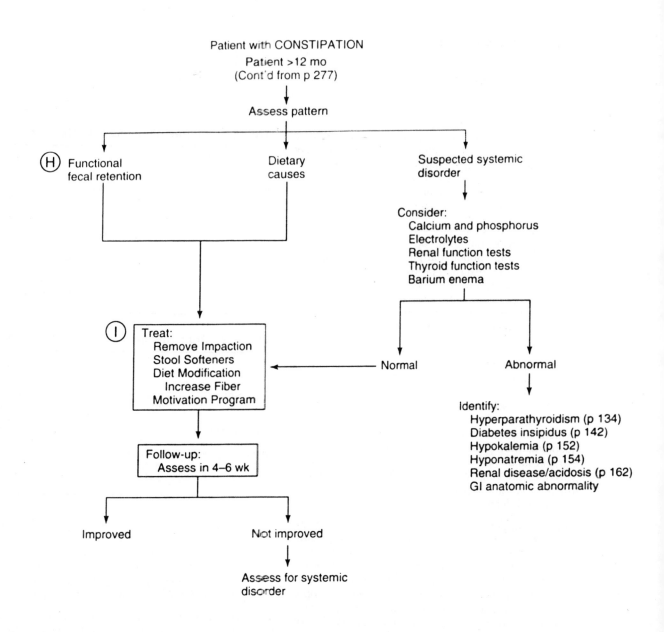

Patient with CONSTIPATION
Patient >12 mo
(Cont'd from p 277)

↓

Assess pattern

(H) Functional
fecal retention

Dietary
causes

Suspected systemic
disorder

↓

Consider:
   Calcium and phosphorus
   Electrolytes
   Renal function tests
   Thyroid function tests
   Barium enema

Normal   Abnormal

(I) Treat:
   Remove Impaction
   Stool Softeners
   Diet Modification
   Increase Fiber
   Motivation Program

↓

Follow-up:
   Assess in 4–6 wk

Improved   Not improved

↓

Assess for systemic
disorder

Identify:
   Hyperparathyroidism (p 134)
   Diabetes insipidus (p 142)
   Hypokalemia (p 152)
   Hyponatremia (p 154)
   Renal disease/acidosis (p 162)
   GI anatomic abnormality

CROHN DISEASE

Stephen Berman, M.D.

Crohn disease, an immune-mediated inflammation of the GI tract of unknown origin, can be categorized by the pattern of involvement: ileocolitis (52%), diffuse small intestine (20%), ileitis (19%), and colitis (9%). Common presenting manifestations include diarrhea, abdominal pain, bloody stools, weight loss, growth failure, and fever.

A. In the history note any anorexia, weight loss, nausea, vomiting, abdominal pain, or diarrhea. Right lower quadrant crampy abdominal pain may mimic appendicitis. Severe anorexia and protracted vomiting suggest intestinal obstruction. The degree of bleeding and diarrhea depends on the involvement of the colon. Systemic extraintestinal symptoms include fever, poor growth, jaundice, delayed puberty, arthritis, conjunctivitis, and rash.

B. Note any aphthous ulcers of the mouth and anal fissures, ulcerations, abscess, fistula, and skin tags. Document signs of chronic malnutrition and hypoalbuminemia (muscle wasting, peripheral edema, clubbing of the fingers and toes) and signs of vitamin deficiency. Matted loops of bowel, especially in right lower quadrant, may present as an abdominal mass. Note extraintestinal manifestations such as arthritis, hepatitis, gallstones, cholangitis, uveitis, episcleritis, enterovesical fistulas, urethritis, nephrolithiasis, anemia, growth retardation, and delayed puberty.

C. Obtain an upper GI series, small bowel follow-through, and barium enema. Characteristic findings include thickened mucosa, ulcerations, pseudopolypoid formation with cobblestoning, and stenotic areas with proximal dilatation. Colonoscopy may show colitis or ulcerations separated by normal mucosa (skip areas). Biopsy shows through and through acute and chronic inflammation and noncaseating granulomas (in <25% of cases). The rectum is usually spared. Consider endoscopy with biopsy of the upper GI tract to distinguish gastric Crohn disease from peptic ulcer disease.

D. Manage moderately ill patients with a caloric intake at least 40% over baseline, supplemented with vitamins (fat-soluble folic acid, B_{12}), minerals (calcium, magnesium), and trace metals (zinc, copper, and iron). Supplementation is required because steatorrhea and involvement of the terminal ileum impair absorption of these substances. Iron supplementation is often required because of chronic intestinal blood loss. Methods to increase caloric intake include high caloric supplements and nighttime intragastric infusion. When lactose intolerance is documented with a hydrogen breath test, avoid lactose-containing foods. A low-residue diet may reduce diarrhea and abdominal pain.

E. Consider sulfasalazine in patients with ileocolitis or colitis who have no extraintestinal manifestations. Maintenance sulfasalazine therapy is not indicated. Treat other patients with prednisone for 6 to 8 weeks, followed by an alternate-day regimen and then gradual tapering by

TABLE 1 Degree of Illness in Crohn Disease

Moderate	Severe	Very Severe
Feeding tolerated despite anorexia and abdominal pain	Marked malnutrition or dehydration and Inability to tolerate oral feedings because of abdominal pain, vomiting, and intermittent partial intestinal obstruction	Toxic appearance (sepsis or toxic megacolon) or Complication requiring surgery

TABLE 2 Drug Therapy for Crohn Disease In Children

Agent	Dosage	Product Availability
Prednisone	1–1.5 mg/kg/day (max 60 mg)	Solution: 5 mg/5 ml Tabs: 1, 2.5, 5, 10, 20, 50 mg
Sulfasalazine	50–75 mg/kg/day divided q.i.d.	Susp: 250 mg/5 ml Tabs: 500 mg
Metronidazole (Flagyl)	15–30 mg/kg/day divided t.i.d. (max 750 mg/day)	Tabs: 250, 500 mg

reducing the drug by 5 mg a week. Steroid-dependent patients may respond to a 3 to 6 month trial of 6-mercaptopurine or azathioprine, allowing a decreased steroid dose. Complications of these drugs include leukopenia, acute pancreatitis, and renal failure. Treat perianal lesions with metronidazole.

F. When necessary, consider enteral alimentation with an elemental formula. Nasogastric feeding for 3 weeks followed by a low-residue diet may be required. Elemental diets can treat such GI complications as fistulas and perianal disease. Treat patients who have severe disease and cannot tolerate enteral alimentation with an elemental formula with parenteral hyperalimentation.

G. Consider surgery for the following: repeated episodes of intestinal obstruction, abscess unresponsive to antibiotic therapy, enterovesicular fistula, toxic megacolon, massive hemorrhage, and progressive disease despite 2 years of adequate steroid therapy. Growth failure is not a clear indication for surgery; surgery is successful in only 20% to 50% of cases. Adult patients with Crohn disease have an increased risk of cancer early in the disease, but the risk does not increase linearly with disease duration, as it does in ulcerative colitis.

References

Balistreri WF. Minimizing the effects of idiopathic IBD. Contemp Pediatr 1985; July:24.

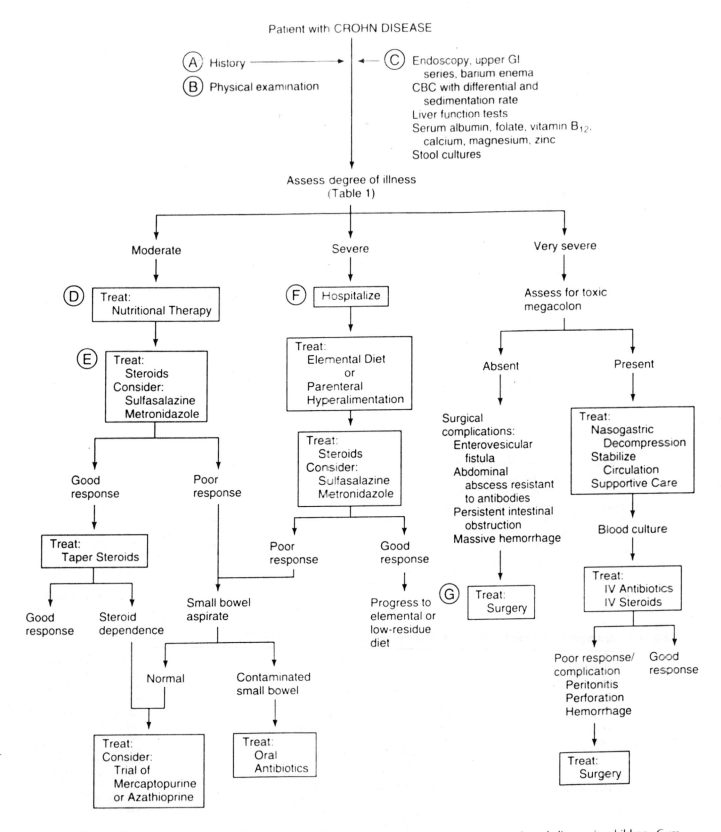

Patient with CROHN DISEASE

(A) History
(B) Physical examination

(C) Endoscopy, upper GI
series, barium enema
CBC with differential and
sedimentation rate
Liver function tests
Serum albumin, folate, vitamin B$_{12}$,
calcium, magnesium, zinc
Stool cultures

Assess degree of illness
(Table 1)

Moderate

(D) Treat:
Nutritional Therapy

(E) Treat:
Steroids
Consider:
Sulfasalazine
Metronidazole

Good response

Poor response

Treat:
Taper Steroids

Good response

Steroid dependence

Small bowel aspirate

Normal

Contaminated small bowel

Treat:
Consider:
Trial of
Mercaptopurine
or Azathioprine

Treat:
Oral
Antibiotics

Severe

(F) Hospitalize

Treat:
Elemental Diet
or
Parenteral
Hyperalimentation

Treat:
Steroids
Consider:
Sulfasalazine
Metronidazole

Poor response

Good response

Progress to
elemental or
low-residue
diet

Very severe

Assess for toxic
megacolon

Absent

Surgical
complications:
Enterovesicular
fistula
Abdominal
abscess resistant
to antibodies
Persistent intestinal
obstruction
Massive hemorrhage

(G) Treat:
Surgery

Present

Treat:
Nasogastric
Decompression
Stabilize
Circulation
Supportive Care

Blood culture

Treat:
IV Antibiotics
IV Steroids

Poor response/
complication
Peritonitis
Perforation
Hemorrhage

Good response

Treat:
Surgery

Crohn BB, Ginsburg L, Oppenheimer GD. Regional ileitis. A pathologic and clinical entity. JAMA 1984; 251:73.

Gryboski JD. Crohn's disease in children. Pediatr Rev 1981; 2:239.

Lenaerts C, Roy CC, Vaillancourt M, et al. High incidence of upper gastrointestinal tract involvement in children with Crohn disease. Pediatrics 1989; 83:777.

MacDonald TT. Inflammatory bowel disease in children. Curr Opin Pediatr 1994; 6:547.

O'Gorman M, Lake AM. Chronic inflammatory bowel disease in childhood. Pediatr Rev 1993; 14:475.

Steffen RM, Wyllie R, Sivak MV, et al. Colonoscopy in the pediatric patient. J Pediatr 1989; 115:507.

DIARRHEA—ACUTE

Stephen Berman, M.D.

Acute diarrhea is an increase in the number of stools and alteration in consistency in relation to the patient's normal stooling pattern. Acute diarrhea is caused by any of several viral, bacterial, and parasitic agents. Rotavirus and Norwalk-like virus are the most common agents, causing up to 50% of acute diarrhea during the winter. Diarrhea can be classified by the underlying pathogenic mechanism. Noninflammatory watery diarrhea results when the infection (or enterotoxin) promotes secretion of fluid and electrolytes or reduces absorption in the small bowel. Pathogens that cause noninflammatory diarrhea are rotaviruses, Norwalklike viruses, *Giardia*, toxigenic *Escherichia coli*, *Staphylococcus aureus*, *Clostridium perfringens*, *Cryptosporidium*, and *Vibrio cholerae*. Inflammatory diarrhea, caused by invasion of the bowel mucosa, often presents with blood, mucus and pus in the stool, tenesmus, severe cramps, and fever. Pathogens that invade the mucosa are *Shigella*, *Campylobacter*, *Salmonella*, invasive *E. coli*, *C. perfringens*, *Aeromonas*, *Yersinia*, and *Entamoeba histolytica*. Systemic bacteremic infections related to intracellular multiplication and penetration occur with *Salmonella typhi* (typhoid fever), *Yersinia*, and *Campylobacter*.

A. In the history ask about the onset, duration, frequency, pattern, and severity of the diarrhea. Ask if the stools contain blood or mucus. Document type and amount of food intake and frequency of urination. Note associated GI symptoms such as vomiting, abdominal pain, and anorexia. Note systemic symptoms such as fever, cough, coryza, rash, weight loss, mental status, and decreased activity level. Identify any precipitating factors such as medications (antibiotics) and ingestions. Ask if other family members have recently had diarrhea.

   In the physical examination assess hydration and circulatory status by documenting blood pressure, pulse, respiratory rate, skin color and turgor, capillary refill, tears, fullness of the fontanelle, and urine output. Assess mental status, noting any irritability, lethargy, seizures, or focal neurologic signs. Watch the child drink and note whether the child drinks normally, eagerly, or poorly (not able to drink). Note extraintestinal signs such as rash, hepatomegaly, splenomegaly, lymphadenopathy, and arthritis.

B. Assess the risk of bacterial or parasitic enteritis. *High-risk* patients have a dysentery-like presentation with fever, toxic appearance, and bloody stools. Tenesmus and crampy abdominal pain may be present. Seizures suggest a *Shigella* infection. Patients at *moderate risk* have a rapid onset of diarrhea without vomiting and more than four diarrheal stools a day with blood or mucus. This clinical presentation has a sensitivity of 86% and positive predictive value of 27% for bacterial enteritis. *Other risk* factors include exposure at home or in day care to bacterial enteritis, raw seafood *(Vibrio)*, raw milk *(Salmonella* and *Campylobacter)*, exposure to a sick dog or cat *(Yersinia)*, recent antibiotics *(Clostridium difficile)*, or travel to a developing country (toxigenic *E. coli*, *Shigella*, *E. histolytica*). Staphylococcal food poisoning presents within 6 hours of ingestion and *C. perfringens* food poisoning presents within 12 to 18 hours of ingestion. Patients under 3 months of age, immunocompromised children, and patients with sickle cell disease also have a higher risk of bacterial infection.

C. The goal of treatment is clinical improvement and shortened duration of fecal shedding to reduce transmission. Treat *Shigella* infections to achieve clinical improve-

(Continued on page 284)

TABLE 1 Antibiotic Therapy for Bacterial and Parasitic Diarrhea in Children

Antibiotic	Dosage	Product Availability
Amoxicillin	15 mg/kg/dose t.i.d. × 5 days	Chewables: 125 mg Tabs: 250, 500 mg
Ampicillin	25 mg/kg/dose q.i.d. × 5 days	Liquid: 125, 250 mg/5 ml
Cefixime (Suprax)	8 mg/kg/dose once daily × 7 days	Liquid: 100 mg/5 ml
Chloramphenicol	10–20 mg/kg/dose q6h	Vial: 1 g
Erythromycin	10 mg/kg/dose q.i.d. × 5–7 days	Liquid: 200, 400 ml/5 ml Chewables: 200 mg Tabs, caps: 250, 500 mg
Furazolidone (Furoxone)	1.5–2 mg/kg/dose q.i.d. × 7 days	Tabs: 100 mg Liquid: 50 mg/15 ml
Gentamicin	<7 days of age 2.5 mg/kg/dose IV q12h >7 days of age 2.5 mg/kg/dose IV q8h	Vials: 20, 80 mg
Metronidazole (Flagyl)	5–13 mg/kg/dose t.i.d. × 7 days (max 750 mg/day)	Tabs: 250 mg
Quinacrine hydrochloride (Atabrine)	2 mg/kg/dose t.i.d. × 7 days (max 300 mg)	Tabs: 100 mg
TMP-SMX	5 mg T/kg/dose b.i.d. or 0.5 ml/kg/dose b.i.d. × 5 days	Liquid: 40 mg T/5 ml Tabs: 80, 160 mg
Vancomycin (Vancocin)	2.5–10 mg/kg/dose q.i.d.	Liquid: 500 mg/6 ml

T, trimethoprim component.

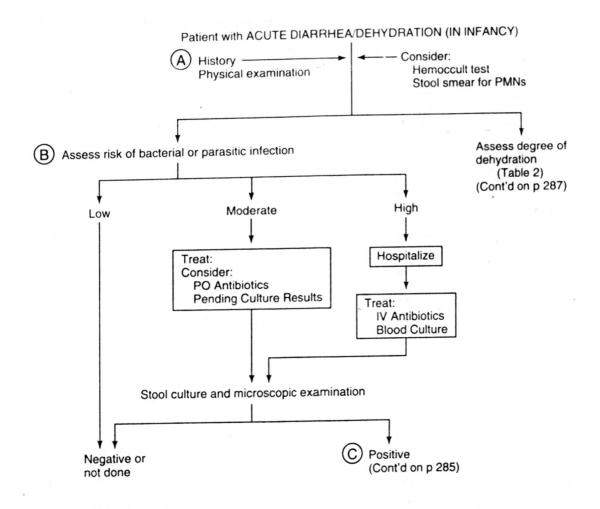

Patient with ACUTE DIARRHEA/DEHYDRATION (IN INFANCY)

(A) History ⟶ ◄── Consider:
Physical examination   Hemoccult test
                            Stool smear for PMNs

Assess degree of
dehydration
(Table 2)
(Cont'd on p 287)

(B) Assess risk of bacterial or parasitic infection

Low   Moderate   High

                              Hospitalize

Treat:
Consider:
  PO Antibiotics
  Pending Culture Results

                         Treat:
                           IV Antibiotics
                           Blood Culture

Stool culture and microscopic examination

Negative or   (C) Positive
not done   (Cont'd on p 285)

ment and stop transmission. Treatment of *Campylobacter* shortens duration of shedding but may not alter the clinical course. In many cases of *Salmonella* infection, antibiotics will not result in clinical improvement and may prolong the carrier state. However, patients at risk for bacteremia or disseminated suppurative disease should be treated. These include infants less than 6 to 12 months of age and patients with sickle cell disease, immunosuppression, or congenital heart disease. Treat enteropathogenic *E. coli* in neonates to prevent necrotizing enterocolitis. The effectiveness of antibiotic therapy in *Yersinia* and *Aeromonas* infections is unclear. In most cases of antibiotic-associated *C. difficile* diarrhea, discontinuation of antibiotics results in clinical improvement. Treat only persistent severe infection. Treat *Giardia* and *E. histolytica* infections with antibiotics (Table 1).

D. For infants with mild illness, have the parents alternate oral rehydrating solutions (ORS) (Hydra-Lyte, Pedialyte, Resol) with breast-feeding or formula or low-sodium fluids without high carbohydrate content. Give as much of these fluids as the infant will take. If the patient is older than 6 months, encourage the eating of solid food. Avoid soft drinks and juices that have a large amount of sugar (Jell-O water, Gatorade) because of their high osmotic load. For patients with moderate illness, have parents give ORS at 15 to 20 ml/kg/hour for 4 hours. Solutions with sodium concentrations of 50 to 90 mEq/L with 2% glucose are equally safe and effective (Table 3). Then begin breast-feeding or formula at 6 ml/kg/hour. If the patient is vomiting, give 1 to 2 teaspoons of ORS every 5 minutes and gradually increase the amount. If the patient refuses to drink, consider a nasogastric tube as an alternative to IV hydration. Continue breast-feeding during the diarrhea episode; it reduces the severity of the episode. The optimal formula is less clear.

TABLE 2 Degree of Dehydration in Acute Diarrhea

Mild	Moderate	Severe
Alert, active	Restless, irritable	Lethargic, unresponsive
Drinks normally	Drinks eagerly	Unable to drink or drinks poorly
Eyes are not sunken	Eyes are sunken	Signs of shock such as hypotension, poor peripheral perfusion, delayed capillary refill (>2 sec), cool pale extremities, thready pulse
Tears are present	Tears are absent	
Mouth and tongue are moist	Mouth and tongue are dry	
Skin does not tent	Skin goes back slowly	Skin goes back very slowly (tents)

Most infants will tolerate their usual formula given as either half or full strength. Those who do not may be switched to a nonlactose soy formula. For children who eat solids, recommend rice, noodles, and potatoes. Slowly reinstitute a normal diet without high-carbohydrate juices or soft drinks.

E. Admit moderately ill patients with acidosis (pH <7.3, HCO_3 <13), azotemia (BUN >20), or an electrolyte abnormality (sodium <130 or >150).

F. Management of hospitalized patients with moderate or severe dehydration requires the correction of fluid deficit and electrolyte abnormalities. Rehydration during the 24 hour period is accomplished in three phases: circulatory stabilization (1 to 2 hours), deficit replacement (next 8 hours), and the maintenance replacement (16 hours). Always treat patients with severe dehydra-

(Continued on page 286)

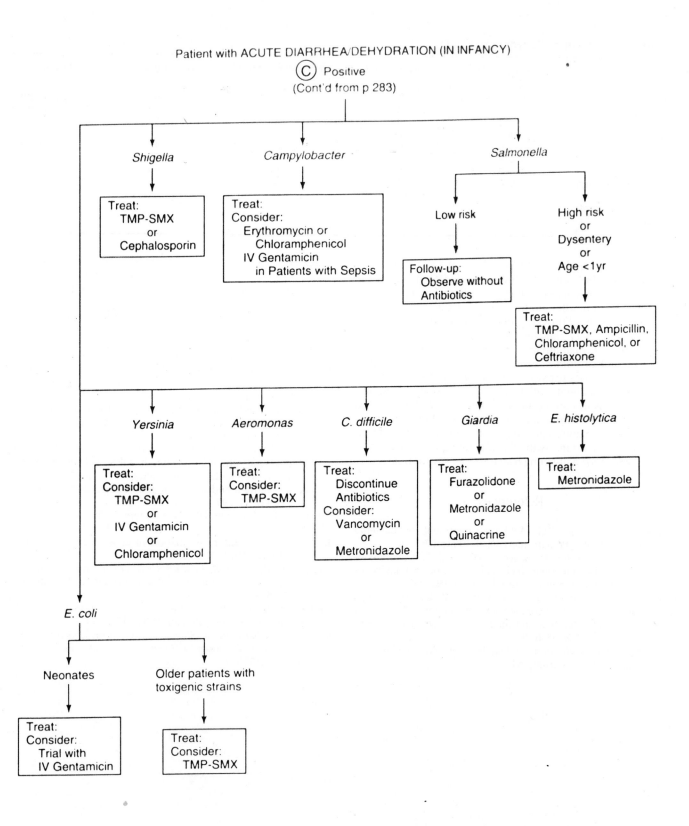

Patient with ACUTE DIARRHEA/DEHYDRATION (IN INFANCY)
Ⓒ Positive
(Cont'd from p 283)

Shigella

Treat:
  TMP-SMX
    or
  Cephalosporin

Campylobacter

Treat:
Consider:
  Erythromycin or
    Chloramphenicol
  IV Gentamicin
    in Patients with Sepsis

Salmonella

Low risk

Follow-up:
  Observe without
  Antibiotics

High risk
  or
Dysentery
  or
Age <1yr

Treat:
  TMP-SMX, Ampicillin,
  Chloramphenicol, or
  Ceftriaxone

Yersinia

Treat:
Consider:
  TMP-SMX
    or
  IV Gentamicin
    or
  Chloramphenicol

Aeromonas

Treat:
Consider:
  TMP-SMX

C. difficile

Treat:
  Discontinue
  Antibiotics
Consider:
  Vancomycin
    or
  Metronidazole

Giardia

Treat:
  Furazolidone
    or
  Metronidazole
    or
  Quinacrine

E. histolytica

Treat:
  Metronidazole

E. coli

Neonates

Treat:
Consider:
  Trial with
  IV Gentamicin

Older patients with
toxigenic strains

Treat:
Consider:
  TMP-SMX

TABLE 3 Content of Rehydrating Fluids

Solution	Glucose (g/dl)	Sodium (mEq/L)	Potassium (mEq/L)	Chloride (mEq/L)	Base (mEq/L)
WHO solution	2.0	90	20	80	30 bicarb
Hydra-Lyte	1.2	84	10	59	70 bicarb
Pedialyte-RS	2.5	75	20	65	30 citrate
Pedialyte	2.5	45	20	35	30 citrate
Lytren	2.0	50	25	45	30 citrate
Resol	2.0	50	20	50	34 citrate
Infalyte	2.0	50	20	40	30 bicarb
Bouillon (1 cube/qt)	2.0	72	12	—	—
Jell-O water (one 3-oz pkg/qt)	5.6	45	18	—	—
Gatorade	4.6	23	3	17	—

tion and shock with 20 ml/kg/hour of isotonic IV fluids. Repeat the isotonic bolus as needed to maintain the circulatory volume. After the patient has been stabilized, administer fluids to replace the deficit over 8 hours without providing maintenance fluid. This can be done with IV fluid or ORS. During the following 16 hours of maintenance replacement, administer the amount of fluid needed for 24 hours of maintenance fluid for patients with isotonic or hypotonic dehydration. For patients with hypertonic dehydration administer fluids to correct the total deficit over 48 hours and lower the serum sodium 0.5 to 1 mEq/L/hour. During or after the maintenance replacement phase, institute refeeding of infants with ORS alternating with breast milk, formula, or half-strength lactose-free soy formula.

References

Ashkenazi S, Cleary TG. Antibiotic treatment of bacterial gastroenteritis. Pediatr Infect Dis J 1991; 10:140.

Brown KH, Gastanduy AS, Saavedra JM, et al. Effectiveness of continued oral feeding on clinical and nutritional outcomes of acute diarrhea in children. J Pediatr 1988; 112:191.

Cohen MB, Mezoff AG, Laney DW Jr, et al. Use of a single solution for oral rehydration and maintenance therapy of infants with diarrhea and mild to moderate dehydration. Pediatrics 1995; 95:639.

Finberg L. Oral rehydration: Finding the right solution. Contemp Pediatr 1987; February:61.

Fontana M, Zuin G, Paccagnine S, et al. Simple clinical score and laboratory-based method to predict bacterial etiology of acute diarrhea in childhood. Pediatr Infect Dis J 1987; 6:1088.

Guerrant RL, Lohr JA, Williams EK. Acute infectious diarrhea: Diagnosis, treatment and prevention. Pediatr Infect Dis J 1986; 5:458.

Hoogkamp-Korstanje JAA, Stolk-Engelaar VMM. Yersina enterocolitica infection in children. Pediatr Infect Dis J 1995; 14:771.

Huskins WC, Griffiths JK, Faruque ASG, et al. Shigellosis in neonates and young infants. J Pediatr 1994; 125:14.

Lieberman JM. Rotavirus and other viral causes of gastroenteritis. Pediatr Ann 1994; 23:529.

Molina S, Vettorazzi C, Peerson JM, et al. Clinical trial of glucose-oral rehydration solution (ORS), rice dextrin-ORS, and rice flour-ORS for the management of children with acute diarrhea and mild or moderate dehydration. Pediatrics 1995; 95:191.

Northaup RS, Flanigan TP. Gastroenteritis. Pediatr Rev 1994; 15:461.

Radetsky M. Laboratory evaluation of acute diarrhea. Pediatr Infect Dis J 1986; 5:230.

Santosham M, Brown K, Sack RB. Oral rehydration therapy and dietary therapy for acute childhood diarrhea. Pediatr Rev 1987; 8:273.

Santosham M, Greenough WB. Oral rehydration therapy: A global perspective. J Pediatr 1991; 118:S44.

Stutman HR. Salmonella, Shigella, and Campylobacter: Common bacterial causes of infectious diarrhea. Pediatr Ann 1994; 23:538.

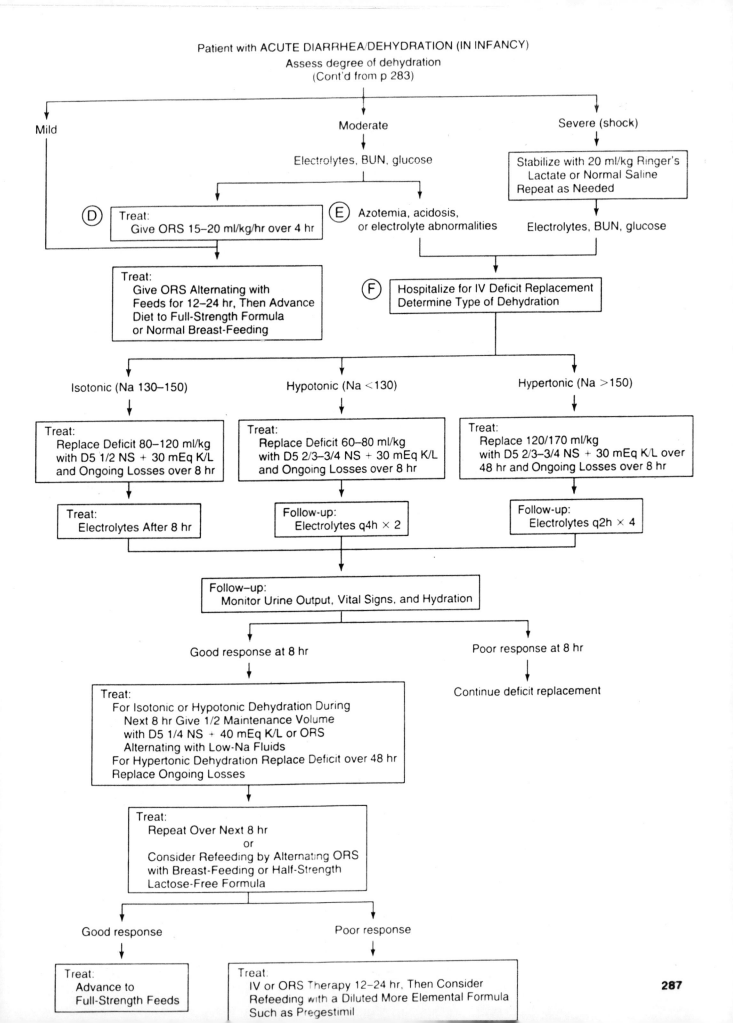

Patient with ACUTE DIARRHEA/DEHYDRATION (IN INFANCY)
Assess degree of dehydration
(Cont'd from p 283)

Mild

Moderate

Electrolytes, BUN, glucose

Severe (shock)

Stabilize with 20 ml/kg Ringer's
Lactate or Normal Saline
Repeat as Needed

Ⓓ Treat:
   Give ORS 15–20 ml/kg/hr over 4 hr

Ⓔ Azotemia, acidosis,
   or electrolyte abnormalities

Electrolytes, BUN, glucose

Treat:
   Give ORS Alternating with
   Feeds for 12–24 hr, Then Advance
   Diet to Full-Strength Formula
   or Normal Breast-Feeding

Ⓕ Hospitalize for IV Deficit Replacement
   Determine Type of Dehydration

Isotonic (Na 130–150)

Treat:
   Replace Deficit 80–120 ml/kg
   with D5 1/2 NS + 30 mEq K/L
   and Ongoing Losses over 8 hr

Hypotonic (Na <130)

Treat:
   Replace Deficit 60–80 ml/kg
   with D5 2/3–3/4 NS + 30 mEq K/L
   and Ongoing Losses over 8 hr

Hypertonic (Na >150)

Treat:
   Replace 120/170 ml/kg
   with D5 2/3–3/4 NS + 30 mEq K/L over
   48 hr and Ongoing Losses over 8 hr

Treat:
   Electrolytes After 8 hr

Follow-up:
   Electrolytes q4h × 2

Follow-up:
   Electrolytes q2h × 4

Follow–up:
   Monitor Urine Output, Vital Signs, and Hydration

Good response at 8 hr

Poor response at 8 hr

Continue deficit replacement

Treat:
   For Isotonic or Hypotonic Dehydration During
   Next 8 hr Give 1/2 Maintenance Volume
   with D5 1/4 NS + 40 mEq K/L or ORS
   Alternating with Low-Na Fluids
   For Hypertonic Dehydration Replace Deficit over 48 hr
   Replace Ongoing Losses

Treat:
   Repeat Over Next 8 hr
      or
   Consider Refeeding by Alternating ORS
   with Breast-Feeding or Half-Strength
   Lactose-Free Formula

Good response

Poor response

Treat:
   Advance to
   Full-Strength Feeds

Treat:
   IV or ORS Therapy 12–24 hr, Then Consider
   Refeeding with a Diluted More Elemental Formula
   Such as Pregestimil

DIARRHEA — CHRONIC

Stephen Berman, M.D.

Chronic diarrhea is an increase in the frequency, fluidity, or volume of the bowel movement, compared with the normal pattern, for longer than 14 to 21 days. Stool output in excess of 10 g/kg/day in infants and more than 200 g/day in children indicates diarrhea. Pathogenic mechanisms that produce chronic diarrhea include osmotic disorders (excessive carbohydrate intake or malabsorption); secretory disorders (infection, hormone-secreting tumors); bacterial overgrowth with bile acid and fatty acid malabsorption; abnormal sodium (Na) and chlorine (Cl) ion absorption; mucosal damage (infection, malnutrition, immune-mediated); reduction in intestinal area (short bowel syndrome); and abnormal intestinal motility (systemic diseases, inflammatory bowel disease, malnutrition, dysfunctional or irritable bowel syndromes).

A. In the history ask about amount and consistency of any blood and frequency of stooling. Obtain a thorough dietary history including the type, frequency, and amount of meals. Ask about vomiting and prior GI disease and surgery. Ask parents to do a 3 day dietary analysis, listing the total intake for three representative 24 hour periods over 2 weeks. A dietitian will calculate the total 24 hour caloric intake for these 3 days.

B. In the physical examination assess nutritional status by plotting growth. Note abdominal distention (disaccharide malabsorption, Hirschsprung, constipation, obstructive disorder), bruising (vitamin K deficiency), a palpable thyroid (hyperthyroidism), respiratory findings (cystic fibrosis), clubbing (cystic fibrosis, Crohn disease, celiac disease), rectal prolapse (celiac disease, cystic fibrosis), perianal tags, fissures, or fistulae (Crohn disease), and signs of systemic disease.

C. Screen a fresh stool sample for ova and parasites, pH, reducing substances, white blood cells, blood, and fats. If sucrose intolerance is suspected, hydrolyze the stool with hydrochloric acid before testing with a Clinitest tablet. Use a Sudan red stain to identify fat droplets before and after acid hydrolysis of the stool samples.

D. Irritable bowel syndrome causes intermittent or persistent diarrhea, cramping, mouth breathing, and excessive flatus *without failure to thrive*. Foods with high osmotic properties or high levels of disaccharides produce diarrhea. Irritable bowel syndrome may follow viral gastroenteritis.

(Continued on page 290)

Patient with CHRONIC DIARRHEA

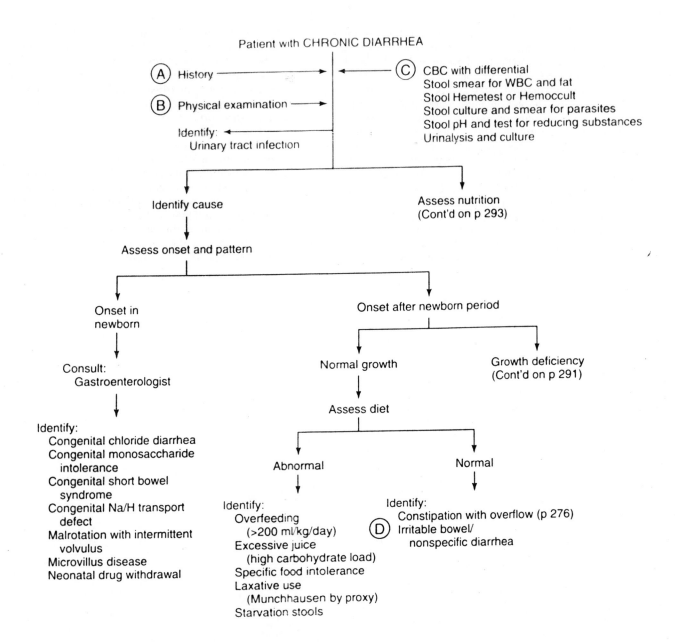

(Cont'd on p 293)

Growth deficiency
(Cont'd on p 291)

E. Infection can cause persistent diarrhea by several mechanisms, including invasion and mucosal damage, secretory diarrhea, and bacterial overgrowth in the small bowel producing malabsorption. Diagnosis and management of the bacterial, viral, and parasitic agents are reviewed in the chapter on acute diarrhea (see p 282). *Cryptosporidium* infection may be common in children with severe malnutrition. The D-xylose absorption test appears to be the best predictor of small intestine mucosal disease (sensitivity 80%, specificity 75%, negative predictive value 86%). It is performed after an overnight fast using a 10% solution at a dose of 0.5 g/kg (maximum 25 g). Blood xylose obtained 60 minutes later is higher than 20 mg/dl in normals. Systemic diseases associated with persistent diarrhea include Shwachman syndrome, (pancreatic insufficiency with cyclic neutropenia), acrodermatitis enteropathica, ad-renal insufficiency, AIDS/HIV, immunodeficiency disorders, cystic fibrosis, Hirschsprung disease, inflammatory bowel disease, malignancy, hyperthyroidism, celiac disease, and eosinophilic gastroenteritis. Infectious causes of chronic diarrhea include bacterial enteritis, parasite enteritis, viral enteritis, and pseudomembranous *Clostridium difficile* colitis.

F. Celiac disease is caused by sensitivity to gluten that produces enteropathy. The severity and extent of mucosal involvement vary greatly. The toxic substance is gliadin, an extract from gluten. The diarrhea has secretory and malabsorption components. Diagnosis can be made with IgA and IgAG antigliadin antibodies. Elimination of gluten from the diet by eliminating products made with wheat, barley, and rye results in rapid clinical improvement. Rice, soy, and corn flours are substituted.

(Continued on page 292)

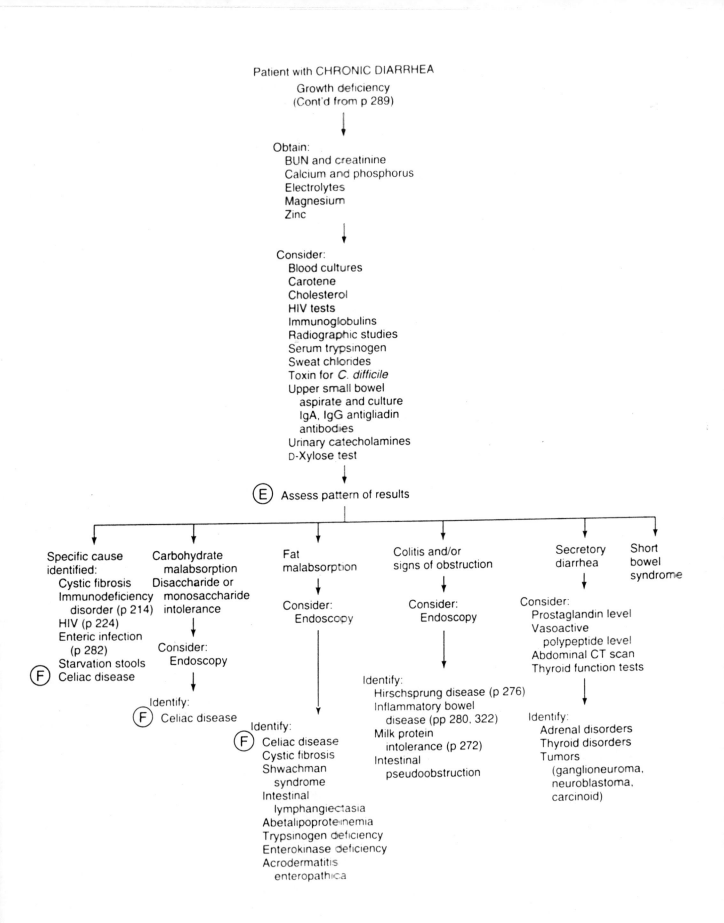

Patient with CHRONIC DIARRHEA
Growth deficiency
(Cont'd from p 289)

Obtain:
    BUN and creatinine
    Calcium and phosphorus
    Electrolytes
    Magnesium
    Zinc

Consider:
    Blood cultures
    Carotene
    Cholesterol
    HIV tests
    Immunoglobulins
    Radiographic studies
    Serum trypsinogen
    Sweat chlorides
    Toxin for *C. difficile*
    Upper small bowel
      aspirate and culture
      IgA, IgG antigliadin
      antibodies
    Urinary catecholamines
    D-Xylose test

(E) Assess pattern of results

Specific cause identified:
Cystic fibrosis
Immunodeficiency
    disorder (p 214)
HIV (p 224)
Enteric infection
    (p 282)
Starvation stools
(F) Celiac disease

Carbohydrate malabsorption
Disaccharide or
monosaccharide
intolerance

Consider:
    Endoscopy

Identify:
(F) Celiac disease

Fat malabsorption

Consider:
    Endoscopy

Identify:
(F) Celiac disease
    Cystic fibrosis
    Shwachman
      syndrome
    Intestinal
      lymphangiectasia
    Abetalipoproteinemia
    Trypsinogen deficiency
    Enterokinase deficiency
    Acrodermatitis
      enteropathica

Colitis and/or signs of obstruction

Consider:
    Endoscopy

Identify:
    Hirschsprung disease (p 276)
    Inflammatory bowel
      disease (pp 280, 322)
    Milk protein
      intolerance (p 272)
    Intestinal
      pseudoobstruction

Secretory diarrhea

Consider:
    Prostaglandin level
    Vasoactive
      polypeptide level
    Abdominal CT scan
    Thyroid function tests

Identify:
    Adrenal disorders
    Thyroid disorders
    Tumors
      (ganglioneuroma,
      neuroblastoma,
      carcinoid)

Short bowel syndrome

G. Patients with altered motility may benefit from a diet modified to increase polyunsaturated fats. A low-osmolar formula with corn syrup appears to help in some cases. In older children avoid frequent feedings of liquids, especially those with high sugar content. Avoid hot, cold, or spicy foods.

H. Treat infants who appear to be recovering from an acute GI insult with adequate calories provided by a low-osmolar formula without lactose. Consider the use of aluminum hydroxide (Amphogel), which binds bile acid and prevents irritation of the colonic mucosa. It may be necessary to tolerate some transient worsening of the diarrhea in patients with starvation stools prior to observing a good response. In difficult cases consider a more elemental formula such as Pregestimil. Avoid the use of absorbents such as kaolin pectin suspension (Kaopectate) and intestinal paralytic agents such as Lomotil.

I. Pediatric semielemental formulas include Pregestimil and Alimentum. These formulas contain casein hydrolysate (short-chain polypeptide), medium-chain triglycerides, and sucrose or glucose polymers. Due to the high osmotic load, the formulas may have to be diluted initially (usually half to two thirds strength). Volume and concentration are gradually increased according to stool output. If semielemental formulas are not available, the World Health Organization recommends an initial diet of either dilute animal milk or yogurt or a soy product with small frequent feedings (at least 6 times a day) of locally available staples such as rice with some vegetable oil and sugar. If diarrhea continues and weight gain remains inadequate, consider a diet of chicken, egg, or other protein and carbohydrate as a mixture of rice and glucose. If this also fails, consider IV glucose plus a chicken-based oral feeding. Provide supplementary vitamins and minerals, in particular folate, vitamin B_{12}, vitamin A, zinc, and iron.

J. Short bowel syndrome can be congenital (intestinal atresia, omphalocele, gastroschisis, vascular anomalies of the superior mesenteric artery) or acquired postnatally (necrotizing enterocolitis, Crohn disease, vascular injury/ischemia). Loss of the ileum prevents reabsorption of fluid secreted by the jejunum in response to the solute load.

K. Continuous enteral infusion enhances absorption of nutrients by allowing continuous saturation of transport carrier proteins in the small intestine. Patients with short bowel syndrome should receive at least 20% of their total calories by enteral feedings to prevent atrophy of the enteral mucosa and reduce the risk of parenteral nutrition liver disease.

(Continued on page 294)

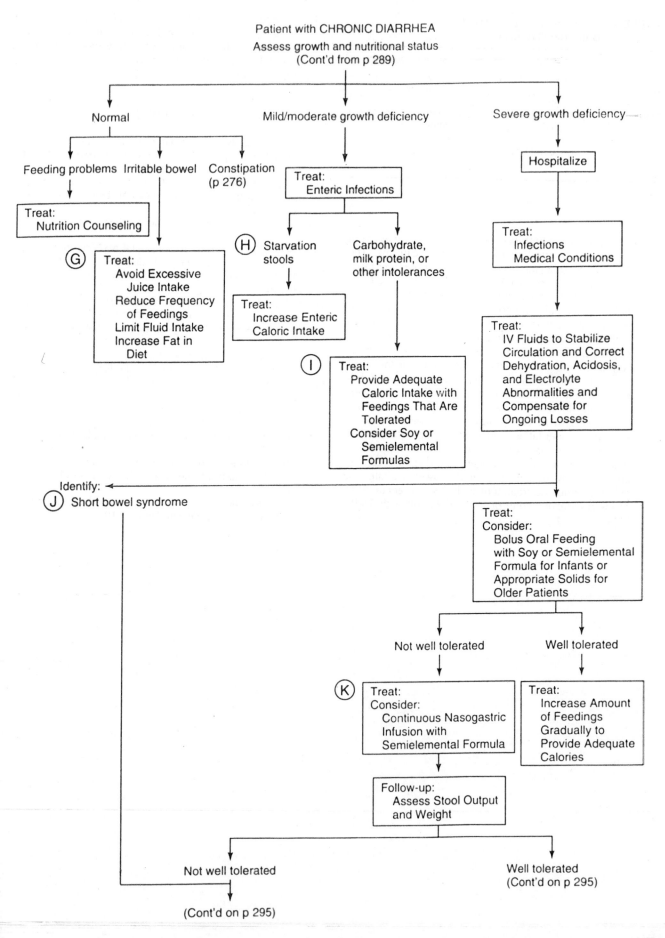

Patient with CHRONIC DIARRHEA
Assess growth and nutritional status
(Cont'd from p 289)

Normal

Feeding problems   Irritable bowel   Constipation (p 276)

Treat:
Nutrition Counseling

(G) Treat:
Avoid Excessive Juice Intake
Reduce Frequency of Feedings
Limit Fluid Intake
Increase Fat in Diet

Mild/moderate growth deficiency

Treat:
Enteric Infections

(H) Starvation stools

Carbohydrate, milk protein, or other intolerances

Treat:
Increase Enteric Caloric Intake

(I) Treat:
Provide Adequate Caloric Intake with Feedings That Are Tolerated
Consider Soy or Semielemental Formulas

Severe growth deficiency

Hospitalize

Treat:
Infections
Medical Conditions

Treat:
IV Fluids to Stabilize Circulation and Correct Dehydration, Acidosis, and Electrolyte Abnormalities and Compensate for Ongoing Losses

Identify:
(J) Short bowel syndrome

Treat:
Consider:
Bolus Oral Feeding with Soy or Semielemental Formula for Infants or Appropriate Solids for Older Patients

Not well tolerated   Well tolerated

(K) Treat:
Consider:
Continuous Nasogastric Infusion with Semielemental Formula

Treat:
Increase Amount of Feedings Gradually to Provide Adequate Calories

Follow-up:
Assess Stool Output and Weight

Not well tolerated
(Cont'd on p 295)

Well tolerated
(Cont'd on p 295)

TABLE 1   Antibiotics Used to Treat Bacterial Overgrowth

Drug	Dosage	Product Availability
Metronidazole	5 mg/kg/dose q6h	Sol: 50 mg/ml
TMP-SMX	0.5 ml/kg/dose b.i.d.	Susp: trimethoprim 40 mg sulfamethoxazole 200 mg/5 ml
Gentamicin	3–10 mg/kg/dose q8h	Vials: 40 mg/ml

L. Bacterial overgrowth occurs when the bacterial count in the small intestine exceeds 10^5 organisms. The bacteria deconjugate bile salts and promote their rapid reabsorption. The decrease in bile salts results in malabsorption of fat and fat-soluble vitamins. In addition, bacterial overgrowth can produce muscosal inflammation. Bacterial overgrowth occurs in patients with short bowel syndrome because of reflux of colonic bacteria when the ileocecal valve is absent as well as the altered motility and dilatation of the small intestine. This condition is associated with exacerbations of diarrhea, abdominal pain, or colitis with intestinal blood loss. D-Lactic acidosis caused by bacterial overgrowth can produce neurologic problems such as disorientation and coma. Diagnostic studies include a hydrogen or glucose breath hydrogen test that document excess hydrogen. The diagnosis can be confirmed by obtaining a small bowel aspirate for culture. Antibiotic treatment includes oral gentamicin or metronidazole alone or in combination with TMP-SMX (Table 1).

M. Monitor patients with short bowel syndrome for vitamins A, D, and E, as well as iron, zinc, calcium, and magnesium deficiencies every 3 to 6 months. Consider monthly parenteral vitamin B_{12} when the ileum has been removed.

References

Boyne LJ, Kerzner B, McClung HJ. Chronic nonspecific diarrhea: The value of a preliminary observation period to assess diet therapy. Pediatrics 1985; 76:557.

Donowitz M, Kokke FT, Saidi R. Current concepts: Evaluation of patients with chronic diarrhea. N Engl J Med 1995; 332:725.

Gryboski J. The child with chronic diarrhea. Contemp Pediatr 1993; May:71.

Holmberg C, Perheentupa J. Congenital Na$^+$/diarrhea: A new type of secretory diarrhea. J Pediatr 1985; 106:56.

Hutt PJ, Tunnessen WW. Very important passages. Contemp Pediatr 1994; 11:97.

Levine JJ, Seidman E, Walker WA. Screening tests for enteropathy in children. Am J Dis Child 1987; 141:35.

Murphy MS, Walker WA. Celiac disease. Pediatr Rev 1991; 12:325.

Not T, Ventura A, Peticarari S, et al. A new, rapid, noninvasive screening test for celiac disease. J Pediatr 1993; 123:425.

Orenstein SR. Enteral versus parenteral therapy for intractable diarrhea of infancy: A prospective, randomized trial. J Pediatr 1986; 109:277.

Sallon S, Deckelbaum RJ, Schmid II, et al. *Cryptosporidium*, malnutrition, and chronic diarrhea in children. Am J Child 1988; 142:312.

Sutphen J, Grand RJ, Flores A, et al. Chronic diarrhea associated with *Clostridium difficile* in children. Am J Dis Child 1983; 137:275.

Vanderhoof JA. Short bowel syndrome: Smoothing the road to recovery. Contemp Pediatr 1992; 9:19.

Patient with CHRONIC DIARRHEA

Short bowel syndrome
(Cont'd from p 293)

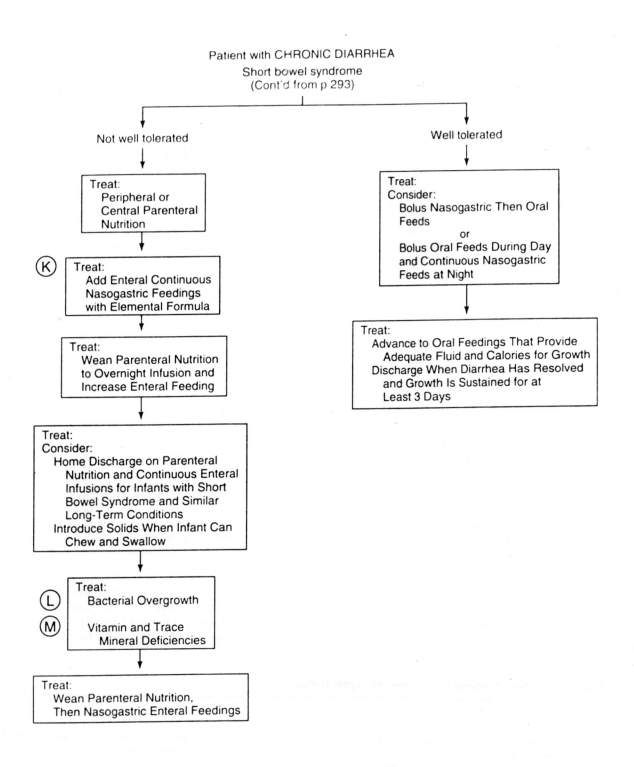

Not well tolerated

Treat:
    Peripheral or
    Central Parenteral
    Nutrition

(K) Treat:
    Add Enteral Continuous
    Nasogastric Feedings
    with Elemental Formula

Treat:
    Wean Parenteral Nutrition
    to Overnight Infusion and
    Increase Enteral Feeding

Treat:
Consider:
    Home Discharge on Parenteral
    Nutrition and Continuous Enteral
    Infusions for Infants with Short
    Bowel Syndrome and Similar
    Long-Term Conditions
    Introduce Solids When Infant Can
    Chew and Swallow

(L) Treat:
    Bacterial Overgrowth
(M)
    Vitamin and Trace
    Mineral Deficiencies

Treat:
    Wean Parenteral Nutrition,
    Then Nasogastric Enteral Feedings

Well tolerated

Treat:
Consider:
    Bolus Nasogastric Then Oral
    Feeds
            or
    Bolus Oral Feeds During Day
    and Continuous Nasogastric
    Feeds at Night

Treat:
    Advance to Oral Feedings That Provide
        Adequate Fluid and Calories for Growth
    Discharge When Diarrhea Has Resolved
        and Growth Is Sustained for at
        Least 3 Days

GASTROESOPHAGEAL REFLUX

Stephen Berman, M.D.

DEFINITION

Gastroesophageal reflux (GER), also called chalasia, is the passage of gastric contents through the lower esophageal sphincter (LES). The reasons for reflux include transient relaxation of the LES, increased intragastric pressure, and decreased basal LES tone. Clinical consequences depend on the degree of reflux, ability of the esophagus to clear the acid contents, duration of contact with acid, and amount of injury to the esophageal mucosa.

A. In the history ask about the onset, frequency, and severity (quantity, degree of forcefulness, presence of bile) of the vomiting. Determine the type of formula, manner of preparation, quantity ingested, and feeding position and technique. Establish the time of vomiting in relation to the feeding. Spitting up or regurgitation of small amounts of formula during or soon after feeding suggests an improper feeding technique such as bottle propping or GER. Note associated symptoms such as fever, cough, coryza, respiratory distress, diarrhea, altered mental status, seizures, and failure to thrive. Inquire about perinatal deaths in the family that suggest inborn errors of metabolism and adrenal insufficiency.

B. In the physical examination assess hydration and circulatory status by determining blood pressure, pulse, respiratory rate, capillary refill, skin color and turgor, tears, fullness of the fontanelle, and urine output. Plot the infant's height, weight, and head circumference on a growth grid to identify failure to thrive or rapid head growth. Assess mental status. Note any acute otitis media, irritability, lethargy, seizures, or focal neurologic signs. Observe a feeding and note the peristaltic waves. Palpation of an abdominal mass (olive) suggests pyloric stenosis.

C. The best approach to evaluating a patient with signs of reflux should be individualized to the clinical presentation. Obtain an upper GI series when growth deficiency is present and an anatomic abnormality or problem with esophageal mobility is suspected. Barium studies will fail to identify about 40% of patients with esophagitis secondary to reflux. A nuclear scan following a feeding with technetium-99 may be useful in identifying pulmonary aspiration and is helpful in assessing the rate of gastric emptying. Endoscopy will assess the extent and severity of esophagitis and identify any bleeding, strictures, peptic and ulcer disease. Esophageal pH monitoring is the most sensitive method of confirming reflux and correlating reflux with apneic events and episodes of respiratory distress.

(Continued on page 298)

TABLE 2 Drug Therapy for Gastroesophageal Reflux in Children and Adolescents

Drug	Dosage	Product Availability
Bethanecol (Urocholine)	0.5–0.75 mg/kg/day 15–30 min before feeding Use with caution if CNS disease, RAD, or cardiac disease is present	Tabs: 5, 10, 25 mg Sol: 1 mg/ ml
Cisapride (Propulsid)	0.2–0.3 mg/kg/dose 3–4 times qd	Susp: 1 mg/ml
Metoclopramide (Reglan)	0.1–0.2 mg/kg/dose 4–6 times/day before loading	Susp: 5 mg/5 ml Tabs: 10 mg

TABLE 1 Degree of Illness in Gastroesophageal Reflux

Mild	Moderate	Severe	Very Severe
No signs of growth failure during infancy and No limitation of normal activities and No complications of reflux	Symptoms of esophagitis (pain) or Signs of aspiration pneumonia/reactive airway disease or Growth failure or Anemia, asymptomatic upper GI bleeding	A life-threatening event, near miss sudden infant death or Active upper GI bleeding or Severe pain that limits normal activities or Severe dehydration or Malnutrition or Electrolyte/serum pH abnormality	Signs of shock or Altered mental status with coma or seizures

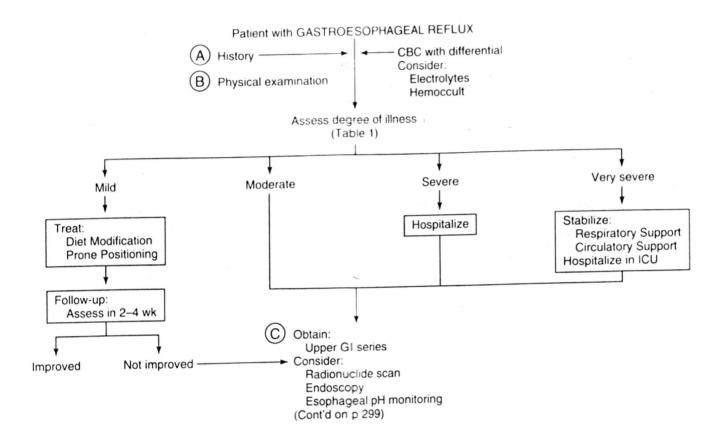

Patient with GASTROESOPHAGEAL REFLUX

(A) History ⟶ ← CBC with differential
Consider:
  Electrolytes
  Hemoccult

(B) Physical examination

Assess degree of illness
(Table 1)

Mild   Moderate   Severe   Very severe

Treat: Hospitalize   Stabilize:
  Diet Modification   Respiratory Support
  Prone Positioning   Circulatory Support
                                                                       Hospitalize in ICU

Follow-up:
  Assess in 2–4 wk

Improved   Not improved ⟶   (C) Obtain:
                                     Upper GI series
                                   Consider:
                                     Radionuclide scan
                                     Endoscopy
                                     Esophageal pH monitoring
                                   (Cont'd on p 299)

D. When GER is identified, change the infant's feeding schedule. Small volumes of formula given more frequently reduce gastric distention. Consider adding cereal to the formula. If necessary, attempt to position the infant's body prone at a 30-degree incline throughout most of the day. This can best be accomplished when the infant straddles a padded post or uses a chalasia harness. When severe symptoms are associated with failure to thrive, consider the use of bethanecol, which decreases vomiting by increasing LES pressure, or metoclopramide (Reglan), which increases gastric emptying, or cisapride (Table 2). If esophagitis is present, consider using antacids and/or H_2 receptor antagonists (see p 316). Patients with severe esophagitis who fail to respond may benefit from sucralfate or omeprazole. Continuous nasogastric or nasoduodenal feedings may be used in an attempt to avoid surgery. The duration of pharmacologic therapy varies from 6 weeks to 3 months. Consider surgery (Nissen fundoplication) if severe symptoms persist after 2 months of therapy or if an esophageal stricture develops.

References

Gunasekaran TS, Hassall EG. Efficacy and safety of omeprazole for severe gastroesophageal reflux in children. J Pediatr 1993; 123:148.

Hebra A, Hoffman MA. Gastroesophageal reflux in children. Pediatr Clin North Am 1993; 40:1233.

Machida HM, Forbes DA, Gall DG, et al. Metoclopramide in gastroesophageal reflux in infancy. J Pediatr 1988; 112:483.

Orenstein SR. Controversies in pediatric gastroesophageal reflux. J Pediatr Gastroenterol Nutr 1992; 14:338.

Orenstein SR, Magill HL, Brooks P. Thickening of infant feedings for therapy of gastroesophageal reflux. J Pediatr 1987; 110:181.

Sutphen JL. Pediatric gastroesophageal reflux disease. Gastroenterol Clin North Am 1990; 19:617.

Tolia V, Calhoun J, Kuhns L, et al. Randomized, prospective, double-blind trial of metoclopramide and placebo for gastroesophageal reflux in infants. J Pediatr 1989; 115:141.

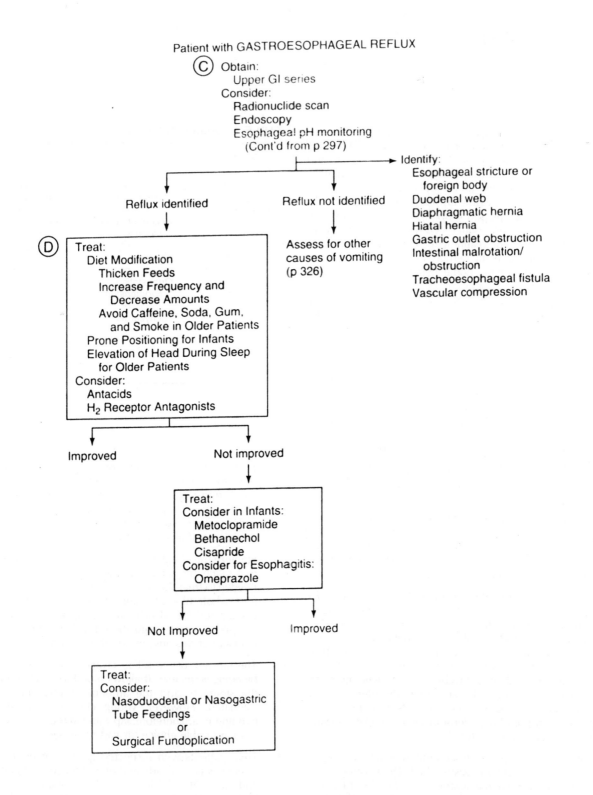

Patient with GASTROESOPHAGEAL REFLUX

C Obtain:
    Upper GI series
  Consider:
    Radionuclide scan
    Endoscopy
    Esophageal pH monitoring
    (Cont'd from p 297)

Identify:
    Esophageal stricture or
      foreign body
    Duodenal web
    Diaphragmatic hernia
    Hiatal hernia
    Gastric outlet obstruction
    Intestinal malrotation/
      obstruction
    Tracheoesophageal fistula
    Vascular compression

Reflux identified

Reflux not identified

Assess for other
causes of vomiting
(p 326)

D Treat:
    Diet Modification
      Thicken Feeds
      Increase Frequency and
        Decrease Amounts
      Avoid Caffeine, Soda, Gum,
        and Smoke in Older Patients
    Prone Positioning for Infants
    Elevation of Head During Sleep
      for Older Patients
  Consider:
    Antacids
    H₂ Receptor Antagonists

Improved

Not improved

Treat:
Consider in Infants:
    Metoclopramide
    Bethanechol
    Cisapride
Consider for Esophagitis:
    Omeprazole

Not Improved

Improved

Treat:
Consider:
    Nasoduodenal or Nasogastric
    Tube Feedings
        or
    Surgical Fundoplication

HEMATEMESIS

Stephen Berman, M.D.

GI bleeding above the ligament of Treitz may manifest as hematemesis. The most common causes of upper GI bleeding by age are as follows: infancy—esophagitis, gastric and duodenal ulcers, and gastric erosions; age 1 to 6 years—gastric ulcers, duodenitis, and esophagitis; age 7 to 18 years—duodenal ulcers, gastric erosions, varices, and esophagitis. Causes of gastritis and esophagitis include infection, aspirin ingestion, gastric outlet obstruction secondary to pyloric stenosis, web or diaphragm, and gastroesophageal reflux (with or without hiatal hernia). Esophageal varices can be caused by extrahepatic portal hypertension (congenital anomalies, omphalitis, umbilical vein catheterization) or intrahepatic portal hypertension (cirrhosis). A large quantity (cupful) of bright red blood suggests extensive hemorrhage. Blood that has been in prolonged contact with stomach acid is dark brown or black (like coffee grounds).

A. In the history ask about the onset of hematemesis and the volume of blood loss. Identify possible precipitating factors and predisposing conditions such as protracted vomiting, peptic ulcer disease, chronic liver disease, current medications (aspirin, steroid, or anticoagulants), corrosive ingestions, bleeding disorders, and recent major stress (difficult delivery, burns, surgery, traumatic injury, dehydration, shock, serious infection). Ask about recent possible oropharyngeal sites of bleeding (epistaxis, dental work, tonsillectomy, sore throat) and ingestion of a foreign body, which may have lodged in the esophagus or stomach. Systemic diseases associated with upper GI bleeding include immunodeficiency disorders, pulmonary or GI infections, malignancy, collagen vascular disease, CNS disease, renal failure, and congenital heart disease.

B. On physical examination evaluate the circulatory status and document any orthostatic blood pressure changes. A drop in orthostatic blood pressure of 10 mm Hg indicates a 10% to 20% intravascular volume loss. Tachycardia and hypotension indicate more than a 30% acute loss of blood volume. Examine the mouth and oropharynx to identify possible sites of bleeding. Note signs of a generalized coagulation disorder such as petechiae, bruising, or ecchymosis. Note signs of liver disease and portal hypertension such as hepatomegaly, splenomegaly, and ascites.

C. The Hemoccult (guaiac) test identifies heme protein but may not be accurate in gastric fluid. The Gastroccult is a better test for blood in gastric fluid. The Kleihauer and Apt-Downey tests distinguish between fetal and maternal red blood cells and are useful in the newborn to identify cases with hematemesis secondary to swallowed maternal blood.

D. Vomited materials that can be mistaken for blood include Jell-O, beets, KoolAid, food dyes, red candy, and some antibiotic syrups.

TABLE 1 Degree of Illness in Hematemesis

Moderate	Severe	Very Severe
Small amount of coffee ground material and No anemia and No orthostatic hypotension, or signs of impaired circulation	Active bleeding with gastric aspirate or History of large blood loss or Anemia or Orthostatic hypotension or Tachycardia	Continuing large blood loss or Signs of shock, acidosis, circulatory instability or Severe anemia or Signs of heart failure or Signs of kidney, liver, bowel ischemia or dysfunction

E. Factors indicating a poor prognosis include an initial hematocrit less than 20% or hemoglobin level less than 7 g/dl, transfusion requirements that exceed 85 ml/kg of blood without surgical intervention, failure to identify an active source of bleeding, a coexisting coagulation disorder, and associated systemic disease.

F. Stabilize the circulation. Initially infuse 20 ml/kg of normal saline or lactated Ringer's solution as rapidly as needed to treat shock. With continued hemorrhage, use fresh whole blood to support the circulation. Consider packed red blood cell transfusion after bleeding has stopped. Correct coagulation disorders with vitamin K, platelet transfusions, and/or fresh frozen plasma.

G. The efficacy of ice saline lavage in controlling active bleeding is unclear. It allows blood to be cleared from the stomach, and the amount of bleeding can be estimated. However, young children may develop hypothermia. Therefore, tap water at room temperature is a reasonable choice for gastric lavage.

H. Treat patients with suspected gastritis or peptic ulcer disease with antacids and/or H_2 receptor antagonists and sucralfate (Table 2, p 316). Patients should be treated with magnesium and aluminum hydroxide preparations, 0.5 ml/kg to maximum 30 ml every 1 to 2 hours to maintain gastric pH at 5 or greater for the initial 48 hours, then at 1 and 3 hours after meals.

I. Consider treatment of massive acute hemorrhage from esophageal varices with a vasopressin infusion to decrease portal venous pressure by reducing splanchnic

(Continued on page 302)

Patient with HEMATEMESIS/UPPER GASTROINTESTINAL BLEEDING

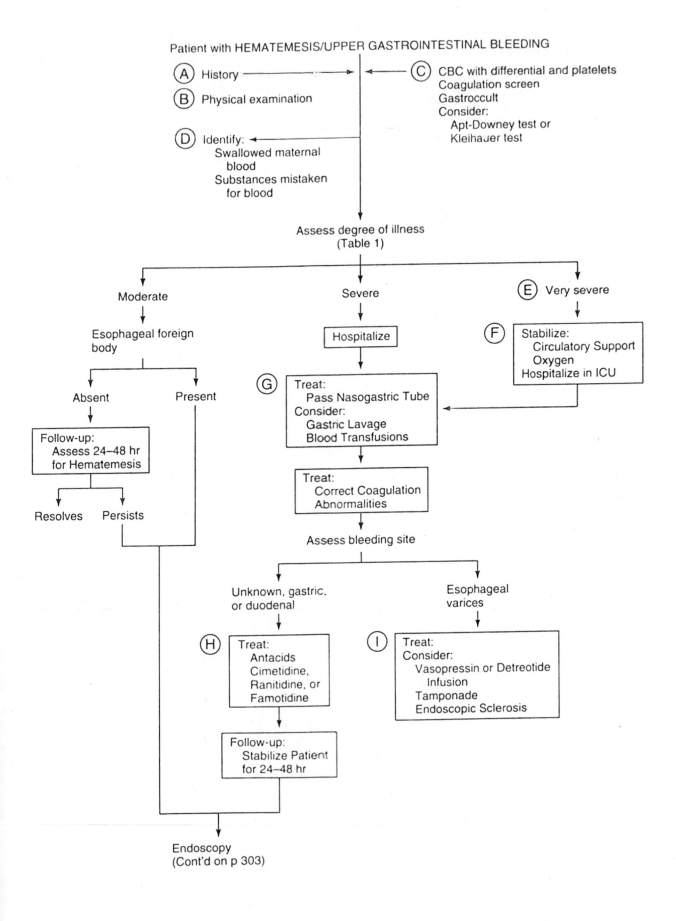

(A) History

(B) Physical examination

(C) CBC with differential and platelets
Coagulation screen
Gastroccult
Consider:
    Apt-Downey test or
    Kleihauer test

(D) Identify:
Swallowed maternal
    blood
Substances mistaken
    for blood

Assess degree of illness
(Table 1)

Moderate

Severe

(E) Very severe

Esophageal foreign
body

Hospitalize

(F) Stabilize:
    Circulatory Support
    Oxygen
    Hospitalize in ICU

Absent   Present

(G) Treat:
    Pass Nasogastric Tube
Consider:
    Gastric Lavage
    Blood Transfusions

Follow-up:
    Assess 24–48 hr
    for Hematemesis

Treat:
    Correct Coagulation
    Abnormalities

Resolves   Persists

Assess bleeding site

Unknown, gastric,
or duodenal

Esophageal
varices

(H) Treat:
    Antacids
    Cimetidine,
    Ranitidine, or
    Famotidine

(I) Treat:
Consider:
    Vasopressin or Detreotide
        Infusion
    Tamponade
    Endoscopic Sclerosis

Follow-up:
    Stabilize Patient
    for 24–48 hr

Endoscopy
(Cont'd on p 303)

blood flow. Failure to control hemorrhage is an indication for endoscopic sclerotherapy or tamponade. Inability to control bleeding is an indication for portocaval shunt surgery. The efficacy of prophylactic endoscopic sclerotherapy to prevent initial bleeding in patients with varices is unclear. Complications of the procedure, which occur in 2% to 15% of cases, include bleeding, stricture, ulceration, perforation, and infection.

J.   Endoscopy identifies the cause of hemorrhage in approximately 90% of patients, and upper GI examination identifies the underlying causes in approximately 50%. Perform endoscopy after the patient has been stabilized. It can provide information about the site and amount of bleeding and the risk of rebleeding. Rebleeding occurs from peptic ulcers in 25% of cases. Endoscopic findings that suggest an increased risk of rebleeding include a vessel visible in the ulcer base or margin and evidence of fresh bleeding from the ulcer. Superficial lesions of esophagitis, gastritis, or duodenitis rarely rebleed. Consider angiography, which will diagnose possible aneurysms of the hepatic artery or gastropancreatic duplication cyst, when bleeding is massive or when endoscopy and upper GI series have failed to reveal the cause in recurrent bleeding.

References

Ament ME. Diagnosis and management of upper gastrointestinal tract bleeding in the pediatric patient. Pediatr Rev 1990; 12:107.

Caulfield M, Wyllie R, Sivak MV, et al. Upper gastrointestinal tract endoscopy in the pediatric patient. J Pediatr 1989; 115:339.

Gryboski JD. Peptic ulcer disease in children. Pediatr Rev 1990; 12:15.

Hyams JS, Leichtner AM, Schwartz AN. Recent advances in diagnosis and treatment of gastrointestinal hemorrhage in infants and children. J Pediatr 1985; 106:1.

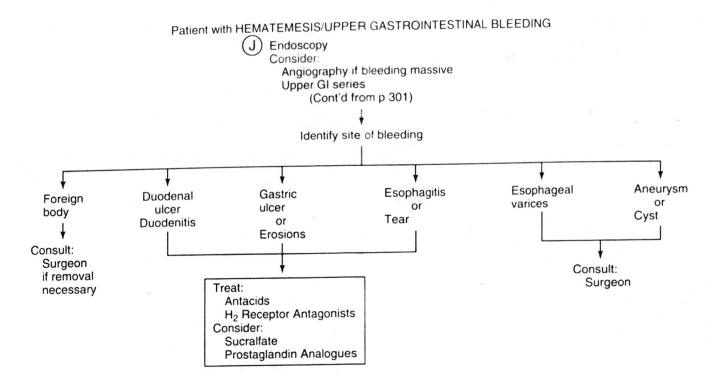

Patient with HEMATEMESIS/UPPER GASTROINTESTINAL BLEEDING

(J) Endoscopy
Consider:
    Angiography if bleeding massive
    Upper GI series
      (Cont'd from p 301)

Identify site of bleeding

Foreign body	Duodenal ulcer Duodenitis	Gastric ulcer or Erosions	Esophagitis or Tear	Esophageal varices	Aneurysm or Cyst

Consult:
Surgeon
if removal
necessary

Treat:
    Antacids
    H$_2$ Receptor Antagonists
Consider:
    Sucralfate
    Prostaglandin Analogues

Consult:
Surgeon

HEPATITIS

Stephen Berman, M.D.

DEFINITIONS

Hepatitis A, a single-stranded RNA virus, used to be known as infectious hepatitis because of its association with epidemics of jaundice. The form that produces fulminant hepatic necrosis was called acute yellow atrophy of the liver. The incubation period is 15 to 40 days, and there is no carrier state or chronic infection. **Hepatitis B,** a double-stranded DNA virus, used to be called serum hepatitis because it was transmitted through contaminated blood and blood products. Additional modes of transmission include oral-oral, sexual, and perinatal routes. Its incubation period is 50 to 180 days, and there is a carrier state and chronic infection. Hepatitis B can cause fulminant liver failure or progress to cirrhosis or hepatocellular carcinoma (HCC). Infants born to infected mothers have about a 60% chance of developing a chronic disease; 3% to 13% of infected adults develop chronic disease. **Hepatitis C,** a single-stranded RNA virus, used to be called non–A, non–B hepatitis and is parenterally transmitted post transfusion. The incubation period is 30 to 150 days, and there is a carrier state. Chronic infection, which develops in about 50% of patients, can progress to cirrhosis or HCC. **Hepatitis D** is a defective RNA virus that cannot replicate without a coexisting infection with hepatitis B. The incubation period is 21 to 90 days, and there is a carrier state and chronic infection. Combined hepatitis D infection is more severe than hepatitis B alone, progressing more rapidly to liver failure, cirrhosis, and portal hypertension. **Hepatitis E,** a single-stranded RNA virus, used to be called enterically transmitted non–A, non–B hepatitis. The incubation period is 14 to 63 days, and there is no carrier state or chronic infection. Infection can be very severe in pregnant women. The characteristics and terminology of associated antigens and antibodies for hepatitis viruses are reviewed in Table 1. **Carrier state** is a persistent infection without biochemical or clinical signs of ongoing hepatic injury. Carriers can transmit the infection to susceptible persons. Hepatitis B carriers can become superinfected with hepatitis D and develop severe acute or chronic disease. **Chronic hepatitis** is defined by persistence of hepatic dysfunction with elevation of enzymes (ALT) or clinical signs of disease for more than 6 months. Chronic disease occurs when the immune response fails to eliminate infected hepatocytes. The two forms are chronic persistent and chronic active hepatitis. **Chronic persistent hepatitis** is defined by a biopsy that shows a lymphocytic infiltrate limited to the portal areas without necrosis or fibrosis. **Chronic active hepatitis** is defined by a biopsy that shows spread of the lymphocytic infiltrate to the periportal regions with piecemeal and bridging necrosis. Fibrosis may be present or absent.

ETIOLOGY

Causes of hepatitis include viral infections (hepatitis A, B, C, D, and E, Epstein-Barr virus, cytomegalovirus, herpes simplex virus, varicella virus, adenoviruses, enteroviruses, rubella virus and arboviruses), bacterial infections (leptospirosis, syphilis, gonorrhea, *Chlamydia*), and parasitic infections (malaria, amoeba). Drug or toxic hepatitis can be associated with phenothiazines, oral contraceptives, valproic acid, erythromycin estolate, indomethacin, and gold. Severe hypoxia, hypotension, right heart failure, and mushroom or acetaminophen intoxications may result in fulminant hepatic necrosis.

A. In the history ask about any fever, anorexia, malaise, vomiting, abdominal pain, jaundice, dark urine, or clay-colored stools. Ask whether there has been travel, blood product transfusions, or exposure to jaundiced individuals. Ask whether the child has begun to feel better when the jaundice increases. Failure of symptoms to improve after the onset of jaundice is a poor prognostic sign. Urticaria and arthritis suggest hepatitis B infection.

B. In the physical examination note any jaundice, tender hepatomegaly, splenomegaly, or abdominal mass. Suspect infectious mononucleosis when exudative tonsillitis, adenopathy, or splenomegaly is present. Signs of chronic liver disease include acne, ascites, digital clubbing, and gynecomastia. Note signs of chronic active disease such as arthritis, polyarthralgia, amenorrhea, colitis, thyroiditis, glomerulonephritis, diabetes, or pleurisy.

C. Hepatitis A is typically characterized by clinical improvement with the onset of jaundice and a normalization of bilirubin and transaminases within 4 to 6

TABLE 1 The Hepatitis Viruses: Characteristics and Terminology of Associated Antigens and Antibodies

Serologic Markers of HAV		
Anti-HAV	Total antibody (IgM and IgG subclasses) directed against HAV	Indicates recent (IgM) or past HAV infection (IgG) Confirms exposure and immunity to HAV
Anti-HAV IgM	IgM antibody to HAV	Indicates recent acute infection
Serologic Markers of HBV		
HBsAg	hepatitis B surface antigen found on the surface of the intact virus and in serum as free particles (tubular or spherical)	Indicates infection with HBV (either acute or chronic)
HBcAg	Hepatitis B core antigen found within the core of the intact virus	Not detectable in serum (found only in liver tissue)
HBeAg	Hepatitis B e antigen (soluble antigen produced during self-cleavage of HBcAg)	Indicates active HBV infection Signifies high infectivity Persistence for 6–8 wk suggests chronic carrier and/or chronic liver disease

(Continued on page 306)

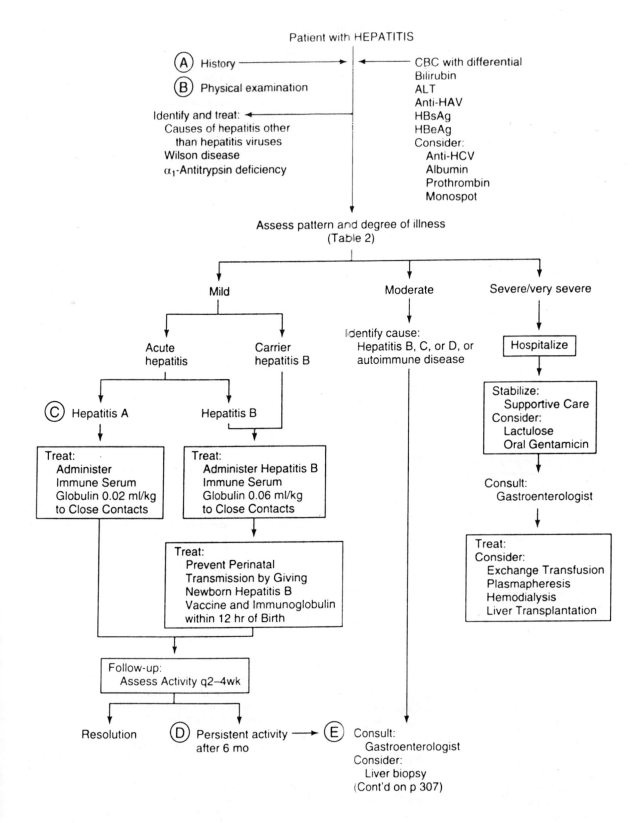

Patient with HEPATITIS

(A) History

(B) Physical examination

CBC with differential
Bilirubin
ALT
Anti-HAV
HBsAg
HBeAg
Consider:
    Anti-HCV
    Albumin
    Prothrombin
    Monospot

Identify and treat:
    Causes of hepatitis other
        than hepatitis viruses
    Wilson disease
    α_1-Antitrypsin deficiency

Assess pattern and degree of illness
(Table 2)

Mild

Moderate

Severe/very severe

Acute
hepatitis

Carrier
hepatitis B

Identify cause:
    Hepatitis B, C, or D, or
    autoimmune disease

Hospitalize

(C) Hepatitis A

Hepatitis B

Stabilize:
    Supportive Care
Consider:
    Lactulose
    Oral Gentamicin

Treat:
    Administer
    Immune Serum
    Globulin 0.02 ml/kg
    to Close Contacts

Treat:
    Administer Hepatitis B
    Immune Serum
    Globulin 0.06 ml/kg
    to Close Contacts

Consult:
    Gastroenterologist

Treat:
    Prevent Perinatal
    Transmission by Giving
    Newborn Hepatitis B
    Vaccine and Immunoglobulin
    within 12 hr of Birth

Treat:
Consider:
    Exchange Transfusion
    Plasmapheresis
    Hemodialysis
    Liver Transplantation

Follow-up:
    Assess Activity q2–4wk

Resolution

(D) Persistent activity
after 6 mo

(E) Consult:
    Gastroenterologist
Consider:
    Liver biopsy
(Cont'd on p 307)

weeks. Slight elevation of unconjugated bilirubin and serum transaminases may persist for up to 3 months. A mild relapse often occurs after 10 to 12 weeks.

D. Acute hepatitis associated with hepatitis A virus rarely has a complicated course. Persistence of clinical symptoms and markedly elevated serum transaminases and bilirubin after 4 weeks suggest persistent hepatitis.

Approximately 10% of children with hepatitis B or C may have persistent disease. Ongoing liver damage is indicated by persistently elevated transaminases, a serum albumin less than 3.5 mg/dl, and a prolonged prothrombin time.

E. Consider early liver biopsy when the clinical presentation is atypical for benign viral hepatitis or includes a

Serologic Markers of HBV — cont'd

HBV DNA	DNA of HBV	Indicates active HBV infection (acute and chronic) Indicates high levels of viral replication, infectivity, and high probability of liver disease
Anti-HBs	Antibody to HBsAg; subclasses IgM (early) and IgG	Indicates clinical recovery from HBV infection and immunity Protective
Anti-HBc	Total antibody to HBcAg	Indicates active HBV infection (acute and chronic)
Anti-HBc IgM	IgM antibody to HBcAg	Early index of acute HBV infection Rises during acute phase, then declines
Anti-HBe	Antibody to HBeAg	Indicates resolution of infection

Serologic Markers of HCV

Anti-HCV	Antibody to nonstructural portion of the HCV genome	Indicates active infection with HCV Present in acute and chronic infection Not protective
HCV RNA	RNA of the hepatitis C virus	Detectable in serum and liver by PCR Best means of confirming infection with HCV

Serologic Markers of HDV

HDAg	Hepatitis D antigen	Detected in acute HDV infections by RIA and EIA
Anti-HDV	Total antibody to the hepatitis D virus	Indicates exposure to HDV Patient may transmit HDV infection
HDV RNA	RNA of the hepatitis D virus	Present in serum

Serologic Markers of HEV

HEAg	Hepatitis E antigen	Research tool; can be found in liver, bile, and stool during incubation period and symptomatic phase of infection
Anti-HEV	Antibody to the hepatitis E virus	Research tool; found in serum during acute illness Immunity to infection may not be complete

HAV, hepatitis A virus; HBV, hepatitis B virus; HBcAg, hepatitis B core antigen; HBsAg, hepatitis B surface antigen; HBeAg, hepatitis B e antigen; HCV, hepatitis C virus; PCR, polymerase chain reaction; HDV, hepatitis D virus; RIA, radioimmunoassay; EIA, enzyme immunoassay; HEV, hepatitis E virus.
Modified from Nowicki MJ, Balistreri WF. Viral hepatitis. In: Oski FA, McMillan JA, eds. Principles and practice of pediatrics updates. Philadelphia: JB Lippincott, 1993:1.

TABLE 2   Pattern and Degree of Illness in Hepatitis

Acute or Carrier/Mild	*Chronic/Moderate*	*Fulminant/Severe*
Uncomplicated acute hepatitis or Carrier state without evidence of ongoing hepatic dysfunction	Extrahepatic signs of chronic hepatitis such as arthritis, serum sickness reactions, glomerulonephritis, infantile papular acrodermatitis (Gianotti-Crosti), or polyarteritis nodosa or Evidence of chronic infection	Signs of hepatic failure such as altered mental status, rapid deterioration, increased serum ammonia, increased prothrombin time resistant to vitamin K, bilirubin > 20 mg/ml, serum transaminase > 3000, ascites, hypoglycemia, and shrinking liver

positive antinuclear antibody test or extrahepatic manifestations. When signs of inflammation (elevated serum transaminases and bilirubin) persist beyond 3 to 6 months, biopsy is indicated.

F.   Treatment of chronic hepatitis B and C infections with α-interferon is effective in about 50% of patients. However, half of the patients who respond relapse when therapy is discontinued. Treatment with acyclovir and corticosteroids does not appear to be effective.

References

Franks AL, Berg CJ, Kane MA, et al. Hepatitis B virus infection among children born in the United States to Southeast Asian refugees. N Engl J Med 1989; 321:1301.

Halsey NA. Discussion of immunization practices: Advisory Committee/American Academy of Pediatrics recommendations for universal infant hepatitis B vaccination. Pediatr Infect Dis J 1993; 12:446.

Kay MH, Wyllie R, Deimler C, et al. Alpha-interferon therapy in children with chronic active hepatitis B and delta virus infection. J Pediatr 1993; 123:1001.

Krugman S. Viral hepatitis: A, B, C, D, and E infections. Pediatr Rev 1992; 13:203.

Mosley JW, Aach RD, Blaine-Hollinger F, et al. Non-A, non-B hepatitis and antibody to hepatitis C virus. JAMA 1990; 263:77.

Nowicki MJ, Balistreri WF. Hepatitis A to E: Building up the alphabet. Contemp Pediatr 1992; November:118.

Nowicki MJ, Balistreri WF. The C's, D's, and E's of viral hepatitis. Contemp Pediatr 1992; December:23.

Russel GJ, Fitzgerald JF, Clark JH. Fulminant hepatic failure. J Pediatr 1987; 111:313.

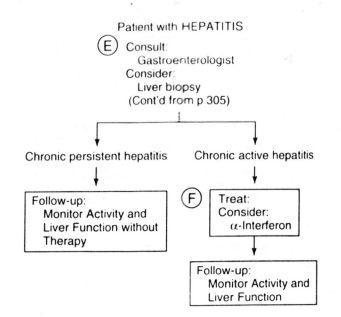

Patient with HEPATITIS

(E) Consult:
  Gastroenterologist
Consider:
  Liver biopsy
(Cont'd from p 305)

Chronic persistent hepatitis   Chronic active hepatitis

Follow-up: (F) Treat:
  Monitor Activity and   Consider:
  Liver Function without   α-Interferon
  Therapy

                                  Follow-up:
                                    Monitor Activity and
                                    Liver Function

HEPATOMEGALY

Perla Santos Ocampo, M.D.
Stephen Berman, M.D.

A. In the history ask about trauma, abdominal distention, pain, fever, appetite, weight loss, jaundice, and symptoms of excessive catecholamine activity. Note exposure to hepatotoxins, infections (hepatitis, mononucleosis, tuberculosis, amebiasis, other protozoal parasites). Ask about underlying conditions such as sickle cell disease and other hematologic disorders, cardiac disease, collagen vascular disorders, and storage diseases.

B. Perform a complete physical examination. Determine liver size by using percussion to identify the upper and lower borders of the liver. The mean span changes from 4.5 to 5 cm at 1 week of age to 6 to 7 cm in early adolescence. If the upper margin of the liver is percussed near the fifth intercostal space in the midclavicular line, the lower edge of the liver should not extend below the costal margin more than 2 cm in infancy or 1 cm in childhood. However, associated conditions that may displace a normal liver downward include pulmonary hyperinflation, pneumothorax, retroperitoneal mass, and subdiaphragmatic abscess. Riedel lobe, a normal anatomic elongation of the right lobe, may be mistaken for hepatomegaly. Determine the liver's contour and consistency. Does the surface feel smooth, irregular, or nodular, and is the edge rounded or sharp? Is palpation of the liver painful? Listen for a bruit or friction rub over the liver. Note any associated ascites and/or splenomegaly, which suggests increased portal venous pressure, tissue infiltration, or reticuloendothelial cell hyperplasia. In newborns perform a funduscopic examination for chorioretinitis (congenital infection). Note skin lesions, subcutaneous nodules, lymphadenopathy, spider angiomata. Note stigmata of storage diseases.

C. Elevated levels of α-fetoprotein and carcinoembryonic antigen suggest a malignancy. Tests for liver damage and of liver function are nonspecific and reflect the amount of inflammation or injury and level of liver function. Prolongation of clotting time, elevation of serum ammonia, and decreased serum albumin indicate liver failure. Elevations in bilirubin, bile acids, lipids, and alkaline phosphatase suggest a problem with bile secretion. Elevations in ALT and AST reflect the amount of acute damage to hepatocyte cells.

D. Hepatomegaly may be caused by extramedullary hematopoiesis, as erythropoietic tissue is present within the liver sinusoids of term infants. Causes of excessive extramedullary hematopoiesis include erythroblastosis fetalis and other severe neonatal anemias.

E. Congenital infections that can produce hepatomegaly include toxoplasmosis, rubella, herpes simplex, cytomegalovirus, and syphilis.

F. Pyogenic and mycotic abscesses are commonly multiple, and amebic abscess is usually solitary. Radiologic examination may show calcification in tuberculosis. Helminthic infections include *Ascaris* in the common bile duct, hydatid disease, and liver flukes. Mycotic infections are actinomycosis and cryptococcosis.

G. Fatty infiltration of the liver can result from malnutrition and vitamin deficiencies. Malnutrition can be related to inadequate protein and caloric intake or malabsorption (cystic fibrosis, celiac disease).

H. Hepatoblastoma and hepatocellular carcinoma account for most primary hepatic malignancies. Hepatoblastomas are most frequent in children under 5 years, and hepatocellular carcinoma has peaks of incidence in children under 4 and between 12 and 15 years. Disorders that predispose to hepatocellular carcinoma include hepatitis B, C, and D; biliary atresia; cirrhosis; storage diseases; and tyrosinemia. The only effective treatment for these malignancies is surgical resection of the tumor (approximately 33% survival).

I. Storage disorders related to inborn errors of metabolism include glycogen storage disease, galactosemia, lipid storage disease, Gaucher disease, mucopolysaccharidosis, Wolman disease, amyloidosis and α_1-antitrypsin deficiency. Hemosiderosis and hemochromatosis are caused by iron deposition in the liver.

References

Callahan CW. Simultaneous percussion auscultation technique for the determination of liver span. Arch Pediatr Adolesc Med 1994; 148:873.

Gentil-Kocher S, Bernard O, Brunelle F, et al. Budd-Chiari syndrome in children: Report of 22 cases. J Pediatr 1988; 113:30.

Harrison HR, Crowe DP, Fulginiti VA. Amebic liver abscess in children: Clinical and epidemiologic features. Pediatrics 1979; 64:923.

Tunnessen WW JR. A 10-year-old boy with hepatomegaly. Contemp Pediatr 1987; March:121.

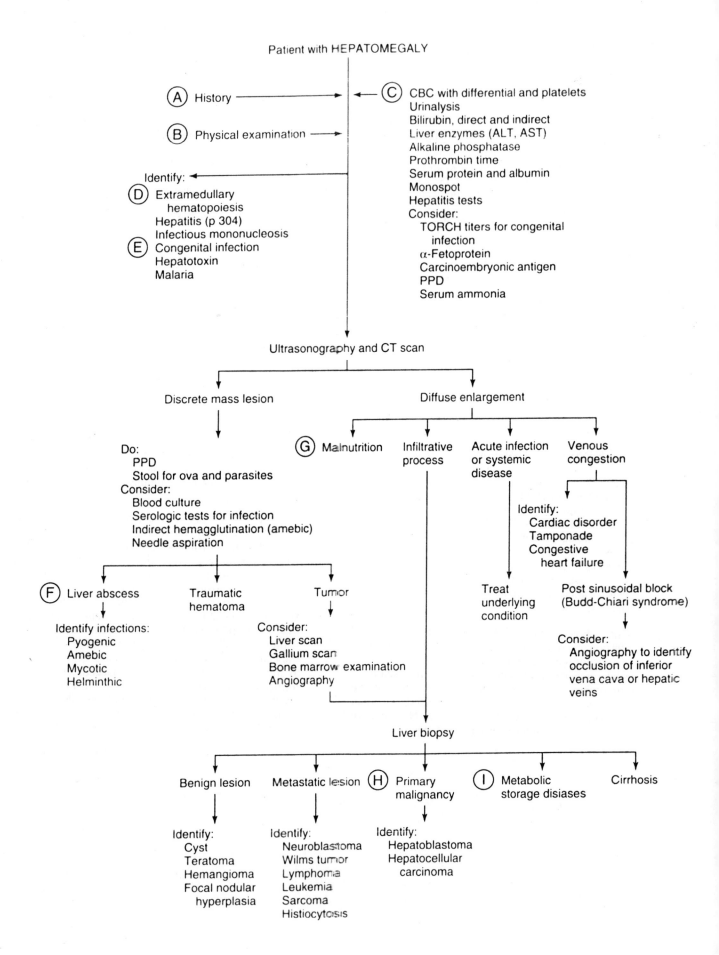

Patient with HEPATOMEGALY

(A) History

(B) Physical examination

(C) CBC with differential and platelets
Urinalysis
Bilirubin, direct and indirect
Liver enzymes (ALT, AST)
Alkaline phosphatase
Prothrombin time
Serum protein and albumin
Monospot
Hepatitis tests
Consider:
    TORCH titers for congenital
      infection
    α-Fetoprotein
    Carcinoembryonic antigen
    PPD
    Serum ammonia

Identify:
(D) Extramedullary
    hematopoiesis
Hepatitis (p 304)
Infectious mononucleosis
(E) Congenital infection
Hepatotoxin
Malaria

Ultrasonography and CT scan

Discrete mass lesion

Diffuse enlargement

Do:
  PPD
  Stool for ova and parasites
Consider:
  Blood culture
  Serologic tests for infection
  Indirect hemagglutination (amebic)
  Needle aspiration

(G) Malnutrition

Infiltrative process

Acute infection or systemic disease

Venous congestion

(F) Liver abscess

Traumatic hematoma

Tumor

Identify:
  Cardiac disorder
  Tamponade
  Congestive
    heart failure

Identify infections:
  Pyogenic
  Amebic
  Mycotic
  Helminthic

Consider:
  Liver scan
  Gallium scan
  Bone marrow examination
  Angiography

Treat underlying condition

Post sinusoidal block
(Budd-Chiari syndrome)

Consider:
  Angiography to identify
  occlusion of inferior
  vena cava or hepatic
  veins

Liver biopsy

Benign lesion

Metastatic lesion

(H) Primary malignancy

(I) Metabolic storage disiases

Cirrhosis

Identify:
  Cyst
  Teratoma
  Hemangioma
  Focal nodular
    hyperplasia

Identify:
  Neuroblastoma
  Wilms tumor
  Lymphoma
  Leukemia
  Sarcoma
  Histiocytosis

Identify:
  Hepatoblastoma
  Hepatocellular
    carcinoma

JAUNDICE AFTER 6 MONTHS OF AGE

Stephen Berman, M.D.

A. In the history ask about the feeding pattern, color of stools, and any fever, malaise, vomiting, abdominal pain, jaundice, pruritus, and dark urine. Document exposure to a hepatitis carrier or person with acute hepatitis or to blood products, medications, or illicit drugs. Note whether the child attends a large child-care or residential facility. Identify hematologic abnormalities such as hemolytic anemia, sickle cell disease, or thalassemia. Identify preexisting liver disease that causes elevations in indirect bilirubin (hepatitis, Gilbert disease, Crigler-Najjar syndrome) and direct bilirubin (Rotor syndrome, Dubin-Johnson syndrome, hepatitis). Note extrahepatic symptoms such as arthritis, polyarthralgia, amenorrhea, colitis, thyroiditis, glomerulonephritis, pleurisy, or rash.

B. In the physical examination note any right upper quadrant abdominal mass or tender hepatomegaly. Exudative tonsillitis, adenopathy, or splenomegaly suggests mononucleosis. Signs of chronic liver disease include acne, ascites, cushingoid facies, digital clubbing, and gynecomastia.

C. The degree of cholestasis and obstructive jaundice is reflected by the level of direct bilirubin and the degree of elevation of alkaline phosphatase and γ-glutamyltranspeptidase (GGT). Hepatocyte membrane disruption is correlated with the levels of the serum transaminases (ALT, AST). With extensive hepatocyte damage, serum albumin is depressed and the prothrombin time prolonged. Anemia associated with burr cells or severe thrombocytopenia suggests severe liver disease. A Coombs-positive hemolytic anemia, aplastic anemia, or pancytopenia may complicate hepatitis.

D. Acute cholecystitis can be caused by a bacterial infection (Salmonella, Shigella, Escherichia coli), virus, or parasites (Giardia and Ascaris). Sclerosing cholangitis usually associated with inflammatory bowel disease is a rare progressive disease that causes stenosis of the extrahepatic bile ducts; when it is suspected, obtain an endoscopic retrograde cholangiogram. No effective therapy is available for sclerosing cholangitis.

TABLE 1 Degree of Illness in Jaundice

Mild	Moderate	Severe
Minimal or no evidence of liver damage or acute infection	Acute hepatitis or Cholestasis or Signs of chronic liver disease	Signs of liver failure or Complication requiring hospitalization

E. Suspect acute hydrops of the bladder in children with Kawasaki disease when ultrasonography demonstrates distention of the gallbladder without calculi and with normal extrahepatic bile ducts. Attempt treatment with supportive care (IV fluids) followed by a low-fat diet before considering surgery in the latter condition.

F. Choledochal cyst is a congenital dilation of the common bile duct. The degree of jaundice, abdominal pain, vomiting, and alteration in stool color are variable. The scintiscan documents continuity of the cyst with the biliary tree.

G. Cholelithasis, or gall stones, may be related to prolonged total parenteral nutrition, disease of the terminal ileum, dehydration, prematurity, hemolytic disease, immaturity of liver glucuronosyltransferase, or ceftriaxone therapy. However, no associated cause is found in approximately half the cases. The stones consist of calcium bilirubinate and/or cholesterol crystals. In some children biliary sludge rather than stones may be responsible for the gallbladder dysfunction. Ultrasonography usually identifies dilation of the intrahepatic and extrahepatic bile ducts even if stones in the common duct are not visualized. Endoscopic retrograde cholangiopancreatography (ERCP) can identify the cause of the obstruction and may also remove sludge or stones. Cholecystectomy is indicated for symptomatic patients, especially when strictures or

(Continued on page 312)

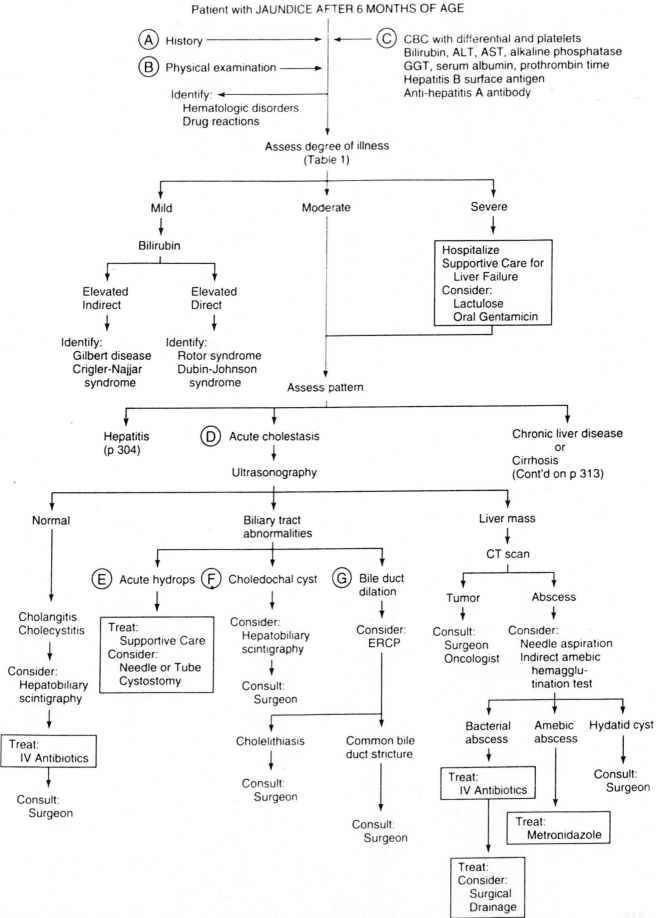

Patient with JAUNDICE AFTER 6 MONTHS OF AGE

(A) History

(B) Physical examination

(C) CBC with differential and platelets
Bilirubin, ALT, AST, alkaline phosphatase
GGT, serum albumin, prothrombin time
Hepatitis B surface antigen
Anti-hepatitis A antibody

Identify:
Hematologic disorders
Drug reactions

Assess degree of illness
(Table 1)

Mild   Moderate   Severe

Bilirubin

Hospitalize
Supportive Care for
Liver Failure
Consider:
Lactulose
Oral Gentamicin

Elevated
Indirect

Elevated
Direct

Identify:
Gilbert disease
Crigler-Najjar
syndrome

Identify:
Rotor syndrome
Dubin-Johnson
syndrome

Assess pattern

Hepatitis
(p 304)

(D) Acute cholestasis

Chronic liver disease
or
Cirrhosis
(Cont'd on p 313)

Ultrasonography

Normal   Biliary tract
abnormalities   Liver mass

CT scan

(E) Acute hydrops   (F) Choledochal cyst   (G) Bile duct
dilation

Tumor   Abscess

Cholangitis
Cholecystitis

Consider:
Hepatobiliary
scintigraphy

Treat:
IV Antibiotics

Consult:
Surgeon

Treat:
Supportive Care
Consider:
Needle or Tube
Cystostomy

Consider:
Hepatobiliary
scintigraphy

Consult:
Surgeon

Cholelithiasis

Consult:
Surgeon

Consider:
ERCP

Common bile
duct stricture

Consult:
Surgeon

Consult:
Surgeon
Oncologist

Consider:
Needle aspiration
Indirect amebic
hemagglu-
tination test

Bacterial
abscess

Amebic
abscess

Hydatid cyst

Treat:
IV Antibiotics

Treat:
Metronidazole

Consult:
Surgeon

Treat:
Consider:
Surgical
Drainage

anatomic anomalies of the common bile duct are present. Cholelitholytics (ursodeoxycholic acid) and lithotripsy have not been approved for children in the United States.

H. A Kayser-Fleischer ring revealed by slit-lamp examination, reduced serum copper and ceruloplasmin, and elevated urine and liver tissue copper identify patients with Wilson disease, an autosomal recessive disorder associated with excessive copper in the liver, brain, kidneys, and cornea. Treat with penicillamine to chelate copper. Liver transplantation can be performed in patients with liver failure. Galactosemia presents with vomiting, diarrhea, failure to thrive, hypoglycemia, cataracts, development delays, and seizures. It is associated with a deficiency of galactose-1-phosphate uridyl transferase. α_1-Antitrypsin deficiency presents with neonatal cholestatic jaundice and hepatomegaly in association with elevated transaminases. In hereditary fructose intolerance the child is deficient in fructose-1-phosphate aldolase or fructose-1, 6-diphosphatase. Test urine for amino and organic acids to identify cases of hereditary tyrosinemia, an autosomal recessive disorder. The chronic form is characterized by cirrhosis, vitamin D–resistant rickets, failure to thrive, and Fanconi syndrome. Obtain a sweat test to identify cystic fibrosis.

References

Ghishan FK. Trimethoprim-sulfamethoxazole-induced intrahepatic cholestasis. Clin Pediatr 1983; 22:212.

Hadide A. Types I and III choledochal cyst. Preoperative diagnosis by ultrasound. Am J Dis Child 1983; 137:663.

Holcomb GW, Holcomb GW. Cholelithiasis in infants, children, and adolescents. Pediatr Rev 1990; 11:268.

June CH, Benjamin SB. Bright yellow — the extended spectrum of Gilbert's syndrome. Am J Gastroenterol 1984; 79:482.

Lake AM, Truman JT, Bode HH, et al. Marked hyperbilirubinemia with Gilbert syndrome and immunochemolytic anemia. J Pediatr 1978; 93:812.

Mews C, Sinatra F. Chronic liver disease in children. Pediatr Rev 1993; 14:436.

Pineiro-Carrero VM, Andres AM. Morbidity and mortality in children with pyogenic liver disease. Am J Dis Child 1991; 143:991.

Schaad UB, Wedgewood-Krucko J, Tschaeppeler H. Reversible ceftriaxone-associated biliary pseudolithiasis in children. Lancet 1988; 2:1411.

Sternlieb I. Perspectives on Wilson's disease. Hepatology 1990; 12:1234.

Thompson JE, Forlenza S, Verma R. Amebic liver abscess: A therapeutic approach. Rev Infect Dis 1985; 7:171.

Whitington PF, Balistreri WF. Liver transplantation in pediatrics: Indications, contraindications, and pretransplant management. J Pediatr 1991; 118:169.

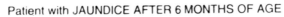

Patient with JAUNDICE AFTER 6 MONTHS OF AGE

Chronic liver disease
or
Cirrhosis
(Cont'd from p 311)

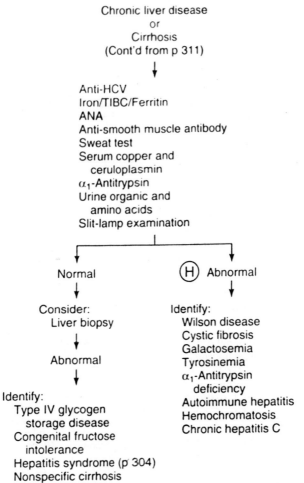

Anti-HCV
Iron/TIBC/Ferritin
ANA
Anti-smooth muscle antibody
Sweat test
Serum copper and
  ceruloplasmin
α_1-Antitrypsin
Urine organic and
  amino acids
Slit-lamp examination

Normal

Consider:
  Liver biopsy

Abnormal

Identify:
  Type IV glycogen
    storage disease
  Congenital fructose
    intolerance
  Hepatitis syndrome (p 304)
  Nonspecific cirrhosis

(H) Abnormal

Identify:
  Wilson disease
  Cystic fibrosis
  Galactosemia
  Tyrosinemia
  α_1-Antitrypsin
    deficiency
  Autoimmune hepatitis
  Hemochromatosis
  Chronic hepatitis C

PANCREATITIS

Stephen Berman, M.D.

DEFINITION

Pancreatitis is an inflammation of the pancreas with intrapancreatic activation of enzymes that cause pain, vomiting, and nausea.

ETIOLOGY

Causes of pancreatitis include acquired and congenital structural defects (biliary tract, cholelithiasis), infections (viral and mycoplasmal), systemic disorders (Kawasaki disease, AIDS, collagen vascular diseases, hemolytic uremic syndrome, cystic fibrosis, diabetes mellitus), metabolic diseases, medications, toxins, trauma, and surgery.

A. In the history ask about acute abdominal pain that radiates to the back or right upper quadrant and is associated with vomiting.

B. In the physical examination note abdominal distention, ascites, and peritoneal signs. There may be signs of an ileus with absent bowel sounds. Discoloration around the umbilicus or flank suggests pancreatic necrosis. Note signs of respiratory distress associated with pleural effusions or pneumonitis. Assess circulatory status and peripheral perfusion to identify intravascular volume loss secondary to third spacing. Note purpura or bleeding that suggests disseminated intravascular coagulation.

C. Laboratory findings of pancreatitis include elevations in serum amylase and lipase levels. Liver function tests may be abnormal when choledocholithiasis or hepatitis is present. Glucose may be increased and calcium decreased with severe disease. The WBC is often elevated, 10,000 to 25,000.

D. Treated by placing a nasogastric tube and providing appropriate fluids intravenously. Pain medication with meperidine is recommended. Correction of hyperglycemia or hypocalcemia may be needed. When pain and vomiting have resolved and bowel sounds are present, start feedings with small amounts of high-carbohydrate, low-fat, low-protein foods and advance as tolerated. Consider using an H_2 receptor antagonist (Table 2) with feedings to reduce gastric acid and increase the availability of pancreatic enzymes.

TABLE 1 Severity of Illness in Pancreatitis

Severe	Very Severe
Severe abdominal pain with nausea and vomiting and	Signs of shock or
Elevated serum amylase or lipase	Disseminated intravascular coagulation or
	Severe respiratory distress/ impending respiratory failure
	Signs of pancreatic necrosis or
	Signs of peritonitis

TABLE 2 Drug Therapy for Peptic Ulcer Disease or Gastritis in Children

Agent	Dosage	Product Availability
Cimetidine (Tagamet)	5 – 10 mg/kg/dose q.i.d. (max 300 mg/dose b.i.d.)	Liquid: 300 mg/5ml Tabs: 200, 300, 400, 800 mg
Famotidine (Pepcid)	40 mg qd for adults	Tabs: 20, 40 mg Liquid: 40 mg/5 ml
Ranitidine (Zantac)	1.25 – 2.5 mg/kg/dose b.i.d. (max 150 mg/ dose b.i.d.)	Tabs: 150, 300 mg Liquid: 15 mg/ml

E. Consider a three-way abdominal series to identify pulmonary complications and signs of ileus. Ultrasonography may demonstrate pancreatic inflammation or a pseudocyst. It is important to diagnose acute surgical problems such as appendicitis and intussusception.

Reference

Steinberg W, Tanner S. Acute pancreatitis. N Engl J Med 1994; 330:1198.

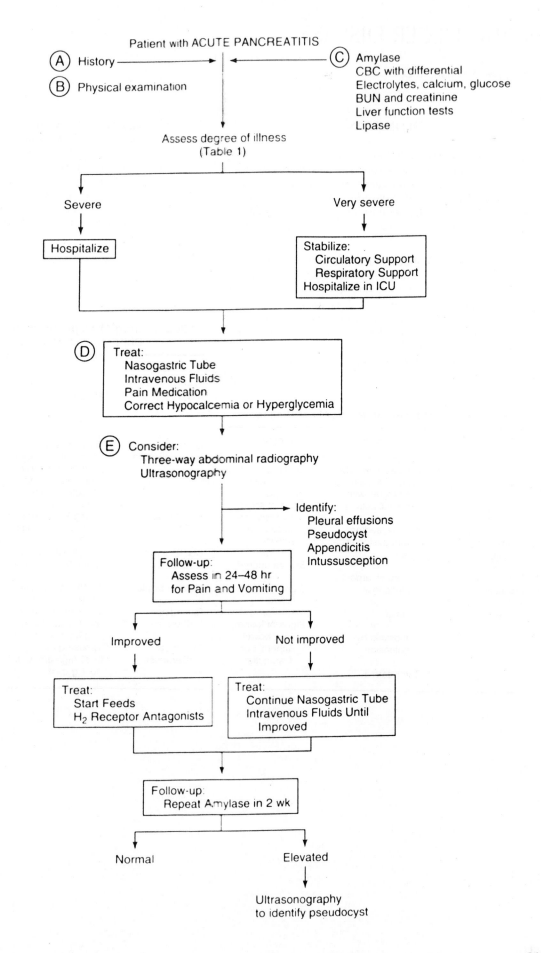

Patient with ACUTE PANCREATITIS

(A) History

(B) Physical examination

(C) Amylase
CBC with differential
Electrolytes, calcium, glucose
BUN and creatinine
Liver function tests
Lipase

Assess degree of illness
(Table 1)

Severe

Very severe

Hospitalize

Stabilize:
  Circulatory Support
  Respiratory Support
Hospitalize in ICU

(D) Treat:
  Nasogastric Tube
  Intravenous Fluids
  Pain Medication
  Correct Hypocalcemia or Hyperglycemia

(E) Consider:
  Three-way abdominal radiography
  Ultrasonography

Identify:
  Pleural effusions
  Pseudocyst
  Appendicitis
  Intussuception

Follow-up:
  Assess in 24–48 hr
  for Pain and Vomiting

Improved

Not improved

Treat:
  Start Feeds
  H$_2$ Receptor Antagonists

Treat:
  Continue Nasogastric Tube
  Intravenous Fluids Until
  Improved

Follow-up:
Repeat Amylase in 2 wk

Normal

Elevated

Ultrasonography
to identify pseudocyst

PEPTIC ULCER DISEASE

Stephen Berman, M.D.

DEFINITION

Peptic ulcer disease with loss of mucosal tissue of the stomach or duodenum results from disorders in acid production and/or mucosal tissue resistance. Secondary peptic ulcers are associated with systemic disorders, acute stress, or drug therapy (salicylates and other nonsteroidal antiinflammatory drugs). *Helicobacter pylori* colonization is associated with peptic ulcer disease.

A. In the history ask about clinical manifestations of peptic ulcer disease, including abdominal pain (82%), nausea (20%), vomiting (25%), hematemesis (16%), and melena (9%). In older patients the classic characteristic of ulcer disease is epigastric pain relieved by eating or antacids and/or nocturnal pain that may awaken the patient from sleep. Vomiting may be the only presenting symptom in children younger than 4 years of age.

B. The initial radiologic work-up in a case of suspected peptic ulcer disease without a history of an upper GI bleed is an upper GI series with a double-contrast technique. If an ulcer crater is not revealed, a small-bowel series should be done to identify inflammatory bowel disease. Spasm of the duodenal bulb, pylorospasm, and delayed gastric emptying are nonspecific findings. Upper GI endoscopy is recommended for children with

(Continued on page 318)

TABLE 1   Degree of Illness in Peptic Ulcer Disease

Moderate	Severe	Very Severe
Abdominal pain that does not interfere with activity and No anemia and No signs of active bleeding and No orthostatic hypotension or signs of impaired circulation	Incapacitating abdominal pain that interferes with normal activity or Active bleeding with gastric aspirate or History of large blood loss or Anemia or Orthostatic hypotension or Tachycardia	Continuing large blood loss or Signs of shock, acidosis, circulatory instability or Severe anemia or Signs of heart failure or Signs of kidney, liver, bowel ischemia or dysfunction

TABLE 2   Drug Therapy for Peptic Ulcer Disease in Children and Adolescents

Drug	Dosage	Product Availability
Amoxicillin	15 mg/kg/dose t.i.d. (max 500 mg/dose)	Liquid: 125, 250 mg/5 ml Tabs: 125, 250, 500 mg
Bismuth subsalicylate	7.5 ml or ½ tablet t.i.d. before meals and at bedtime for children < 10 yr; double dosage for those > 10 yr	
Cimetidine (Tagamet)	5–8 mg/kg/dose q.i.d. (max 300 mg/dose q.i.d.)	Liquid: 300 mg/5 ml Tabs: 200, 300, 400, 800 mg
Clarithromycin (Biaxin)	15 mg/kg/day b.i.d. (max 500 mg/dose)	Liquid: 125, 250 mg/5 ml Tabs: 250, 500 mg
Metronidazole	7.5–10 mg/kg/dose b.i.d.	Tabs: 250, 500 mg
Ranitidine (Zantac)	1.25–2 mg/kg/dose b.i.d. (max 150 mg/kg/dose b.i.d.)	Tabs: 150, 300 mg
Sucralfate (Carafate)	1 g/dose q.i.d. 40–80 mg/kg/day up to 1 g q.i.d.	Tabs: 1 g Liquid: 100 mg/ml

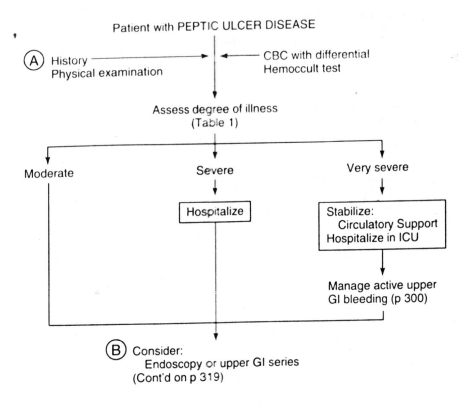

Patient with PEPTIC ULCER DISEASE

(A) History ————————→ ←——— CBC with differential
    Physical examination   Hemoccult test

Assess degree of illness
(Table 1)

Moderate   Severe   Very severe

                      | Hospitalize | | Stabilize: |
                                           | Circulatory Support |
                                           | Hospitalize in ICU |

                                           Manage active upper
                                           GI bleeding (p 300)

(B) Consider:
    Endoscopy or upper GI series
    (Cont'd on p 319)

TABLE 3 Abbreviated List of Antacid Preparations

Antacid	Composition	Neutralizing Capacity (mEq/ml)	Dose to Neutralize 80 mEq of HCl (ml)	Sodium Content (mg/ml)	Approximate Cost/Day ($)
Maalox TC	Al and Mg hydroxides	5.7	14	0.16	1.50
Mylanta II	Al and Mg hydroxides, simethicone	5.0	16	0.22	1.71
Gelusil II	Al and Mg hydroxides	4.8	17	0.26	1.66
Camalox	Al and Mg hydroxides, CA carbonate	3.6	22	0.50	1.88
Alternagel	Al hydroxide gel	3.2	25	0.40	2.03
Maalox	Al and Mg hydroxides	2.7	30	0.27	1.57
Riopan	Al and Mg hydroxides	3.0	27	0.02	1.40
Mylanta	Al and Mg hydroxides, simethicone	2.5	32	0.14	1.26
Gelusil	Al and Mg hydroxides, simethicone	2.4	33	0.14	1.34

Al, aluminum; Mg, magnesium.
From Byrne WJ. Diagnosis and treatment of peptic ulcer disease in children. Pediatr Rev 1985; 7:182.

upper GI bleeding (when stable) and cases with a non-diagnostic upper GI series whose symptoms persist and require further therapy.

C. *H. pylori* is best diagnosed with a histologic study of a biopsy sample of the greater curvature of the antrum obtained by endoscopy. It is identified most frequently in children with duodenal ulcers and antritis and less frequently when a gastric ulcer is present. Treatment with double or triple combination therapy with bismuth subsalicylate and amoxicillin or clarithromycin (Biaxin) with or without metronidazole for 6 weeks appears to be effective (Table 2). Clarithromycin may be administered to adolescents.

D. Manage peptic ulcer disease in children initially with regular-strength antacids 1 ml/kg/dose (maximum 30 ml) given 1 to 3 hours after meals and 2 ml/kg/dose (maximum 60 ml) at bedtime for 6 to 8 weeks (Table 3). Consider cimetidine for children 3 to 12 years of age and ranitidine for adolescents. Experience with famotidine or nizatidine is limited in children. Sucralfate, a coating agent, can be used as an alternative to treat duodenal ulcers in adolescents. Consider using omeprazole, a proton pump inhibitor that reduces acid secretion in gastric parietal cells, when patients fail to respond to conventional therapy.

References

Chong SKF, Lou Q, Asnicar MA, et al. *Helicobacter pylori* infection in recurrent abdominal pain in childhood: Comparison of diagnostic tests and therapy. Pediatrics 1995; 96:211.

Gryboski JD. Peptic ulcer disease in children. Pediatr Rev 1990; 12:15.

Gunasekaran TS, Hassall EG. Efficacy and safety of omeprazole for severe gastroesophageal reflux in children. J Pediatr 1993; 123:151.

Israel DM, Hassall E. Treatment and long term follow-up of *Helicobacter pylori*–associated duodenal ulcer disease in children. J Pediatr 1993; 123:53.

Maton PN. Omeprazole. N Engl J Med 1991; 324:965.

Mezoff AG, Balisteri WF. Peptic ulcer disease in children. Pediatr Rev 1995, 16:257.

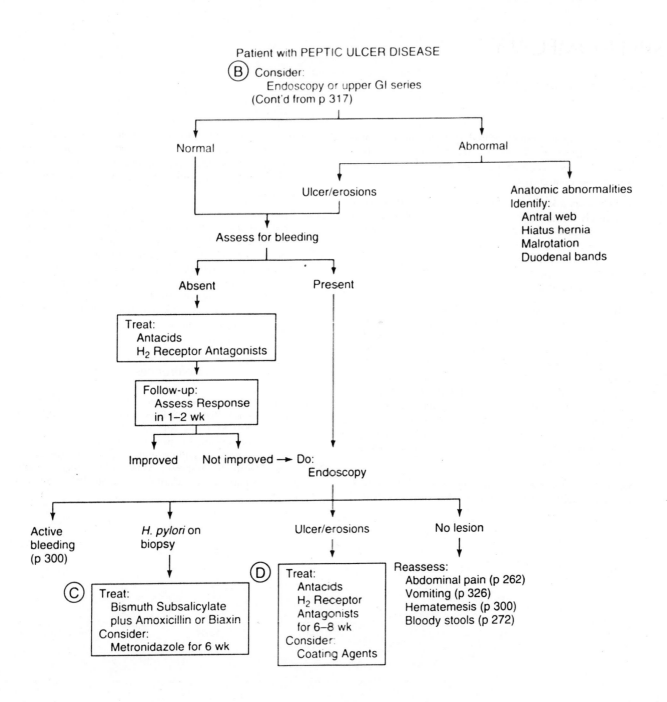

Patient with PEPTIC ULCER DISEASE

(B) Consider:
    Endoscopy or upper GI series
(Cont'd from p 317)

Normal ————— Abnormal

Ulcer/erosions ————— Anatomic abnormalities
Identify:
    Antral web
    Hiatus hernia
    Malrotation
    Duodenal bands

Assess for bleeding

Absent ————— Present

Treat:
    Antacids
    H₂ Receptor Antagonists

Follow-up:
    Assess Response
    in 1–2 wk

Improved   Not improved → Do:
                              Endoscopy

Active   H. pylori on   Ulcer/erosions   No lesion
bleeding   biopsy
(p 300)

(C) Treat: (D) Treat: Reassess:
    Bismuth Subsalicylate   Antacids   Abdominal pain (p 262)
    plus Amoxicillin or Biaxin   H₂ Receptor   Vomiting (p 326)
Consider: Antagonists   Hematemesis (p 300)
    Metronidazole for 6 wk   for 6–8 wk   Bloody stools (p 272)
                              Consider:
                                  Coating Agents

319

SPLENOMEGALY

Perla Santos Ocampo, M.D.

The tip of the spleen is normally palpable in premature infants and in about a third of full-term infants. It may be felt up to 3 to 5 years of age. Thereafter a palpable spleen may be presumed to be enlarged.

A. In the history ask about acute illness, associated personal and family hematologic disorders, and possible food or drug exposure precipitating the episode. Ask about presence or recurrence of systemic symptoms such as fever, jaundice, pallor, bleeding, tea-colored urine, bone and joint pains, weight loss, abnormal sweating, anorexia, and abdominal enlargement.

B. Perform a thorough physical examination. The abdomen of the patient should be well relaxed. If the spleen is huge, its edge may extend well down into the left lower quadrant. Palpation of the splenic notch is helpful in identification. Note size and consistency. Auscultate to detect a bruit or friction rub. Other masses on the left side of the abdomen that should be differentiated from the spleen are a large kidney, pancreatic cyst, ovarian cyst, omental mass, mesenteric cyst, retroperitoneal tumor, and adrenal neoplasm. Ascertain whether lymph nodes and/or the liver are enlarged. Note any ascites and signs of storage diseases.

C. Signs of a hematologic disorder are pallor and jaundice associated with anemia, an abnormal smear, elevated indirect bilirubin, and reticulocytosis. Hemolytic anemias that can cause splenomegaly include hemoglobinopathies, thalassemia, enzyme defects, hereditary spherocytosis, and other autoimmune hemolytic anemias.

D. Acute or chronic infection causes splenomegaly. Bacterial causes include sepsis, bacterial endocarditis, typhoid fever, tuberculosis, cat-scratch disease, brucellosis, typhus syphilis, and Lyme disease *(Borrelia burgdorferi)*. Viral agents include Epstein-Barr virus (mononucleosis), cytomegalovirus, HIV, and hepatitis viruses. Protozoans include malaria, toxoplasmosis, schistosomiasis, kala-azar and visceral larva migrans. Mycotic agents are histoplasmosis and coccidioidomycosis.

References

Lanzkowsky P, Nelson NM, Seidel HM. Splenomegaly. In: Hoekelman RA, Blatman S, Friedman SB, et al, eds. Primary pediatric care. St. Louis: Mosby, 1987:1092.

Pearson HA. The spleen. In: Behrman RE, Vaughan VC, eds. Textbook of pediatrics. Philadelphia: Saunders, 1987:1075.

Pearson SJ, Dennis S, Tunnessen WW. Splenomegaly: Something's bad in the air. Contemp Pediatr 1992; September:49.

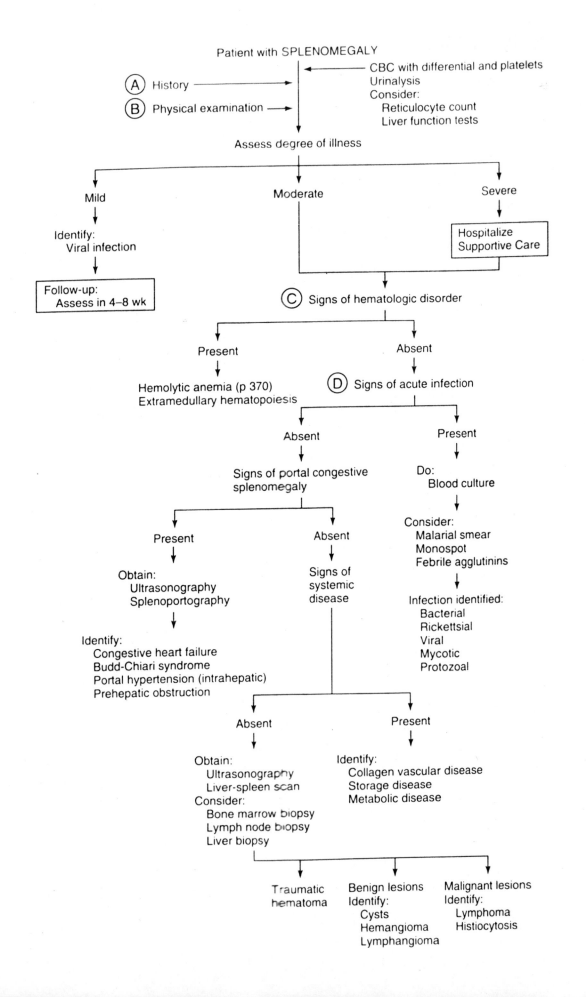

Patient with SPLENOMEGALY

(A) History

(B) Physical examination

CBC with differential and platelets
Urinalysis
Consider:
    Reticulocyte count
    Liver function tests

Assess degree of illness

Mild

Identify:
    Viral infection

Follow-up:
    Assess in 4–8 wk

Moderate

Severe

Hospitalize
Supportive Care

(C) Signs of hematologic disorder

Present

Hemolytic anemia (p 370)
Extramedullary hematopoiesis

Absent

(D) Signs of acute infection

Absent

Signs of portal congestive
splenomegaly

Present

Obtain:
    Ultrasonography
    Splenoportography

Identify:
    Congestive heart failure
    Budd-Chiari syndrome
    Portal hypertension (intrahepatic)
    Prehepatic obstruction

Absent

Signs of
systemic
disease

Present

Do:
    Blood culture

Consider:
    Malarial smear
    Monospot
    Febrile agglutinins

Infection identified:
    Bacterial
    Rickettsial
    Viral
    Mycotic
    Protozoal

Absent

Obtain:
    Ultrasonography
    Liver-spleen scan
Consider:
    Bone marrow biopsy
    Lymph node biopsy
    Liver biopsy

Present

Identify:
    Collagen vascular disease
    Storage disease
    Metabolic disease

Traumatic
hematoma

Benign lesions
Identify:
    Cysts
    Hemangioma
    Lymphangioma

Malignant lesions
Identify:
    Lymphoma
    Histiocytosis

ULCERATIVE COLITIS

Stephen Berman, M.D.

Ulcerative colitis, an immune-mediated inflammation of the colon of unknown origin, can be categorized by the patterns of involvement: pancolitis or limited disease. Patients present with diarrhea, bloody stools, tenesmus, and abdominal pain. Patients with pancolitis have more severe disease, a higher incidence of extraintestinal manifestations, and an increased risk of toxic megacolon and cancer. Chronic colonic blood loss may lead to hypochromic microcytic anemia. A protein-losing enteropathy results in hypoalbuminemia.

A. In the history note the onset, pattern (nocturnal diarrhea), severity (blood and mucus), and frequency of diarrhea. In ulcerative colitis stools usually contain blood and mucus. Document associated symptoms, including urgency and tenesmus, abdominal pain, fecal incontinence, anorexia, chronic fever, and weight loss. Perianal disease such as fistulas or fissures usually suggests Crohn disease rather than ulcerative colitis. Extraintestinal manifestations of ulcerative colitis include growth retardation, delayed puberty, mucocutaneous lesions, urethritis, arthritis, arthralgias, conjunctivitis, anemia, chronic active hepatitis, and pericholangitis.

B. Endoscopic findings of ulcerative colitis range from colonic erythema and edema to friable mucosa with ulceration. The barium enema may be unremarkable or may show segmental pseudostrictures in the distal colon, with the loss of haustral markings and mucosal mottling. When a narrow, short colon without haustral markings is visualized, suspect chronic long-term disease.

C. Suspect toxic megacolon in a toxic patient with abdominal distention and peritoneal signs. When shock is present, treat toxic megacolon with nasogastric decom-

(Continued on page 324)

TABLE 1   Degree of Illness in Ulcerative Colitis

Moderate	Severe	Very Severe
Minimal systemic symptoms or intestinal complaints of pain or diarrhea	Incapacitating systemic symptoms or abdominal pain or Bloody diarrhea associated with dehydration, marked weight loss, or severe anemia	Toxic appearance (sepsis or toxic megacolon) or Signs of acute intestinal obstruction, peritonitis, or massive hemorrhage

Patient with ULCERATIVE COLITIS

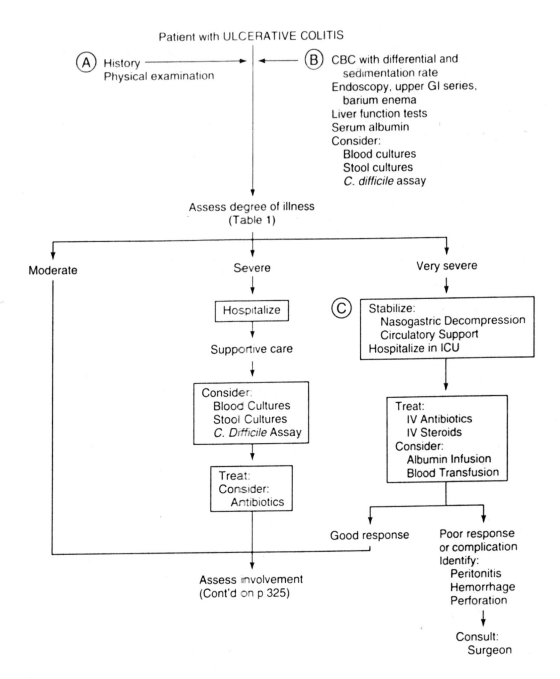

Ⓐ History ——————→ ←—————— Ⓑ CBC with differential and
Physical examination   sedimentation rate
                                    Endoscopy, upper GI series,
                                       barium enema
                                    Liver function tests
                                    Serum albumin
                                    Consider:
                                       Blood cultures
                                       Stool cultures
                                       C. difficile assay

Assess degree of illness
(Table 1)

Moderate   Severe   Very severe

                     | Hospitalize | Ⓒ | Stabilize: |
                                            | Nasogastric Decompression |
                     Supportive care | Circulatory Support |
                                            | Hospitalize in ICU |

                     | Consider: |
                     | Blood Cultures | | Treat: |
                     | Stool Cultures | | IV Antibiotics |
                     | *C. Difficile* Assay | | IV Steroids |
                                            | Consider: |
                     | Treat: | | Albumin Infusion |
                     | Consider: | | Blood Transfusion |
                     | Antibiotics |

                                         Good response   Poor response
                                                          or complication
                                                          Identify:
                                                             Peritonitis
                                                             Hemorrhage
Assess involvement   Perforation
(Cont'd on p 325)
                                                          Consult:
                                                             Surgeon

pression and infusions of salt-poor albumin and blood transfusions. Avoid barium studies and initiate therapy with antibiotics and steroids.

D. Treat ulcerative colitis with sulfasalazine (Azulfidine), which is split by bacterial action in the colon into sulfapyridine and 5-aminosalicylic acid, the active ingredient. Sulfapyridine is absorbed and excreted in the bile. Avoid oral antibiotics that will alter intestinal flora and prevent cleavage of the drug. Give the patient folic acid supplementation. Monitor the patient's blood count weekly for the first month, since neutropenia, a Heinz body hemolytic anemia, or a serum sickness reaction can occur. Anorexia, nausea, and headache are common side effects. Consider steroid-retention enemas in patients with left-sided colitis or proctitis. Treat patients with unresponsive disease or extraintestinal manifestations with 6 to 8 weeks of prednisone 1 to 2 mg/kg/day (maximum 60 mg). Consider azathioprine for patients who cannot be weaned from steroids after 8 weeks of daily therapy without relapse.

E. Consider surgery when prolonged high-dose steroid therapy is necessary, severe growth retardation is present prior to epiphyseal closure, the colitis has failed to respond after 2 years of medical therapy, or biopsy reveals evidence of a precancerous dysplastic mucosa. The risk of cancer is low during the first 10 years of the disease but increases approximately 1% to 2% every year thereafter. Yearly follow-up visits and endoscopy are essential to monitor the course of the disease and detect dysplastic changes early.

References

Ament M. Inflammatory disease of the colon: Ulcerative colitis and Crohn's colitis. J Pediatr 1975; 86:322.

Balistreri WF. Minimizing the effects of idiopathic IBD. Contemp Pediatr 1985; July:24.

Devroede G, Taylor WF, Sauer WG, et al. Cancer risk and life expectancy of children with ulcerative colitis. N Engl J Med 1971; 285:17.

Gryboski JD. Ulcerative colitis in children 10 years or younger. J Pediatr Gastroenterol Nutr 1993; 12:24.

MacDonald TT. Inflammatory bowel disease in children. Curr Opin Pediatr 1994; 6:547.

Noll RA, Ferry GD. Pediatric inflammatory bowel disease. Curr Opin Gastroenterol 1992; 8:676.

O'Gorman MO, Lake AM. Chronic inflammatory bowel disease in childhood. Pediatr Rev 1993; 14:475.

Silverman A, Roy CC. Pediatric clinical gastroenterology. 3rd ed. St. Louis: Mosby, 1983:353.

Steffen RM, Wyllie R, Sivak MV Jr, et al. Colonoscopy in the pediatric patient. J Pediatr 1989; 115:507.

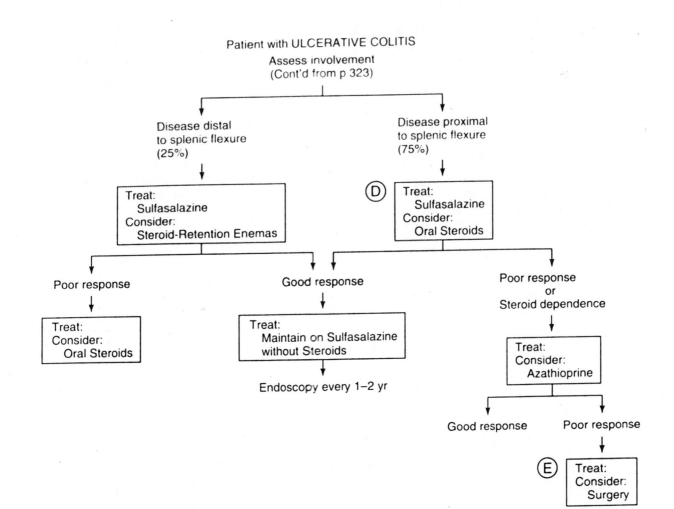

Patient with ULCERATIVE COLITIS
Assess involvement
(Cont'd from p 323)

Disease distal
to splenic flexure
(25%)

Disease proximal
to splenic flexure
(75%)

Treat:
  Sulfasalazine
Consider:
  Steroid-Retention Enemas

Ⓓ Treat:
  Sulfasalazine
Consider:
  Oral Steroids

Poor response

Good response

Poor response
or
Steroid dependence

Treat:
Consider:
  Oral Steroids

Treat:
  Maintain on Sulfasalazine
  without Steroids

Endoscopy every 1–2 yr

Treat:
Consider:
  Azathioprine

Good response

Poor response

Ⓔ Treat:
Consider:
  Surgery

VOMITING AFTER INFANCY

Stephen Berman, M.D.

A. In the history ask about the onset, frequency, severity (quantity and forcefulness), and timing of vomiting. Identify precipitating factors such as feeding, cough, or activity. Note associated symptoms such as abdominal pain, alterations in mental status, bloody stools, coryza, cough, diarrhea, dysuria, failure to thrive, fever, headache, jaundice, polydipsia, and urinary frequency. A recent history of chickenpox or influenza syndrome suggests Reye syndrome. Vomiting associated with bloody stools and intermittent abdominal pain suggests intussusception. Nighttime vomiting suggests a CNS disorder or possible exposure to a toxin (CO poisoning). Identify predisposing conditions such as hepatitis, inflammatory bowel disease, necrotizing enterocolitis, pregnancy, prior abdominal surgery, and sickle cell disease. Precipitating factors include current medications, ingestions (salicylate), and toxins. In adolescence suspect bulimia or superior mesenteric artery syndrome when vomiting is associated with marked weight loss.

B. In the physical examination assess the circulatory and hydration status by ascertaining blood pressure, pulse, respiratory rate, capillary refill, skin color and turgor, tears, fullness of the fontanelle, and urine output. Plot the child's height, weight, and head circumference on a growth grid to identify cases with failure to thrive or rapid head growth. Assess the mental status and note any irritability, lethargy, seizures, papilledema, retinal hemorrhage, ataxia, and focal neurologic signs. Document extraintestinal manifestations such as rash, arthritis, lymphadenopathy, hepatosplenomegaly, and infections.

C. Consider a diagnostic work-up for infection, systemic disorders, and CNS disorders. Infections that can result in persistent vomiting include acute otitis media, urinary tract infection, pneumonia, sepsis, and meningitis. Systemic disorders with persistent vomiting include hepatobiliary disorders (hepatitis, cholangitis, choledochal cyst, cholecystitis), cystic fibrosis (meconium ileus equivalent), inborn errors of metabolism, and CNS abnormalities (hydrocephalus, tumors, cerebral edema, increased intracranial pressure).

D. Suspect acute pancreatitis when acute abdominal pain radiates to the back or right upper quadrant and is associated with vomiting. Ascites, abdominal distention, and peritoneal signs may be present. Elevation

TABLE 1 Degree of Illness in Vomiting After Infancy

Mild	Moderate	Severe	Very Severe
Previously healthy child with no signs of bacterial infection, systemic disorder, or dehydration	Signs of bacterial infection or Systemic disorder or Vomiting longer than 1 wk or Growth failure/weight loss	Signs of severe dehydration or Intestinal obstruction or Acidosis or Electrolyte abnormalities or Altered mental status: lethargy, confusion, disorientation	Signs of shock or Altered mental status: unresponsive, too weak to feed, seizures, signs of meningeal irritation

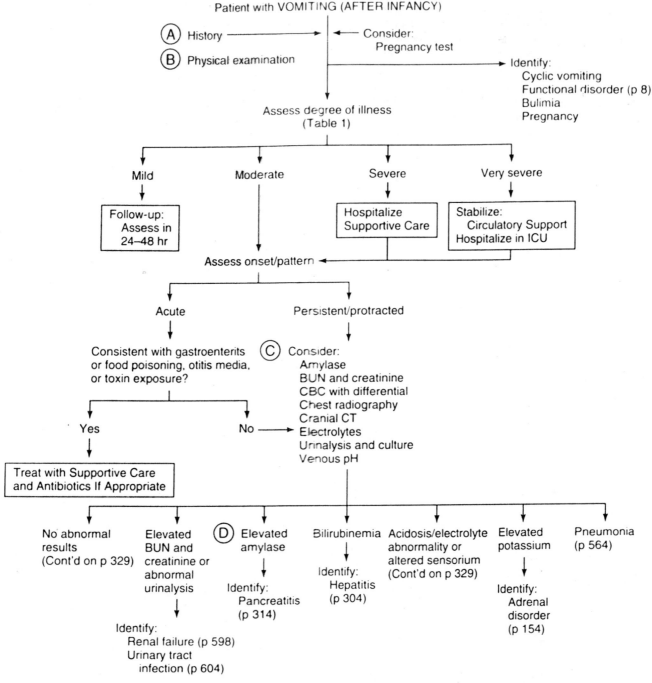

Patient with VOMITING (AFTER INFANCY)

(A) History ⟶ ← Consider:
                    Pregnancy test

(B) Physical examination

⟶ Identify:
    Cyclic vomiting
    Functional disorder (p 8)
    Bulimia
    Pregnancy

Assess degree of illness
(Table 1)

| Mild | Moderate | Severe | Very severe |

Mild: Follow-up: Assess in 24–48 hr

Severe: Hospitalize Supportive Care

Very severe: Stabilize: Circulatory Support Hospitalize in ICU

Assess onset/pattern ←

Acute

Persistent/protracted

Consistent with gastroenterits or food poisoning, otitis media, or toxin exposure?

(C) Consider:
    Amylase
    BUN and creatinine
    CBC with differential
    Chest radiography
    Cranial CT
    Electrolytes
    Urinalysis and culture
    Venous pH

Yes

No ⟶

Treat with Supportive Care and Antibiotics If Appropriate

No abnormal results (Cont'd on p 329)

Elevated BUN and creatinine or abnormal urinalysis

Identify:
Renal failure (p 598)
Urinary tract infection (p 604)

(D) Elevated amylase

Identify:
Pancreatitis (p 314)

Bilirubinemia

Identify:
Hepatitis (p 304)

Acidosis/electrolyte abnormality or altered sensorium (Cont'd on p 329)

Elevated potassium

Identify:
Adrenal disorder (p 154)

Pneumonia (p 564)

327

of serum amylase or a radioimmune assay of pancreatic trypsinogen suggests pancreatitis. Ultrasonography may show findings of inflammation or a pseudocyst. Causes of pancreatitis include acquired or congenital structural defects, trauma, metabolic disorders, infection, hemolytic uremia syndrome, and drug toxicity.

E. Suspect Reye-like syndrome when the patient has persistent vomiting, hyperventilation, and altered mental status (confusion, combativeness, disorientation, stupor, coma) in association with hepatic dysfunction (elevated serum transaminases and ammonia).

References

Carraccio C, Tunnessen WW Jr. Recurrent vomiting: What's obstructing the diagnosis? Contemp Pediatr 1989; August:151.

Fuchs S, Jaffe D. Vomiting. Pediatr Emerg Care 1990; 6:164.

Ramos AG, Tuchman DN. Persistent vomiting. Pediatr Rev 1994; 15:24.

Patient with VOMITING (After Infancy)

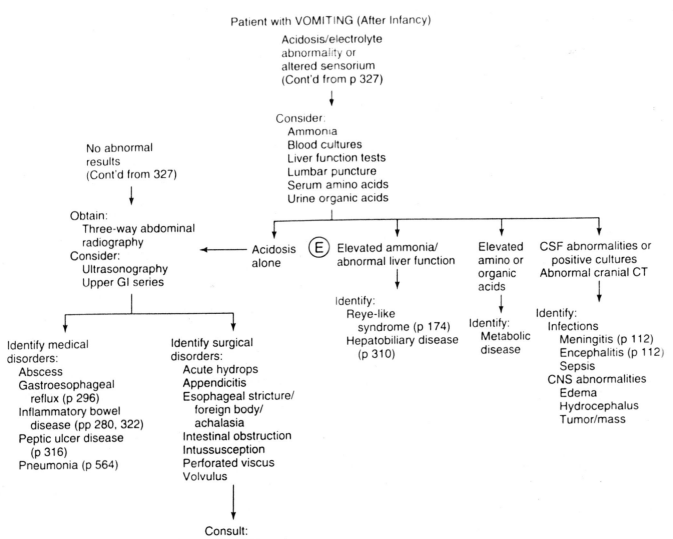

Acidosis/electrolyte
abnormality or
altered sensorium
(Cont'd from p 327)

Consider:
Ammonia
Blood cultures
Liver function tests
Lumbar puncture
Serum amino acids
Urine organic acids

No abnormal
results
(Cont'd from 327)

Obtain:
Three-way abdominal
radiography
Consider:
Ultrasonography
Upper GI series

Acidosis
alone

(E) Elevated ammonia/
abnormal liver function

Elevated
amino or
organic
acids

CSF abnormalities or
positive cultures
Abnormal cranial CT

Identify:
Reye-like
syndrome (p 174)
Hepatobiliary disease
(p 310)

Identify:
Metabolic
disease

Identify:
Infections
Meningitis (p 112)
Encephalitis (p 112)
Sepsis
CNS abnormalities
Edema
Hydrocephalus
Tumor/mass

Identify medical
disorders:
Abscess
Gastroesophageal
reflux (p 296)
Inflammatory bowel
disease (pp 280, 322)
Peptic ulcer disease
(p 316)
Pneumonia (p 564)

Identify surgical
disorders:
Acute hydrops
Appendicitis
Esophageal stricture/
foreign body/
achalasia
Intestinal obstruction
Intussusception
Perforated viscus
Volvulus

Consult:
Surgeon

VOMITING DURING INFANCY

Stephen Berman, M.D.

A. In the history ask about the onset, frequency, and severity (quantity, degree of forcefulness, presence of bile) of the vomiting. Determine the type of formula, manner of preparation, quantity ingested, and feeding position and technique. Establish the timing of vomiting in relation to the feeding. Spitting up, or regurgitation of small amounts of formula during or soon after feeding, suggests an improper feeding technique such as bottle propping or mild gastroesophageal reflux. Note associated symptoms such as fever, cough, coryza, respiratory distress, diarrhea, altered mental status, seizures, and failure to thrive. Inquire about perinatal deaths in the family that suggest inborn errors of metabolism and adrenal insufficiency. Any infant with a history of necrotizing enterocolitis or bilious vomiting should be considered to have a possible intestinal obstruction.

B. In the physical examination assess hydration and circulatory status by determining blood pressure, pulse, respiratory rate, capillary refill, skin color and turgor, presence of tears, fullness of the fontanelle, and urine output. Plot the infant's height, weight, and head circumference on a growth grid to identify cases of failure to thrive or rapid head growth. Assess the mental status. Note any acute otitis media, irritability, lethargy, seizures, and focal neurologic signs. Observe a feeding and note the peristaltic waves. Palpation of abdominal mass (olive) suggests pyloric stenosis.

C. Protracted vomiting may result in significant loss of stomach acid, causing hypochloremic alkalosis. Hypochloremic alkalosis is often associated with a paradoxically acid urine because of intracellular potassium deficits. Treat these patients with normal saline and replace the potassium deficit; alkalinization of the urine indicates that the potassium has been replaced.

D. Systemic illnesses that can cause persistent vomiting during infancy include adrenal insufficiency, metabolic disorders, CNS disorders with increased intracranial pressure, hepatobiliary disorders, and renal disease. Acidosis, vomiting, and failure to thrive suggest an endocrine or metabolic disorder such as diabetic ketoacidosis, adrenal insufficiency, adrenogenital syndrome, aminoaciduria, galactosemia, glycogen storage disease, lysosomal disease, and fructose intolerance.

TABLE 1 Degree of Illness in Vomiting Infant

Mild	Moderate	Severe	Very Severe
Previously healthy infant with no signs of bacterial infection, growth deficiency, systemic disorder, or dehydration	Signs of bacterial infection or Systemic disorder or Vomiting >1 wk or Growth failure/weight loss or Aspiration pneumonia	Signs of severe dehydration or Intestinal obstruction (bilious vomiting) or Acidosis or Electrolyte abnormalities or Altered mental status: lethargy, confusion, disorientation or Too weak to feed	Signs of shock or Altered mental status: unresponsive or Seizures or Signs of meningeal irritation

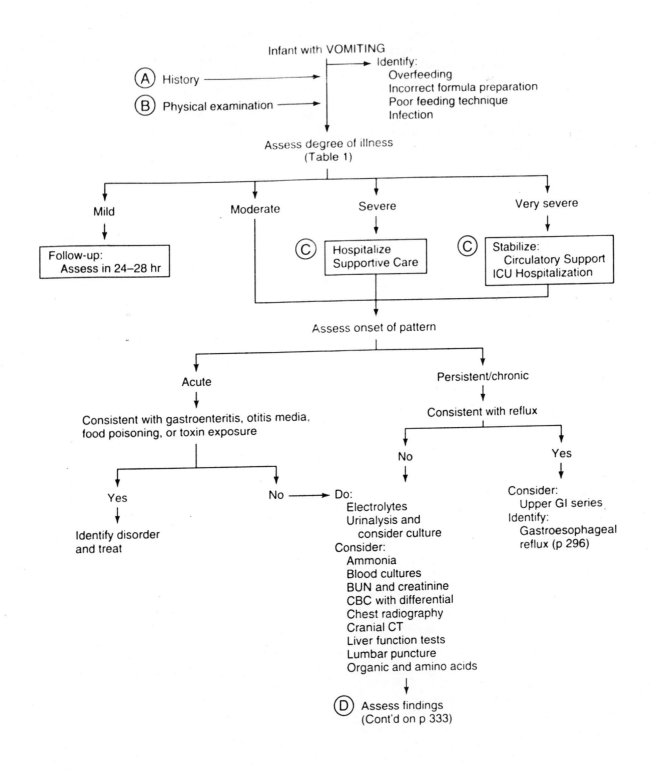

Infant with VOMITING

(A) History

(B) Physical examination

Identify:
Overfeeding
Incorrect formula preparation
Poor feeding technique
Infection

Assess degree of illness
(Table 1)

Mild

Moderate

Severe

Very severe

Follow-up:
Assess in 24–28 hr

(C) Hospitalize
Supportive Care

(C) Stabilize:
Circulatory Support
ICU Hospitalization

Assess onset of pattern

Acute

Consistent with gastroenteritis, otitis media,
food poisoning, or toxin exposure

Yes

No ——→ Do:
Electrolytes
Urinalysis and
consider culture
Consider:
Ammonia
Blood cultures
BUN and creatinine
CBC with differential
Chest radiography
Cranial CT
Liver function tests
Lumbar puncture
Organic and amino acids

Identify disorder
and treat

(D) Assess findings
(Cont'd on p 333)

Persistent/chronic

Consistent with reflux

No

Yes

Consider:
Upper GI series
Identify:
Gastroesophageal
reflux (p 296)

Acute infections associated with vomiting are gastroenteritis, acute otitis media, urinary tract infection, respiratory infections (pneumonia), and sepsis.

References

Breaux CW, Georgeson KE, Royal SA, et al. Changing patterns in the diagnosis of hypertrophic pyloric stenosis. Pediatrics 1988; 81:213.

Caty MG, Azizkhan RG. Acute surgical conditions of the abdomen. Pediatr Ann 1994; 23:192.

Hoekelman RA. Pyloric stenosis is a pediatrician's diagnosis. Pediatr Ann 1994; 23:181.

Lilien LD, Srinivasan G, Pyati SP, et al. Green vomiting in the first 72 hours in normal infants. Am J Dis Child 1986; 140:662.

Swischuk LE. Infant with acute vomiting. Pediatr Emerg Care 1991; 7:305.

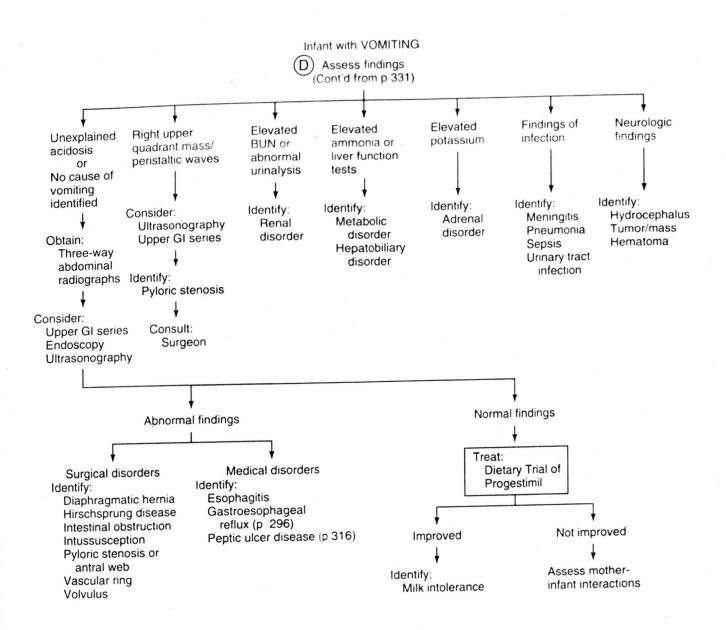

Infant with VOMITING

(D) Assess findings
(Cont'd from p 331)

Unexplained
acidosis
or
No cause of
vomiting
identified
↓
Obtain:
Three-way
abdominal
radiographs
↓
Consider:
Upper GI series
Endoscopy
Ultrasonography

Right upper
quadrant mass/
peristaltic waves
↓
Consider:
Ultrasonography
Upper GI series
↓
Identify:
Pyloric stenosis
↓
Consult:
Surgeon

Elevated
BUN or
abnormal
urinalysis
↓
Identify:
Renal
disorder

Elevated
ammonia or
liver function
tests
↓
Identify:
Metabolic
disorder
Hepatobiliary
disorder

Elevated
potassium
↓
Identify:
Adrenal
disorder

Findings of
infection
↓
Identify:
Meningitis
Pneumonia
Sepsis
Urinary tract
infection

Neurologic
findings
↓
Identify:
Hydrocephalus
Tumor/mass
Hematoma

Abnormal findings

Surgical disorders
Identify:
Diaphragmatic hernia
Hirschsprung disease
Intestinal obstruction
Intussusception
Pyloric stenosis or
antral web
Vascular ring
Volvulus

Medical disorders
Identify:
Esophagitis
Gastroesophageal
reflux (p 296)
Peptic ulcer disease (p 316)

Normal findings
↓
Treat:
Dietary Trial of
Progestimil

Improved
↓
Identify:
Milk intolerance

Not improved
↓
Assess mother-
infant interactions

GYNECOLOGIC DISORDERS

Breast Lump in Adolescent Girls
Breast Pain in Adolescent Girls
Dysfunctional Uterine Bleeding
Galactorrhea (Nipple Discharge) in Adolescent
  Girls

Pelvic Inflammatory Disease
Pelvic Pain and Dysmenorrhea
Primary Amenorrhea
Secondary Amenorrhea
Vulvovaginitis

BREAST LUMP IN ADOLESCENT GIRLS

Roberta K. Beach, M.D., M.P.H.

Breast growth prior to 8 years of age is considered precocious. Pubertal breast budding occurs usually between 9 and 12 years of age, is often unilateral at first, and requires only observation. Never biopsy a breast bud since removal will prevent future breast growth. Once fatty and glandular tissue has developed, a palpable breast lump requires evaluation.

A. Note how and when the lump was discovered, progression of its size, any pain, date of last menses, and relation of symptoms to menstrual cycle. Determine history of breast problems or family history of breast disease. Look for predisposing factors of trauma or drug use, including prescription drugs, oral contraceptives, marijuana, and other street drugs. Assess diet for large amounts of methylxanthines (caffeine, theophylline, or theobromine found in coffee, tea, cola, and chocolate), although their association with breast symptoms is debatable. Exclude pregnancy in any adolescent girl with breast symptoms.

B. Palpate both breasts carefully. Assess location, size, margins, mobility, and tenderness of lesions. Check for nipple discharge and lymphadenopathy in axillary or supraclavicular regions. Diagram size and location of lesion in chart. Note Tanner stage of breast development.

C. Assessment is based primarily on physical findings. Almost all lesions in teenagers are fibroadenomas or simple cysts. Malignancy cannot be excluded by age, however, since about 150 cases of adenocarcinoma are reported annually in American women under 25 years of age. Mammography is not useful in adolescents because their breast tissue is too dense for accurate interpretation. Ultrasound, fine-needle aspiration cytology (FNAC), or biopsy may facilitate diagnosis.

D. Suspicious lesions warrant prompt surgical referral. Adenocarcinoma presents as a hard, nonmobile, usually painless lump. Cystosarcoma phylloides in young patients is a rapidly growing, firm mass sometimes accompanied by skin retraction or necrosis. It is rarely malignant, and excision is curative. Giant fibroadenoma, although benign, may cause breast atrophy due to size and should be excised. Intraductal papilloma presents as a unilateral cylindric mass under the areola with bloody nipple discharge. Juvenile papillomatosis, first described in 1980, is diagnosed by biopsy of the solid tumor and treated with excision due to uncertain potential for malignancy. Lipomas, if firm and encapsulated, can mimic more serious lesions.

E. Fibroadenoma accounts for 90% of lesions in biopsy studies of teenagers and 40% in office practice. Characteristic findings are a firm, mobile, well-demarcated lump less than 5 cm in diameter. Some 60% are in the upper outer quadrant. Since one fourth will regress over time, observe for 2 to 3 months. If it persists or enlarges, definitive diagnosis is needed.

F. Breast ultrasonography, now widely available, differentiates a cyst from a solid tumor. Cysts in teenagers do not require biopsy. Since ultrasonography cannot reliably distinguish between benign and malignant solid tumors, a biopsy should be performed on persistent solid lesions. A solid mass on ultrasound is unlikely to resolve spontaneously.

G. Cysts, which account for 60% of the breast lumps in teenagers, tend to be tender, spongy, and single or multiple. Symptoms and size are greater just prior to menses and subside afterward. Half will resolve spontaneously in 2 to 3 months. A number of drugs, including most street drugs and perhaps methylxanthines in certain women, have been associated with breast pain and swelling. The effects are reversible when the drugs are stopped.

H. Needle aspiration is a simple, safe office procedure. Local anesthetic is not necessary. Immobilize the cyst between thumb and forefinger and insert a 20 gauge needle while pulling on the syringe to create negative pressure. Removal of serous watery fluid will confirm the diagnosis and reduce the cyst. FNAC, in which the fluid is examined for malignant cells, is seldom indicated for teenagers.

References

Beach RK. Breast disorders. In: McAnarney ER, Kreipe RE, Orr DP, Comerci GD, eds. Textbook of adolescent medicine. Philadelphia: Saunders, 1992:720.

Greydanus DE, Parks DS, Farrell EG. Breast disorders in children and adolescents. Pediatr Clin North Am 1989; 36:601.

Hindle WH, Pan EY. Breast disorders in female adolescents. Adolescent Medicine: State of the Arts Reviews 1994; 5:123.

Laufer J, Augarten A, Szeinberg A, Engelberg S. Pathological case of the month: Cystosarcoma phylloides in an adolescent female. Arch Pediatr Adolesc Med 1994; 148:1067.

McSweeney MD, Egan RL. Breast cancer in the younger patient: Recent results. Cancer Res 1984; 90:36.

Neinstein LS, Atkinson J, Diament M. Prevalence and longitudinal study of breast masses in adolescents. J Adolesc Health 1993; 13:227.

Patient with BREAST LUMP

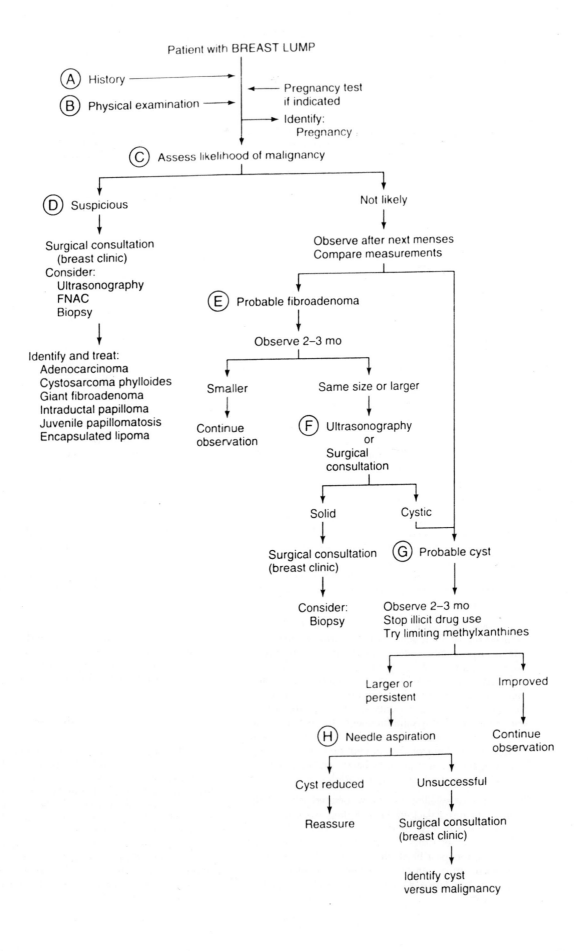

(A) History

(B) Physical examination

Pregnancy test
if indicated

Identify:
    Pregnancy

(C) Assess likelihood of malignancy

(D) Suspicious

Surgical consultation
(breast clinic)
Consider:
    Ultrasonography
    FNAC
    Biopsy

Identify and treat:
    Adenocarcinoma
    Cystosarcoma phylloides
    Giant fibroadenoma
    Intraductal papilloma
    Juvenile papillomatosis
    Encapsulated lipoma

Not likely

Observe after next menses
Compare measurements

(E) Probable fibroadenoma

Observe 2–3 mo

Smaller

Continue
observation

Same size or larger

(F) Ultrasonography
    or
    Surgical
    consultation

Solid

Surgical consultation
(breast clinic)

Consider:
    Biopsy

Cystic

(G) Probable cyst

Observe 2–3 mo
Stop illicit drug use
Try limiting methylxanthines

Larger or
persistent

Improved

(H) Needle aspiration

Continue
observation

Cyst reduced

Reassure

Unsuccessful

Surgical consultation
(breast clinic)

Identify cyst
versus malignancy

BREAST PAIN IN ADOLESCENT GIRLS

Roberta K. Beach, M.D., M.P.H.

Breast pain (mastalgia or mastodynia) is a common complaint in adolescents. It may be cyclic and related to the menstrual cycle, noncyclic (often due to drug use), associated with breast masses, or the earliest sign of inflammation. It may be the precursor to benign breast disease, a syndrome of breast nodularity, cysts, swelling, and pain. The pain may not be in the breast at all but rather in the underlying muscles or chest wall. Breast pain is one of the earliest signs of pregnancy, which must always be excluded in adolescent girls.

A. In the history ask about onset, location, pattern, relationship to menstrual cycles, and history of any masses or skin lesions. Document the date of the last menses. Note use of any hormonal contraception (oral contraceptives, Depo-Provera, Norplant). Explore the possibility of pregnancy or drug use (assure confidentiality). Identify associated breast-feeding, trauma, or muscle strain (e.g., weight lifting or new exercise). Check diet for excessive methylxanthines (caffeine, tea, cola, chocolate). Elicit any personal or family history of breast disorders. Ask about patient's underlying fears (e.g., cancer).

B. Perform a complete breast examination. Palpate for any breast masses or lymphadenopathy. Check for nipple discharge. Note any inflammation (swelling, heat, tenderness, erythema). Distinguish pectoral or chest wall pain from breast tissue pain.

C. The presumptive diagnosis is based on history and physical findings. Associated breast masses and galactorrhea should be evaluated first. In the absence of such findings, breast pain is classified as physiologic, musculoskeletal, or inflammatory. Duct ectasia, associated with breast pain in perimenopausal women, is not common in adolescents.

D. Physiologic pain is due to fluid retention and hormone-induced breast tissue sensitivity to estrogens, progesterone, and prolactin. Cyclic pain just prior to menses is normal. Young adolescents need only an explanation and reassurance. A mild analgesic, such as ibuprofen, heat, and a supportive bra, can be recommended. Although studies in adolescents are inadequate, limiting salt or dietary methylxanthines seem to help some patients. Severe breast pain in adult women has been treated with danazol, bromocriptine, or tamoxifen; however, these are expensive, have significant side effects, and have not been tested in adolescents.

E. Painful breast swelling can be associated with all the drugs that cause galactorrhea, including exogenous hormones, tranquilizers, antidepressants, phenothiazines, and many street drugs, including marijuana. Through dopamine receptor blockade or catecholamine depletion, these drugs can produce low levels of prolactin secretion. Avoidance of the drug will result in resolution of symptoms.

TABLE 1 Drugs Used in the Treatment of Breast Pain in Adolescent Girls

Drug	Maximum Dosage
Antibiotics	
Dicloxacillin	250 mg q.i.d. × 3–4 wk
Cephalexin	250 mg q.i.d. × 3–4 wk
Analgesics	
Ibuprofen	600 mg t.i.d. (if not pregnant)
Acetaminophen	700–1000 mg q4h

F. Examination may reveal the pain to be in the pectoral muscles, intercostal spaces, or costochondral junctions. Muscle strain may come from sports, weight lifting, or horseplay. Tietze syndrome is a postviral inflammation of localized costochondral junctions. Trauma may result in bruising or hematomas. Treatment depends on the specific cause and usually includes analgesics, heat, and rest.

G. Cellulitis, mastitis, and true breast abscess may first present as breast pain. Look for tenderness, erythema, warmth, and possibly a mass. Breast-feeding is the most common cause, but spread of cutaneous infection from superficial skin lesions, folliculitis, or trauma is possible.

H. *Staphylococcus aureus* is present in 80% to 90% of breast infections in teenagers. Other aerobic or anaerobic organisms cause the remainder. A vigorous course of antistaphylococcal antibiotics, such as dicloxacillin or an appropriate cephalosporin, is continued for 3 to 4 weeks or until the infection is completely resolved. Repeat examinations to confirm resolution are essential. Breast-feeding may be continued unless there is frank purulent discharge.

I. If a fluctuant abscess is found, refer the patient for surgical drainage. Do not attempt an office procedure. The abscess is often more extensive than it appears, and the procedure is best done under general anesthesia.

References

Beach RK. Breast disorders. In: McAnarney ER, Kreipe RE, Orr DP, Comerci GD, eds. Textbook of adolescent medicine. Philadelphia: Saunders, 1992:720.

Greydanus DE, Parks DS, Farrell EG. Breast disorders in children and adolescents. Pediatr Clin North Am 1989; 36:601.

Pye JK, Mansel RE, Hughes LE. Clinical experience of drug treatments for mastalgia. Lancet 1985; 2:373.

Schwartz GF. Benign neoplasms and inflammations of the breast. Clin Obstet Gynecol 1982; 25:373.

Vorherr H. Fibrocystic breast disease: Pathophysiology, pathomorphology, clinical picture, and management. Am J Obstet Gynecol 1986; 154:161.

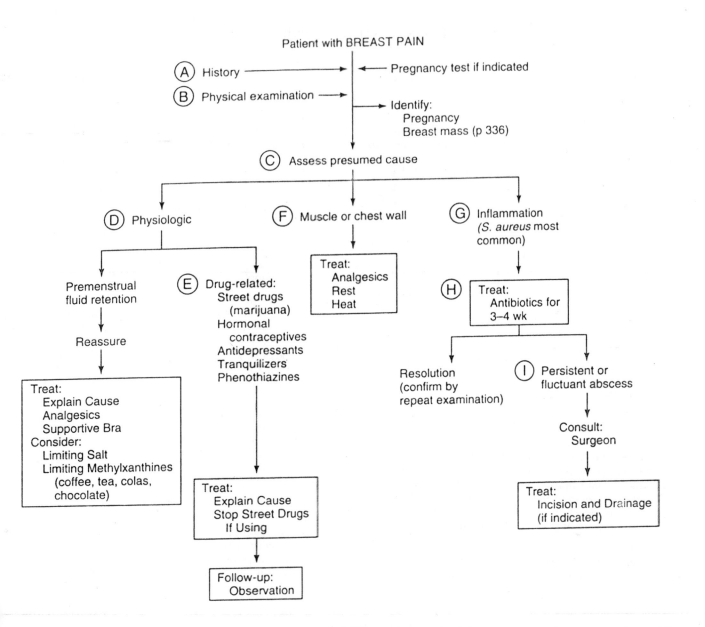

Patient with BREAST PAIN

(A) History ──────→ ←── Pregnancy test if indicated

(B) Physical examination ──→

→ Identify:
   Pregnancy
   Breast mass (p 336)

(C) Assess presumed cause

(D) Physiologic

(F) Muscle or chest wall

(G) Inflammation
   (*S. aureus* most common)

Premenstrual
fluid retention

(E) Drug-related:
   Street drugs
      (marijuana)
   Hormonal
      contraceptives
   Antidepressants
   Tranquilizers
   Phenothiazines

Treat:
   Analgesics
   Rest
   Heat

(H) Treat:
   Antibiotics for
   3–4 wk

Reassure

Treat:
   Explain Cause
   Analgesics
   Supportive Bra
Consider:
   Limiting Salt
   Limiting Methylxanthines
      (coffee, tea, colas,
      chocolate)

Treat:
   Explain Cause
   Stop Street Drugs
   If Using

Follow-up:
   Observation

Resolution
(confirm by
repeat examination)

(I) Persistent or
   fluctuant abscess

Consult:
   Surgeon

Treat:
   Incision and Drainage
   (if indicated)

DYSFUNCTIONAL UTERINE BLEEDING

Stephen Berman, M.D.

Dysfunctional uterine bleeding (DUB), which is excessive, painless, irregular menstrual bleeding related to anovulatory cycles, is most common during the first 2 years after menarche. A normal menstrual period is 2 to 7 days with heavy bleeding for 1 to 2 days. The normal cycle range is 21 to 35 days. Bleeding is excessive if an adolescent soaks six or more full-size pads. Secondary causes of excessive bleeding, occurring in approximately 5% of cases, include gonorrheal or chlamydial genital infections, coagulation disorders, ectopic pregnancy, threatened abortion, hypo- or hyperthyroidism, polycystic ovary syndrome, and mass lesions of the uterus.

A. In the history ask about age of menarche, pattern of menstrual cycle, duration and amount of bleeding, cramps, pain, nausea, and vomiting. Ask about sexual activity and if appropriate, method of contraception and possibility of pregnancy. Obtain a family history of bleeding disorders, bleeding with prior surgical or dental procedures, bruising, petechiae, use of aspirin. Note symptoms of thyroid disease and other endocrine disorders.

B. Do a complete physical examination. In nonvirginal adolescents perform a pelvic examination and obtain cultures for *Neisseria gonorrhoeae,* rapid tests for *Chlamydia,* and wet preps on any discharge. Virginal girls less than 2 years beyond menarche with painless, excessive bleeding without significant anemia do not require an internal pelvic examination. Virginal girls with significant anemia or pain should have a pelvic by a skilled, experienced clinician.

C. Immediately begin treatment of mild and moderate cases with iron supplementation and continue therapy for 3 months after the anemia has resolved. Consider adding a stool softener for constipation.

D. Treat moderate cases of DUB with a low-dose combined estrogen and synthetic progestin oral contraceptive pill (OCP). Continue the OCPs until the anemia has resolved with appropriate iron therapy. When therapy is started during bleeding, consider administering a higher dose (up to four tablets) until the bleeding stops, then taper the dose by one tablet every 2 days down to one tablet per day. Advise the adolescent that the medication can cause nausea and breast tenderness.

E. To stop massive uterine bleeding, consider giving IV Premarin (a water-soluble equine estrogen) in combination with an oral high-dose combination estrogen and synthetic progestin (Enovid 5 mg or Ovral or ethinyl estradiol 0.5 mg plus medroxyprogesterone [Provera] 20 mg). The Premarin can be given every 6 hours up to a maximum four doses. Initially, the Enovid is given every 6 hours until bleeding is controlled, then tapered over 7 to 10 days to one pill daily. Keep the patient on Enovid for one 21 day cycle; then discontinue and allow a withdrawal bleed; then start low-dose combination OCPs as described for moderate cases.

References

Coupey SM, Ahlstrom P. Common menstrual disorders. Pediatr Clin North Am 1989; 36:551.

Cowan BD, Morrison JC. Management of abnormal genital bleeding in girls and women. N Engl J Med 1991; 324:1710.

TABLE 1 Degree of Illness in Dysfunctional Uterine Bleeding

Mild	Moderate	Severe	Very Severe
Minimal bleeding without pain or discomfort and Hemoglobin >11 g/dl and hematocrit >35%	Moderate bleeding with a hemoglobin between 9 and 11 g/dl and hematocrit 25%–35%	Severe bleeding or Signs of circulatory compromise with tachycardia, orthostatic hypotension, or Hemoglobin <9 g/dl and hematocrit <25%	Signs of shock with poor peripheral perfusion and/or hypotension

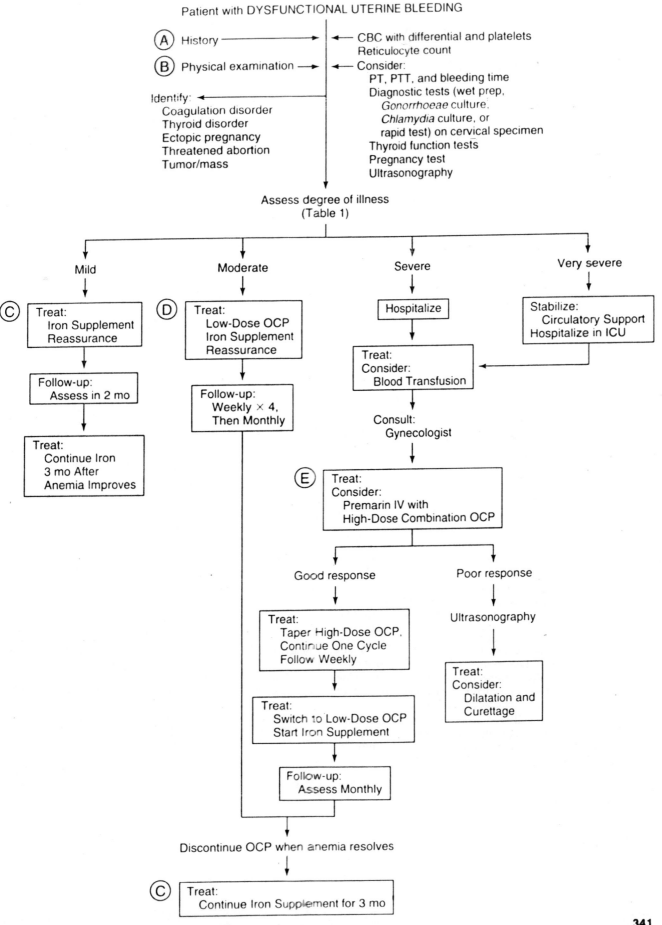

Patient with DYSFUNCTIONAL UTERINE BLEEDING

(A) History ⎯⎯⎯⎯→ ⎯ CBC with differential and platelets
Reticulocyte count

(B) Physical examination ⎯→ ⎯ Consider:
PT, PTT, and bleeding time
Diagnostic tests (wet prep,
Gonorrhoeae culture,
Chlamydia culture, or
rapid test) on cervical specimen
Thyroid function tests
Pregnancy test
Ultrasonography

Identify: ⎯◄⎯
Coagulation disorder
Thyroid disorder
Ectopic pregnancy
Threatened abortion
Tumor/mass

Assess degree of illness
(Table 1)

Mild | Moderate | Severe | Very severe

(C) Treat:
Iron Supplement
Reassurance

(D) Treat:
Low-Dose OCP
Iron Supplement
Reassurance

Hospitalize

Stabilize:
Circulatory Support
Hospitalize in ICU

Follow-up:
Assess in 2 mo

Follow-up:
Weekly × 4,
Then Monthly

Treat:
Consider:
Blood Transfusion

Treat:
Continue Iron
3 mo After
Anemia Improves

Consult:
Gynecologist

(E) Treat:
Consider:
Premarin IV with
High-Dose Combination OCP

Good response | Poor response

Treat:
Taper High-Dose OCP,
Continue One Cycle
Follow Weekly

Ultrasonography

Treat:
Consider:
Dilatation and
Curettage

Treat:
Switch to Low-Dose OCP
Start Iron Supplement

Follow-up:
Assess Monthly

Discontinue OCP when anemia resolves

(C) Treat:
Continue Iron Supplement for 3 mo

341

GALACTORRHEA (NIPPLE DISCHARGE) IN ADOLESCENT GIRLS

Roberta K. Beach, M.D., M.P.H.

Nipple discharge in adolescent girls is almost always galactorrhea, usually due to recent pregnancy or drug use but occasionally from neuroendocrine disorders.

A. Reassurance about confidentiality may be necessary to obtain an accurate history. Document date of last menses and any possibility of pregnancy or early spontaneous abortion (late heavy menses). Elicit a thorough drug history, including hormonal contraceptives, all prescription or nonprescription medications, and any street drugs. Note any neuroendocrine symptoms (headache, visual disturbance, polydipsia, goiter, oligomenorrhea).

B. Perform a full breast examination. To express nipple discharge, press firmly around areolae and strip milk ducts with firm lengthwise strokes from periphery to nipple. If no fluid is obtained, have the patient wear a white gauze sponge in her bra and bring it in if any discharge occurs.

C. If the history is consistent with galactorrhea, no laboratory tests are needed. A smear of discharge on a glass slide can be sent to cytology for a Pap test to detect abnormal cells. A stain for fat globules will confirm galactorrhea. A β–human chorionic gonadotropin (HCG) pregnancy test will remain positive (> 25 IU) for 2 to 4 weeks after pregnancy termination and can confirm a recent pregnancy.

D. A bloody nipple discharge may indicate intraductal papilloma. Refer the patient for surgical consultation. A serous (yellow, gray, brown, or greenish-black) fluid is usually caused by benign duct ectasia. A Pap smear of the fluid is done for reassurance to rule out malignant cells. A purulent discharge signals an abscess. A white or tan discharge from Montgomery tubercles on the areola may be produced for several weeks or months during puberty or pregnancy. It is benign and resolves spontaneously.

E. Many drugs are implicated in a variety of breast symptoms, including pain, swelling, cysts, and galactorrhea. The mechanisms usually involve dopamine receptor blockade or catecholamine depletion, both of which stimulate low levels of prolactin production. In teenagers hormonal contraceptives, regular marijuana use, and antidepressant therapy are the most frequent causes. Galactorrhea will resolve within 2 to 3 months after drugs are discontinued.

F. Postpartum colostrum or milk production may follow any form of pregnancy termination, including induced or spontaneous abortion. Such galactorrhea will usually resolve within 3 months. After a term delivery it may persist for more than 1 year, especially if hormonal contraceptives are used.

G. If no history of pregnancy or drug use is obtained, neuroendocrine problems should be considered. Hyperprolactinemia and hypothyroidism are the most likely disorders in adolescents. Excessive manual stimulation of the nipple may produce low levels of prolactin. Obtain a prolactin level and thyroid-stimulating hormone (TSH). High TSH confirms hypothyroidism, in which prolactinemia is a secondary association. High prolactin levels otherwise suggest a CNS lesion, most likely a pituitary adenoma or microadenoma.

H. If prolactin levels are normal, further evaluation depends on the menstrual history. If menses are regular, repeat assessment of prolactin levels every 6 months to rule out a slow-growing pituitary microadenoma. Usually the galactorrhea resolves spontaneously and the cause is unknown. Patients with galactorrhea and amenorrhea need evaluation for uncommon disorders such as renal, adrenal, and ovarian tumors, polycystic ovary syndrome, hypothalamic lesions, and neurogenic causes such as severe emotional distress or anorexia.

I. If neuroendocrine causes are suspected, consultation is indicated. CT or MRI can detect pituitary adenomas or microadenomas. Treatment is surgical removal or suppression with bromocriptine. Other causes require sophisticated laboratory assessment. Patients with galactorrhea require persistent follow-up until a cause is identified or the problem resolves.

References

Beach RK. Breast disorders. In: McAnarney ER, Kreipe RE, Orr DP, Comerci GD, eds. Textbook of Adolescent Medicine. Philadelphia: Saunders, 1992:720.

Devitt JE. Management of nipple discharge by clinical findings. Am J Surg 1985; 149:789.

Greydanus DE, Parks DS, Farrell EG. Breast disorders in children and adolescents. Pediatr Clin North Am 1989; 36:601.

Rohr RD. Galactorrhea in the adolescent. J Adolesc Health Care 1984; 5:37.

Simmons PS. Diagnostic considerations in breast disorders of children and adolescents. Pediatr Adolesc Gynecol 1992; 19:91.

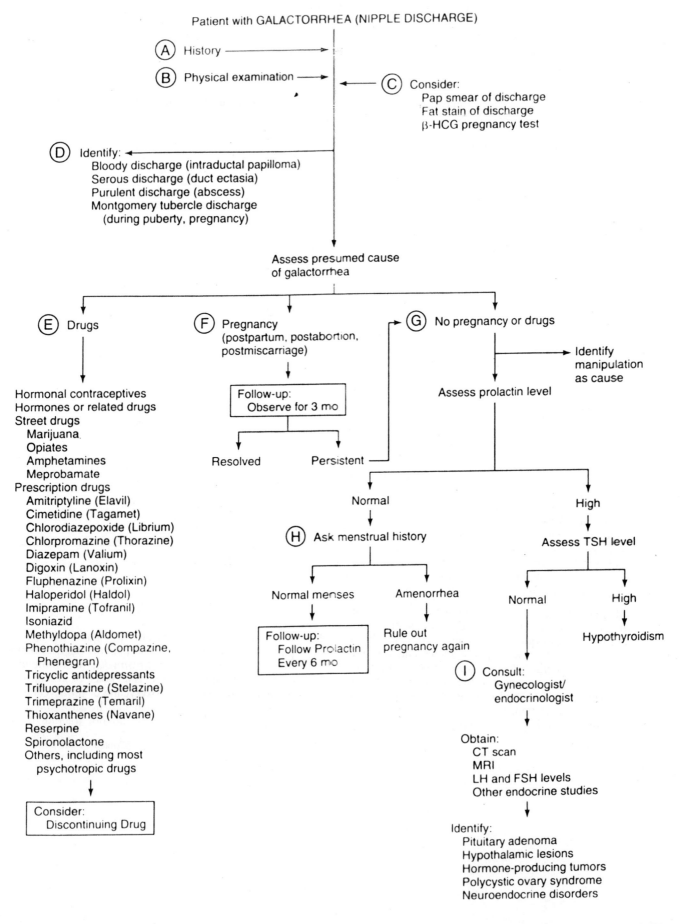

Patient with GALACTORRHEA (NIPPLE DISCHARGE)

(A) History

(B) Physical examination

(C) Consider:
Pap smear of discharge
Fat stain of discharge
β-HCG pregnancy test

(D) Identify:
Bloody discharge (intraductal papilloma)
Serous discharge (duct ectasia)
Purulent discharge (abscess)
Montgomery tubercle discharge
(during puberty, pregnancy)

Assess presumed cause
of galactorrhea

(E) Drugs

Hormonal contraceptives
Hormones or related drugs
Street drugs
    Marijuana
    Opiates
    Amphetamines
    Meprobamate
Prescription drugs
    Amitriptyline (Elavil)
    Cimetidine (Tagamet)
    Chlorodiazepoxide (Librium)
    Chlorpromazine (Thorazine)
    Diazepam (Valium)
    Digoxin (Lanoxin)
    Fluphenazine (Prolixin)
    Haloperidol (Haldol)
    Imipramine (Tofranil)
    Isoniazid
    Methyldopa (Aldomet)
    Phenothiazine (Compazine,
        Phenegran)
    Tricyclic antidepressants
    Trifluoperazine (Stelazine)
    Trimeprazine (Temaril)
    Thioxanthenes (Navane)
    Reserpine
    Spironolactone
    Others, including most
        psychotropic drugs

Consider:
Discontinuing Drug

(F) Pregnancy
(postpartum, postabortion,
postmiscarriage)

Follow-up:
Observe for 3 mo

Resolved   Persistent

(G) No pregnancy or drugs

→ Identify
    manipulation
    as cause

Assess prolactin level

Normal   High

(H) Ask menstrual history   Assess TSH level

Normal menses   Amenorrhea   Normal   High

Follow-up: Rule out   Hypothyroidism
Follow Prolactin pregnancy again
Every 6 mo

(I) Consult:
    Gynecologist/
    endocrinologist

Obtain:
    CT scan
    MRI
    LH and FSH levels
    Other endocrine studies

Identify:
    Pituitary adenoma
    Hypothalamic lesions
    Hormone-producing tumors
    Polycystic ovary syndrome
    Neuroendocrine disorders

PELVIC INFLAMMATORY DISEASE

Stephen Berman, M.D.

Pelvic inflammatory disease (PID), or infection of the uterus and fallopian tubes (upper genital tract), is common in sexually active adolescents (one in eight sexually active 15 year olds). Pathogens that cause PID include *Neisseria gonorrhoeae* (25% to 50%), *Chlamydia* (25% to 43%), anaerobic bacteria, *Ureaplasma urealyticum*, *Mycoplasma hominis*, *Haemophilus influenzae*, and gram-negative enterics. Mixed bacterial infection is common. Additional risk factors for PID are multiple sex partners, history of a sexually transmitted disease (STD), and use of an intrauterine device (IUD). Complications of PID are perihepatitis (Fitz-Hugh-Curtis syndrome) (5% to 10%), tuboovarian abscess (7% to 19%), subsequent ectopic pregnancy (5%), chronic pelvic pain (21%), and infertility (21%).

A. Suspect PID when a sexually active adolescent has lower abdominal pain, increased vaginal discharge, increased menstrual flow or intermenstrual spotting, fever, dysmenorrhea, dysuria, malaise, nausea, or vomiting. Symptoms often worsen within the first week after menses begin. Obtain a history of sexual activity (number of partners), contraceptive use, prior STDs, and treatment.

B. Perform a pelvic examination. Patients with PID usually have lower abdominal tenderness, cervical motion tenderness, and adnexal tenderness.

C. Laboratory findings that support PID are an increase in the absolute neutrophil count over 10,000, erythrocyte sedimentation rate greater than 15 mm/hour, a positive Gram stain of cervical discharge for *N. gonorrhoeae* or more than 5 white blood cells per high-power field, and positive rapid test for *Chlamydia*. However, these studies may be normal. Pelvic ultrasonography identifies adnexal enlargement and tuboovarian abscess with greater sensitivity than clinical examination.

D. Adequate follow-up of adolescents with PID is necessary to assess response to therapy, to identify persistent cases, and to reduce sequelae; however, a study has shown that approximately two thirds of adolescents with PID fail to return for follow-up appointments. Consider hospitalizing all adolescents with PID. Additional factors that compromise compliance and follow-up include lack of transportation, homelessness, limited parental involvement, and lack of a telephone.

TABLE 1 Degree of Illness in Pelvic Inflammatory Disease

Moderate	Severe	Very Severe
Afebrile or low grade fever and	Fever >38.4° C (101° F) or	Signs of sepsis or septic shock or
No vomiting and	Persistent vomiting or severe abdominal pain or	Altered mental status or
Able to take medication and	Inability to take medication, poor compliance, poor follow-up or	Poor peripheral perfusion or hypotension or
Likely to be compliant with good follow-up	Pregnancy or	Respiratory distress (adult respiratory distress syndrome)
	Suspected or identified pelvic abscess or	
	IUD in place or	
	Uncertain diagnosis with possible appendicitis or ectopic pregnancy or	
	History of recurrent PID episodes or	
	Failure to respond to outpatient therapy	

IUD, intrauterine device.

E. It is not possible to clinically distinguish the specific pathogens causing PID, so all patients need coverage for *N. gonorrhoeae* and *Chlamydia*. Recommended outpatient treatment of PID is a choice of IM cefoxitin or ceftriaxone *plus* oral doxycycline or tetracycline for 10 to 14 days. Erythromycin can be substituted for doxycycline for patients who do not tolerate doxy-

(Continued on page 346)

Patient with PELVIC INFLAMMATORY DISEASE

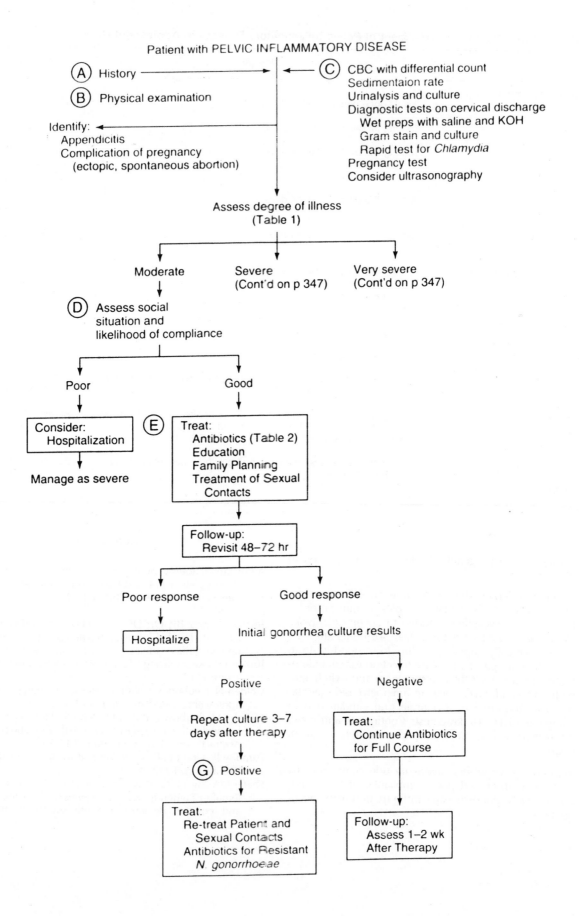

(A) History

(B) Physical examination

(C) CBC with differential count
Sedimentaion rate
Urinalysis and culture
Diagnostic tests on cervical discharge
    Wet preps with saline and KOH
    Gram stain and culture
    Rapid test for *Chlamydia*
Pregnancy test
Consider ultrasonography

Identify:
Appendicitis
Complication of pregnancy
    (ectopic, spontaneous abortion)

Assess degree of illness
(Table 1)

Moderate

Severe
(Cont'd on p 347)

Very severe
(Cont'd on p 347)

(D) Assess social
situation and
likelihood of compliance

Poor

Good

Consider:
Hospitalization

Manage as severe

(E) Treat:
Antibiotics (Table 2)
Education
Family Planning
Treatment of Sexual
    Contacts

Follow-up:
Revisit 48–72 hr

Poor response

Good response

Hospitalize

Initial gonorrhea culture results

Positive

Negative

Repeat culture 3–7
days after therapy

Treat:
Continue Antibiotics
for Full Course

(G) Positive

Treat:
Re-treat Patient and
    Sexual Contacts
Antibiotics for Resistant
    N. gonorrhoeae

Follow-up:
Assess 1–2 wk
After Therapy

TABLE 2 Drugs Used in the Treatment of Pelvic Inflammatory Disease in Adolescent Girls

Drug	Dosage	Product Availability
Outpatient Treatment		
Cefoxitin	2 g IM once plus probenecid 1 g PO	Vials: 1, 2 g
or		
Ceftriaxone	250 mg IM once	Vials: 0.25, 5, 1 g
plus		
Doxycycline	100 mg PO b.i.d. × 10–14 days	Tabs, caps: 50, 100 mg
		Susp: 25 mg/5 ml
		Syrup: 50 mg/5 ml
or		
Tetracycline	500 mg PO q.i.d. × 10–14 days	Caps: 100, 250, 500 mg
		Tabs: 250, 500 mg
or		
Erythromycin	500 mg PO q.i.d. × 10–14 days	Susp: 200, 400 mg/5 ml
		Tabs: 250, 500 mg
Alternative		
Ofloxacin (for patients > 18 yr)	400 mg PO q.i.d. × 14 days	
plus		
Clindamycin	450 mg PO q.i.d. × 14 days	Caps: 75, 150 mg
		Liquid: 75 mg/5 ml
or		
Metronidazole	500 mg PO q.i.d. × 14 days	Tabs: 250, 500 mg
Inpatient Treatment of Choice		
Cefoxitin	2 g IV q6h × minimum 4 days	Vials: 1, 2 g
plus		
Doxycycline	100 mg IV q12h × 48 hr after clinical improvement; then 100 mg PO b.i.d. to complete 10–14 days	Injection: 100, 200 mg/vial
		Tabs, caps: 50, 100 mg
Alternative		
Clindamycin	900 mg IV q8h (15–40 mg/kg/dose) × 48 hr after clinical improvement; then 450 mg PO q.i.d. to complete 10–14 days, or complete the course with doxycycline 100 mg PO b.i.d.	Amps: 0.15, 0.3, 0.6 g
plus		
Gentamicin	2 mg/kg IV in one dose, then 1.5 mg/kg q8h (in patients with normal renal function)	Sol: 10, 40 mg/ml
or		
Tobramycin		

cycline or are pregnant. (Table 2 lists drugs used in the treatment of PID.)

F. Recommended inpatient IV treatment of PID is cefoxitin plus doxycycline or clindamycin *plus* gentamicin or tobramycin. Doxycycline is added to cover *Chlamydia*. Continue IV antibiotics for at least 48 hours after the patient clinically improves. Failure to respond in 48 to 72 hours is a sign of a resistant infection (often anaerobic) or an abscess. Obtain a sonogram and switch antibiotics to clindamycin plus an aminoglycoside (gentamicin or tobramycin). Continue oral clindamycin to complete a 10 to 14 day course. Continue IV antibiotics for at least 4 days, until the patient is afebrile for 48 hours.

G. Reasons for treatment failure include reinfection by a sexual partner and poor compliance. Penicillinase-producing *N. gonorrhoeae* can be treated with spectinomycin.

References

American Academy of Pediatrics. Gonococcal infections. In: Peter G, ed. 1994 Red Book: Report of the committee on infectious diseases. 23rd ed. Elk Grove Village, IL: 1994:351.

Blythe MJ, Katz BP, Orr DP, et al. Historical and clinical factors associated with *Chlamydia trachomatis* genitourinary infection in female adolescents. J Pediatr 1988; 112:6:1000.

Brown HP. Recognizing STDs in adolescents. Contemp Pediatr 1989; 6:17.

Golden N, Neuhoff S, Cohen H. Pelvic inflammatory disease in adolescents. J Pediatr 1989; 114:138.

Murphy M, Shubow J, Wise PH. Pelvic inflammatory disease: Is hospitalization necessary to ensure therapeutic compliance? Abstract. Am J Dis Child 1983; 137:540.

Paradise JE, Grant L. Pelvic inflammatory disease in adolescents. Pediatr Rev 1992; 13:216.

Shafer MA, Sweet RL. Pelvic inflammatory disease in adolescent females: Epidemiology, pathogenesis, diagnosis, treatment, and sequelae. Pediatr Clin North Am 1989; 36:513.

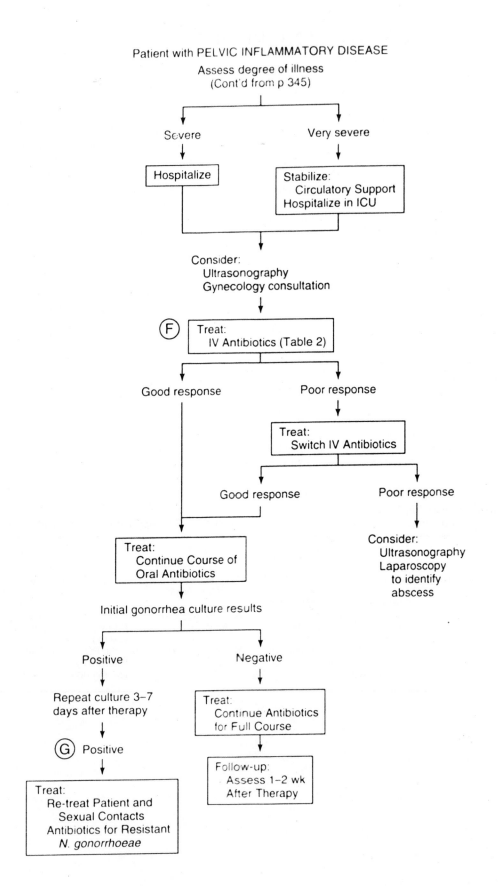

Patient with PELVIC INFLAMMATORY DISEASE
Assess degree of illness
(Cont'd from p 345)

Severe

Very severe

Hospitalize

Stabilize:
Circulatory Support
Hospitalize in ICU

Consider:
Ultrasonography
Gynecology consultation

F Treat:
IV Antibiotics (Table 2)

Good response

Poor response

Treat:
Switch IV Antibiotics

Good response

Poor response

Treat:
Continue Course of
Oral Antibiotics

Consider:
Ultrasonography
Laparoscopy
to identify
abscess

Initial gonorrhea culture results

Positive

Negative

Repeat culture 3–7
days after therapy

Treat:
Continue Antibiotics
for Full Course

G Positive

Treat:
Re-treat Patient and
Sexual Contacts
Antibiotics for Resistant
N. gonorrhoeae

Follow-up:
Assess 1–2 wk
After Therapy

PELVIC PAIN AND DYSMENORRHEA

Stephen Berman, M.D.

DEFINITION

Chronic pelvic pain is constant or cyclic pain present for at least 3 months. Causes can be gynecologic (dysmenorrhea, mittelschmerz, endometriosis, chronic pelvic inflammatory disease [PID], ovarian cyst, pelvic serositis), urinary (infection, hydronephrosis, retention), GI (constipation, dysfunctional bowel syndrome, adhesions, inflammatory bowel disease, lactose intolerance), or psychogenic. Dysmenorrhea presents as lower abdominal or back pain associated with menses. In the United States approximately 60% of girls 12 to 17 years of age have menstrual pain or discomfort. It results from prostaglandin $F_{2\alpha}$ and E_2 activity in the myometrium. Primary dysmenorrhea is related to anovulatory menstrual cycles. The pain starts the same day as the blood flow and rarely continues more than 3 days. Secondary dysmenorrhea can be caused by genital tract infections (PID), endometriosis, malformations of the genital tract (bicornate uterus, uterine horn), pelvic masses, and intrauterine devices.

A. In the history determine the onset, frequency, severity, pattern, and location of pain as well as sexual activity. Note associated symptoms such as fever, nausea, vomiting, rash, jaundice, arthritis, organomegaly, change in bowel pattern, and weight loss. Inquire as to symptoms of urinary tract infection such as dysuria, urgency, or frequency and gynecologic symptoms such as dysmenorrhea and vaginal discharge. Document the timing and relation of pain to menstrual periods and sexual relations. Note history of sexually transmitted disease and abdominal surgery. Obtain a psychosocial history to identify stress in the patient's life and level of anxiety (family and school). Determine how pain alters daily lifestyle and routine.

B. Perform an appropriate pelvic examination, which includes a speculum examination of the vagina, a bimanual rectovaginal abdominal palpation and a wet prep, Gram stain, gonococcal (GC) culture, and *Chlamydia* rapid test of cervical discharge. Consider as indicative of infection any discharge other than a normal thin, clear to partially opaque fluid with less than 5 white blood cells per high-power field. Adnexal tenderness with or without a cervical discharge suggests PID or tubal pregnancy. It is not necessary to do an internal pelvic examination in virginal adolescents with mild pain of typical primary dysmenorrhea unless it does not respond to a trial of two different prostaglandin inhibitors.

(Continued on page 350)

TABLE 1 Degree of Illness in Pelvic Pain/Dysmenorrhea

Mild	Moderate
Pain consistent with primary dysmenorrhea or mittelschmerz	Pain that alters normal routine *or* Characteristics suggesting secondary dysmenorrhea (onset of pain several days before menses, severe pain not relieved by prostaglandin inhibitors, or abnormal pelvic examination)

TABLE 2 Therapy for Dysmenorrhea in Adolescents

Drug	Dosage	Product Availability
Ibuprofen (Motrin, Advil)	400 mg PO q6h	Tabs: 200, 300, 400, 600, 800 mg Liquid: 100 mg/5 ml
Naproxen sodium (Anaprox)	500 mg PO followed by 250 mg q12h	Tabs: 250, 375, 500 mg Liquid: 125 mg/5 ml
Mefenamic acid (Ponstel)	500 mg PO followed by 250 mg q6h	Tabs: 250, 500 mg

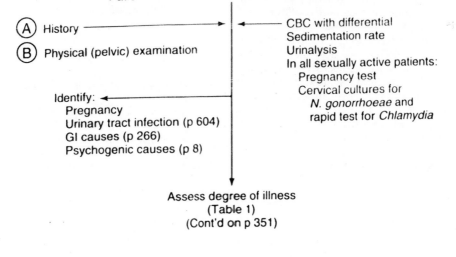

Patient with PELVIC PAIN/DYSMENORRHEA

(A) History ⎯⎯⎯⎯⎯⎯⎯⎯ → ← ⎯⎯ CBC with differential
Sedimentation rate
Urinalysis
(B) Physical (pelvic) examination
In all sexually active patients:
Pregnancy test
Cervical cultures for
N. gonorrhoeae and
Identify: ←⎯⎯
rapid test for Chlamydia
Pregnancy
Urinary tract infection (p 604)
GI causes (p 266)
Psychogenic causes (p 8)

Assess degree of illness
(Table 1)
(Cont'd on p 351)

C. Treat dysmenorrhea with ibuprofen, naproxen, or mefenamic acid (Table 2). Begin therapy at the first sign of menstrual cramps or flow and continue for 1 to 3 days. Ibuprofen and naproxen are available over the counter. Naproxen has a longer half-life and can be given twice a day. Mefenamic acid may have the fastest onset of action, since it blocks prostaglandins already synthesized. Consider a low-dose combination oral contraceptive in sexually active adolescents needing contraception. It may take 2 to 3 months for contraceptives to become effective. Failure of the pain to respond to therapy requires a pelvic examination if not done previously and a gynecology consultation for laparoscopy to rule out pelvic pathology such as endometriosis.

D. Laparoscopy is indicated when (1) it is necessary to confirm clinical findings and/or ultrasound studies that suggest significant pathology; (2) the cause of chronic pelvic pain remains unknown despite an appropriate work-up (functional and organic), and pain causes major alterations in lifestyle; or (3) dysmenorrhea fails to respond to medical therapy. Findings of laparoscopy (present in approximately 75% of those without a diagnosis by the third visit) include endometriosis, postoperative adhesions, pelvic serositis, ovarian cyst, uterine malformations, and ileitis.

References

Barr RG. Abdominal pain in the female adolescent. Pediatr Rev 1983; 4:281.

Beach RK. Menstrual cramps need not be a "curse." Contemp Pediatr 1989; October:41.

Coupey SM, Ahlstrom P. Common menstrual disorders. Pediatr Clin North Am 1989; 36:551.

Emans SJ. Pelvic examination of the adolescent patient. Pediatr Rev 1983; 4:307.

Emans SJ, Goldstein DP. Pediatric and adolescent gynecology. 2nd ed. Boston: Little, Brown, 1982.

Gidwani GP. Endometriosis: More common than you think. Contemp Pediatr 1989; October:99.

Goldstein DP. Acute and chronic pelvic pain. Pediatr Clin North Am 1989; 36:573.

Goldstein DP, de Cholnoky C, Emans SJ, et al. Laparoscopy in the diagnosis and management of pelvic pain in adolescents. J Reprod Med 1980; 24:251.

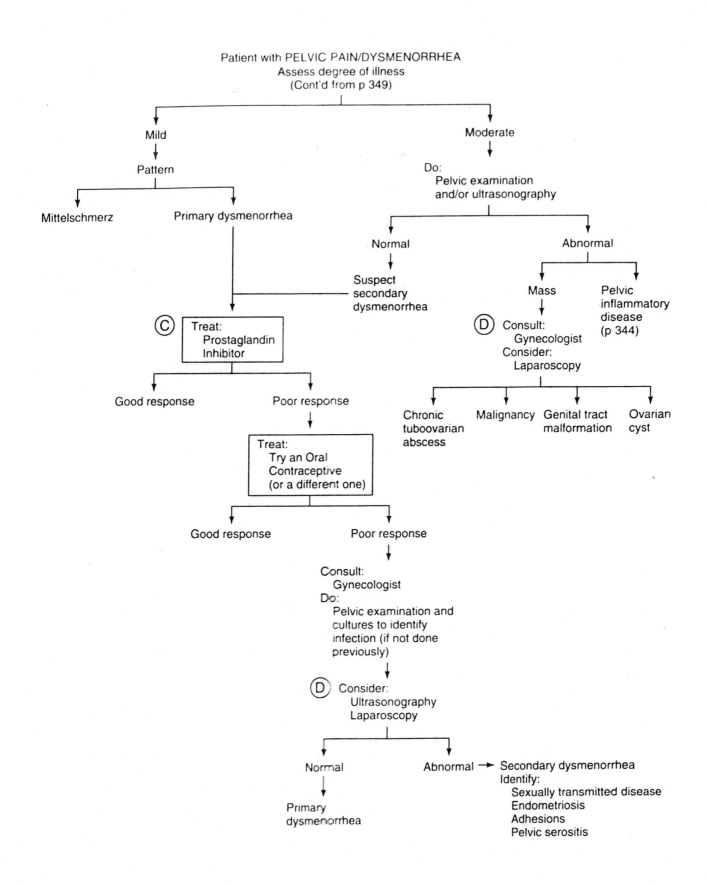

Patient with PELVIC PAIN/DYSMENORRHEA
Assess degree of illness
(Cont'd from p 349)

Mild → Pattern

Mittelschmerz

Primary dysmenorrhea

Moderate → Do:
Pelvic examination and/or ultrasonography

Normal → Suspect secondary dysmenorrhea

Abnormal

Mass → ⒹConsult: Gynecologist Consider: Laparoscopy

Pelvic inflammatory disease (p 344)

Chronic tuboovarian abscess

Malignancy

Genital tract malformation

Ovarian cyst

ⒸTreat: Prostaglandin Inhibitor

Good response

Poor response → Treat: Try an Oral Contraceptive (or a different one)

Good response

Poor response → Consult: Gynecologist
Do: Pelvic examination and cultures to identify infection (if not done previously)

ⒹConsider: Ultrasonography Laparoscopy

Normal → Primary dysmenorrhea

Abnormal → Secondary dysmenorrhea
Identify:
Sexually transmitted disease
Endometriosis
Adhesions
Pelvic serositis

PRIMARY AMENORRHEA

Kathleen A. Mammel, M.D.

DEFINITION

Primary amenorrhea is the failure to begin menstruation. Lack of menses and secondary sex characteristics by 14 years of age, or lack of menses in the presence of secondary sex characteristics by 16 years of age, is cause for concern. Primary amenorrhea may be due to anatomic abnormalities (imperforate hymen, transverse vaginal septum, vaginal agenesis, agenesis of the cervix, absent uterus), physiologic delay (familial, hypogonadotropic hypogonadism, chronic disease, stress, obesity, or weight loss), or chromosomal abnormalities (Turner syndrome, mosaicism, testicular feminization). Do not wait for the specified age to begin the evaluation when pregnancy is suspected or the patient has an anatomic defect or stigmata of Turner syndrome.

A. History should include whether puberty has begun, any weight loss or gain, level of exercise, presence of stressors, and the age of menarche of female relatives. Review systems for symptoms of chronic illness or endocrinopathies, including headaches, vision change, and galactorrhea. Always perform a pregnancy test, as the history for sexual activity may not be reliable.

B. Perform a careful physical examination, noting the percent of ideal body weight for height and age, Tanner stage, vaginal patency, presence of the uterus, signs of virilization (acne, clitoromegaly > 5 mm, hirsutism), or stigmata of Turner syndrome (< 60 inches tall, shield-like chest, widespread nipples, webbed neck, wide carrying angle of the arms, and so on). Assess presence of the uterus through rectoabdominal examination or ultrasound if pelvic examination is not appropriate.

C. Constitutional delay is normal pubertal progression at a slow rate. Early signs of puberty may be found on examination. Reassure the patient about a normal outcome and monitor for pubertal changes every 3 to 6 months.

TABLE 1 Drug Therapy for Primary Amenorrhea in Adolescent Girls

Drug	Dosage
Medroxyprogesterone acetate (Provera)	10 mg orally b.i.d. × 5 days to test for estrogenization
Demulen 28 day	Cycle 1 tab orally qd

(Continued on page 354)

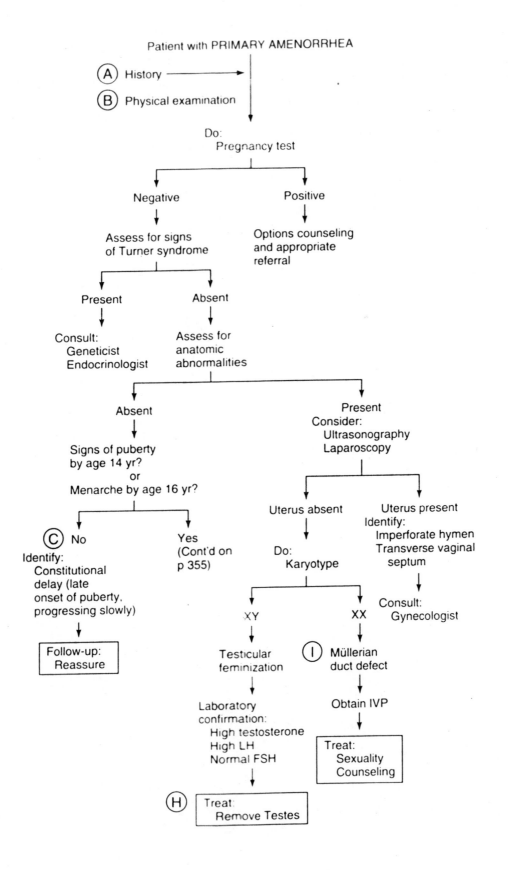

Patient with PRIMARY AMENORRHEA

(A) History ⟶

(B) Physical examination

Do:
Pregnancy test

Negative — Positive

Negative:
Assess for signs
of Turner syndrome

Positive:
Options counseling
and appropriate
referral

Present — Absent

Present:
Consult:
Geneticist
Endocrinologist

Absent:
Assess for
anatomic
abnormalities

Absent — Present

Absent:
Signs of puberty
by age 14 yr?
or
Menarche by age 16 yr?

Present:
Consider:
Ultrasonography
Laparoscopy

Uterus absent — Uterus present

(C) No

No:
Identify:
Constitutional
delay (late
onset of puberty,
progressing slowly)

Follow-up:
Reassure

Yes
(Cont'd on
p 355)

Uterus absent:
Do:
Karyotype

Uterus present:
Identify:
Imperforate hymen
Transverse vaginal
septum

Consult:
Gynecologist

XY — XX

XY:
Testicular
feminization

Laboratory
confirmation:
High testosterone
High LH
Normal FSH

(H) Treat:
Remove Testes

(I) Müllerian
duct defect

Obtain IVP

Treat:
Sexuality
Counseling

353

D. In the normal girl with secondary sex characteristics options are vaginal smear for estrogen influence and a challenge of medroxyprogesterone (Provera) 10 mg orally b.i.d. for 5 days. If the uterine lining has been adequately primed with estrogen, withdrawal flow should occur 5 to 7 days after finishing the medroxyprogesterone. Draw follicle-stimulating hormone (FSH) and luteinizing hormone (LH) levels in patients with low estrogen to distinguish hypergonadotropic from hypogonadotropic causes.

E. Severe hypothalamic repression may be caused by anorexia nervosa, chronic systemic disease, or severe emotional stress. A gynecologist, endocrinologist, or both are helpful at this point.

F. Obtaining testosterone (T) and dihydroepiandrostenedione sulfate (DHAS) will help to separate polycystic ovaries from adrenal causes of virilization and amenorrhea. Polycystic ovarian disease is a spectrum of disorders and does not necessarily include the classic symptoms of obesity, hirsutism, oligomenorrhea, and infertility. Up to 20% of patients do not have elevated LH levels, but LH and FSH may confirm the diagnosis. Progesterone may be given as 10 mg daily for the first 10 days of each month to allow withdrawal flow if there is no evidence of progressive hirsutism and the ovaries are normal in size. Oral contraceptive pills with a low androgenic profile (e.g., Demulen) are an alternative treatment.

G. Consult an endocrinologist to discover whether the cause is an androgen-producing adrenal or ovarian tumor, adrenal hyperplasia, or Cushing syndrome or disease. (Polycystic ovaries can be seen as a part of these more complex conditions.)

H. Testicular feminization requires removal of the testes, as they may undergo malignant degeneration.

I. The patient with a Müllerian duct defect should have an intravenous pyelogram (IVP) to rule out an associated renal anomaly.

References

Emans SJH, Goldstein DP. Pediatric and adolescent gynecology. 3rd ed. Boston: Little, Brown, 1990.

Kaplan DW, Mammel KA. Adolescence. In: Hay WW, Groothius JR, Haywood AR, Levin MJ, eds. Current pediatric diagnosis and treatment. 12th ed. Norwalk, CT: Appleton & Lange, 1995:113

Litt IF. Menstrual problems during adolescence. Pediatr Rev 1983; 4:203.

Rogol A, Blizzard R. Variations and disorders of pubertal development. In: Kappy MS, Blizzard RM, Migeon CJ, eds. The diagnosis and treatment of endocrine disorders in childhood and adolescence. 4th ed. Springfield, IL: Charles C. Thomas, 1994:868.

Speroff L, Glass RH, Kase NG. Clinical gynecologic endocrinology and infertility. 4th ed. Baltimore: Williams & Wilkins, 1989.

Strasburger VC, ed. Adolescent gynecology. Pediatr Clin North Am 1989; 38:3.

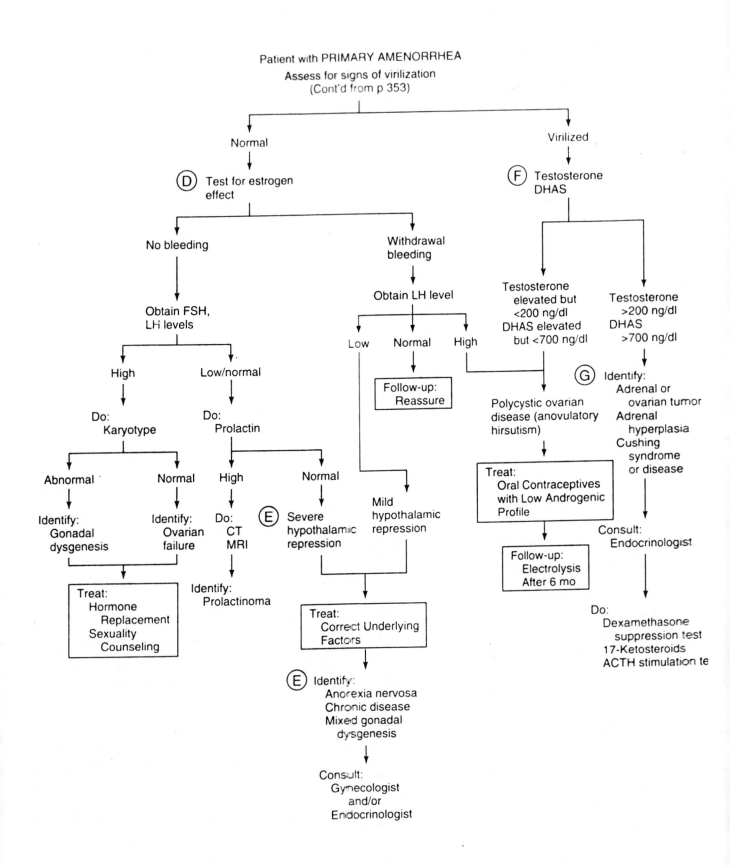

Patient with PRIMARY AMENORRHEA

Assess for signs of virilization
(Cont'd from p 353)

Normal

Ⓓ Test for estrogen effect

No bleeding

Obtain FSH, LH levels

High

Do: Karyotype

Abnormal

Identify: Gonadal dysgenesis

Normal

Identify: Ovarian failure

Treat:
Hormone
Replacement
Sexuality
Counseling

Low/normal

Do: Prolactin

High

Do: CT MRI

Identify: Prolactinoma

Normal

Ⓔ Severe hypothalamic repression

Treat:
Correct Underlying Factors

Ⓔ Identify:
Anorexia nervosa
Chronic disease
Mixed gonadal dysgenesis

Consult:
Gynecologist
and/or
Endocrinologist

Withdrawal bleeding

Obtain LH level

Low

Normal

Follow-up: Reassure

High

Mild hypothalamic repression

Virilized

Ⓕ Testosterone DHAS

Testosterone elevated but <200 ng/dl DHAS elevated but <700 ng/dl

Polycystic ovarian disease (anovulatory hirsutism)

Treat:
Oral Contraceptives with Low Androgenic Profile

Follow-up:
Electrolysis After 6 mo

Testosterone >200 ng/dl DHAS >700 ng/dl

Ⓖ Identify:
Adrenal or ovarian tumor
Adrenal hyperplasia
Cushing syndrome or disease

Consult: Endocrinologist

Do:
Dexamethasone suppression test
17-Ketosteroids
ACTH stimulation te

SECONDARY AMENORRHEA

Kathleen A. Mammel, M.D.

DEFINITION

Secondary amenorrhea is the absence of menses for three consecutive cycles after the establishment of regular menstrual periods. Do not wait for the lapse of three cycles before performing a pregnancy test, however. Indeed, this is the necessary first step in the evaluation of secondary amenorrhea. Secondary amenorrhea results when estrogen is unopposed by progesterone, maintaining the endometrium in the proliferative phase. The most common causes in teenagers are pregnancy, stress, and polycystic ovaries.

A. In the history ask about the previous menstrual pattern, recent stresses (illness, weight loss or gain, significant exercise, emotional turmoil, chronic disease), any sexual activity, date of last intercourse, and contraceptive use. Note any headaches, visual changes, or galactorrhea.

B. In the physical examination do a funduscopic examination, check visual fields, palpate the thyroid, obtain vital signs, compress the areola to check for galactorrhea, and look for signs of androgen excess (hirsutism, acne, clitoromegaly, ovarian enlargement).

C. After a negative pregnancy test, a progesterone challenge can ascertain whether the endometrium has been estrogen primed. If so, a withdrawal bleed should occur 5 to 7 days after the last dose.

D. If withdrawal flow occurs after progesterone and the patient is not hirsute, mild hypothalamic suppression resulting from stress, weight change, athletics, and so on is the likely diagnosis. Polycystic ovaries need not cause hirsutism; hence, this is still in the differential diagnosis. Thyroid disease or other chronic illness should be investigated with the appropriate laboratory studies as indicated by history and physical examination. The treatment of mild hypothalamic suppression includes correcting underlying factors (e.g., maintaining ideal body weight, reducing athletics if the patient is agreeable, counseling for stress or depression), monitoring of the menstrual pattern, and treatment with progesterone every 3 months to allow withdrawal flow (to prevent later risk of endometrial cancer).

E. Polycystic ovaries (see p 352) may be managed with oral contraceptive pills to reduce androgenic signs and allow regular cycles. Clomiphene citrate may be necessary when the patient desires pregnancy.

F. Endocrinology consultation is appropriate if testosterone (T) and dihydroepiandrostenedione sulfate (DHAS) are significantly elevated to differentiate androgen-producing tumor of the ovary or adrenal gland from adrenal hyperplasia and Cushing syndrome or disease.

TABLE 1 Drug Therapy for Secondary Amenorrhea in Adolescent Girls

Drug	Dosage
Medroxyprogesterone acetate (Provera)	5–10 mg/day × 5 days for progesterone challenge
Demulen 28 day or Orthocept	Cycle 1 tab PO qd

G. For patients who fail to have a withdrawal bleed, obtain serum estradiol, follicle-stimulating hormone (FSH), luteinizing hormone (LH), and prolactin levels. Patients with elevated prolactin may have a pituitary microadenoma or hyperplasia, which can be assessed further on CT scan or MRI.

H. Severe hypothalamic dysfunction is unlikely to respond to progesterone with a withdrawal flow. This may result from severe weight loss or weight gain or other severe stressors. Other disorders can be differentiated on the basis of history, physical, and laboratory studies.

I. Elevated gonadotropins imply ovarian failure, which may be the result of chemotherapy, pelvic irradiation, viral illness, chromosomal abnormality (in primary amenorrhea), or autoimmune process. Antiovarian antibodies should be obtained and laparoscopy considered. A gynecology-endocrinology consultation is particularly useful to evaluate the cause and institute hormone replacement therapy.

References

Emans SJH, Goldstein DP. Pediatric and Adolescent Gynecology. 3rd ed. Boston: Little, Brown, 1990.

Kaplan DW, Mammel KA. Adolescence. In: Haywood AR, Hay WW, Groothuis JR, Levin MJ, eds. Current Pediatric Diagnosis and Treatment. 12th ed. Norfolk, CT: Appleton & Lange, 1995:85.

Litt IF. Menstrual problems during adolescence. Pediatr Rev 1983; 4:203.

Rogol A, Blizzard R. Variations and disorders of pubertal development. In: Kappy MS, Blizzard RM, Migeon CJ, eds. The diagnosis and treatment of endocrine disorders in childhood and adolescence. 4th ed. Springfield, IL: Thomas, 1994:857.

Shangold MM. Causes, evaluation, and management of athletic oligo-/amenorrhea. Med Clin North Am 1985; 69:83.

Speroff L, Glass RH, Kase NG. Clinical gynecologic endocrinology and infertility. 4th ed. Baltimore: Williams & Wilkins, 1989.

Strasburger VC, ed. Adolescent gynecology. Pediatr Clin North Am 1989; 38:3.

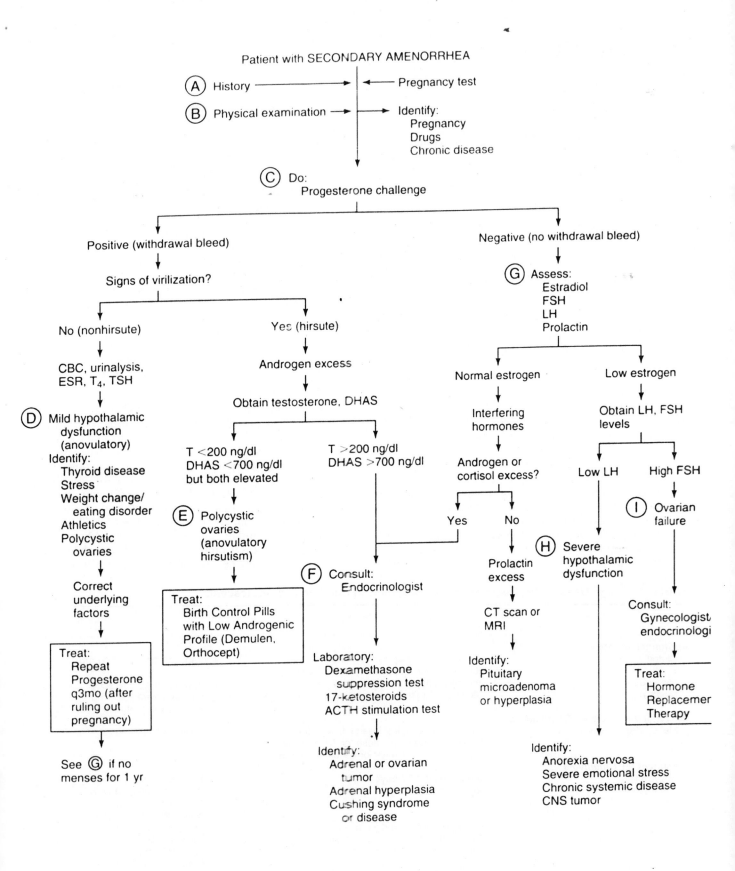

Patient with SECONDARY AMENORRHEA

(A) History ——————→ ←—— Pregnancy test

(B) Physical examination ——→ —→ Identify:
Pregnancy
Drugs
Chronic disease

(C) Do:
Progesterone challenge

Positive (withdrawal bleed)

Signs of virilization?

No (nonhirsute)

CBC, urinalysis,
ESR, T$_4$, TSH

(D) Mild hypothalamic
dysfunction
(anovulatory)
Identify:
Thyroid disease
Stress
Weight change/
eating disorder
Athletics
Polycystic
ovaries

Correct
underlying
factors

Treat:
Repeat
Progesterone
q3mo (after
ruling out
pregnancy)

See (G) if no
menses for 1 yr

Yes (hirsute)

Androgen excess

Obtain testosterone, DHAS

T <200 ng/dl
DHAS <700 ng/dl
but both elevated

T >200 ng/dl
DHAS >700 ng/dl

(E) Polycystic
ovaries
(anovulatory
hirsutism)

Treat:
Birth Control Pills
with Low Androgenic
Profile (Demulen,
Orthocept)

(F) Consult:
Endocrinologist

Laboratory:
Dexamethasone
suppression test
17-ketosteroids
ACTH stimulation test

Identify:
Adrenal or ovarian
tumor
Adrenal hyperplasia
Cushing syndrome
or disease

Negative (no withdrawal bleed)

(G) Assess:
Estradiol
FSH
LH
Prolactin

Normal estrogen

Interfering
hormones

Androgen or
cortisol excess?

Yes   No

Prolactin
excess

CT scan or
MRI

Identify:
Pituitary
microadenoma
or hyperplasia

Low estrogen

Obtain LH, FSH
levels

Low LH   High FSH

(H) Severe
hypothalamic
dysfunction

(I) Ovarian
failure

Consult:
Gynecologist/
endocrinologi

Treat:
Hormone
Replacemen
Therapy

Identify:
Anorexia nervosa
Severe emotional stress
Chronic systemic disease
CNS tumor

VULVOVAGINITIS

Stephen Berman, M.D.

Vulvovaginitis, infection of the vaginal mucosa and/or the cervix, presents with a vaginal discharge and vulvar irritation. The causes of and clinical approaches to this condition differ between prepubertal girls and postpubertal adolescents. Most cases of prepubertal vulvovaginitis are related to poor personal hygiene and are caused by gram-negative enteric organisms such as *Escherichia coli*. Other enteric pathogens that can infect the vaginal area are *Shigella* and *Yersinia*. *Haemophilus influenzae* and *Staphylococcus aureus* can be present as normal flora or can be responsible for vaginitis. Most cases of vulvovaginitis in adolescents are infections with *Candida, Trichomonas,* or bacterial vaginosis. This is caused by an increase in the concentration of *Gardnerella vaginalis* and anaerobes and a decrease in lactobacilli in the vaginal flora. The sexually transmitted pathogens, *Neisseria gonorrhoeae, Trichomonas, Chlamydia,* herpes simplex, and condyloma acuminatum, are more common in adolescents; their identification in younger children requires an evaluation for sexual abuse. Allergic or contact vulvovaginitis can be caused by many irritants such as soaps, bubble bath, douches, and deodorants. A retained foreign body or tampon can be a predisposing reason for persistent discharge.

A. In the history ask about the onset, duration, quantity, color, and odor of the vaginal discharge. Identify associated symptoms such as abdominal pain, pruritus, dysuria, and fever. Identify precipitating factors such as poor perianal hygiene (wiping from back to front), trauma, masturbation, recent antibiotics, possible foreign body, bubble baths, harsh soaps, and nylon tights. In the preadolescent explore the possibility of sexual abuse. In the adolescent determine sexual activity and menstrual history.

B. In the physical examination inspect the external genitalia for redness or excoriation of labia majora, labia minora, clitoris, and introitus. Note any signs of trauma (bruising, hematoma, tear). Examine the prepubertal child in the knee-chest position to best visualize the vagina and cervix. In the adolescent perform an appropriate pelvic examination, which includes a speculum examination of the vagina, a bimanual rectovaginal abdominal palpation and a wet prep. In the prepubertal child obtain specimens with a moistened (nonbacteriostatic saline) cotton-tipped applicator. Inflammation of the vulva with fissures or excoriations suggests a monilial infection. Herpes simplex infections cause a vesicular eruption. Note cervical erosion, ectropion, or discharge. Adnexal tenderness suggests pelvic inflammatory disease or salpingitis.

C. Diagnostic tests should include the following: wet preps with saline and 10% potassium hydroxide (KOH), vaginal pH in adolescents to screen for bacterial vaginosis, culture for *N. gonorrhoeae* for all cases (Thayer-Martin agar), respiratory-type pathogens in preadolescents (blood and chocolate agar), gram-negative enterics in preadolescents (MacConkey agar), and fungus in adolescents (Biggy agar). In adolescents and in cases of suspected sexual abuse, do a rapid test for *Chlamydia* (Micro trak) and/or culture (McCoy cells). When vulvar or anal pruritus is present in a prepubertal child, consider a morning cellophane tape specimen to identify

TABLE 1 Drugs Used in the Treatment of Vulvovaginitis in Children and Adolescents

Drug	Dosage	Product Availability
Antifungal Agents		
Clotrimazole	500 mg vaginal suppository, once	Vaginal tabs: 100, 500 mg
	200 mg vaginal suppository qd × 3 days	
Miconazole	2% cream, apply at bedtime × 7 days	Vaginal cream 1%: 45 g
Nystatin	100,000 U vaginal suppositories b.i.d. × 14 days	Vaginal cream 2%: 45 g
		Vaginal suppositories: 100, 200 mg
Bacterial Vaginosis or *Trichomonas*		
Metronidazole (Flagyl)	Prepubertal 5 mg/kg/dose t.i.d. × 7 days	Tabs: 250, 500 mg
	Adolescent 2 g single dose for *Trichomonas* or	
	500 mg b.i.d. × 7 days for bacterial vaginosis	
Treatment for *Chlamydia*		
Doxycycline	100 mg b.i.d. × 7 days	Tabs, caps: 50, 100 mg
Tetracycline	500 mg q.i.d.	Caps: 100, 250, 500 mg
		Tabs: 250, 500 mg
		Liquid: 200, 400 mg/5 ml
Erythromycin	Adolescent: 500 mg/dose q.i.d. × 7 days	Chewable: 200 mg
	Prepubertal child: 10 mg/kg/dose PO q.i.d. × 10 days	Tabs: 400 mg
Azithromycin	Adolescent: 1 g PO single dose	Caps: 250 mg
		Susp: 100, 200 mg/5 ml
Treatment for *N. gonorrhoeae*		
Cefixime	400 mg PO single dose	Liquid: 100 mg/5 ml
Ciprofloxacin	500 mg PO single dose (age ≥ 18 yr)	Tabs: 250, 500, 750 mg
Ofloxacin	400 mg PO single dose (age ≥ 18 yr)	Tabs: 200, 300, 400 mg
Spectinomycin	40 mg/kg (max 2 g) IM single dose	Vials: 2, 4 g

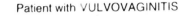

Patient with VULVOVAGINITIS

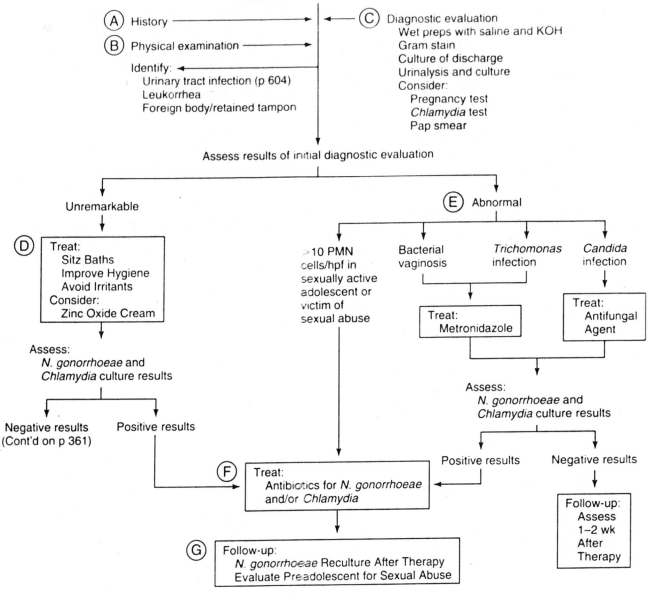

pinworms. *Trichomonas* infections are identified when flagellated, motile organisms are seen on wet prep. Budding hyphae seen with a KOH prep indicate *Monilia* infection. Clue cells or epithelial cells coated with refractile bacteria on wet prep are consistent with *G. vaginalis* infections. Sheets of epithelial cells seen on wet prep indicate leukorrhea, a normal variant. More than 10 polymorphonuclear (PMN) cells per high-power field (hpf) in the discharge of a sexually active adolescent suggests gonorrheal and/or chlamydial infection.

D. Most cases of prepubertal vulvovaginitis are related to poor perianal hygiene. Manage cases with nonspecific vaginitis with sitz baths and improved perianal hygiene (cotton underpants, front-to-back wiping, avoidance of

nylon tights and tight-fitting pants). Consider a trial of zinc oxide cream three times a day. Failure to respond is an indication for an oral antibiotic such as ampicillin or a cephalosporin.

E. Suspect bacterial vaginosis in a sexually active adolescent when an adherent grayish white discharge is present, the vaginal pH is above 4.5, clue cells are increased, and a characteristic odor is present when the KOH prep is done. Treat bacterial vaginosis infections (*G. vaginalis*) or presumed anaerobes with metronidazole (Table 1). Amoxicillin is a less effective alternative. Treat *Trichomonas vaginalis* with metronidazole. Infection with *Candida* is infrequent in the prepubertal child. When present, it is usually associated with recent antibiotic therapy or diabetes mellitus. Treat *Candida vaginalis* with clotrimazole or nystatin suppositories or miconazole 2% (Monostat). Consider the use of 1% hydrocortisone cream if inflammation is severe.

F. Recommended antibiotic therapy for uncomplicated gonococcal vulvovaginitis and presumed concomitant chlamydial infection varies with the age and weight of the patient (Table 1). Treat prepubertal girls who weigh less than 100 lb (45 kg) with ceftriaxone IM or spectinomycin IM plus erythromycin. Treat children who weigh more than 100 lb or are 9 years of age or older with ceftriaxone IM or cefixime orally or spectinomycin IM. Patients 18 years of age or older can also be treated with ciprofloxacin orally or ofloxacin orally. All the gonococcal treatment options listed above should be combined with either doxycycline orally or azithromycin orally for treatment of chlamydia.

G. When a prepubertal girl has a sexually transmitted agent, perform a thorough evaluation for possible sexual abuse. All contacts (extended family, babysitter, parents) should be interviewed. The patient should have repeated interviews, with trained personnel using play therapy when appropriate. Consider hospitalization to carry out the evaluation.

References

American Academy of Pediatrics. Gonococcal infections. In: Peter G, ed. 1994 Red Book: Report of the committee on infectious diseases. 23rd ed. Elk Grove Village, IL: 1994:195.

Brunham RC, Paavonen J, Steven CE, et al. Mucopurulent cervicitis: The ignored counter-part in women of urethritis in men. N Engl J Med 1984; 311:1.

Emans SJ. Vulvovaginitis in the child and adolescent. Pediatr Rev 1986; 8:12.

Ingram DL. *Neisseria gonorrhoeae* in children. Pediatr Ann 1994; 23:341.

O'Connor PA, Oliver WJ. Group A β-hemolytic streptococcal vulvovaginitis: A recurring problem. Pediatr Emerg Care 1985; 1:94.

Rosenfeld WD, Clark J. Vulvovaginitis and cervicitis. Pediatr Clin North Am 1989; 36:489.

Shafer MA, Sweet RL, Ohm-Smith MJ, et al. Microbiology of the lower genital tract in postmenarchal adolescent girls: Differences by sexual activity, contraception, and presence of nonspecific vaginitis. J Pediatr 1985; 107:974.

Sirotnak AP. Testing sexually abused children for sexually transmitted diseases: Who to test, when to test, and why. Pediatr Ann 1994; 23:370.

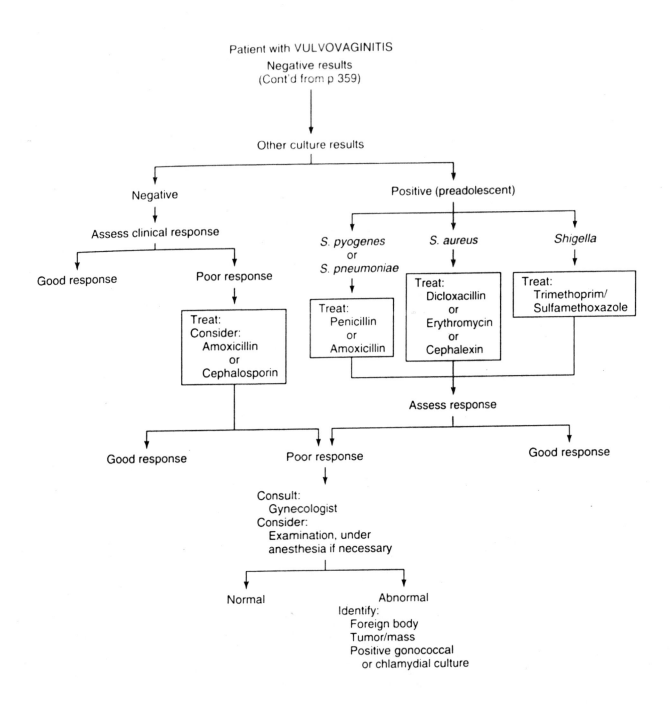

Patient with VULVOVAGINITIS
Negative results
(Cont'd from p 359)

Other culture results

Negative

Assess clinical response

Good response   Poor response

Treat:
Consider:
Amoxicillin
or
Cephalosporin

Good response   Poor response

Consult:
  Gynecologist
Consider:
  Examination, under
  anesthesia if necessary

Normal   Abnormal
                          Identify:
                            Foreign body
                            Tumor/mass
                            Positive gonococcal
                              or chlamydial culture

Positive (preadolescent)

S. pyogenes   S. aureus   Shigella
or
S. pneumoniae

Treat: Treat: Treat:
Penicillin   Dicloxacillin   Trimethoprim/
or   or   Sulfamethoxazole
Amoxicillin   Erythromycin
                    or
                    Cephalexin

Assess response

Good response

HEMATOLOGIC DISORDERS

Bleeding Disorders
Generalized Lymphadenopathy
Hemolytic Anemia
Microcytic Anemia

Neutropenia
Normocytic or Macrocytic Anemia
Thrombocytopenia

BLEEDING DISORDERS

Rachelle Nuss, M.D.
Peter A. Lane, M.D.

A. In the history ask about the type and extent of bruising or bleeding as well as the frequency and duration of these symptoms. Epistaxis is common in children, but recurrent nose bleeds longer than 10 minutes suggest thrombocytopenia or a platelet function defect. Oral mucous membrane bleeding in infancy suggests hemophilia. Note jaundice (liver disease), poor weight gain (uremia, malabsorption with secondary vitamin K deficiency), recurrent joint pain or swelling (hemophilia, collagen vascular disease), or recent abdominal or joint pain (Henoch-Schönlein purpura). Breast-fed infants may be at risk for vitamin K deficiency, particularly after a bout of diarrhea. Inquire about excessive bleeding following any operations, especially circumcision, tonsillectomy, or tooth extraction. Note all drug use; ask specifically about aspirin. Consider the possibility of physical abuse (see p 18). Review the family history for any clues to congenital bleeding disorders.

B. Perform a complete physical examination. Note petechiae (thrombocytopenia or platelet dysfunction), jaundice (liver disease), lymphadenopathy or hepatosplenomegaly (leukemia, malignancy), rash or joint swelling (collagen vascular disease, Henoch-Schönlein purpura, hemophilia), and abnormal skin (Ehlers-Danlos syndrome).

C. Bleeding is a frequent complication of systemic disease such as sepsis, liver disease, and uremia. Consider other diagnoses such as Henoch-Schönlein purpura and physical abuse.

D. Children with known coagulopathies require expeditious therapy for significant episodes of bleeding: factor VIII concentrates or desmopressin acetate for factor VIII deficiency (classic hemophilia), desmopressin acetate or factor VIII containing von Willebrand factor concentrate for von Willebrand disease, and desmopressin acetate or platelet transfusions for platelet function defects. Less common hereditary deficiencies of clotting factors are treated with factor concentrates or fresh frozen plasma.

E. A normal bleeding screen does not exclude a coagulopathy; significant unexplained bleeding requires a hematology consultation and further evaluation.

(Continued on page 366)

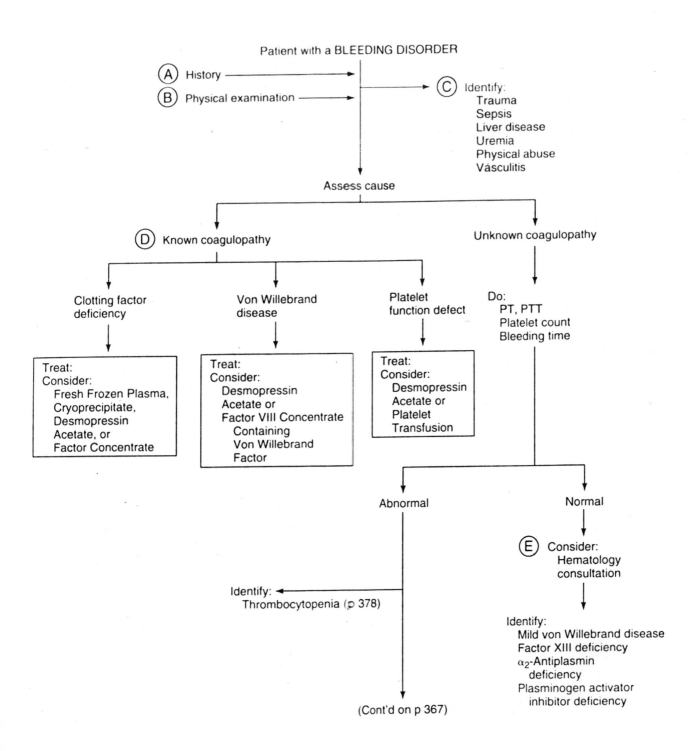

Patient with a BLEEDING DISORDER

(A) History ————————————→

(B) Physical examination ——————→

(C) Identify:
  Trauma
  Sepsis
  Liver disease
  Uremia
  Physical abuse
  Vasculitis

Assess cause

(D) Known coagulopathy

Unknown coagulopathy

Clotting factor deficiency

Von Willebrand disease

Platelet function defect

Do:
PT, PTT
Platelet count
Bleeding time

Treat:
Consider:
  Fresh Frozen Plasma,
  Cryoprecipitate,
  Desmopressin
  Acetate, or
  Factor Concentrate

Treat:
Consider:
  Desmopressin
  Acetate or
  Factor VIII Concentrate
  Containing
  Von Willebrand
  Factor

Treat:
Consider:
  Desmopressin
  Acetate or
  Platelet
  Transfusion

Abnormal

Normal

Identify: ←
Thrombocytopenia (p 378)

(E) Consider:
  Hematology
  consultation

Identify:
  Mild von Willebrand disease
  Factor XIII deficiency
  α_2-Antiplasmin
    deficiency
  Plasminogen activator
    inhibitor deficiency

(Cont'd on p 367)

F. Repeating the partial thromboplastin time (PTT) after 1:1 mixing with normal plasma may help differentiate a factor deficiency from an inhibitor of coagulation.

G. Desmopressin acetate may be efficacious in uremia, some cases of von Willebrand disease, or platelet function defects. Individuals with von Willebrand disease unresponsive to desmopressin should receive factor VIII containing von Willebrand factor concentrates, whereas individuals with platelet defects unresponsive to desmopressin may require platelet transfusion.

H. An isolated prolongation of the prothrombin time (PT) is rare and suggests factor VII deficiency, mild vitamin K deficiency, or liver disease.

I. Prolongation of both PT and PTT suggests a diffuse coagulopathy such as that caused by severe vitamin K deficiency, heparin excess, liver disease, disseminated intravascular coagulation (DIC), afibrinogenemia, dysfibrinogenemia, or hypofibrinogenemia. A factor II, V, or X deficiency or an inhibitor may be present. Consider giving vitamin K; treat serious bleeding with fresh frozen plasma.

References

Hathaway WE. New insights on vitamin K. Hematol Oncol Clin North Am 1987; 1:367.

Holmberg L, Nilsson IM. Von Willebrand's disease. Eur J Haematol 1992; 48:127.

Hoyer L. Hemophilia A. N Engl J Med 1994; 330:38.

Mannucci PM. Desmopressin: A nontransfusional form of treatment for congenital and acquired bleeding disorders. Blood 1988; 72:1449.

Manno C. Difficult pediatric diagnoses: Bruising and bleeding. Pediatr Clin North Am 1991; 38:637.

Patient with BRUISING OR BLEEDING
Abnormal
(Cont'd from p 365)

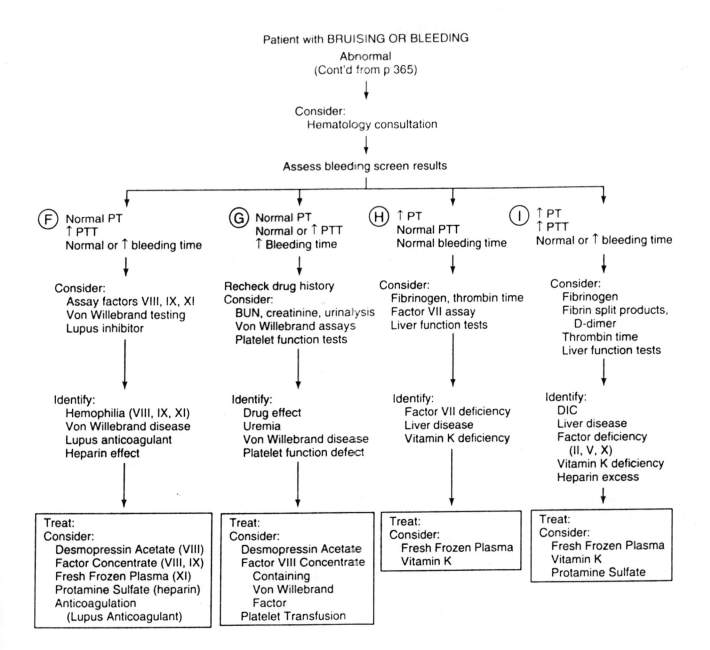

Consider:
Hematology consultation

Assess bleeding screen results

F Normal PT
↑ PTT
Normal or ↑ bleeding time

Consider:
Assay factors VIII, IX, XI
Von Willebrand testing
Lupus inhibitor

Identify:
Hemophilia (VIII, IX, XI)
Von Willebrand disease
Lupus anticoagulant
Heparin effect

Treat:
Consider:
Desmopressin Acetate (VIII)
Factor Concentrate (VIII, IX)
Fresh Frozen Plasma (XI)
Protamine Sulfate (heparin)
Anticoagulation
(Lupus Anticoagulant)

G Normal PT
Normal or ↑ PTT
↑ Bleeding time

Recheck drug history
Consider:
BUN, creatinine, urinalysis
Von Willebrand assays
Platelet function tests

Identify:
Drug effect
Uremia
Von Willebrand disease
Platelet function defect

Treat:
Consider:
Desmopressin Acetate
Factor VIII Concentrate
Containing
Von Willebrand
Factor
Platelet Transfusion

H ↑ PT
Normal PTT
Normal bleeding time

Consider:
Fibrinogen, thrombin time
Factor VII assay
Liver function tests

Identify:
Factor VII deficiency
Liver disease
Vitamin K deficiency

Treat:
Consider:
Fresh Frozen Plasma
Vitamin K

I ↑ PT
↑ PTT
Normal or ↑ bleeding time

Consider:
Fibrinogen
Fibrin split products,
D-dimer
Thrombin time
Liver function tests

Identify:
DIC
Liver disease
Factor deficiency
(II, V, X)
Vitamin K deficiency
Heparin excess

Treat:
Consider:
Fresh Frozen Plasma
Vitamin K
Protamine Sulfate

GENERALIZED LYMPHADENOPATHY

Peter A. Lane, M.D.
Rachelle Nuss, M.D.

DEFINITION

Generalized lymphadenopathy is abnormal enlargement of more than two noncontiguous lymph node regions.

A. In the history ask about systemic symptoms such as persistent or recurrent fever (infection, malignancy, collagen vascular disease), sore throat (infectious mononucleosis), cough (tuberculosis or fungal infection), epistaxis or easy bruising (leukemia), limp, or limb pain (juvenile rheumatoid arthritis, leukemia, neuroblastoma). Note duration and severity of any systemic symptoms and assess whether they are improving or progressing. Obtain a complete history of travel and animal exposures. Note all recent immunizations and medications (serum sickness, drug reaction, phenytoin-induced lymphadenopathy). Document routine immunizations; inquire about possible exposure to tuberculosis. Identify risk for infection with HIV.

B. In the physical examination note the degree and extent of lymphadenopathy. Discrete, mobile, nontender lymph nodes are palpable in most healthy children. Small inguinal or high cervical nodes (1 cm or less) and occipital, submandibular, or axillary nodes (3 mm or less) are normal. Note thyromegaly (hyperthyroidism), massive hepatosplenomegaly (malignancy, storage disease, infection), arthritis (collagen vascular disease, leukemia), or a characteristic rash or conjunctivitis (viral exanthem, juvenile rheumatoid arthritis, systemic lupus, Kawasaki disease, leptospirosis, histiocytosis).

C. Atypical lymphocytes are frequently associated with many viral illnesses. A differential count with 10% to 20% atypical lymphocytes suggests infectious mononucleosis, cytomegalovirus (CMV), toxoplasmosis, viral hepatitis, or drug hypersensitivity.

D. False-negative monospot tests frequently occur early in the course of infectious mononucleosis and are common in very young children with Epstein-Barr virus (EBV) infection.

E. Children with moderate or severe illness have prolonged fever, unexplained weight loss, persistent cough, known exposure to tuberculosis, risk factors for HIV, or significant systemic toxicity.

F. Severe anemia, neutropenia, or thrombocytopenia accompanying generalized lymphadenopathy suggests a malignancy, severe infection, or storage disease. Obtain a hematology/oncology consultation prior to performing a bone marrow examination to avoid omitting important special studies (biopsy, chromosomes, lymphoid markers, fungal and viral cultures).

References

Burns JC, Mason WH, Glode MP, et al. Clinical and epidemiologic characteristics of patients referred for evaluation of possible Kawasaki disease. J Pediatr 1991; 118:680.

Grossman M, Shiramizu B. Evaluation of lymphadenopathy in children. Curr Opin Pediatr 1994; 6:68.

Knight PJ, Mulne AF, Vassy LE. When is lymph node biopsy indicated in children with enlarged peripheral nodes? Pediatrics 1982; 69:391.

Schuster V, Kreth HW. Epstein-Barr virus infection and associated diseases in children: I. Pathogenesis, epidemiology, and clinical aspects. Eur J Pediatr 1992; 151:718.

Zuelzer WW, Kaplan J. The child with lymphadenopathy. Semin Hematol 1975; 12:323.

Patient with GENERALIZED LYMPHADENOPATHY

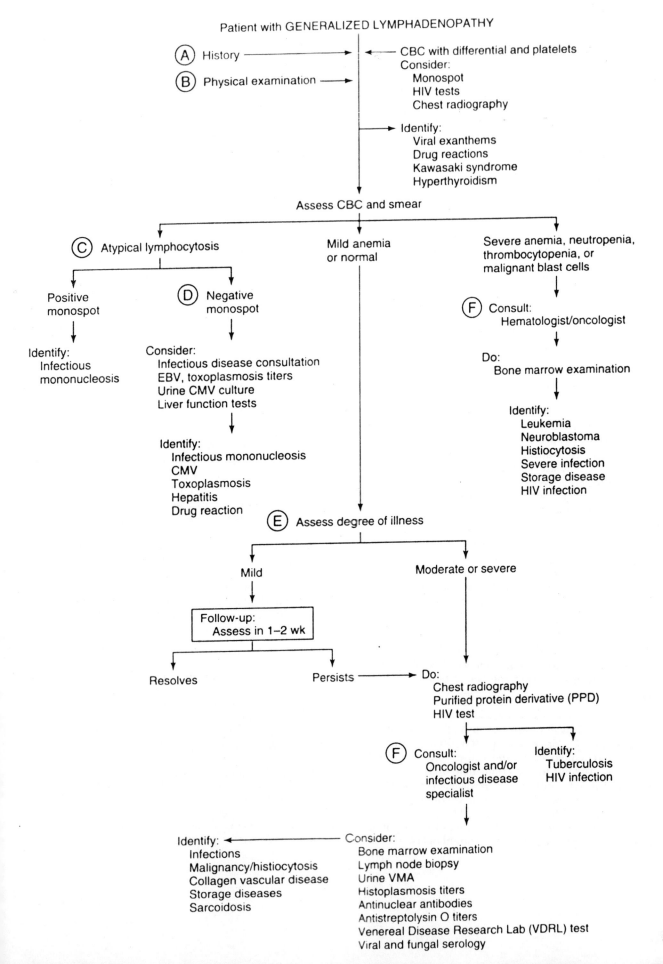

(A) History ──────────→ ←── CBC with differential and platelets
                              Consider:
(B) Physical examination ──→   Monospot
                                  HIV tests
                                  Chest radiography

                        ──→ Identify:
                                Viral exanthems
                                Drug reactions
                                Kawasaki syndrome
                                Hyperthyroidism

Assess CBC and smear

(C) Atypical lymphocytosis   Mild anemia   Severe anemia, neutropenia,
                                    or normal   thrombocytopenia, or
                                                        malignant blast cells

Positive   (D) Negative   (F) Consult:
monospot   monospot   Hematologist/oncologist

Identify: Consider: Do:
Infectious   Infectious disease consultation   Bone marrow examination
mononucleosis   EBV, toxoplasmosis titers
                    Urine CMV culture
                    Liver function tests   Identify:
                                                             Leukemia
                Identify: Neuroblastoma
                    Infectious mononucleosis   Histiocytosis
                    CMV   Severe infection
                    Toxoplasmosis   Storage disease
                    Hepatitis   HIV infection
                    Drug reaction
                                (E) Assess degree of illness

                        Mild   Moderate or severe

                   ┌─────────────────────┐
                   │ Follow-up: │
                   │ Assess in 1–2 wk   │
                   └─────────────────────┘

        Resolves   Persists ────→ Do:
                                             Chest radiography
                                             Purified protein derivative (PPD)
                                             HIV test

                                        (F) Consult: Identify:
                                             Oncologist and/or   Tuberculosis
                                             infectious disease   HIV infection
                                             specialist

Identify: ←──────────────── Consider:
    Infections   Bone marrow examination
    Malignancy/histiocytosis   Lymph node biopsy
    Collagen vascular disease   Urine VMA
    Storage diseases   Histoplasmosis titers
    Sarcoidosis   Antinuclear antibodies
                                Antistreptolysin O titers
                                Venereal Disease Research Lab (VDRL) test
                                Viral and fungal serology

HEMOLYTIC ANEMIA

Peter A. Lane, M.D.
Rachelle Nuss, M.D.

A. In the history ask about symptoms that suggest severe hemolysis such as headache, dizziness, syncope, fever, chills, and abdominal or back pain. Inquire about neonatal and recurrent jaundice. Note possible precipitating factors such as viral illness and the use of medications. A history of recurrent infections, arthritis, rash, mouth ulcers, thrombosis, or thyroid disease suggests autoimmune hemolysis. African, Mediterranean, or Arab ancestry suggests the possibility of a sickle cell syndrome or glucose-6-phosphate dehydrogenase (G6PD) deficiency (in a boy). G6PD deficiency also occurs in Asians. Obtain a family history of anemia, jaundice, splenectomy, and unexplained gallstones.

B. In the physical examination assess the circulatory status. If the hemoglobin is greater than 6 g/dl, significant tachypnea or tachycardia suggests a rapidly falling hemoglobin or shock secondary to sepsis with disseminated intravascular coagulation (DIC) or to a splenic sequestration. Note fever (intravascular hemolysis, acute infection, collagen-vascular disease) or growth retardation (longstanding anemia or diseases associated with autoimmune hemolysis). Note splenomegaly. Splenomegaly is unusual in older children with homozygous sickle cell anemia but common in sickle-hemoglobin C disease, sickle β-thalassemia, and hereditary spherocytosis. Moderate to massive splenomegaly suggests a splenic sequestration. Note petechiae or bruising (DIC, hemolytic-uremic syndrome [HUS]) and arthritis or rash (collagen vascular disease).

C. Perform a CBC and a reticulocyte count. A normal hemoglobin does not exclude hemolysis, since an increased production of red cells may completely compensate for their increased destruction. Microcytosis (see p 372) suggests a thalassemia syndrome, hemoglobin C or E disease, hereditary pyropoikilocytosis, or coexistent iron deficiency. A low or normal reticulocyte count suggests a hypoplastic crisis.

D. Perform both direct and indirect Coombs tests. Coombs-negative autoimmune hemolytic anemias are rare in children.

E. Determine the thermal amplitude (warm or cold) and antigen specificity (e.g., Rh, I) of the antibody, as well as whether IgG, C_3, or both are present on the red cells. These studies help clarify the cause, treatment, and prognosis. Attempt to find compatible units of packed RBCs but avoid transfusions if possible. Most cases of autoimmune hemolytic anemia in children are idiopathic or related to infection (e.g., Epstein-Barr virus, mycoplasma) and are transient. Neutropenia, thrombocytopenia, a prolonged partial thromboplastin time (PTT), or positive antinuclear antibodies (ANA) suggest other autoantibodies and an underlying collagen vascular disease.

F. Spherocytes and elliptocytes occur in many clinical settings. Obtain CBC, reticulocyte counts, and blood smears from family members; hereditary spherocytosis and elliptocytosis are usually autosomal dominant.

G. In the absence of microcytosis or liver disease, target cells suggest a hemoglobinopathy. A sickle solubility test (e.g., sickle prep) confirms the presence of sickle hemoglobin but is *negative* in infants with sickle cell anemia owing to high levels of fetal hemoglobin. Older children with sickle cell trait have a positive sickle solubility test but do not have hemolysis or an abnormal blood smear. Obtain a hemoglobin electrophoresis to diagnose a sickle cell syndrome accurately.

H. Red cell fragmentation suggests a microangiopathic hemolytic process. Consider DIC or HUS in the acutely ill child. DIC is most commonly associated with overwhelming infection.

I. In some cases red cell morphology does not suggest a specific diagnosis. G6PD (X-linked recessive) and pyruvate kinase (autosomal recessive) deficiencies are the most common inherited defects of red cell metabolism. Unstable hemoglobins usually show autosomal dominant inheritance because heterozygotes are affected. Oxidant-mediated hemolysis may be induced by infection or by oxidant medications (e.g., sulfamethoxazole, nitrofurantoin) in patients with G6PD deficiency or with some unstable hemoglobinopathies; in such cases there may be blister cells or bite cells on the peripheral blood smear and a Heinz body preparation may be positive. Unstable hemoglobins are best detected by the isopropanol precipitation test.

References

Becker PS, Lux SE. Disorders of the red cell membrane. In: Nathan DG, Oski FA, eds. Hematology of Infancy and Childhood. 4th ed. Philadelphia: Saunders, 1993:526.

Beutler E. Glucose-6-phosphate dehydrogenase deficiency. N Engl J Med 1991; 324:169.

Lane PA, Nuss R, Ambruso DR. Autoimmune hemolytic anemia. In: Hay WW Jr, Groothuis JR, Hayward AR, Levin MJ, eds. Current Pediatric Diagnosis and Treatment. 12th ed. Norwalk, CT: Appleton & Lange, 1995:837.

Mentzer WC, Wagner GM. The Hereditary Hemolytic Anemias. New York: Churchill Livingstone, 1989.

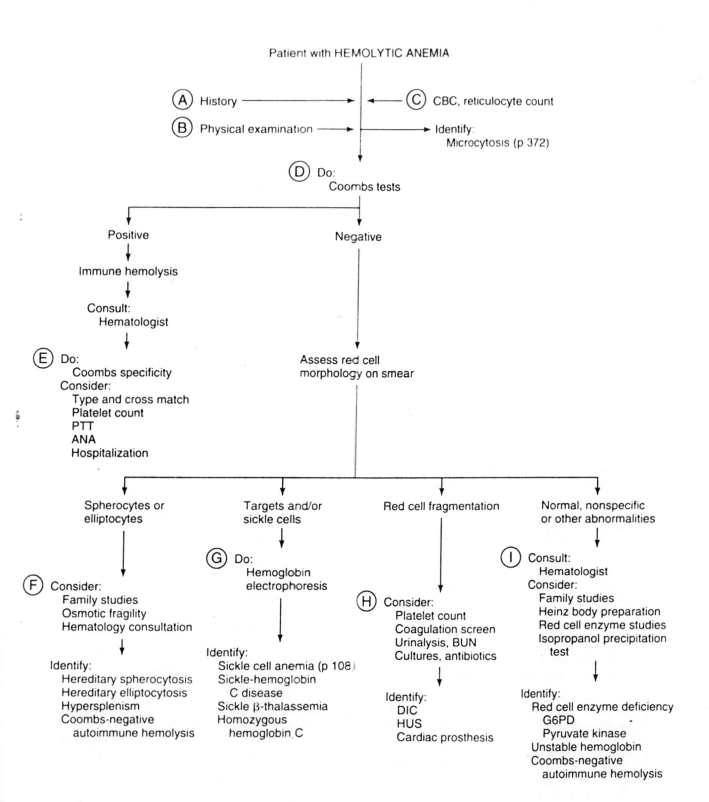

Patient with HEMOLYTIC ANEMIA

(A) History ──────────────→ ←────── (C) CBC, reticulocyte count

(B) Physical examination ──────→ ──→ Identify:
　　　　　　　　　　　　　　　　　　　Microcytosis (p 372)

(D) Do:
　　Coombs tests

Positive

Immune hemolysis

Consult:
　Hematologist

(E) Do:
　　Coombs specificity
Consider:
　Type and cross match
　Platelet count
　PTT
　ANA
　Hospitalization

Negative

Assess red cell
morphology on smear

Spherocytes or elliptocytes

(F) Consider:
　Family studies
　Osmotic fragility
　Hematology consultation

Identify:
　Hereditary spherocytosis
　Hereditary elliptocytosis
　Hypersplenism
　Coombs-negative
　　autoimmune hemolysis

Targets and/or sickle cells

(G) Do:
　　Hemoglobin
　　electrophoresis

Identify:
　Sickle cell anemia (p 108)
　Sickle-hemoglobin
　　C disease
　Sickle β-thalassemia
　Homozygous
　　hemoglobin C

Red cell fragmentation

(H) Consider:
　Platelet count
　Coagulation screen
　Urinalysis, BUN
　Cultures, antibiotics

Identify:
　DIC
　HUS
　Cardiac prosthesis

Normal, nonspecific or other abnormalities

(I) Consult:
　Hematologist
Consider:
　Family studies
　Heinz body preparation
　Red cell enzyme studies
　Isopropanol precipitation
　　test

Identify:
　Red cell enzyme deficiency
　　G6PD
　　Pyruvate kinase
　Unstable hemoglobin
　Coombs-negative
　　autoimmune hemolysis

MICROCYTIC ANEMIA

Peter A. Lane, M.D.
Rachelle Nuss, M.D.

A. In the history ask about chronic illness, recurrent infections, and fever (anemia of chronic disease), irritability and pica (iron deficiency or lead poisoning), and blood loss (iron deficiency). A diet deficient in iron may cause iron deficiency anemia in children age 6 to 36 months, particularly if large volumes of cow's milk are consumed. Note any family history of anemia or jaundice. Consider the possibility of a hemoglobinopathy in children of African, Mediterranean, and Arab ancestry (α-thalassemia, β-thalassemia, sickle β-thalassemia, homozygous hemoglobin C disease) and in south or southeast Asian children (α-thalassemia, β-thalassemia, hemoglobin E disease).

B. In the physical examination note jaundice or splenomegaly (thalassemia, homozygous hemoglobin C) and delayed growth and development (chronic disease). Assess the circulatory status, and note signs of high-output congestive heart failure.

C. Normal values for hemoglobin, hematocrit (Hct), and mean corpuscular volume (MCV) vary with age: in the newborn, Hct is above 45% and MCV is above 94; at 6 months, Hct is over 33% and MCV is over 70; at 2 years, Hct is above 34% and MCV is over 72; at 5 years, Hct is above 35% and MCV is over 75. Thereafter, normal values for Hct and MCV gradually increase until they reach adult normal levels after puberty. The red blood cell count (RBC) and the relative distribution width (RDW) of red cell size may help differentiate thalassemia from iron deficiency. The RBC is often elevated in thalassemia, and the index of MCV divided by RBC usually is below 13; with iron deficiency the RBC is not elevated, and the MCV divided by RBC usually is above 13. The RDW is usually elevated in iron deficiency but normal in mild thalassemia. Review peripheral smear for red cell morphology.

D. Institute a trial of oral iron (3 mg/kg/day of elemental iron). Do not give with milk or formula. A response to oral iron is the best single test of iron deficiency.

E. In the face of moderately severe microcytic anemia, a presumptive diagnosis of iron deficiency should be made only with a history of an iron-poor diet (age 6 to 36 months) or explained blood loss (older than 36 months) and a history and physical examination that do not suggest another cause of microcytosis or anemia. The prevalence of anemia resulting from iron deficiency has declined markedly in the United States in the past 2 decades, so other causes of anemia now have a proportionately greater likelihood.

F. Obtain a hematology consultation. Consider hospitalization and cautious transfusion if the hemoglobin is less than 5 g/dl or if there are signs of cardiac decompensation.

G. In iron deficiency, oral iron therapy causes a reticulocytosis within 5 to 7 days. Documentation of this reticulocyte response is a relatively inexpensive way to confirm the diagnosis and assess the efficacy of therapy.

H. Severe microcytosis and hypochromia suggest significant iron deficiency or β-thalassemia; numerous target cells suggest thalassemia (including sickle β-thalassemia) or homozygous hemoglobin C or E disease. Basophilic stippling is often present with lead poisoning but is not specific for this diagnosis (see I, below). The erythrocyte protoporphyrin is mildly elevated in iron deficiency and markedly elevated with lead poisoning. The serum ferritin is typically low in iron deficiency (low serum iron) but high in the anemia of chronic disease (low serum iron). The serum ferritin may be falsely normal or elevated if measured during an acute illness. The absence of microcytosis in both parents usually excludes the diagnosis of β-thalassemia or sickle β-thalassemia, but not α-thalassemia, in their child. A quantitative hemoglobin electrophoresis shows an elevated A_2 and/or F hemoglobin in β-thalassemia, a hemoglobin S level greater than the hemoglobin A level in sickle β-thalassemia, and hemoglobin C or E in hemoglobin C or E diseases. The hemoglobin electrophoresis is usually normal in α-thalassemia trait, except in the newborn in whom Bart's hemoglobin is detected.

I. Lead poisoning has been associated with microcytic anemia, but recent evidence indicates that lead levels below 40 μg/dl are not causally associated with anemia. Most of the anemia associated with lead poisoning is due to coexistent iron deficiency.

J. Iron therapy should be continued until body stores are replenished. The possibility of blood loss should be thoroughly investigated when iron deficiency occurs in children over 3 years of age.

References

Clark M, Royal J, Seeler R. Interaction of iron deficiency and lead and the hematologic findings in children with severe lead poisoning. Pediatrics 1988; 81:247.

Dallman PR, Siimes MA. Percentile curves for hemoglobin and red cell volume in infancy and childhood. J Pediatr 1979; 94:26.

Dallman PR, Yip R. Changing characteristics of childhood anemia. J Pediatr 1989; 114:161.

Giardina PJ, Hilgartner MW. Update on thalassemia. Pediatr Rev 1992; 13:55.

Hurst D, Tittle B, Kleman KM, et al. Anemia and hemoglobinopathies in Southeast Asian refugee children. J Pediatr 1983; 102:692.

Oski FA. Iron deficiency in infancy and childhood. N Engl J Med 1993; 329:190.

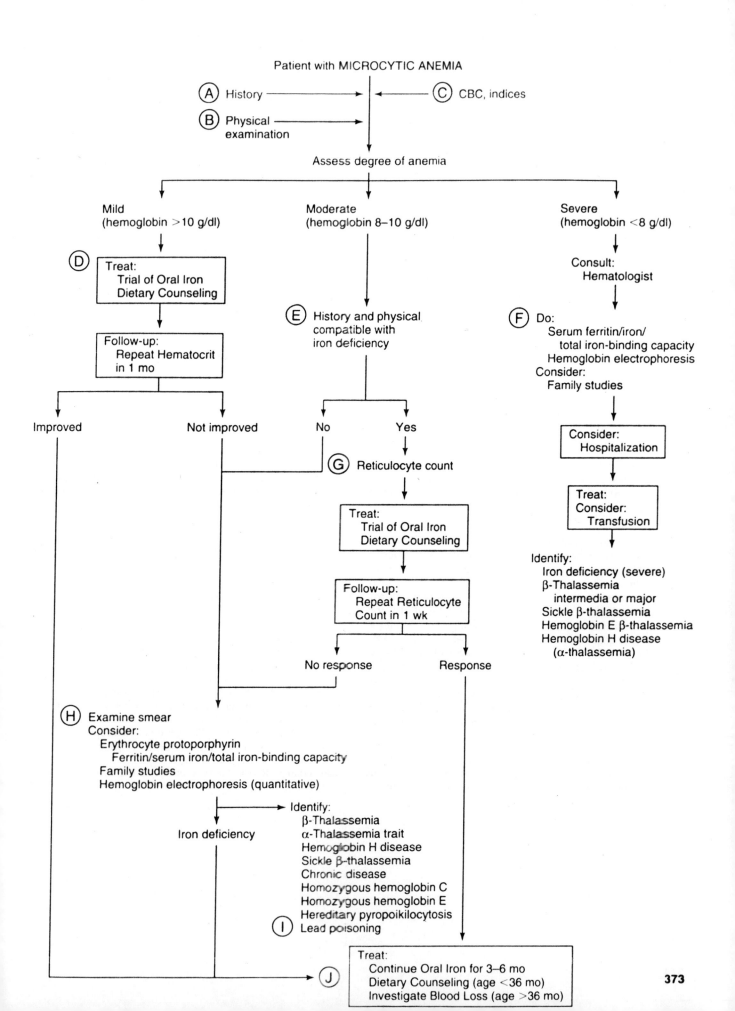

Patient with MICROCYTIC ANEMIA

(A) History ──────────→ ←────── (C) CBC, indices

(B) Physical ──────────→
examination

Assess degree of anemia

Mild
(hemoglobin >10 g/dl)

(D) Treat:
Trial of Oral Iron
Dietary Counseling

Follow-up:
Repeat Hematocrit
in 1 mo

Improved   Not improved

Moderate
(hemoglobin 8–10 g/dl)

(E) History and physical
compatible with
iron deficiency

No   Yes

(G) Reticulocyte count

Treat:
Trial of Oral Iron
Dietary Counseling

Follow-up:
Repeat Reticulocyte
Count in 1 wk

No response   Response

Severe
(hemoglobin <8 g/dl)

Consult:
Hematologist

(F) Do:
Serum ferritin/iron/
total iron-binding capacity
Hemoglobin electrophoresis
Consider:
Family studies

Consider:
Hospitalization

Treat:
Consider:
Transfusion

Identify:
Iron deficiency (severe)
β-Thalassemia
intermedia or major
Sickle β-thalassemia
Hemoglobin E β-thalassemia
Hemoglobin H disease
(α-thalassemia)

(H) Examine smear
Consider:
Erythrocyte protoporphyrin
Ferritin/serum iron/total iron-binding capacity
Family studies
Hemoglobin electrophoresis (quantitative)

Identify:
β-Thalassemia
α-Thalassemia trait
Hemoglobin H disease
Sickle β-thalassemia
Chronic disease
Homozygous hemoglobin C
Homozygous hemoglobin E
Hereditary pyropoikilocytosis
(I) Lead poisoning

Iron deficiency

Treat:
Continue Oral Iron for 3–6 mo
Dietary Counseling (age <36 mo)
Investigate Blood Loss (age >36 mo)

(J)

373

NEUTROPENIA

Rachelle Nuss, M.D.
Peter A. Lane, M.D.

DEFINITION

Neutropenia is an absolute decrease in the number of circulating neutrophils in the blood. The absolute neutrophil count (ANC) is determined by multiplying the total white blood cell count by the percentage of neutrophils plus bands. Neutropenia is mild if the ANC is between 1000 and 1500, moderate if between 500 and 1000, and severe if less than 500. For children 2 weeks to 1 year of age the lower limit of normal is 1000 rather than 1500. In general the severity of neutropenia correlates with risk of pyogenic infection.

ETIOLOGY

Most cases of childhood neutropenia are self-limited and associated with a viral illness or drug therapy. Influenza, hepatitis, rubella, adenovirus, coxsackie, measles, mumps, Epstein-Barr, and cytomegalovirus (CMV) have all been associated with neutropenia.

A. In the history ask about previous and current infections. A family history of recurrent infection or unexplained childhood deaths suggests a congenitally acquired immunodeficiency. Risk factors for human immunodeficiency virus should be determined.

B. In the physical examination note the nutritional status of the child; marasmus and B_{12}, folate, and copper deficiencies are associated with neutropenia. Fanconi anemia, osteopetrosis, and aminoacidurias may have physical stigmata and may also have associated neutropenia. Children with neutropenia may be at risk for pyogenic bacterial infection with endogenous skin flora such as *Staphylococcus aureus* and gram-negative rods. The skin should be examined for signs of cellulitis or abscess formation. Note gingivostomatitis, perirectal cellulitis, otitis media, and signs of pneumonia and septicemia. Lymphadenopathy, hepatomegaly, and splenomegaly suggest an underlying malignancy or immunodeficiency. Arthritis suggests a collagen vascular disease.

C. A moderately or severely ill child has one or more of the following findings: (1) abnormal nutrition, growth, and development; (2) severe, chronic, or recurrent infec-tion; (3) unexplained hepatosplenomegaly or lymph-adenopathy; (4) signs of collagen vascular disease; (5) immature white blood cells, anemia, or throm-bocytopenia; or (6) a family history of neutropenia or recurrent infection.

D. If the child remains well, another CBC can be obtained in 6 to 8 weeks. If in the interim the child develops signs of moderate or severe illness, a CBC should be obtained sooner. A normal neutrophil count during a febrile illness suggests a benign cause of the neutropenia.

E. Otherwise healthy children with isolated, transient neutropenia discovered during a minor acute illness or routine preoperative screening are at little risk for serious infectious complications. Once a normal count is obtained, no further counts are indicated.

F. Chronic neutropenia may be benign, cyclic, severe, or associated with metabolic or immune diseases. In an otherwise well child obtaining biweekly blood counts for 4 to 6 weeks is indicated to determine whether cyclic neutropenia occurs. Most individuals with cyclic neutropenia become neutropenic every 12 to 21 days and the count remains low for 3 to 10 days, during which time they may have fever, stomatitis, pharyngitis, and cervical adenopathy. If this 4 to 6 week evaluation does not reveal cycling or the child's condition becomes worrisome, hematology consultation is warranted to exclude a more serious etiology for the neutropenia.

References

Atario A, O'Shea J. Risk of infectious complications in well-appearing children with transient neutropenia. Am J Dis Child 1989; 143:973.

Baranski B, Young N. Hematologic consequences of viral infections. Hematol Oncol Clin North Am 1987; 1:167.

Hammond IV W, Price T, Souza L, et al. Treatment of cyclic neutropenia with granulocyte colony–stimulating factor. N Engl J Med 1989; 320:1306.

Jonsson OG, Buchanan GR. Chronic neutropenia during childhood: A 13 year experience in a single institution. Am J Dis Child 1991; 145:232.

Valiaveedan R, Rao S, Miller S, et al. Transient neutropenia of childhood. Clin Pediatr 1987; 26:639.

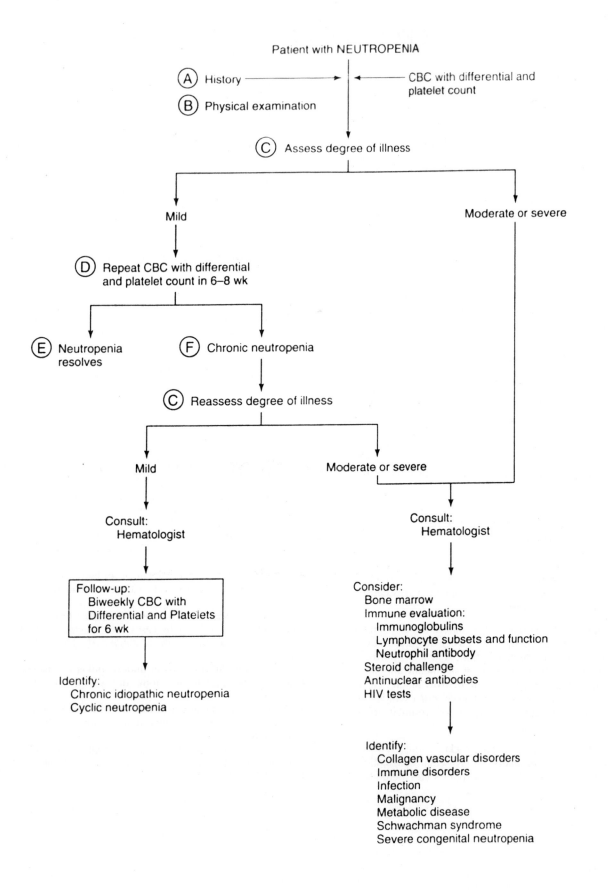

Patient with NEUTROPENIA

(A) History ——————→ | ←————— CBC with differential and platelet count

(B) Physical examination

(C) Assess degree of illness

Mild   Moderate or severe

(D) Repeat CBC with differential and platelet count in 6–8 wk

(E) Neutropenia resolves   (F) Chronic neutropenia

(C) Reassess degree of illness

Mild   Moderate or severe

Consult: Hematologist   Consult: Hematologist

Follow-up:
Biweekly CBC with
Differential and Platelets
for 6 wk

Consider:
  Bone marrow
  Immune evaluation:
    Immunoglobulins
    Lymphocyte subsets and function
    Neutrophil antibody
  Steroid challenge
  Antinuclear antibodies
  HIV tests

Identify:
  Chronic idiopathic neutropenia
  Cyclic neutropenia

Identify:
  Collagen vascular disorders
  Immune disorders
  Infection
  Malignancy
  Metabolic disease
  Schwachman syndrome
  Severe congenital neutropenia

NORMOCYTIC OR MACROCYTIC ANEMIA

Peter A. Lane, M.D.
Rachelle Nuss, M.D.

A. Note symptoms such as jaundice (hemolysis or liver disease), persistent or recurrent fever (chronic infection, juvenile rheumatoid arthritis [JRA], malignancy, human immunodeficiency virus [HIV]), epistaxis or easy bruising (leukemia, aplastic anemia, hemolytic uremic syndrome [HUS]), limp or limb pain (JRA, leukemia, neuroblastoma, sickle cell disease), chronic diarrhea (malabsorption), or acute diarrhea (HUS). Note any medications, such as anticonvulsants (e.g., dilantin, valproate) or antimetabolites (e.g., AZT), that cause anemia. The dietary history may suggest B_{12} or folate deficiency. Obtain a family history of any anemia, jaundice, splenomegaly, and unexplained gallstones (hereditary hemolytic disorders).

B. Document short stature (severe chronic anemia, renal disease, hypothyroidism, Diamond-Blackfan anemia, Fanconi anemia) and microcephaly or congenital anomalies (Fanconi anemia, Diamond-Blackfan anemia). Note signs of systemic diseases such as hypertension or edema (renal disease), petechiae and bruising (leukemia, aplastic anemia, HUS), jaundice (hemolysis or liver disease), generalized lymphadenopathy (JRA, leukemia, HIV), and splenomegaly (leukemia, sickle syndromes, hereditary spherocytosis, liver disease, hypersplenism).

C. Note the mean corpuscular volume (MCV) and use age-adjusted normal values for determining the presence or absence of microcytosis (see p 372) or macrocytosis. Macrocytosis suggests a megaloblastic anemia, a bone marrow failure state (Fanconi anemia, Diamond-Blackfan anemia, preleukemia), liver disease, hypothyroidism, or a significant reticulocytosis caused by hemolysis or hemorrhage.

D. The reticulocyte count helps differentiate anemias caused by increased peripheral red cell destruction from those caused by underproduction. A low or "normal" reticulocyte count in the face of significant anemia is inappropriate and suggests bone marrow failure. However, a low reticulocyte count does *not* exclude hemolysis; hemolytic anemias sometimes present in aplastic or hypoplastic crisis.

E. Review the peripheral smear. Sickle forms, red cell fragmentation (disseminated intravascular coagulation, hemolytic uremic syndrome), or spherocytes (hereditary spherocytosis, autoimmune hemolytic anemia) suggest hemolysis.

F. Consider the possibility of malignancy or aplastic anemia when a low neutrophil and/or platelet count coexists with the anemia of underproduction. A normal or elevated neutrophil and platelet count suggests a pure red cell aplasia.

G. Consult a hematologist/oncologist before performing a bone marrow examination to avoid omitting important special studies (e.g., biopsy, chromosomes, lymphoid markers).

H. Pure red cell aplasia of unknown origin often requires a bone marrow examination. However, if the history, physical examination, and laboratory results are all consistent with transient erythroblastopenia of childhood, the bone marrow examination may be delayed and the child followed closely with weekly examinations and CBCs.

References

Alter BP. Fanconi's anemia: Current concepts. Am J Pediatr Hematol Oncol 1992; 14:170.

Alter BP, Young NS. The bone marrow failure syndromes. In: Nathan DG, Oski FA, eds. Hematology of infancy and childhood. 4th ed. Philadelphia: Saunders, 1993:216.

Boineau FG, Lewy JE, Roy S, et al. Prevalence of anemia and correlations with mild and chronic renal insufficiency. J Pediatr 1990; 116:S60.

Dallman PR, Siimes MA. Percentile curves for hemoglobin and red cell volume in infancy and childhood. J Pediatr 1979; 94:26.

Hays T, Lane PA, Shafer F. Transient erythroblastopenia of childhood: A review of 26 cases and reassessment of indications for bone marrow aspiration. Am J Dis Child 1989; 143:605.

Means RT Jr, Krantz SB. Progress in understanding the pathogenesis of the anemia of chronic disease. Blood 1992; 80:1639.

Meyers PA. Megaloblastic anemias. In: Miller DR, Baehner RL, eds. Blood diseases of infancy and childhood. 6th ed. St. Louis: Mosby, 1989:199.

Scadden DT, Zon LI, Groopman JE. Pathophysiology and management of HIV-associated hematologic disorders. Blood 1989; 74:1455.

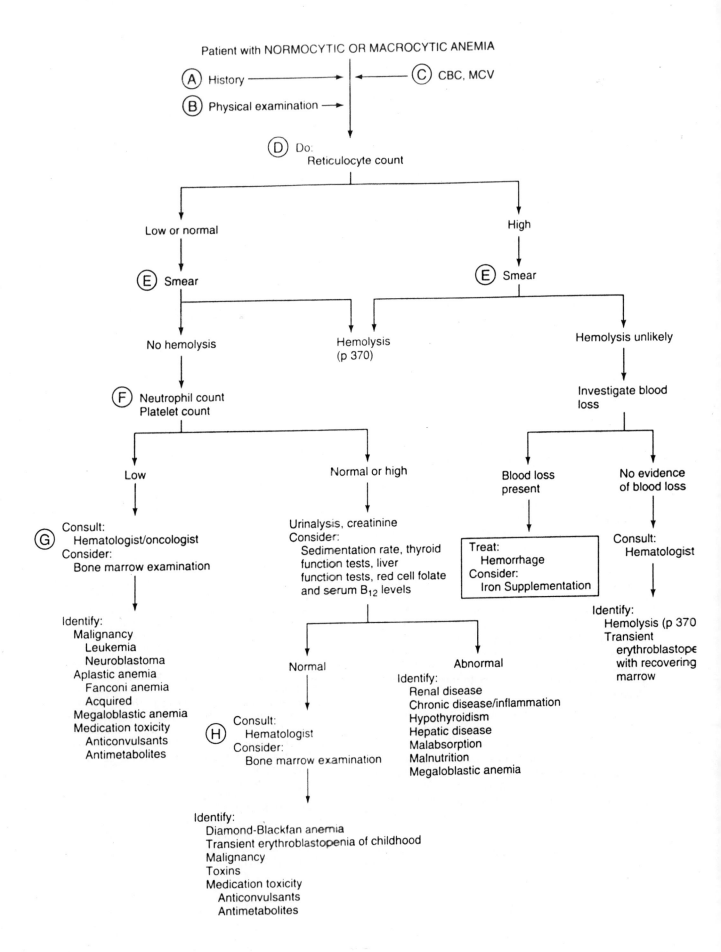

Patient with NORMOCYTIC OR MACROCYTIC ANEMIA

(A) History ————————→   ←———— (C) CBC, MCV

(B) Physical examination ——→

(D) Do:
    Reticulocyte count

Low or normal

(E) Smear

No hemolysis

(F) Neutrophil count
    Platelet count

Low

(G) Consult:
    Hematologist/oncologist
    Consider:
    Bone marrow examination

Identify:
  Malignancy
    Leukemia
    Neuroblastoma
  Aplastic anemia
    Fanconi anemia
    Acquired
  Megaloblastic anemia
  Medication toxicity
    Anticonvulsants
    Antimetabolites

Normal or high

Urinalysis, creatinine
Consider:
  Sedimentation rate, thyroid
  function tests, liver
  function tests, red cell folate
  and serum B$_{12}$ levels

Normal

(H) Consult:
    Hematologist
    Consider:
    Bone marrow examination

Identify:
  Diamond-Blackfan anemia
  Transient erythroblastopenia of childhood
  Malignancy
  Toxins
  Medication toxicity
    Anticonvulsants
    Antimetabolites

Abnormal

Identify:
  Renal disease
  Chronic disease/inflammation
  Hypothyroidism
  Hepatic disease
  Malabsorption
  Malnutrition
  Megaloblastic anemia

**Hemolysis
(p 370)**

High

(E) Smear

Hemolysis unlikely

Investigate blood
loss

**Blood loss
present**

Treat:
  Hemorrhage
Consider:
  Iron Supplementation

**No evidence
of blood loss**

Consult:
  Hematologist

Identify:
  Hemolysis (p 370
  Transient
    erythroblastope
    with recovering
    marrow

THROMBOCYTOPENIA

Peter A. Lane, M.D.
Rachelle Nuss, M.D.

A. In the history ask about the type and duration of bruising, bleeding, or petechiae. Note recent illnesses such as diarrhea (hemolytic uremic syndrome) and sore throat (infectious mononucleosis, acute poststreptococcal glomerulonephritis). Document associated symptoms such as fever (infection, leukemia, collagen vascular disease), limp, and limb pain (leukemia, collagen vascular disease). Note any medications. Obtain a family history of bleeding disorders. Assess risk for HIV or other immunodeficiency disorder.

B. In the physical examination note fever and assess the degree of illness. Acutely ill and toxic-appearing children with thrombocytopenia require expeditious evaluation (disseminated intravascular coagulation [DIC], sepsis, hemolytic-uremic syndrome [HUS], severe hemorrhage). Note the extent and type of manifestations of bleeding. Short stature, microcephaly, skeletal anomalies, hyperpigmentation, hypogenitalism (Fanconi anemia), absent radii with normal thumbs (thrombocytopenia with absent radii), and chronic eczema and recurrent infections in a boy (Wiskott-Aldrich syndrome) are all clues to congenital thrombocytopenia. Splenomegaly or generalized lymphadenopathy suggests leukemia, malignancy, infection such as HIV or infectious mononucleosis, a storage disease, or hypersplenism. Typically, children with idiopathic thrombocytopenic purpura (ITP) do *not* have splenomegaly. Arthritis, mouth ulcers, or a characteristic rash may suggest a collagen vascular disease.

C. Order a CBC with differential and platelet count. The finding of anemia or neutropenia (absolute neutrophil count <1500/mm^3) in association with thrombocytopenia helps direct the subsequent work-up. While neutropenia may occur with infection, its association with significant thrombocytopenia also suggests bone marrow failure. Anemia suggests bone marrow failure, intravascular hemolysis, autoimmune disease, HIV infection, or blood loss secondary to thrombocytopenic bleeding.

D. Review the peripheral blood smear. Red cell fragmentation suggests intravascular hemolysis. Spherocytes (autoimmune hemolysis) or macrocytes (bone marrow failure, Fanconi anemia, or brisk reticulocytosis) are also helpful clues. Note platelet size and morphology. Boys with Wiskott-Aldrich syndrome have tiny platelets; large platelets suggest rapid platelet turnover, as seen in ITP, or a familial thrombocytopenia such as Bernard-Soulier syndrome or May-Hegglin anomaly.

E. Consult a hematologist prior to performing a bone marrow examination to avoid omitting important special studies (biopsy, chromosomes, lymphoid markers). The absence of lymphadenopathy, organomegaly, and leukemic blasts on the blood smear does not exclude leukemia.

F. Although ITP is the most common cause of acute thrombocytopenia in an otherwise well child, other diagnostic possibilities must always be entertained. A positive antinuclear antibody (ANA) or Coombs test indicates other autoantibodies and suggests an underlying collagen vascular disease. The decision to perform a bone marrow examination may be individualized. Children who are thought to have ITP sometimes are observed with serial CBCs and platelet counts. However, if clinical features atypical of ITP (lymphadenopathy, splenomegaly, neutropenia, or anemia) are present or if steroid therapy is planned, a bone marrow evaluation should be performed.

G. Because splenomegaly and lymphadenopathy are unusual in children with ITP, these findings in a child with significant thrombocytopenia (lacking a clear alternative explanation [e.g., long-standing splenomegaly with portal hypertension suggesting hypersplenism or tests indicating HIV infection]) dictate an early bone marrow examination.

References

Baker RC, Seguin JH, Leslie N, et al. Fever and petechiae in children. Pediatrics 1989; 84:1051.

Blanchette V, Imbach P, Andrew M, et al. Randomized trial of intravenous immunoglobulin G, intravenous anti-D, and oral prednisone in childhood acute immune thrombocytopenic purpura. Lancet 1994; 344:703.

Bussel JB. Autoimmune thrombocytopenic purpura. Hematol Oncol Clin North Am 1990; 4:179.

Dubansky AS, Boyett JM, Falletta J, et al. Isolated thrombocytopenia and acute lymphoblastic leukemia. Pediatrics 1989; 84:1068.

Ellaurie M, Burns ER, Bernstein LJ, et al. Thrombocytopenia and human immunodeficiency virus in children. Pediatrics 1988; 82:905.

Halperin DS, Doyle JJ. Is bone marrow examination justified in idiopathic thrombocytopenic purpura? Am J Dis Child 1988; 142:508.

Manco-Johnson MJ. Disseminated intravascular coagulation and other hypercoagulable syndromes. Int J Pediatr Hematol Oncol 1994; 1:1.

Mullen CA, Anderson KD, Blaese RM. Splenectomy and/or bone marrow transplantation in the management of the Wiskott-Aldrich syndrome: Long-term follow-up of 62 cases. Blood 1993; 82:2961.

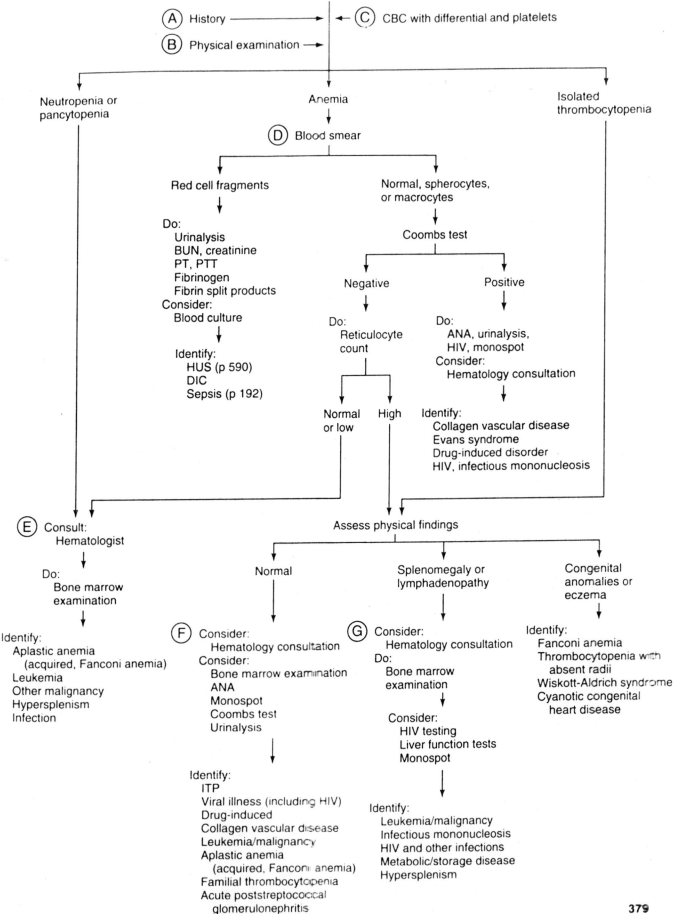

Patient with THROMBOCYTOPENIA

(A) History ⟶ ← (C) CBC with differential and platelets

(B) Physical examination ⟶

Neutropenia or pancytopenia

Anemia

(D) Blood smear

Red cell fragments

Do:
Urinalysis
BUN, creatinine
PT, PTT
Fibrinogen
Fibrin split products
Consider:
Blood culture

Identify:
HUS (p 590)
DIC
Sepsis (p 192)

Normal, spherocytes, or macrocytes

Coombs test

Negative

Do:
Reticulocyte count

Positive

Do:
ANA, urinalysis,
HIV, monospot
Consider:
Hematology consultation

Identify:
Collagen vascular disease
Evans syndrome
Drug-induced disorder
HIV, infectious mononucleosis

Normal or low   **High**

Isolated thrombocytopenia

(E) Consult:
Hematologist

Do:
Bone marrow examination

Identify:
Aplastic anemia
(acquired, Fanconi anemia)
Leukemia
Other malignancy
Hypersplenism
Infection

Assess physical findings

Normal

(F) Consider:
Hematology consultation
Consider:
Bone marrow examination
ANA
Monospot
Coombs test
Urinalysis

Identify:
ITP
Viral illness (including HIV)
Drug-induced
Collagen vascular disease
Leukemia/malignancy
Aplastic anemia
(acquired, Fanconi anemia)
Familial thrombocytopenia
Acute poststreptococcal
glomerulonephritis

Splenomegaly or lymphadenopathy

(G) Consider:
Hematology consultation
Do:
Bone marrow examination

Consider:
HIV testing
Liver function tests
Monospot

Identify:
Leukemia/malignancy
Infectious mononucleosis
HIV and other infections
Metabolic/storage disease
Hypersplenism

Congenital anomalies or eczema

Identify:
Fanconi anemia
Thrombocytopenia with
absent radii
Wiskott-Aldrich syndrome
Cyanotic congenital
heart disease

MUSCULOSKELETAL DISORDERS

EVALUATION OF MUSCULOSKELETAL DISORDERS

Richard C. Fisher, M.D.
Stephen Berman, M.D.

A. In the history ask about systemic factors as well as those pertaining to the specific area of musculoskeletal involvement. Note any precipitating factors such as trauma, systemic illness, bacterial and viral infections, recent immunizations, and overuse. It is important to determine the family's perception of the problem and how it has changed over time. A careful family history should reveal similar or related problems that may have a genetic basis. Predisposing conditions, such as malignancy, immunodeficiency, hemoglobinopathy, osteogenesis imperfecta, and steroid use, are also important. If the disorder is secondary to trauma, determine the type and mechanism of injury and the extent and speed of swelling. Immediate joint swelling suggests a hemarthrosis, which accompanies severe ligament injury and intraarticular fracture. The duration of the symptoms and their change over time are important, especially the way they vary with activities. Many childhood musculoskeletal disorders are not accompanied by pain. Acute trauma and arthritis are usually painful, but overuse syndromes may be painful only with activity. Changes in gait, a limp, and foot problems are often not painful and may only be noticed by observers. Disorders in these categories may be more noticeable at the end of the day, when muscles become fatigued.

B. In the physical examination look for signs of systemic disease, including muscle weakness, abnormal neurologic reflexes, jaundice, enlarged liver or spleen, lymphadenopathy, vaginal discharge, purpura, heart murmurs, bruises, and multiple fractures. The extremity examination includes the vascular system, nerves, skin, muscles, tendons, joints, and bones. The vascular examination includes palpation of the pulses and observation of the color, capillary refill, and temperature of the extremity. Pain with passive stretch of fingers or toes may indicate a forearm or calf compartment syndrome. Note sensation, motor power, and reflexes along with any change in these functions over time. Spasticity, hyperreflexia, and clonus accompany cerebral palsy, a frequent cause of gait changes. Swelling, ecchymosis, abrasions, and point tenderness give clues to underlying injuries. Open wounds accompanying fractures or into joints indicate immediate surgical debridement. Determine the location of all areas of pain and possible joint involvement. The joint examination includes evaluation of active and passive range of motion, presence of effusion, ligamentous stability, and deformity. Loss of motion results from guarding associated with pain or from mechanical impingement resulting from an osteochondral fracture or a cartilage tear. In the presence of acute infection the child usually does not permit any motion of the joint. An effusion is palpable in the region around the joint. In the case of the knee it is most evident on compression of the suprapatellar pouch. Pain with stress of the ligament and no laxity implies a grade I injury. Grade II injuries have moderate laxity with a definite but soft end point to stress. Grade III injuries have total ligament disruption and no resistance when stressed. Ligamentous laxity calls for a stress radiograph to be certain the motion is not occurring through the growth plate. Loss of internal rotation is often the first sign of a hip joint problem.

C. Radiographs are often indicated as an adjunct to the initial evaluation following a careful history and physical examination. These will usually be sufficient for diagnostic purposes. At times special imaging studies may be indicated for a more detailed evaluation. Techniques useful for the musculoskeletal system include the nuclear bone scan (shows areas of increased bone formation and resorption), CT scan (useful for looking at bone detail, as in certain fractures), MRI (allows visualization of bone and soft-tissue, especially the cartilage in the knee and tumors), and ultrasound. The last is used for screening for instability in the newborn hip and evaluating cystic lesions. Other useful techniques include blood and urine examination, synovial fluid analysis, and electromyography and nerve conduction studies.

References

Cackwell GD, Passo MH. Pursuing the source of musculoskeletal pain. Contemp Pediatr 1994; 11:72.

Greene WB, Heckman JD. The clinical measurement of joint motion. Rosemont, IL: American Academy of Orthopaedic Surgeons, 1993.

Holen KJ, Terjesen T, Tegnander A, et al. Ultrasound screening for hip dysplasia in newborns. J Pediatr Orthop 1994; 14:667.

Jackman KV. Acute pediatric orthopedic conditions. Pediatr Ann 1994; 23:240.

Staheli LT. Fundamentals of pediatric orthopedics. New York: Raven Press, 1992.

Tolo VT, Wood B. Pediatric orthopaedics in primary care. Baltimore: Williams & Wilkins, 1993.

Patient with a MUSCULOSKELETAL DISORDER

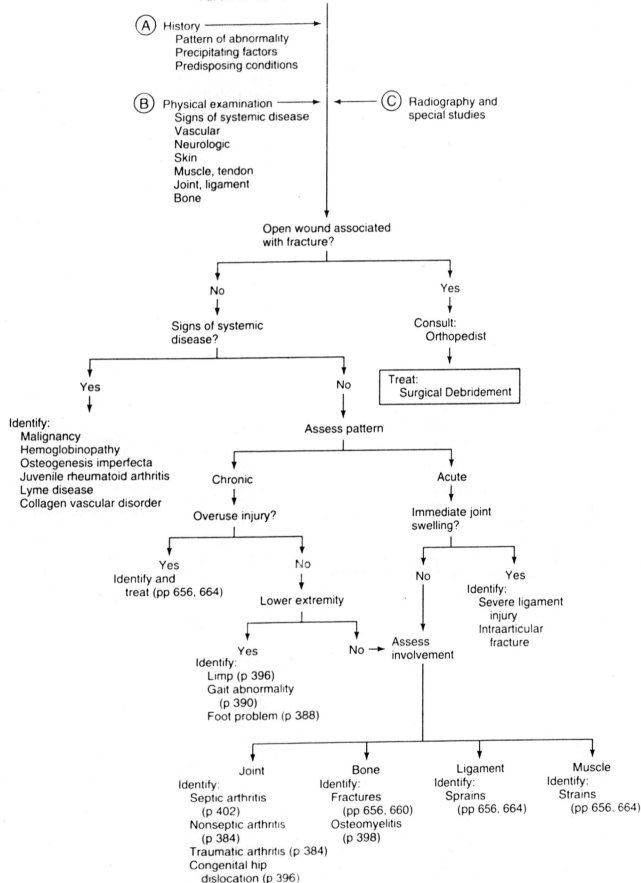

(A) History
    Pattern of abnormality
    Precipitating factors
    Predisposing conditions

(B) Physical examination
    Signs of systemic disease
    Vascular
    Neurologic
    Skin
    Muscle, tendon
    Joint, ligament
    Bone

(C) Radiography and special studies

Open wound associated with fracture?

No

Yes

Signs of systemic disease?

Consult:
    Orthopedist

Treat:
    Surgical Debridement

Yes

No

Identify:
    Malignancy
    Hemoglobinopathy
    Osteogenesis imperfecta
    Juvenile rheumatoid arthritis
    Lyme disease
    Collagen vascular disorder

Assess pattern

Chronic

Acute

Overuse injury?

Immediate joint swelling?

Yes
Identify and treat (pp 656, 664)

No

No

Yes
Identify:
    Severe ligament injury
    Intraarticular fracture

Lower extremity

Yes
Identify:
    Limp (p 396)
    Gait abnormality (p 390)
    Foot problem (p 388)

No →

Assess involvement

Joint
Identify:
    Septic arthritis (p 402)
    Nonseptic arthritis (p 384)
    Traumatic arthritis (p 384)
    Congenital hip dislocation (p 396)

Bone
Identify:
    Fractures (pp 656, 660)
    Osteomyelitis (p 398)

Ligament
Identify:
    Sprains (pp 656, 664)

Muscle
Identify:
    Strains (pp 656, 664)

ARTHRITIS

Stephen Berman, M.D.

Arthritis, an inflammation of a joint space, is associated with joint swelling, pain, and limitation of motion. Causes include rheumatic disorders, infections, reactive effusions, malignancies, trauma, and noninflammatory indications.

A. Determine the time of onset, precipitating factors (trauma, drugs, immunizations, tick bite), duration, pattern of evolution (constant versus intermittent, migratory versus rapidly additive, or slowly cumulative), severity (disruption of normal routine), associated symptoms or illnesses, and family history of arthritis or rheumatic disorders.

B. The CBC with differential may suggest malignancy or sickle cell disease. Anemia or hemolysis may be associated with systemic lupus erythematosus or systemic juvenile rheumatoid arthritis. Leukocytosis is nonspecific and is associated with infection and rheumatoid disorders. Thrombocytosis is consistent with Kawasaki disease. Sedimentation rate greater than 20 mm/hour, C-reactive protein greater than 40 mg/L and temperature higher than 38.5° C suggest acute infection in cases of monoarticular arthritis. An elevated sedimentation rate is a nonspecific finding of inflammation. A normal sedimentation rate does not exclude rheumatoid disease; one third of patients with juvenile rheumatoid arthritis have a normal sedimentation rate.

C. Findings on bone and joint radiographs include effusion, lytic lesions, bone destruction, fracture, periostitis, leukemic lines, avascular necrosis, and osteoporosis. Bone and joint scans can be positive for septic arthritis or osteomyelitis prior to the appearance of radiographic findings.

D. Analyze the effusion from joint aspiration for cell count, differential, glucose, mucin clot formation, Gram stain and counterimmunoelectropheresis. Septic arthritis usually has more than 50,000 WBCs with a predominance of neutrophils (above 90%), a glucose less than 20 mg/100, and a poor mucin clot. Aseptic inflammatory effusions (rheumatoid, postinfectious, and vasculitis) often have 10,000 to 50,000 WBCs with 50% to 80% neutrophils, glucose 20 to 50 mg/100, and a fair to poor mucin clot. Traumatic effusions have fewer than 2000 WBCs with 10% to 30% neutrophils, glucose greater than 50 mg/100, and a good mucin clot. Xanthocromia and crenated red cells suggest old trauma.

E. Signs that suggest systemic disease include jaundice (hepatitis); diarrhea, bloody stools, abdominal pain, perianal disease, and weight loss (bacterial enteritis, inflammatory bowel disease); palpable purpura, abdominal pain, bloody stools, hematuria (Henoch-Schönlein purpura), conjunctivitis, cracked lips, prolonged fever, lymphadenopathy and rash (Kawasaki disease); history of tick bite, erythema chronicum migrans, flulike symptoms, meningeal signs (Lyme disease), iridocyclitis, or carditis (rheumatic disease or vasculitis); hepatosplenomegaly, chronic fevers, weight loss, lymphadenopathy (malignancy); scaly rash and nailbed pitting (psoriasis); polyarthralgias and tendinitis in sexually active adolescents or vaginal discharge, pelvic inflammatory disease (gonorrhea); multiple bruises (coagulation disorders and nonaccidental trauma); and joint hypermobility (Ehlers-Danlos syndrome).

F. Suspect juvenile rheumatoid arthritis when the pattern is symmetric and polyarticular, with cervical spine involvement or arthritis present constantly for more than 6 weeks. Antinuclear antibodies (ANA) are positive in 50% of patients with a pauciarticular pattern. Immunoglobulins and complement are often increased. Uveitis and carditis may be associated findings.

(Continued on page 386)

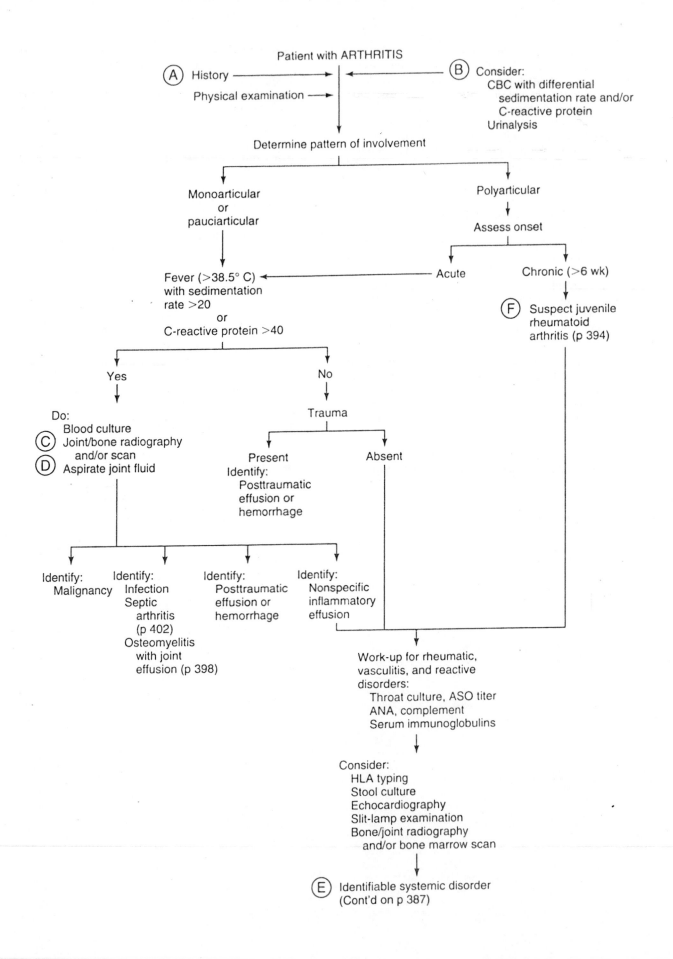

Patient with ARTHRITIS

Ⓐ History ⟶   ⟵ Ⓑ Consider:
                                          CBC with differential
    Physical examination ⟶   sedimentation rate and/or
                                              C-reactive protein
                                          Urinalysis

Determine pattern of involvement

Monoarticular   Polyarticular
or
pauciarticular   Assess onset

Fever (>38.5° C) ⟵   Acute   Chronic (>6 wk)
with sedimentation
rate >20   Ⓕ Suspect juvenile
    or   rheumatoid
C-reactive protein >40   arthritis (p 394)

Yes   No

Do: Trauma
Blood culture
Ⓒ Joint/bone radiography   Present   Absent
    and/or scan   Identify:
Ⓓ Aspirate joint fluid   Posttraumatic
                            effusion or
                            hemorrhage

Identify: Identify: Identify: Identify:
Malignancy   Infection   Posttraumatic   Nonspecific
             Septic   effusion or   inflammatory
             arthritis   hemorrhage   effusion
             (p 402)
             Osteomyelitis
             with joint
             effusion (p 398)

                            Work-up for rheumatic,
                            vasculitis, and reactive
                            disorders:
                                Throat culture, ASO titer
                                ANA, complement
                                Serum immunoglobulins

                            Consider:
                                HLA typing
                                Stool culture
                                Echocardiography
                                Slit-lamp examination
                                Bone/joint radiography
                                    and/or bone marrow scan

                            Ⓔ Identifiable systemic disorder
                                (Cont'd on p 387)

G. An ANA titer greater than 1:80 suggests systemic lupus erythematosus (SLE). The diagnosis of SLE requires the presence of at least four of the following findings: butterfly rash, discoid lesions, alopecia, Raynaud's phenomenon, photosensitivity, oral or nasal pharyngeal ulceration, arthritis, lupus erythematosus cells, false-positive VDRL, proteinuria, urine cellular casts, pleuritis or pericarditis, seizures or psychosis, hemolytic anemia, leukopenia, or thrombocytopenia. Work up suspected SLE with complement, anti-DNA antibodies, and urinalysis.

H. The diagnosis of rheumatic fever requires two major Jones criteria or one major and two minor criteria with evidence of an antecedent streptococcal infection (positive culture, antistreptolysin O [ASO] titer, or scarlet fever). The major Jones criteria include carditis, migratory polyarthritis, chorea, erythema marginatum, and subcutaneous nodules. The minor criteria are fever, arthralgia, prior rheumatic fever, elevated erythrocyte sedimentation rate or C-reactive protein, and a prolonged P-R interval.

I. Ankylosing spondylitis presents in adolescents as intermittent peripheral arthritis associated with chronic low-back pain, sacroiliitis, and limited back and/or chest range of motion. Some 90% of cases in whites are HLA B27–positive. Intermittent episodes of iritis can occur.

J. Reactive arthritis is present when an infection produces a sterile inflammatory effusion in a joint separate from the focus of infection. Organisms that produce reactive arthritis include *Shigella, Salmonella, Yersinia, Campylobacter, Chlamydia,* group A *Streptococcus, Meningococcus, Neisseria gonorrhoeae,* and viruses such as rubella, mumps, influenza, adenovirus, herpesvirus, and hepatitis B.

K. Serum sickness reactions with arthritis can occur with many drugs especially penicillins and cephalosporins (Cefaclor).

L. Toxic or transient synovitis, usually involving the hip, often presents with a painful limp and referred pain to the knee in children between 4 and 9 years of age. Low-grade fever and a slightly elevated sedimentation rate may present. The arthritis normally resolves within 2 weeks. Aseptic necrosis is a rare complication.

References

Brewer EJ, Gedalia A. The child with joint pain: An algorithmic approach. Contemp Pediatr 1985; 2:18.

Fink CW. Reactive arthritis. Pediatr Infect Dis 1988; 7:58.

Kunnamo I, Kallio P, Pelkonen P, et al. Clinical signs and laboratory tests in the differential diagnosis of arthritis in children. Am J Dis Child 1987; 141:34.

Petty RE, Tingle AJ. Arthritis and viral infection. J Pediatr 1988; 113:948.

Rennebohm RM. Rheumatic diseases of childhood. Pediatr Rev 1988; 10D:183.

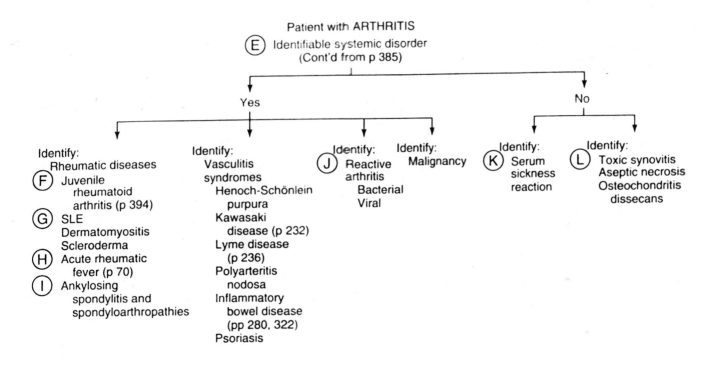

Patient with ARTHRITIS

Ⓔ Identifiable systemic disorder
(Cont'd from p 385)

Yes

Identify:
Rheumatic diseases
Ⓕ Juvenile
    rheumatoid
    arthritis (p 394)
Ⓖ SLE
    Dermatomyositis
    Scleroderma
Ⓗ Acute rheumatic
    fever (p 70)
Ⓘ Ankylosing
    spondylitis and
    spondyloarthropathies

Identify:
Vasculitis
syndromes
    Henoch-Schönlein
    purpura
    Kawasaki
    disease (p 232)
    Lyme disease
    (p 236)
    Polyarteritis
    nodosa
    Inflammatory
    bowel disease
    (pp 280, 322)
    Psoriasis

Identify:
Ⓙ Reactive
    arthritis
    Bacterial
    Viral

Identify:
Malignancy

No

Identify:
Ⓚ Serum
    sickness
    reaction

Identify:
Ⓛ Toxic synovitis
    Aseptic necrosis
    Osteochondritis
    dissecans

FOOT PAIN

Richard C. Fisher, M.D.
Stephen Berman, M.D.

A.   In the physical examination observe the foot with and without weight bearing and the child's gait with and without shoes. A skin or soft-tissue abnormality, such as plantar warts, paronychia, or subungual exostosis, may be the primary problem. Other abnormalities, including blisters and bursae, may be manifestations of underlying structural changes. The foot may appear structurally normal or show obvious abnormality. In either case, if superficial causes for pain are excluded, radiography will aid further evaluation. Although rare, tumor and infection should be ruled out.

B.   A bunion may appear in the adolescent and is usually not symptomatic. Pain, when present, arises over the first metatarsal head as a result of irritation from shoe wear. When present at this age, the hallux valgus deformity (lateral deviation of the great toe) is often secondary to a primary metatarsus varus medial deviation. Standing radiographs are most helpful in evaluating this deformity. Bunionette (tailor's bunion) is a similar deformity of the fifth toe. Treatment consists of altering shoe wear to relieve metatarsal head pressure; postpone surgery as long as possible.

C.   The most common fractures occur in the toes and metatarsals. With little or no displacement these can be treated with a firm-soled shoe or a walking cast until they are no longer tender and new bone is evident on x-rays. Displaced fractures should be reduced, especially if the growth plate is involved. Other nondisplaced fractures can be treated in a cast, but displaced fractures of the calcaneus and talus should be referred for consultation.

D.   Physiologic flatfeet result from a fat pad in the arch of neonates, which disappears by 2 to 3 years of age. Flexible flatfeet, the most common variety, are often familial and may be accompanied by loose joints generally. Examination of the foot in a non–weight bearing position and with toe-walking yields a normal arch in a flexible flatfoot. Treatment consisting of molded heel cups or scaphoid pads should be reserved for severe deformity of symptomatic feet. Rigid flatfeet cannot be passively corrected. They result from either a congenital vertical talus or a tarsal coalition. Vertical talus is usually associated with neuromuscular abnormalities such as arthrogryposis and myelodysplasia. Treatment is surgical. Tarsal coalitions result from a cartilage and eventually a bony bridge between tarsal bones. Most commonly, the calcaneal and navicular bones are involved, and an oblique radiograph of the foot is necessary for diagnosis. Treatment initially should be a trial of plaster, supportive shoes, or activity change. Surgery for resection of the bar or fusion may eventually be indicated for persistent symptoms. The high-arched (calcaneocavus) foot is frequently the result of a central or peripheral neurologic abnormality. Polio is the most common cause worldwide, but other more subtle and progressive causes should be ruled out. Treat foot pain with shoe alterations and inserts. With progression, surgical correction will be necessary.

E.   Kohler disease and Freiberg infarction are both considered to be ischemic necrosis of the tarsal navicular and the second metatarsal head respectively. Both present as pain about the involved bone, and radiographs are usually diagnostic. Treatment consists of restricting activity initially; plaster may be needed for persistent symptoms. Osteochondritis dissecans of the talus commonly involves the medial corner of the talar dome and manifests as pain, joint swelling, and occasionally locking if the fragment becomes mobile. For early cases with a stable fragment, immobilization will be sufficient to allow the process to resolve. If locking occurs, surgery is usually necessary.

F.   Stress fractures are characterized by pain with activity and by point tenderness. A recent increase in activity is frequent. The metatarsals are a common site of stress injuries. Initial radiographs may be normal; the bone scan will be positive earlier. Pain over the Achilles tendon and its insertion into the os calcis apophysis (Sever syndrome) results from a combination of a tight gastrocsoleus mechanism and overuse. Pain at the insertion of the posterior tibial tendon occurs in the presence of an accessory navicular, usually following minimal trauma or overuse. A mass over the medial aspect of the foot distal to the medial malleolus suggests an accessory navicular bone.

References

Coleman SS. Complex foot deformities in children. Philadelphia: Lea & Febiger, 1983.

Staheli LT. Fundamentals of pediatric orthopedics. New York: Raven Press, 1992.

Tolo VT, Wood B. Pediatric orthopaedics in primary care. Baltimore: Williams & Wilkins, 1993.

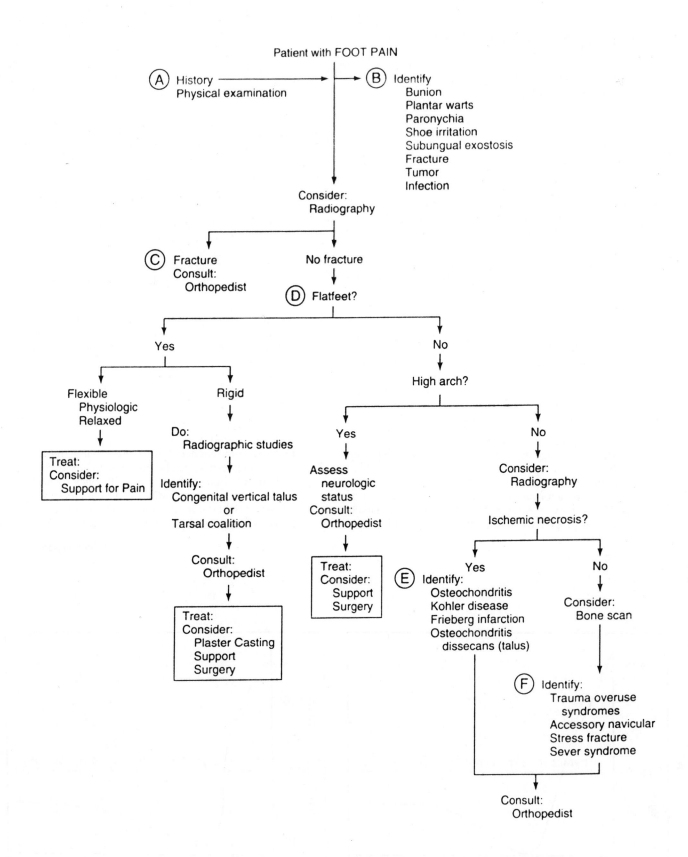

Patient with FOOT PAIN

(A) History ⟶ (B) Identify
Physical examination   Bunion
       Plantar warts
       Paronychia
       Shoe irritation
       Subungual exostosis
       Fracture
       Tumor
       Infection

Consider:
Radiography

(C) Fracture   No fracture
Consult:
Orthopedist

(D) Flatfeet?

Yes   No

Flexible   Rigid   High arch?
Physiologic
Relaxed

        Do: Yes   No
        Radiographic studies

| Treat: |
| Consider: |
| Support for Pain |

Assess   Consider:
        Identify: neurologic   Radiography
        Congenital vertical talus   status
        or   Consult:
        Tarsal coalition   Orthopedist   Ischemic necrosis?

        Consult:
        Orthopedist   Yes   No

| Treat: |
| Consider: |
| Support |
| Surgery |

(E) Identify:
    Osteochondritis
    Kohler disease
    Frieberg infarction
    Osteochondritis
       dissecans (talus)

Consider:
Bone scan

| Treat: |
| Consider: |
| Plaster Casting |
| Support |
| Surgery |

(F) Identify:
    Trauma overuse
       syndromes
    Accessory navicular
    Stress fracture
    Sever syndrome

Consult:
Orthopedist

GAIT ABNORMALITIES

Richard C. Fisher, M.D.
Stephen Berman, M.D.

A. Observe the child walking toward and away from you. Observe the angle the thigh makes with the calf at the knee, the tibiofemoral angle. It varies with age and changes with growth (Fig. 1). Until the child is 18 months of age, it is normally in varus angulation. By age 2 to 3 years valgus angulation develops to an average of 12 degrees. With further growth it gradually declines to the adult value of about 8 degrees.

B. With the child standing or supine measure varus angulation (bow-legs) along the major axis of the femur to the midpatella and distally to the center of the ankle joint. Until 18 months of age, 15 degrees of varus angulation is within the normal range. Significant varus angulation persisting beyond 2 years of age needs further evaluation and possibly surgical correction. Causes include Blount disease, rickets, and injury to the growth plate from infection or trauma. A second peak incidence of genu varum in the teens results from adolescent Blount disease. It is most common in black children, is often unilateral, and usually requires surgical correction.

C. Valgus angulation (knock-knees) is measured the same way as varus angulation. However, it is best measured with the child bearing weight. In children less than 6 years of age values up to 15 degrees are normal. Progressive deformity beyond 6 years and unilateral deformity require further evaluation. The most likely causes of progressive valgus angulation include meta-bolic bone disease (renal disease), paralysis, and trauma to the proximal tibia.

D. Toe walking (equinus) results from either a fixed or a functional deformity. It is the sign of a tight heel cord. A tight Achilles tendon will not yield to passive stretch. If the tendon is tight but yields slowly, look for other signs of spasticity such as clonus and hyperactive reflexes. If the tendon has normal passive motion, consider habitual toe walking, usually seen in a patient 1 to 3 years of age. This gait pattern is self-limiting without treatment.

E. Assess the angle of the foot with the straight line of progression, the foot progression angle (Fig. 2). Define toeing in as a negative angle and toeing out as a positive angle. A normal foot progression angle is 0 to +30 degrees (Fig. 3). Note the position of the patella. Medial deviation indicates the problem may be above the knee.

F. Signs of metatarsus adductus or medial deviation of the forefoot include convexity of the lateral border of the foot and a prominence at the base of the fifth metatarsal. A flexible deformity can be treated with home exercises and an outflared (abductor) shoe. Inability to overcorrect the later convexity easily and a fixed crease suggest a fixed or rigid deformity. These children require serial plaster casting followed by braces or abductor shoes.

(Continued on page 392)

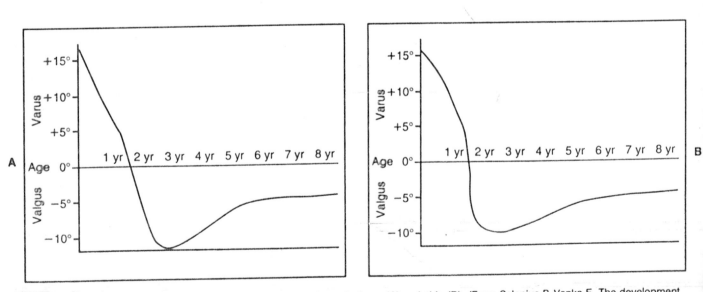

Figure 1 Tibiofemoral angle in children. Mean values are shown for boys **(A)** and girls **(B)**. (From Salenius P, Vanka E. The development of tibiofemoral angle in children. J Bone Joint Surg 1975; 57A:259; with permission.)

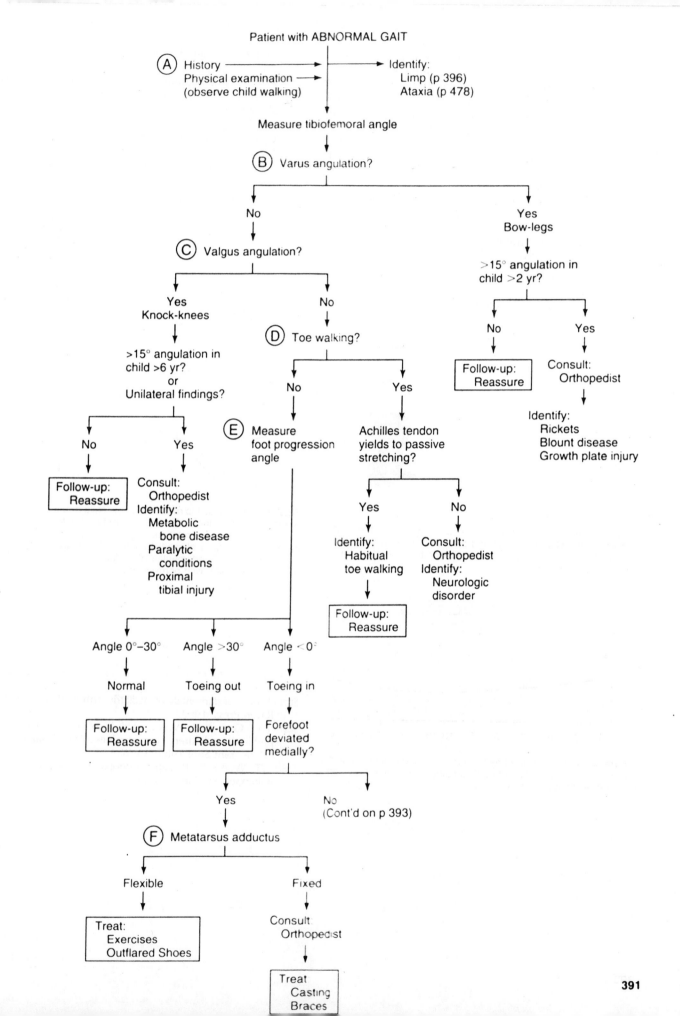

Patient with ABNORMAL GAIT

Ⓐ History ⟶
Physical examination ⟶
(observe child walking)

Identify:
Limp (p 396)
Ataxia (p 478)

Measure tibiofemoral angle

Ⓑ Varus angulation?

No

Ⓒ Valgus angulation?

Yes
Knock-knees

>15° angulation in
child >6 yr?
or
Unilateral findings?

No

Follow-up:
Reassure

Yes

Consult:
Orthopedist
Identify:
Metabolic
bone disease
Paralytic
conditions
Proximal
tibial injury

No

Ⓓ Toe walking?

No

Ⓔ Measure
foot progression
angle

Yes

Achilles tendon
yields to passive
stretching?

Yes

Identify:
Habitual
toe walking

Follow-up:
Reassure

No

Consult:
Orthopedist
Identify:
Neurologic
disorder

Yes
Bow-legs

>15° angulation in
child >2 yr?

No

Follow-up:
Reassure

Yes

Consult:
Orthopedist

Identify:
Rickets
Blount disease
Growth plate injury

Angle 0°–30°

Normal

Follow-up:
Reassure

Angle >30°

Toeing out

Follow-up:
Reassure

Angle <0°

Toeing in

Forefoot
deviated
medially?

Yes

Ⓕ Metatarsus adductus

Flexible

Treat:
Exercises
Outflared Shoes

Fixed

Consult:
Orthopedist

Treat:
Casting
Braces

No
(Cont'd on p 393)

391

G. Internal tibial torsion is common in children under 2 years of age, and it changes to external rotation with normal growth. The extent of internal tibial torsion can be estimated by measuring the angle formed by the axis of the thigh and the foot with child prone and the knee flexed to 90 degrees. The normal range of this angle is between 0 and 30 degrees of external rotation. A severe degree of internal torsion produces an awkward gait and seems to cause affected children to trip over their toes, especially when they are tired. Mild deformities will correct spontaneously; correction may be hastened in young children by preventing them from sitting and sleeping with the feet turned out. A Denis Browne splint may help these children. Rarely, older children need corrective osteotomy.

H. Femoral anteversion produces toeing in because of excessive internal rotation of the hip. Assess the degree of rotation of the hip with the child prone, the pelvis flat on the table, and the hips in a neutral position (Fig. 4). Allow each leg to drop by gravity into full internal and external rotation. Internal rotation should not exceed 70 degrees; the sum of internal and external rotation should approximate 100 degrees. Femoral anteversion should correct spontaneously. The parents should encourage the child to sit cross-legged. Exercises, braces, and orthopedic shoes are not indicated. Consider derotational osteotomy (major surgery) only in children older than 8 years with severe deformity.

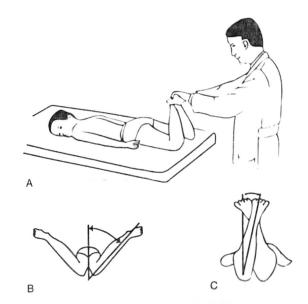

A

B

C

Figure 4 A, Assess hip rotation with the child prone and the knees flexed to a right angle. Allow the legs to fall into a comfortable maximum position in rotation. Level the pelvis and estimate or measure the degree of medial rotation (B) or lateral rotation (C). (From Staheli LT. Fundamentals of pediatric orthopedics. New York: Raven Press, 1992; with permission.)

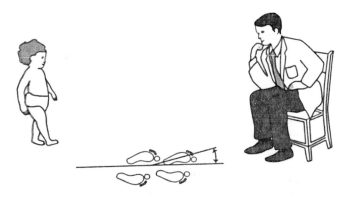

Figure 2 The foot progression angle is the average of the angles formed by the axis of the foot and the line of progression. (From Staheli LT. Fundamentals of pediatric orthopedics. New York: Raven Press, 1992; with permission.)

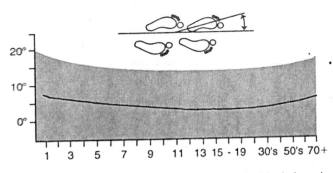

Figure 3 Normal range of foot progression angle (shaded area). (From Staheli LT. Fundamentals of pediatric orthopedics. New York: Raven Press, 1992; with permission.)

References

Craig CL, Goldberg MJ. Foot and leg problems. Pediatr Rev 1993; 14:395.

Staheli LT. Fundamentals of pediatric orthopedics. New York: Raven Press, 1992.

Staheli LT, Corbett M, Wyss C, et al. Lower extremity rotational problems in children: Normal values to guide management. J Bone Joint Surg 1985; 39:67-A.

Tolo VT, Wood B. Pediatric orthopaedics in primary care. Baltimore: Williams & Wilkins, 1993.

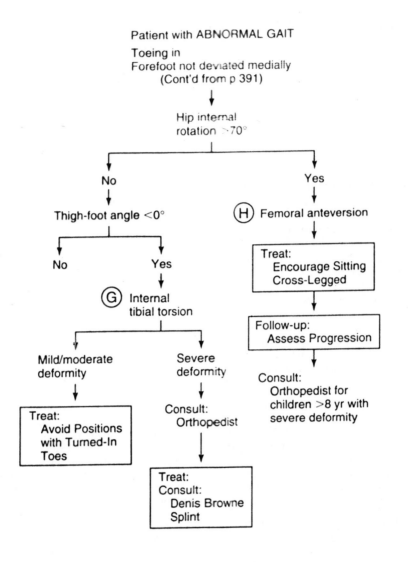

Patient with ABNORMAL GAIT
Toeing in
Forefoot not deviated medially
(Cont'd from p 391)

Hip internal
rotation >70°

No

Thigh-foot angle <0°

No　　Yes

Ⓖ Internal
tibial torsion

Mild/moderate
deformity

Treat:
　Avoid Positions
　with Turned-In
　Toes

Severe
deformity

Consult:
　Orthopedist

Treat:
Consult:
　Denis Browne
　Splint

Yes

Ⓗ Femoral anteversion

Treat:
　Encourage Sitting
　Cross-Legged

Follow-up:
　Assess Progression

Consult:
　Orthopedist for
　children >8 yr with
　severe deformity

JUVENILE RHEUMATOID ARTHRITIS

Stephen Berman, M.D.

CLASSIFICATION

History, physical examination, and laboratory screening are intended to sort children into one of three forms of juvenile rheumatoid arthritis (JRA): systemic, pauciarticular, and polyarticular. Systemic JRA is characterized by spiking fever, hepatosplenomegaly, lymphadenopathy, pericarditis, and cervical spine involvement. The pauciarticular form presents with a history of asymmetric arthritis for more than 72 hours and is often associated with positive antinuclear antibody (ANA) results and/or HLA B27 antigen. Iridocyclitis is most frequently associated with this type of JRA. The polyarticular form is subdivided into rheumatoid factor seronegative and seropositive disease. Seronegative disease has a more favorable prognosis and is characterized by symmetric polyarthritis, low-grade fever, mild anemia, moderate hepatosplenomegaly, and a positive ANA in 25% of cases. Seropositive disease has a poor prognosis and is characterized by destructive symmetric polyarthritis, rheumatoid nodules, and a positive ANA in 75% of cases.

A. In mild cases of JRA the child is afebrile and experiences mild pain with minimal limitation of activity. Moderate involvement is characterized by recurrent fevers and pain with moderate limitation of activity. In severe JRA the child has incapacitating fever, anemia, iridocyclitis, pericarditis, or incapacitating pain. Patients with severe illness may develop hemorrhagic, hepatic, and neurologic manifestations.

B. Salicylate therapy should be instituted and therapeutic blood levels of 20 to 30 mg/100 ml documented (Table 1). Liver function tests should be followed during therapy. A good response is achieved when fever is controlled and pain, joint swelling, and range of motion improve. Definite improvement should occur in 2 to 6 weeks. Treat iridocyclitis with topical steroids. Muscle atrophy and leg length discrepancies may be sequelae of pauciarticular disease, especially of the knee.

C. Use alternative antiinflammatory agents when the desired therapeutic response is not achieved. Consider ibuprofen, naproxen, and tolmetin. Failure of these agents to relieve symptoms sufficiently to allow an acceptable routine is an indication to consider gold therapy, hydroxychloroquine, or possibly steroids or immunosuppressive agents.

D. If symptoms of severe disease (pericarditis, severe anemia, high fever, iridocyclitis) persist with salicylate therapy, consider starting prednisone after obtaining a bone marrow biopsy to rule out occult malignancy. Persistence of systemic symptoms and thrombocytopenia longer than 6 months is associated with an increased risk of developing destructive arthritis. Use systemic steroids with great caution because of their adverse effects on bone mineralization.

References

American Academy of Pediatrics Section on Rheumatology and Section on Ophthalmology. Guidelines for the ophthalmologic examinations in children with juvenile rheumatoid arthritis. Pediatrics 1993; 92:295.

Eichenfield AH, Athreya BH, Doughty RA, Cebul RD. Utility of rheumatoid factor in the diagnosis of juvenile rheumatoid arthritis. Pediatrics 1986; 78:480.

Manners PJ, Ansell BM. Slow-acting antirheumatic drug use in systemic onset juvenile chronic arthritis. Pediatrics 1986; 77:99.

Ostrov BE, Goldsmith DP, Athreya BH. Differentiation of systemic juvenile rheumatoid arthritis from acute leukemia near the onset of disease. J Pediatr 1993; 122:595.

Schneider R, Lang BA, Reilly BJ, et al. Prognostic indicators of joint destruction in systemic-onset juvenile rheumatoid arthritis. J Pediatr 1992; 120:200.

Vostrejs M, Hollister JR. Muscle atrophy and leg length discrepancies in pauciarticular juvenile rheumatoid arthritis. Am J Dis Child 1988; 142:343.

TABLE 1 Drugs Used for the Treatment of Juvenile Rheumatoid Arthritis

Drug	Dosage	Product Availability
Aspirin	Initial: 60 mg/kg/24 hr divided q6–8h p.r.n.; increase 20/mg/kg/24 hr after 5–7 days, then increase 10 mg/kg/24 hr at 5–7 day intervals to max 100 mg/kg/24 hr (therapeutic level 15–30 mg/dl)	Caps: 325 mg Tabs: 65, 81, 325, 500, 650 mg
Gold sodium thiomalate	1 mg/kg IM qwk with 0.1 ml 1% lidocaine (max 50 mg)	Injectable: 10, 25, 50 mg/ml
Hydroxychloroquine sulfate	3–5 mg/kg/24 hr qd or b.i.d. (max 7 mg/kg/24 hr or 400 mg/24 hr)	Tabs: 200 mg
Ibuprofen (Advil, Medeprin, Motrin, Nuprin)	30–50 mg/kg/24 hr divided t.i.d. or q.i.d. (max 2.4 g/kg/24 hr)	Tabs: 200, 300, 400, 600, 800 mg
Naproxen (Naprosyn)	Initial: 10 mg/kg/24 hr divided b.i.d. (max 1 g/24 hr)	Liquid: 125 mg/5 ml Tabs: 250, 375, 500 mg
Prednisone	0.2–2 mg/kg/24 hr divided b.i.d.	Tabs: 1, 2.5, 5, 10, 20, 50 mg Syrup: 5 mg/5 ml
Tolmetin sodium (Tolectin)	Initial: 15 mg/kg/24 hr divided t.i.d. p.r.n.; increase 5 mg/kg/24 hr after 5–7 days (max 30 mg/kg/24 hr)	Tabs: 200, 600 mg Caps: 400 mg

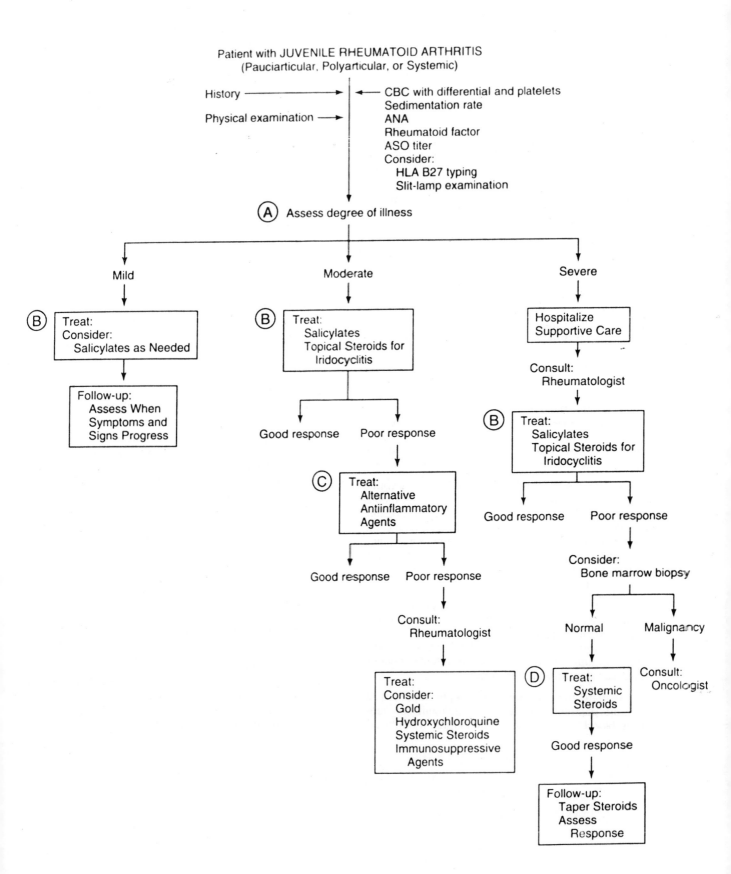

Patient with JUVENILE RHEUMATOID ARTHRITIS
(Pauciarticular, Polyarticular, or Systemic)

History ⟶

Physical examination ⟶

CBC with differential and platelets
Sedimentation rate
ANA
Rheumatoid factor
ASO titer
Consider:
    HLA B27 typing
    Slit-lamp examination

(A) Assess degree of illness

Mild

Moderate

Severe

(B) Treat:
Consider:
    Salicylates as Needed

Follow-up:
    Assess When
    Symptoms and
    Signs Progress

(B) Treat:
    Salicylates
    Topical Steroids for
    Iridocyclitis

Good response   Poor response

(C) Treat:
    Alternative
    Antiinflammatory
    Agents

Good response   Poor response

Consult:
    Rheumatologist

Treat:
Consider:
    Gold
    Hydroxychloroquine
    Systemic Steroids
    Immunosuppressive
        Agents

Hospitalize
Supportive Care

Consult:
    Rheumatologist

(B) Treat:
    Salicylates
    Topical Steroids for
    Iridocyclitis

Good response   Poor response

Consider:
    Bone marrow biopsy

Normal   Malignancy

(D) Treat:
    Systemic
    Steroids

Consult:
    Oncologist

Good response

Follow-up:
    Taper Steroids
    Assess
        Response

LIMP

Richard C. Fisher, M.D.
Stephen Berman, M.D.

A. The characteristics of limps vary with the cause. A limp caused by pain (antalgic gait) has a short stride length on the uninvolved limb and decreased support time on the painful limb. An antalgic gait secondary to spine infection (diskitis or osteomyelitis) will be slow and cautious to avoid jarring motions. Painless limps result from neuromuscular abnormalities or a difference in leg lengths. Foot slap at heel strike is secondary to peroneal nerve weakness. A crouched gait can result from hip and knee contractures or spasticity if the foot is also in the equinus position. An equinus gait can also be seen in idiopathic toe walkers and patients with club feet. A Trendelenburg gait is characterized by a drop of the opposite side of the pelvis with weight bearing on the involved limb. It is seen commonly with hip abductor weakness or hip joint pain and instability. Hip abnormalities that cause a limp generally can be grouped by age. The most common problems in the 1 to 3 year old child are congenital hip abnormalities and septic arthritis, and in the 4 to 10 year old child be alert for leg length differences, toxic synovitis, and Legg-Calve-Perthes syndrome. Slipped capital femoral epiphyses, stress fractures, osteochondritis dissecans, and hip dysplasia become symptomatic at 11 to 16 years of age.

B. Unequal leg lengths can be measured clinically with a tape from the anterosuperior iliac spine to the medial malleolus or more accurately by x-ray scanogram. Congenital abnormalities of the proximal femur include bony malformations (coxa vara, focal deficiencies) and dislocation of the hip. These are associated with asymmetry of the buttock and thigh creases, unequal leg lengths if unilateral, and a Trendelenburg gait.

C. Causes of myalgia and arthralgia that produce limp include trauma, recent immunization, viral infections (coxsackie, influenza), bacterial infections, trichinosis, toxoplasmosis, and collagen vascular diseases (dermatomyositis, lupus erythematosus, polyarteritis nodosa, rheumatoid arthritis, polymyositis).

D. Differentiate toxic synovitis from septic hip. Usually systemic parameters such as the sedimentation rate, white blood count, and fever are helpful. If doubt still exists, aspiration is indicated. The synovitis will spontaneously resolve with protection of the hip through bed rest and crutch walking. Weight-bearing activities are permitted when the hip regains full motion without pain. Stress fractures occur in older patients, and the bone scan will be positive before radiographic changes are seen.

E. Aseptic necrosis of the proximal femoral epiphysis (Legg-Calve-Perthes syndrome) and slipped capital femoral epiphysis both begin as a painless limp but usually have become symptomatic by the time the patient seeks medical care. Anteroposterior and lateral radiographs of both hips are important to the diagnosis. The treatment of Aseptic necrosis is complex, requiring a period of non–weight-bearing and range-of-motion exercises possibly followed by bracing or surgery. Slipping of the proximal femoral epiphysis is a surgical emergency; the patient should immediately begin bed rest with traction until the epiphysis can be stabilized with pin fixation.

F. Hip dysplasia leads to degenerative changes in the involved hip joint late in adolescence. This, like osteochondritis dissecans of the hip, appears as pain following activities. As with many abnormalities of the hip, the first symptoms may be knee pain and loss of internal rotation of the hip joint. Initial treatment for both problems consists of rest and antiinflammatory medication. Surgery is indicated if the response is poor.

References

Henrickson M, Passo MH. Recognizing patterns in chronic limb pain. Contemp Pediatr 1994; 11:33.

Phillips WA. The child with a limp. Orthop Clin North Am 1987; 18:489.

Staheli LT. Fundamentals of pediatric orthopedics. New York: Raven Press, 1992.

Todd FN, Lamoreuax LW, Skinner SR. Variation in the gait of normal children. J Bone Joint Surg 1989; 71-A:196.

Tolo VT, Wood B. Pediatric orthopaedics in primary care. Baltimore: Williams & Wilkins, 1993.

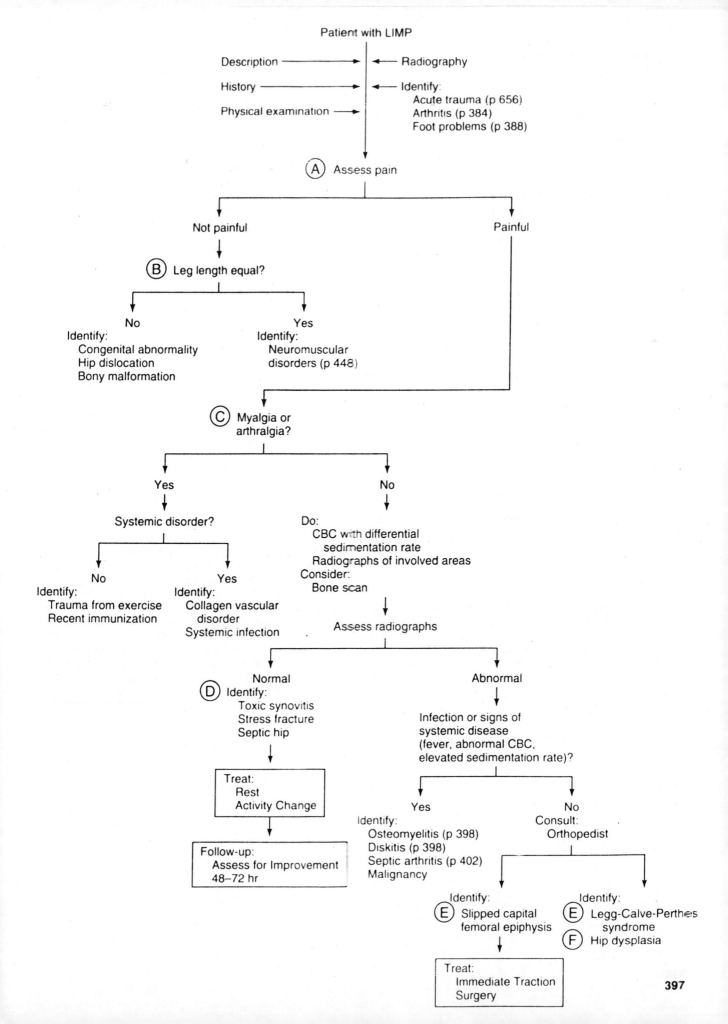

Patient with LIMP

Description ——————→ ←—————— Radiography

History ——————→ ←—————— Identify:
Acute trauma (p 656)
Arthritis (p 384)
Physical examination ——————→ Foot problems (p 388)

Ⓐ Assess pain

Not painful / Painful

Ⓑ Leg length equal?

No
Identify:
Congenital abnormality
Hip dislocation
Bony malformation

Yes
Identify:
Neuromuscular
disorders (p 448)

Ⓒ Myalgia or
arthralgia?

Yes

No
Do:
CBC with differential
sedimentation rate
Radiographs of involved areas
Consider:
Bone scan

Systemic disorder?

No
Identify:
Trauma from exercise
Recent immunization

Yes
Identify:
Collagen vascular
disorder
Systemic infection

Assess radiographs

Normal
Ⓓ Identify:
Toxic synovitis
Stress fracture
Septic hip

Treat:
Rest
Activity Change

Follow-up:
Assess for Improvement
48–72 hr

Abnormal

Infection or signs of
systemic disease
(fever, abnormal CBC,
elevated sedimentation rate)?

Yes
Identify:
Osteomyelitis (p 398)
Diskitis (p 398)
Septic arthritis (p 402)
Malignancy

No
Consult:
Orthopedist

Identify:
Ⓔ Slipped capital
femoral epiphysis

Identify:
Ⓔ Legg-Calve-Perthes
syndrome
Ⓕ Hip dysplasia

Treat:
Immediate Traction
Surgery

397

OSTEOMYELITIS

Richard C. Fisher, M.D.
Stephen Berman, M.D.

DEFINITIONS

Osteomyelitis is a bacterial infection of bone. In children it occurs most frequently as acute or subacute hematogenous infection but may result from open trauma, puncture wound or bite, or contiguous infection in a joint or the skin. The metaphyseal regions of the tibia, femur, and humerus are the long bones most often affected. The calcaneus and talus are also frequently involved. Neonatal osteomyelitis is associated with a septic arthritis in 75% of cases. It may involve multiple sites and will cross the epiphyseal plate to damage the secondary ossification center. **Subacute osteomyelitis** differs from the acute form by having a longer duration of symptoms, less severe systemic signs and symptoms, and positive radiographic findings on presentation. It may follow a short course of antibiotics given for an infection remote from bone.

ETIOLOGY

Hematogenous infections are caused predominantly by *Staphylococcus aureus* (50% of cases), *Haemophilus influenzae* type B (5%), group A streptococcus, *Streptococcus pneumoniae,* and *Bacteroides.* In the neonate group B streptococcus (GBS), *H. influenzae,* and gram-negative species are common in addition to *S. aureus.* Be alert for *Salmonella* in patients with sickle cell disease and *Pseudomonas aeruginosa* after puncture wounds of the foot.

A. A 2 to 4 day history of fever, malaise, refusal to bear weight or move the extremity, and localized pain suggest acute hematogenous osteomyelitis. Preceding respiratory tract infections (75%) and trauma (25%) are common. Local signs include swelling, warmth, and tenderness over the metaphyseal region of the bone. Passive joint motion in this disorder should be only minimally painful, in contrast to that in septic arthritis.

B. A WBC above 15,000 is present about a third of the time, and erythrocyte sedimentation rate (ESR) is above 15 in 90% of children with acute osteomyelitis. Radiographic changes of bone destruction and periosteal new bone formation are seen 10 to 14 days after the onset of infection, but nonspecific soft-tissue swelling may be seen earlier. The 99m Tc bone scan is usually positive before radiographic changes are seen but may be cold (i.e., no uptake) in early severe infections and in neonates.

C. Pelvic osteomyelitis causes systemic signs, few localizing signs, pain with pelvic compression, discomfort with hip motion, and refusal to walk. The diagnosis is best confirmed with blood cultures, a bone scan, and possibly a CT scan, MRI, or ultrasound. Treatment consists of IV and oral antibiotics; surgical drainage is not usually necessary. Disk space infection (diskitis) manifests as back pain with refusal to walk or flex the lumbar spine; abdominal pain may be present. The ESR is elevated but the WBC is usually normal with no fever. Blood cultures may be positive (usually *S. aureus*); disk space aspiration is not indicated unless treatment fails. Beware of other organisms in older children and adolescents in whom drug use is suspected. Treatment consists of antistaphylococcal antibiotics and immobilization using a cast or brace.

D. The diagnosis is confirmed by blood cultures and aspiration of the involved bone. Perform bone aspiration at the site of maximum swelling using a 16 or 18 gauge needle with a stylet. If the infection has broken through the cortex, pus will be aspirated from the subperiosteal abscess. If no pus is encountered, proceed into the medullary cavity. Send pus or tissue fluid for culture and Gram stain. Blood cultures are positive in about 50% of patients, bone cultures in about 90%. Pus indicates an abscess cavity, hence surgical drainage.

(Continued on page 400)

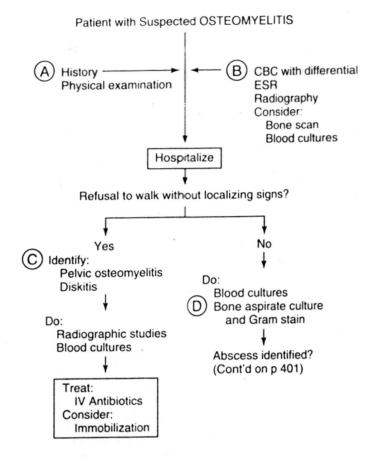

Patient with Suspected OSTEOMYELITIS

Ⓐ History ⟶ ⟵ Ⓑ CBC with differential
Physical examination   ESR
                            Radiography
                            Consider:
                                Bone scan
                                Blood cultures

Hospitalize

Refusal to walk without localizing signs?

Yes   No

Ⓒ Identify:
    Pelvic osteomyelitis
    Diskitis   Do:
                                Blood cultures
                            Ⓓ Bone aspirate culture
Do: and Gram stain
    Radiographic studies
    Blood cultures   Abscess identified?
                            (Cont'd on p 401)

Treat:
    IV Antibiotics
Consider:
    Immobilization

TABLE 1 IV Antibiotic Therapy for Osteomyelitis in Children

Antibiotic	Dosage	Product Availability
Cefotaxime	50 mg/kg q6–8h	Vials: 0.5, 1, 2 g
Ceftriaxone	50 mg/kg q12h	Vials: 0.25, 0.5, 1 g
Chloramphenicol	25 mg/kg q6–8h	Vial: 1 g
Clindamycin	8–13 mg/kg q8h	Vials: 2, 4, 6 ml (150 mg/ml)
Gentamicin	2.5 mg/kg Neonates < 7 days: q12h Neonates > 7 days, infants, children: q8h	Vials: 20, 80 mg
Nafcillin	40–50 mg/kg q6h	Vials: 0.5, 1, 2 g
Oxacillin	40–50 mg/kg q6h	Vials: 0.25, 0.5, 1, 2, 4 g
Ticarcillin	50–75 mg/kg q6h	Vials: 1, 3, 6 g
Vancomycin	10–15 mg/kg q8h	Vials: 0.5, 1 g

if a definite abscess is not formed, begin IV antibiotic treatment in the hospital.

E. The choice of antibiotic therapy (Table 1) is based on the Gram stain and the age of the patient. Neonatal osteomyelitis is usually caused by *S. aureus,* GBS, or gram-negative enteric organisms. A semisynthetic penicillin (oxacillin or nafcillin) and an aminoglycoside (gentamicin) or cephalosporin (cefotaxime) provide the broad-spectrum coverage needed. In older children initial antibiotic coverage should also cover *H. influenzae.* Use a semisynthetic penicillin plus a third-generation cephalosporin (cefotaxime, ceftriaxone) or chloramphenicol. Subsequent IV therapy should be based on culture results. Vancomycin may be needed to treat *S. aureus* infections resistant to semisynthetic penicillin. Clindamycin may be needed for anaerobic infection resistant to penicillin: Children with sickle cell disease should be treated with chloramphenicol or ceftriaxone to cover *Salmonella* infection. Infections following foot puncture wounds should be treated with ticarcillin to cover *Pseudomonas* spp.

F. An adequate response includes a decrease in the swelling, pain, and fever within 1 to 3 days. The ESR will fall slowly over 1 to 3 weeks, and radiographic changes may show deterioration before gradual improvement. If the response is adequate, consider switching to oral antibiotics at 5 to 10 days. This should be done while the patient is hospitalized and being monitored by determination that the peak serum bactericidal level is greater than 1:8. Continue antibiotic treatment for 3 to 6 weeks according to the clinical response. Consider abscess or anaerobic infection if the response is inadequate. Consider surgical debridement and open cultures.

References

Craigen MAC, Watters J, Hackett JS. The changing epidemiology of osteomyelitis in children. J Bone Joint Surg 1992; 74-B:541.

Dagan R. Management of acute hematogenous osteomyelitis and septic arthritis in the pediatric patient. Pediatr Infect Dis J 1993; 12:88.

Dubey L, Krasinski K, Hernanz-Schulman M. Osteomyelitis secondary to trauma or infected contiguous soft tissue. Pediatr Infect Dis J 1988; 7:26.

Prober CG. Current antibiotic therapy of community-acquired bacterial infections in hospitalized children: Bone and joint infections. Pediatr Infect Dis J 1992; 11:156.

Roy DR. Osteomyelitis. Pediatr Rev 1995; 16:380.

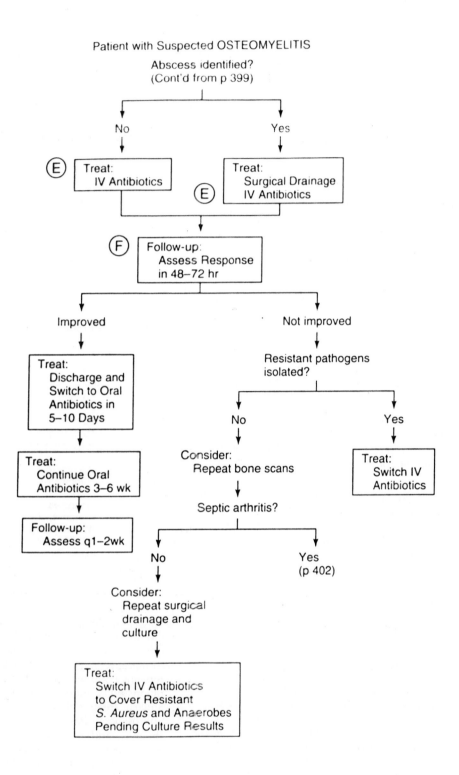

Patient with Suspected OSTEOMYELITIS
Abscess identified?
(Cont'd from p 399)

No

Yes

(E) Treat:
IV Antibiotics

(E) Treat:
Surgical Drainage
IV Antibiotics

(F) Follow-up:
Assess Response
in 48–72 hr

Improved

Not improved

Treat:
Discharge and
Switch to Oral
Antibiotics in
5–10 Days

Resistant pathogens
isolated?

No

Yes

Treat:
Continue Oral
Antibiotics 3–6 wk

Consider:
Repeat bone scans

Treat:
Switch IV
Antibiotics

Follow-up:
Assess q1–2wk

Septic arthritis?

No

Yes
(p 402)

Consider:
Repeat surgical
drainage and
culture

Treat:
Switch IV Antibiotics
to Cover Resistant
S. Aureus and Anaerobes
Pending Culture Results

SEPTIC ARTHRITIS

Richard C. Fisher, M.D.
Stephen Berman, M.D.

DEFINITION

Septic arthritis, a bacterial joint infection, most often involves the knee, hip, and ankle. Other commonly infected sites are the elbow, wrist, and shoulder joint. In 5% to 8% of patients multiple joints are involved; this is usually associated with some type of immune compromise.

ETIOLOGY

Infections with *Staphylococcus aureus* are the most frequent cause of septic arthritis in children older than 5 years. Although *Haemophilus influenza* type B (HIB) used to be the most frequent cause of septic arthritis in children under 5 years of age, the widespread use of HIB vaccine has reduced this infection. Less common pathogens include *Streptococcus pneumoniae*, *Streptococcus pyogenes*, *Neisseria meningitidis*, *Neisseria gonorrhoeae*, *Salmonella*, and other gram-negative organisms. Multiple joint involvement suggests *S. aureus* but can occur with *H. influenzae*, *S. pneumoniae*, and *N. meningitidis*. *N. gonorrhoeae* infections increase in frequency in older children and adolescents. The frequency of involvement from other organisms depends on the age of the child (Table 1).

A. In the history ask about fever, progressive reluctance to use the extremity, and limited range of motion, which suggest an acutely septic joint. Many cases of septic arthritis are associated with recent sore throat, upper respiratory infection, or local trauma.

B. The physical examination shows swelling, redness, and painful motion of the involved joint, which is usually held in a partially flexed position.

C. A negative radiograph usually rules out bony lesions. Always consider occult trauma. Acute septic arthritis shows soft-tissue swelling, distention of the joint capsule, and occasionally increase in the joint space.

D. Perform sterile joint aspiration if septic arthritis is suspected. Fluoroscopic control is useful for hip and shoulder aspirations. Cloudy yellow or white joint fluid with a WBC higher than 50,000 and predominance of neutrophils suggests a pyogenic process. Send the fluid for Gram stain and culture, which are positive in about 60% of cases. Counterimmunoelectrophoresis may help to identify HIB infections in patients who received prior antibiotics and thus may have negative Gram stains and cultures. Blood cultures are positive in 40% to 50% of cases of septic arthritis and are the only method of identifying the pathogen in about 10% of cases. Consider a lumbar puncture for children with signs of meningitis or documented *H. influenzae* infection, since associated *H. influenzae* bacteremia predisposes the child to meningitis.

TABLE 1 Most Frequent Pathogens by Age

Neonate	S. aureus
	GBS
	E. coli
Child <5 yr	S. aureus
	H. influenzae
	GBS
Child >5 yr	S. aureus
Adolescent	S. aureus
	N. gonorrhoeae

GBS, group B streptococcus.

TABLE 2 IV Antibiotic Therapy for Septic Arthritis in Children and Adolescents

Drug	Dosage	Product Availability
Cefotaxime (Claforan)	50 mg/kg q6–8h	Vials: 0.5, 1, 2 g
Ceftriaxone	50 mg/kg q12h	Vials: 0.25, 0.5, 1 g
Chloramphenicol	25 mg/kg q6–8h	Vials: 1 g
Clindamycin (Cleocin)	8–13 mg/kg q18h	Vials: 2, 4, 6 ml (150 mg/ml)
Gentamicin	2.5 mg/kg Neonates <7 days, q12h Neonates >7 days, infants, children, q8h	Vials: 20, 80 mg
Nafcillin	40–50 mg/kg q6h	Vials: 0.5, 1, 2 g
Oxacillin	40–50 mg/kg q6h	Vials: 0.25, 0.5, 1, 2, 4 g
Vancomycin (Vancocin)	10–15 mg/kg q8h	Vials: 500 mg, 1 g

E. Surgical drainage is necessary for septic arthritis of the hip and shoulder joints and should be considered for other *S. aureus* infections that do not respond promptly to therapy. Surgical drainage for other joint infections remains controversial, but usually repeat needle aspiration and IV antibiotics are accepted initial treatments. Surgical treatments can be by open technique or by arthroscopic drainage for joints such as the knee, shoulder, and ankle. Arthroscopic drainage is as effective as open drainage but may have to be repeated if the clinical course does not show rapid improvement. *N. gonorrhoeae* is usually a polyarticular migratory arthritis that rarely requires open drainage.

F. The choice of initial IV antibiotic therapy (Table 2) is based on the Gram stain and the age of the patient. Treat neonatal septic arthritis with the semisynthetic penicillin, oxacillin, or nafcillin and an aminoglycoside or a cephalosporin. In children 1 to 5 years of age initial antibiotic therapy should cover HIB, *S. aureus*, and *S. pneumoniae*. A semisynthetic penicillin plus cepha-

(Continued on page 404)

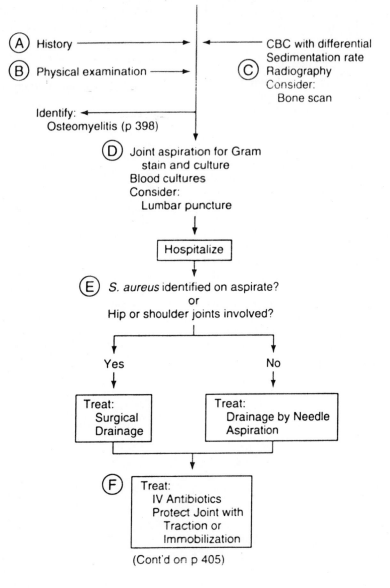

Patient with Suspected SEPTIC ARTHRITIS

(A) History ⟶ ⟵ CBC with differential
Sedimentation rate
(B) Physical examination ⟶ (C) Radiography
Consider:
Bone scan

Identify: ⟵
Osteomyelitis (p 398)

(D) Joint aspiration for Gram
stain and culture
Blood cultures
Consider:
Lumbar puncture

Hospitalize

(E) *S. aureus* identified on aspirate?
or
Hip or shoulder joints involved?

Yes   No

Treat: Treat:
Surgical   Drainage by Needle
Drainage   Aspiration

(F) Treat:
IV Antibiotics
Protect Joint with
Traction or
Immobilization

(Cont'd on p 405)

losporin (cefotaxime, ceftriaxone) or chloramphenicol can be used. In older children and adolescents the most common organisms are *S. aureus, S. pyogenes,* and *N. gonorrhoeae.* A semisynthetic penicillin provides appropriate therapy. Treat children with sickle cell disease with chloramphenicol or ceftriaxone to cover *Salmonella* infections. Adjust antibiotic therapy appropriately when culture results are obtained. Treat *S. aureus* or *S. pneumoniae* resistant to semisynthetic penicillin with vancomycin. Treat anaerobes resistant to penicillin with clindamycin.

G. Signs of adequate response include decreased swelling and pain and increased range of motion of the involved joint. Systemic signs, including erythrocyte sedimentation rate (ESR), fever, and malaise, should also improve. Suspect an associated osteomyelitis when the response to treatment is inadequate. It may be appropriate to repeat the bone scan at this point, as the initial radiograph or bone scan may have failed to reveal the underlying osteomyelitis. Start oral therapy when the response is adequate, adjusting the dose to produce a peak serum bactericidal titer greater than 1:8. Treat *N. gonorrhoeae* for at least 10 days, *H. influenzae* for 14 days, and other bacterial infections for 30 days or until the ESR returns to normal. Factors associated with a poor functional outcome include involvement of the hip joint with osteomyelitis of the proximal femur, *S. aureus* infection, and joint symptoms present for more than 4 days before initiating treatment.

H. Normal activities should be resumed only when the joint has returned to full function with a full range of painless motion, no swelling, and adequate strength in the extremity. Follow-up radiography is indicated to determine the degree of articular damage.

References

Bennett OM, Namnyak SS. Acute septic arthritis of the hip joint in infancy and childhood. Clin Orthop Rel Res 1992; 281:123.

Dagan R. Management of acute hematogenous osteomyelitis and septic arthritis in the pediatric patient. Pediatr Infect Dis J 1993; 12:88.

Hasselbacher P. Synovial fluid examination. In: Schumacher HR, Klippel JH, Robinson DR, eds. Primer on the rheumatoid diseases. 9th ed. Atlanta: Arthritis Foundation, 1988:55.

Prober CG. Current antibiotic therapy of community-acquired bacterial infections in hospitalized children: Bone and joint infections. Pediatr Infect Dis J 1992; 11:156.

Yagupsky P, Bar-Ziv Y, Howard CB, Dagan R. Epidemiology, etiology and clinical features of septic arthritis in children younger than 24 months. Arch Pediatr Adolesc Med 1995; 149:537.

Patient with Suspected SEPTIC ARTHRITIS

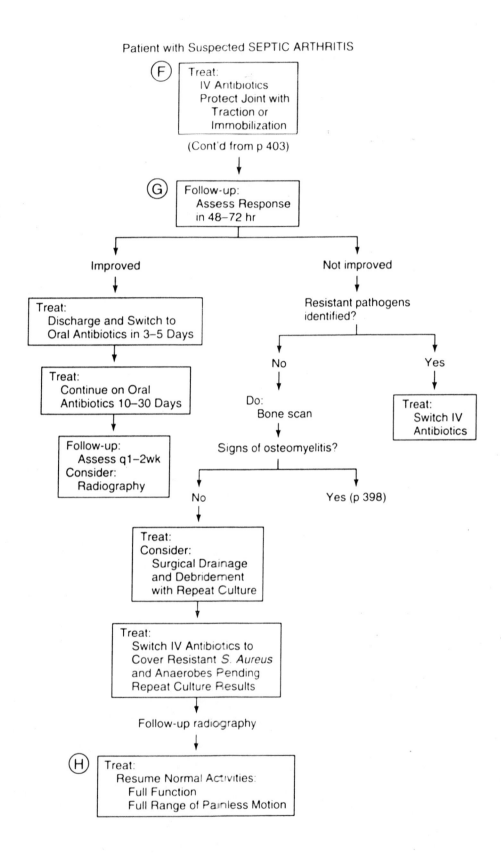

(Cont'd from p 403)

Improved

Not improved

Do:
Bone scan

Signs of osteomyelitis?

No

Yes (p 398)

Follow-up radiography

NEONATAL DISORDERS

ANEMIA IN THE NEWBORN

Peter A. Lane, M.D.
Rachelle Nuss, M.D.

A. In the history document any prenatal infections or drug use. Also note any history of maternal vaginal bleeding, placenta previa, abruptio placentae, or umbilical cord rupture, constriction or velamentous insertion, as well as cesarean, breech, or traumatic delivery. Obtain a family history of neonatal jaundice, anemia, splenomegaly, and unexplained gallstones.

B. In the physical examination note tachypnea, tachycardia, peripheral vasoconstriction (acute blood loss), and hepatosplenomegaly (chronic anemia, intrauterine infection, congenital malignancy). Jaundice appearing before 24 hours of age suggests significant hemolysis.

C. A hematocrit less than 45% during the first 3 days of life is abnormal and requires explanation. The mean corpuscular volume (MCV) at birth is normally above 95. An MCV below 95 suggests α-thalassemia or chronic intrauterine blood loss (as with fetal maternal transfusion). Rarely, a low MCV may be seen with hemolytic disease caused by hereditary elliptocytosis or pyropoikilocytosis. The presence of neutropenia and/or thrombocytopenia (see p 444) suggests the possibility of infection (see p 436). Except in an emergency, no anemic newborn should receive a blood transfusion before adequate diagnostic studies.

D. Normal reticulocyte values are 3% to 7% during the first day of life and 1% to 3% during the second and third days. A low reticulocyte count in the face of significant anemia suggests bone marrow failure.

E. An indirect hyperbilirubinemia, abnormal peripheral blood smear, or ABO or Rh incompatibility between the mother and infant suggests hemolysis.

F. Perform direct and indirect Coombs tests. ABO isoimmunization is usually associated with a negative direct and a positive indirect Coombs test.

G. Infants with immune hemolysis have varying degrees of hemolysis, which may continue for 3 months. Severe, life-threatening anemia may develop in infants with Rh sensitization; such infants require close follow-up with serial hematocrits until the hemolysis resolves.

H. Examine the peripheral blood smear. Spherocytes suggest ABO isoimmunization, hereditary spherocytosis, or infection (e.g., cytomegalovirus). Red cell fragmentation suggests intravascular hemolysis (infection, disseminated intravascular coagulation [DIC]). Consider infection and/or DIC in any ill newborn with hemolysis, particularly if thrombocytopenia is also present.

I. Review the obstetric history and examine the placenta for clues to the cause of fetal blood loss.

J. Perform a Kleihauer-Betke test to detect fetal red cells in the maternal circulation. False-negatives occur when an ABO incompatibility results in the rapid clearance of the infant's red cells from the maternal circulation.

K. Newborns with significant prenatal or perinatal blood loss are at risk for iron deficiency during the first 6 months of life.

L. Anemic infants without evidence of hemolysis or blood loss whose mothers have a negative Kleihauer test may have α-thalassemia, especially if the MCV is below 95. Ethnic groups affected most often include south and southeast Asians, Mediterraneans, and Africans. The diagnosis of α-thalassemia may be confirmed with a hemoglobin electrophoresis that shows Bart's hemoglobin.

References

Ballin A, Brown EJ, Zipursky A. Idiopathic Heinz body hemolytic anemia in newborn infants. Am J Pediatr Hematol Oncol 1989; 11:3.

Blanchette VS, Zipursky A. Assessment of anemia in newborn infants. Clin Perinatol 1984; 11:489.

Oski FA. Anemia in the neonatal period. In: Oski FA, Naiman JL, eds. Hematologic problems in the newborn. 3rd ed. Philadelphia: Saunders, 1982:56.

Oski FA. The erythrocyte and its disorders. In: Nathan DG, Oski FA, eds. Hematology of infancy and childhood. 4th ed. Philadelphia: Saunders, 1993:18.

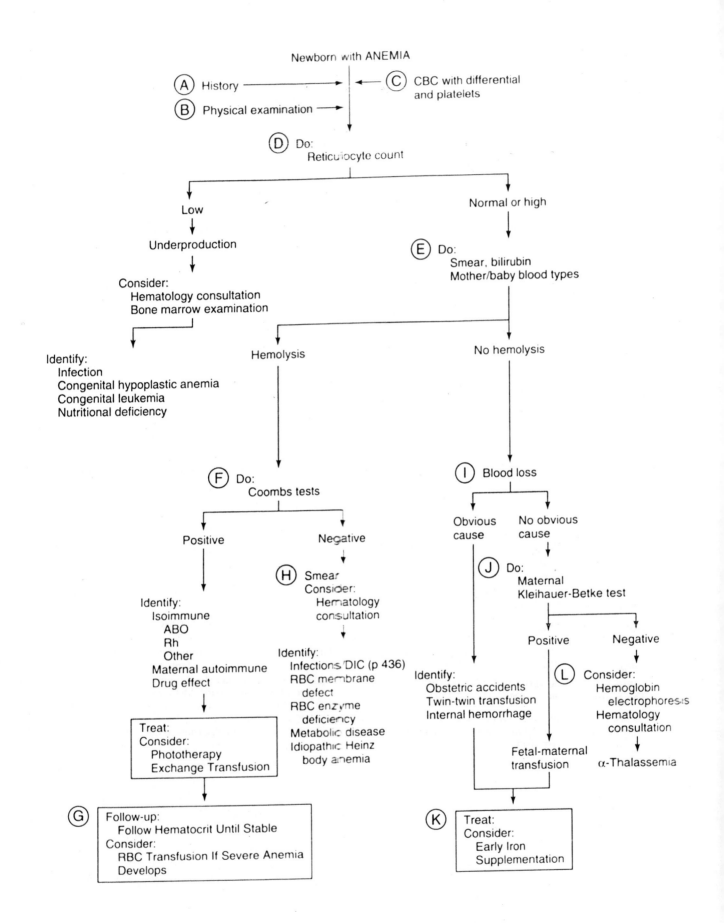

Newborn with ANEMIA

(A) History ——————→ ←—— (C) CBC with differential and platelets

(B) Physical examination ——→

(D) Do:
Reticulocyte count

Low
↓
Underproduction
↓
Consider:
Hematology consultation
Bone marrow examination

Identify:
Infection
Congenital hypoplastic anemia
Congenital leukemia
Nutritional deficiency

Normal or high
↓
(E) Do:
Smear, bilirubin
Mother/baby blood types

Hemolysis

No hemolysis

(F) Do:
Coombs tests

Positive
↓
Identify:
Isoimmune
ABO
Rh
Other
Maternal autoimmune
Drug effect
↓
Treat:
Consider:
Phototherapy
Exchange Transfusion

Negative
↓
(H) Smear
Consider:
Hematology
consultation
↓
Identify:
Infections/DIC (p 436)
RBC membrane
defect
RBC enzyme
deficiency
Metabolic disease
Idiopathic Heinz
body anemia

(I) Blood loss

Obvious
cause

No obvious
cause

(J) Do:
Maternal
Kleihauer-Betke test

Positive

Negative

Identify:
Obstetric accidents
Twin-twin transfusion
Internal hemorrhage

(L) Consider:
Hemoglobin
electrophoresis
Hematology
consultation
↓
α-Thalassemia

Fetal-maternal
transfusion

(G) Follow-up:
Follow Hematocrit Until Stable
Consider:
RBC Transfusion If Severe Anemia
Develops

(K) Treat:
Consider:
Early Iron
Supplementation

BLEEDING IN THE NEWBORN

Rachelle Nuss, M.D.
Peter A. Lane, M.D.

A. In the history ask about significant maternal illnesses such as diabetes (renal vein thrombosis), hypertension, or autoimmune disease (thrombocytopenia). Identify drugs ingested during pregnancy that are associated with platelet dysfunction (salicylates), vitamin K deficiency (anticonvulsants, antituberculous chemotherapy, warfarin), or thrombocytopenia (antihypertensives). Note the gestational history, method of delivery, and Apgar scores. Consider risk factors for bacterial infection such as prematurity, prolonged rupture of membranes, maternal amnionitis, and fetal distress during labor. Take a detailed family history of bleeding. Finally, document with certainty the administration of vitamin K at birth.

B. In the physical examination note the extent and type of bleeding. Assess the cardiovascular status for signs of intravascular volume depletion (rapid blood loss or sepsis). Severe jaundice, hepatosplenomegaly, respiratory distress, or signs of sepsis suggest a generalized acquired bleeding disorder. Congenital hemostatic defects present most typically in an otherwise well-appearing child with unexplained bleeding. Look carefully for a cavernous hemangioma, and consider the possibility of intracranial hemorrhage.

C. Perform a CBC and review the peripheral smear. Leukocytosis or neutropenia suggests sepsis. Significant red cell fragmentation with decreased platelets suggests a consumptive coagulopathy (disseminated intravascular coagulapathy [DIC], necrotizing enterocolitis [NEC], large-vessel thrombosis, cavernous hemangioma). In sick newborns consider cultures, arterial blood gas, chest and abdominal radiography, and urinalysis.

D. Perform a prothrombin time (PT), partial thromboplastin time (PTT), and platelet count. The PT and PTT are physiologically prolonged in normal newborns, so values obtained in a bleeding newborn should be compared with newborn norms in a given laboratory. The normal platelet count is 150,000 or more.

E. A normal coagulation screen does not exclude a coagulopathy. A newborn with unexplained bleeding and normal PT, PTT, and platelet count may be evaluated further with a bleeding time and a hematology consultation.

F. Prolongation of both the PT and PTT with thrombocytopenia suggests a consumptive coagulopathy. Identify the cause of the coagulopathy and order fibrinogen level and fibrin split products (FSP) and/or a D-dimer. Treat serious bleeding with fresh frozen plasma and platelet transfusion. Consider liver function tests and viral cultures if the cause of the coagulopathy is uncertain. In the newborn liver disease may be associated with thrombocytopenia as well as with a prolonged PT and PTT.

G. Treat serious bleeding with fresh frozen plasma. If vitamin K has not been given, it should be ordered immediately, with a repeat PT and PTT 4 to 6 hours later; a marked improvement strongly suggests vitamin K deficiency. DIC may occur without a thrombocytopenia in the asphyxiated newborn. Congenital deficiencies of factor I, II, V, or X are rare. Protamine sulfate reverses heparin excess.

H. An isolated prolongation of the PTT suggests a congenital defect in hemostasis or heparin effect. Order clotting assays for factors VIII, IX, and XI. Treat serious bleeding with fresh frozen plasma (or cryoprecipitate or factor concentrate for confirmed factor VIII or IX deficiency), and consider a hematology consultation.

I. An isolated prolonged PT suggests factor VII deficiency, vitamin K deficiency, or early liver disease.

References

Hathaway WE, Bonnar J. Hemostatic disorders of the pregnant woman and newborn infant. New York: Elsevier, 1987.

Hathaway WE, Goodnight S. Disorders of hemostasis and thrombosis. New York: McGraw-Hill, 1993.

Huysman M, Sauer P. The vitamin K controversy. Curr Op Ped 1994; 6:129.

Pramanik AK. Bleeding disorders in neonates. Pediatr Rev 1992; 13:163.

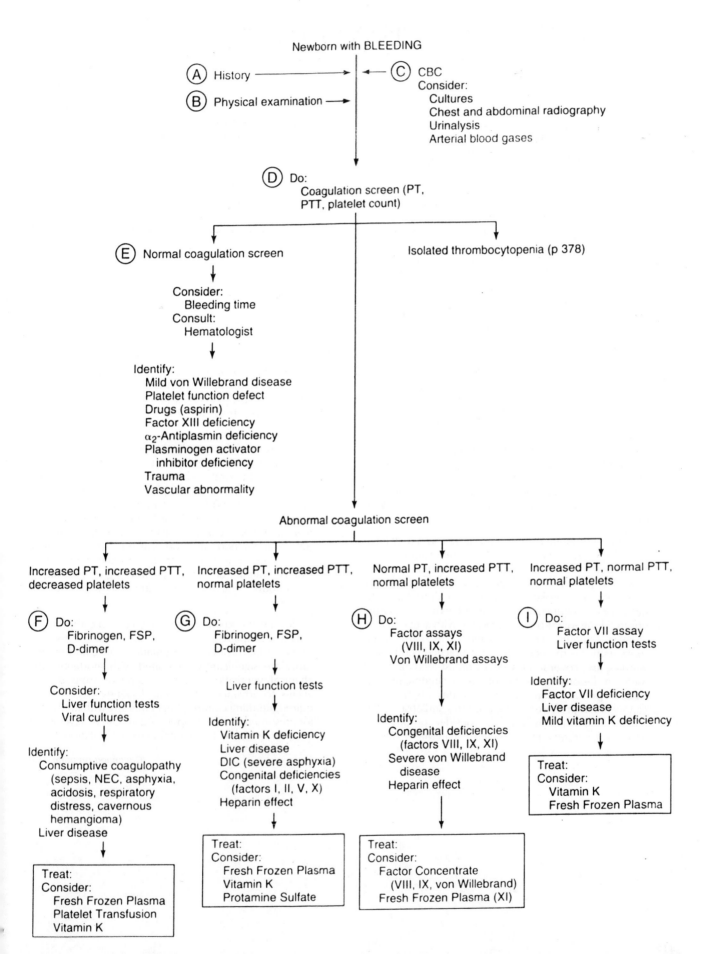

Newborn with BLEEDING

(A) History
(B) Physical examination

(C) CBC
Consider:
  Cultures
  Chest and abdominal radiography
  Urinalysis
  Arterial blood gases

(D) Do:
  Coagulation screen (PT, PTT, platelet count)

(E) Normal coagulation screen

Consider:
  Bleeding time
Consult:
  Hematologist

Identify:
  Mild von Willebrand disease
  Platelet function defect
  Drugs (aspirin)
  Factor XIII deficiency
  α_2-Antiplasmin deficiency
  Plasminogen activator
    inhibitor deficiency
  Trauma
  Vascular abnormality

Isolated thrombocytopenia (p 378)

Abnormal coagulation screen

Increased PT, increased PTT, decreased platelets

(F) Do:
  Fibrinogen, FSP, D-dimer

Consider:
  Liver function tests
  Viral cultures

Identify:
  Consumptive coagulopathy
  (sepsis, NEC, asphyxia, acidosis, respiratory distress, cavernous hemangioma)
  Liver disease

Treat:
Consider:
  Fresh Frozen Plasma
  Platelet Transfusion
  Vitamin K

Increased PT, increased PTT, normal platelets

(G) Do:
  Fibrinogen, FSP, D-dimer

Liver function tests

Identify:
  Vitamin K deficiency
  Liver disease
  DIC (severe asphyxia)
  Congenital deficiencies
  (factors I, II, V, X)
  Heparin effect

Treat:
Consider:
  Fresh Frozen Plasma
  Vitamin K
  Protamine Sulfate

Normal PT, increased PTT, normal platelets

(H) Do:
  Factor assays
  (VIII, IX, XI)
  Von Willebrand assays

Identify:
  Congenital deficiencies
  (factors VIII, IX, XI)
  Severe von Willebrand disease
  Heparin effect

Treat:
Consider:
  Factor Concentrate
  (VIII, IX, von Willebrand)
  Fresh Frozen Plasma (XI)

Increased PT, normal PTT, normal platelets

(I) Do:
  Factor VII assay
  Liver function tests

Identify:
  Factor VII deficiency
  Liver disease
  Mild vitamin K deficiency

Treat:
Consider:
  Vitamin K
  Fresh Frozen Plasma

411

CONGENITAL HERPES SIMPLEX INFECTIONS

Susan Niermeyer, M.D.

Neonatal herpes simplex virus (HSV) infections are uncommon but potentially devastating. No comprehensive maternal screening strategy can predict infants at risk, so early recognition and treatment are keys to reducing morbidity and mortality.

A. Approximately 70% of neonates with HSV infection are born to mothers with no history of genital lesions. Most neonatal cases result from primary maternal HSV infection at delivery. The mother often lacks a distinguishing clinical picture; she may have a nonspecific febrile illness or be entirely asymptomatic. The risk of HSV infection in infants born to mothers with recurrent disease and specific IgG antibody is no more than one tenth that of infants whose mothers have infection during pregnancy but lack type-specific antibody. The risk of neonatal infection resulting from delivery during an episode of primary maternal herpes is estimated to be 50%, and the risk of infection in the setting of recurrent maternal disease is probably less than 3%.

B. Nonspecific clinical signs (fever, lethargy, irritability, respiratory distress, poor feeding, poor tone) are likely more common than typical skin lesions. Because initial symptoms are rarely diagnostic for HSV, include HSV in the differential diagnosis of the sick infant. Search for the characteristic papulovesicular lesions, often with a pustular appearance and erythematous base; these may be single or grouped over the oral mucosa, face, scalp, extremities, or torso.

C. Management of an asymptomatic infant who may have been exposed to HSV varies by maternal history. An infant born to a mother with documented recurrent genital herpes who has no signs or symptoms at delivery does not require isolation and may be cultured at 24 to 48 hours (conjunctiva and nasopharynx) or simply observed. An infant born to a mother with active lesions at delivery requires contact isolation. The infant should room with the mother, who must practice good hand washing and cover lesions. Allow breast-feeding unless there are lesions on the breast. Defer circumcision. In cases of primary maternal infection, delivery by cesarean section is preferred; obtain cultures and observe the infant. If delivery is vaginal, consider prophylactic acyclovir pending culture results. If maternal disease is recurrent, vaginal delivery is acceptable, and the infant should be cultured and observed. When the type of maternal disease is unknown, follow guidelines for primary infection.

D. An asymptomatic infant who is not being treated may be discharged routinely if reliable follow-up is assured. Continue prophylactic treatment for 3 days of negative cultures. Follow-up in both groups should be at least weekly until the patient is 4 to 6 weeks of age. If cultures are positive, treat for 14 days and arrange close follow-up.

E. Symptomatic infants with nonspecific signs or characteristic evidence of herpes infection require complete evaluation for viral and bacterial sepsis. Include viral cultures of conjunctiva, nasopharynx and rectum; blood cultures; urine and CSF for viral and bacterial culture. Reserve an aliquot of CSF for herpes polymerase chain reaction (PCR). Scrape lesions for viral culture; antigen detection methods may be applied to provide rapid information. Shell-vial centrifugation and immunoperoxidase staining of culture specimens give information in 24 hours; 90% of routine cultures show positivity by 3 days.

F. Anticipate the need for intensive care in symptomatic patients. Impaired consciousness, pneumonitis, disseminated intravascular coagulation (DIC), and prematurity are significantly associated with mortality. Mechanical ventilation, fluid and pressor support, and access to advanced diagnostic facilities are often required. Pending cultures, begin therapy with antibiotics for presumed bacterial sepsis, and initiate IV acyclovir or vidarabine (Table 1). Maintain contact isolation.

TABLE 1 Antiviral Therapy for Neonatal HSV

Drug	Dosage
Acyclovir	30 mg/kg/24 hr IV divided q8h for 10–14 days or 1500 mg/m²/day
Vidarabine	15–30 mg/kg/day IV given over 12–24 hr through 0.45-μm filter

(Continued on page 414)

Patient with HERPES SIMPLEX EXPOSURE OR SUSPECTED INFECTION

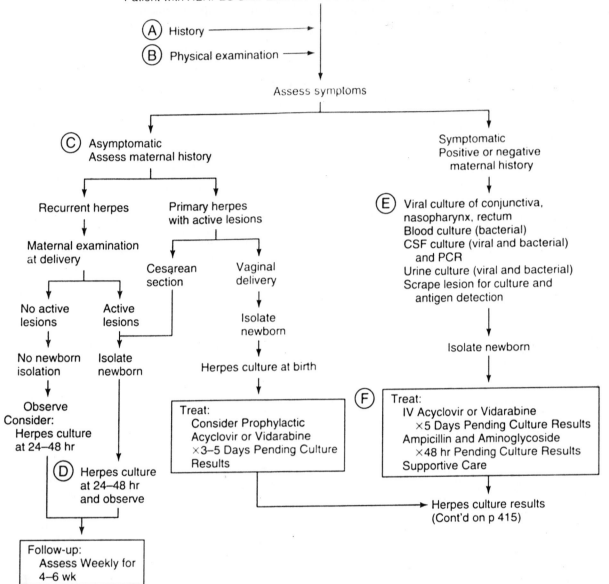

Ⓐ History

Ⓑ Physical examination

Assess symptoms

Ⓒ Asymptomatic
Assess maternal history

Symptomatic
Positive or negative
maternal history

Recurrent herpes

Primary herpes
with active lesions

Ⓔ Viral culture of conjunctiva,
nasopharynx, rectum
Blood culture (bacterial)
CSF culture (viral and bacterial)
and PCR
Urine culture (viral and bacterial)
Scrape lesion for culture and
antigen detection

Maternal examination
at delivery

Cesarean
section

Vaginal
delivery

No active
lesions

Active
lesions

Isolate
newborn

Isolate newborn

No newborn
isolation

Isolate
newborn

Herpes culture at birth

Observe
Consider:
Herpes culture
at 24–48 hr

Ⓕ Treat:
IV Acyclovir or Vidarabine
×5 Days Pending Culture Results
Ampicillin and Aminoglycoside
×48 hr Pending Culture Results
Supportive Care

Ⓓ Herpes culture
at 24–48 hr
and observe

Treat:
Consider Prophylactic
Acyclovir or Vidarabine
×3–5 Days Pending Culture
Results

Herpes culture results
(Cont'd on p 415)

Follow-up:
Assess Weekly for
4–6 wk

G. Assess the clinical pattern of HSV infection to guide management and aid in prognosis. Infants with localized infection may have either cutaneous (skin, mucosa, eye) or CNS disease (meningoencephalitis). Localized skin lesions may spread or progress to disseminated disease. CNS involvement may be accompanied by altered consciousness, focal or multifocal seizures. Consider CT and electroencephalography to define the degree of involvement. CNS involvement may also be part of disseminated disease. This presentation often includes jaundice, hepatomegaly, shock, and DIC. Pneumonitis coupled with hepatitis suggests HSV. Obtain an ophthalmology consultation to identify eye involvement; HSV causes keratoconjunctivitis and chorioretinitis.

H. The prognosis for neonates with localized mucocutaneous disease is far better than for other forms. Survival is the rule; more than 90% develop normally. Approximately 15% of survivors have multiple cutaneous recurrences, a risk factor for subsequent abnormal development. Disseminated disease is fatal in 50% to 60% of cases, even with antiviral treatment. Meningoencephalitis is fatal in 14% of cases despite treatment. Nearly two thirds of survivors of CNS or disseminated disease develop abnormally.

References

Brown ZA, Benedetti J, Ashley R, et al. Neonatal herpes simplex virus infection in relation to asymptomatic maternal infection at the time of labor. N Engl J Med 1991; 324:1247.

Jenkins M, Kohl S. New aspects of neonatal herpes. Infect Dis Clin North Am 1992; 6:57.

Libman MD, Dascal A, Kramer MS, Mendelson J. Strategies for the prevention of neonatal infection with herpes simplex virus: A decision analysis. Rev Infect Dis 1991; 13:1093.

McIntosh D, Isaacs D. Herpes simplex virus infection in pregnancy. Arch Dis Child 1992; 67:1137.

Whitley RJ. Herpes simplex virus infections. In: Remington JS, Klein JO, eds. Infectious diseases of the fetus and newborn infant. 3rd ed. Philadelphia: Saunders, 1990:282.

Whitley RJ, Gnann JW Jr. Acyclovir: A decade later. N Eng J Med 1992; 327:782.

Patient with HERPES SIMPLEX EXPOSURE OR SUSPECTED INFECTION

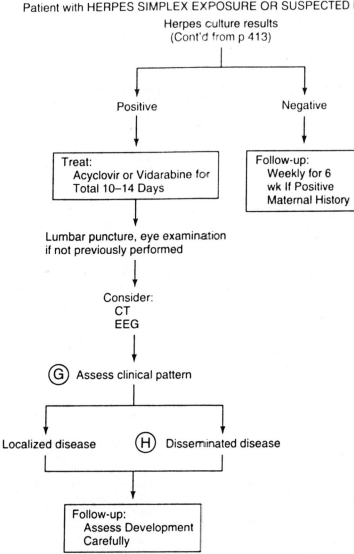

Herpes culture results
(Cont'd from p 413)

Positive

Negative

Treat:
  Acyclovir or Vidarabine for
  Total 10–14 Days

Follow-up:
  Weekly for 6
  wk If Positive
  Maternal History

Lumbar puncture, eye examination
if not previously performed

Consider:
CT
EEG

G Assess clinical pattern

Localized disease   H Disseminated disease

Follow-up:
  Assess Development
  Carefully

INBORN ERROR OF METABOLISM IN A NEWBORN

Carol L. Greene, M.D.

While an individual inborn error of metabolism (IEM) is rare, these diseases as a group are important causes of neonatal morbidity and mortality. Prompt treatment can prevent mental retardation and death. Even in a dying neonate, identification of an IEM and subsequent counseling can prevent further catastrophes for the family. In the neonatal period inborn errors of metabolism present with nonspecific signs suggestive of neonatal sepsis. The most common early symptoms are poor feeding, lethargy, and irritability. These symptoms may begin either before or after introducing specific feedings. An IEM may present with laboratory results similar to asphyxia.

A. Ask about a family history of consanguinity, mental retardation, seizures, sudden death (especially neonatal death or sudden infant death syndrome [SIDS]), recurrent emesis, or altered mental status. Hypertonia in a neonate is highly suggestive of IEM, and unusual odors are also important clues (note the acrid odor of IV ampicillin). Microcephaly and malformations may be due to a maternal IEM. Tachypnea, apnea, hypotonia (occasionally with increased reflexes), altered mental status, hepatomegaly, and jaundice are common in the neonatal presentation of IEM. Macrocephaly, rashes, and cataracts, while rare, are more specific for certain disorders.

B. Investigations to identify sepsis combined with a blood ammonia and urine for reducing substances can provide clues to the presence of IEM. Since there are no reliable clinical findings for IEM, it is important to recognize that an IEM, especially organic acidemia, can cause anemia, neutropenia, and thrombocytopenia. The anion gap must be assessed (a normal anion gap does not rule out an IEM), as renal tublar acidosis may be secondary to IEM (glactosemia and tyrosinemia). Use special handling (no tourniquet and ice for transport) to obtain a blood ammonia. (All errors tend to increase the level, so a normal ammonia rules out hyperammonemia even when the sample was improperly drawn.) Because newborns do not make ketones with starvation, finding positive urine ketones suggests IEM. Since many IV antibiotics can cause a urine 1+ reducing substance, remember to get a urine sample before antibiotic treatment begins. Urine-reducing substances may be negative in galactosemia.

C. Documentation of sepsis (especially with gram-negative enteric organisms) does not exclude IEM, as galactosemia and other disorders can predispose to sepsis. Positive urine-reducing substances, acidosis out of proportion to the degree of systemic illness, or CNS symptoms more severe than suggested by systemic symptoms indicate a need to consider the possibility of IEM. An elevated ammonia needs treatment regardless of the cause and also indicates very high risk of IEM. Documenting other specific causes of symptoms makes IEM less likely.

D. Differential diagnosis of IEM is complicated by the variability in presentation of neonates with the same disorder and by the similarity of presentation of disorders in different categories. For example, both the carbohydrate disorder galactosemia and the amino acid disorder tyrosinemia cause severe liver disease. The algorithm is intended to emphasize the unique features of each presentation, and it is important to remember each neonate with IEM may have several types of clinical and biochemical abnormalities. You may need to follow more than one arm of the algorithm.

E. Laboratory studies may be obtained most rapidly by discussion with appropriate consultant/laboratory; diagnosis can be made in some instances within hours to institute most appropriate therapy.

F. Few neonates (e.g., those rare neonates with severe primary lactic acidemia due to pyruvate dehydrogenase deficiency) will become worse with IV glucose. Since protein cannot be withheld indefinitely, it will need to be resumed cautiously when the infant is stable. Treatment is available for specific conditions such as pyridoxine for responsive seizures, vitamin B_{12} for methylmalonic acidemia, and pharmacologic treatment for hyperammonemia.

References

Burton BK. Inborn errors of metabolisms: The clinical diagnosis in early infancy. Pediatrics 1987; 79:359.

Goodman SI. Inherited metabolic disease in the newborn: Approach to diagnosis and treatment. Adv Pediatr 1985; 33:197.

Goodman SI, Greene CL. Metabolic disorders of the newborn. Pediatr Rev 1994; 15:9.

Greene CL, Goodman SI. Inborn errors of metabolism. In: Haywood AR, Hay WW, Groothius JR, Levin J, eds. Current pediatric diagnosis and treatment. 12th ed. 1995:926.

Surtees R, Leonard JV. Acute metabolic encephalopathy: A review of causes, mechanisms and treatment. J Inher Metab Dis 1989; 12(Suppl 1):42.

Neonate with a Suspected INBORN ERROR OF METABOLISM

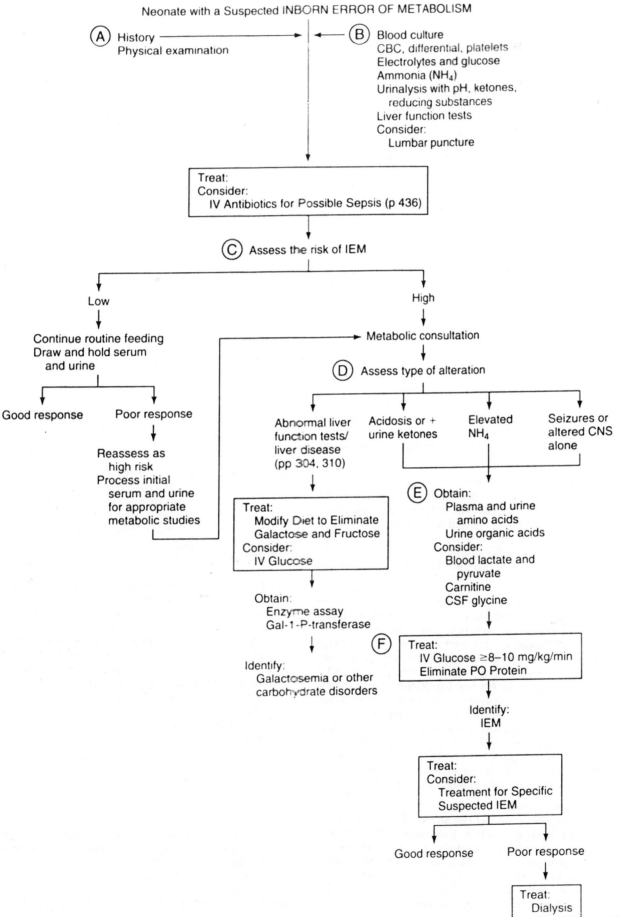

(A) History
Physical examination

(B) Blood culture
CBC, differential, platelets
Electrolytes and glucose
Ammonia (NH₄)
Urinalysis with pH, ketones,
    reducing substances
Liver function tests
Consider:
    Lumbar puncture

Treat:
Consider:
    IV Antibiotics for Possible Sepsis (p 436)

(C) Assess the risk of IEM

Low

High

Continue routine feeding
Draw and hold serum
and urine

Metabolic consultation

(D) Assess type of alteration

Good response   Poor response

Reassess as
    high risk
Process initial
    serum and urine
    for appropriate
    metabolic studies

Abnormal liver
function tests/
liver disease
(pp 304, 310)

Acidosis or +
urine ketones

Elevated
NH₄

Seizures or
altered CNS
alone

Treat:
    Modify Diet to Eliminate
    Galactose and Fructose
Consider:
    IV Glucose

(E) Obtain:
    Plasma and urine
        amino acids
    Urine organic acids
Consider:
    Blood lactate and
        pyruvate
    Carnitine
    CSF glycine

Obtain:
    Enzyme assay
    Gal-1-P-transferase

Identify:
    Galactosemia or other
    carbohydrate disorders

(F) Treat:
    IV Glucose ≥8–10 mg/kg/min
    Eliminate PO Protein

Identify:
IEM

Treat:
Consider:
    Treatment for Specific
    Suspected IEM

Good response   Poor response

Treat:
    Dialysis

JAUNDICE/NEONATAL

Susan Niermeyer, M.D.

Neonatal jaundice is in most cases a normal part of postnatal transition. However, extremely high levels of unconjugated bilirubin may occur with or without hemolysis; elevated direct bilirubin in the neonate always requires investigation.

A. In the history identify maternal conditions such as acute infection or chronic conditions (e.g., diabetes, Rh sensitization) that predisposes to jaundice in the infant. Ask about medications during pregnancy, especially sulfonamides, nitrofurantoins, and antimalarials and early Rhogam administration to Rh-negative mothers. In the labor and delivery history note the use of pitocin, forceps, vacuum extraction (cephalohematoma), and delayed cord clamping. Ask about a family history of jaundice, anemia, or liver disease, especially in siblings.

B. In the physical examination determine whether the infant is premature or small for gestational age. Note signs of extravascular blood such as extensive bruising or cephalohematoma. Note signs of systemic illness such as fever, temperature instability, abdominal distention, vomiting, seizures, and failure to thrive. Palpate carefully for a right upper quadrant mass (choledochal cyst). Microcephaly, petechiae, hepatosplenomegaly, or chorioretinitis suggests intrauterine infection. Pallor and hepatosplenomegaly suggest severe hemolytic anemia.

C. Visible jaundice in a term infant at 24 hours of age or less requires evaluation, as does jaundice extending to the lower extremities at less than 48 hours, intense jaundice or jaundice of the palms and soles at any age. A rapid rise of bilirubin (> 5 mg/dl/day) or a direct bilirubin above 1.5 mg/dl suggests underlying disease. Hemolytic disease or extravascular blood loss may or may not cause anemia.

D. A positive direct and/or indirect Coombs test identifies isoimmunization related to Rh, ABO, or minor blood group antigens or maternal autoimmune hemolytic anemia. Guidelines for phototherapy and exchange transfusion in hemolytic disease are difficult to generalize: some infants with Coombs-positive ABO incompatibility do not need treatment; some infants with Rh isoimmunization require immediate exchange transfusion based on cord bilirubin. Frequent monitoring is vital, as bilirubin can rise rapidly; direct therapy at maintaining the bilirubin at 20 to 22 mg/dl or less. Patients with a positive Coombs test, especially when associated with Rh incompatibility, should be followed carefully for 3 months to identify anemia.

E. A peripheral smear showing red cell fragments, spherocytes, or abnormal red cell shape suggests hemolytic anemia. Such disorders include spherocytosis, elliptocytosis, infantile pyknocytosis, enzyme deficiencies (glucose-6-phosphate dehydrogenase, or G6PD, pyruvate kinase deficiency), congenital viral infections (cytomegalovirus, or CMV), disseminated intravascular coagulation, and α- and γ-thalassemia.

F. Extravascular blood collections often present as a cephalohematoma or facial bruising. Increased enterohepatic circulation of bilirubin occurs in pyloric stenosis, small- or large-bowel obstruction, and swallowing of blood. Metabolic and endocrine disorders that cause elevated unconjugated bilirubin include galactosemia, hypothyroidism, hypopituitarism, and Crigler-Najjar syndrome. Polycythemia (twin-twin transfusion or delayed cord clamping) may be associated with exaggerated jaundice.

G. Exaggerated physiologic jaundice is a diagnosis of exclusion. A greater proportion of breast-fed than formula-fed infants reach high bilirubin concentrations. Exaggerated jaundice in the first 5 days of life in breast-fed infants may be termed breast-feeding jaundice, or lack-of breast-milk jaundice, as opposed to the later, more prolonged jaundice designated breast-milk jaundice. Breast-feeding jaundice is likely the result of unphysiologic management of breast-feeding, especially insufficient frequency (< 9 to 11 feedings/day), delayed initiation of breast-feeding (beyond 1 to 2 hours of life), and supplementation with water or formula in the first days of life. Revised guidelines for treatment of jaundice in healthy term infants were published by the American Academy of Pediatrics in 1994.

H. Cholestatic jaundice in the neonate may result from biliary disease (extra- or intrahepatic biliary obstruction) or hepatocellular disease (infectious, metabolic, or chemical). Ultrasonography is especially useful in detection of extrahepatic biliary obstruction; however, it may be nondiagnostic in biliary atresia. Radionuclide scans evaluate hepatocellular function as well as biliary anatomy. Hepatic imidoacetic acid (HIDA) scans in biliary atresia show normal uptake and absent excretion into the gut, and hepatitis is characterized by slow uptake but normal excretion (unless severe). When extrahepatic biliary atresia is suspected, intraoperative cholangiogram and hepatic portoenterostomy (Kasai procedure) should be performed in the first 8 to 10 weeks of life. If neonatal hepatitis is suspected, perform an α_1-antitrypsin screen, sweat test for cystic fibrosis, urine screen for reducing substances, amino and organic acids, serum bile acids, T_4/TSH, galactose-1-phosphate uridyl transferase, and tests for perinatal infections (CMV, herpes, rubella, toxoplasmosis, syphilis, hepatitis A, B, and C).

References

Gartner LM. On the question of the relationship between breastfeeding and jaundice in the first 5 days of life. Semin Perinatol 1994; 18:502.

Haber BA, Lake AM. Cholestatic jaundice in the newborn. Clin Perinatol 1990; 17:483.

Newman TB, Maisels MJ. Evaluation and treatment of jaundice

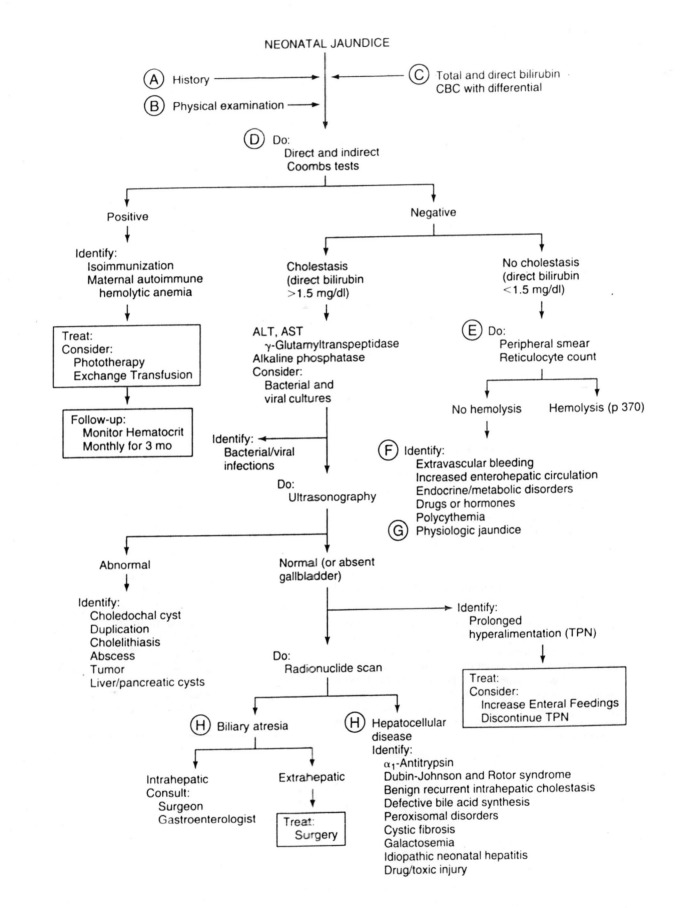

NEONATAL JAUNDICE

Ⓐ History

Ⓑ Physical examination

Ⓒ Total and direct bilirubin
CBC with differential

Ⓓ Do:
Direct and indirect
Coombs tests

Positive

Identify:
  Isoimmunization
  Maternal autoimmune
    hemolytic anemia

Treat:
Consider:
  Phototherapy
  Exchange Transfusion

Follow-up:
  Monitor Hematocrit
  Monthly for 3 mo

Negative

Cholestasis
(direct bilirubin
>1.5 mg/dl)

No cholestasis
(direct bilirubin
<1.5 mg/dl)

ALT, AST
  γ-Glutamyltranspeptidase
Alkaline phosphatase
Consider:
  Bacterial and
  viral cultures

Ⓔ Do:
  Peripheral smear
  Reticulocyte count

No hemolysis   Hemolysis (p 370)

Identify:
  Bacterial/viral
  infections

Ⓕ Identify:
  Extravascular bleeding
  Increased enterohepatic circulation
  Endocrine/metabolic disorders
  Drugs or hormones
  Polycythemia
Ⓖ Physiologic jaundice

Do:
  Ultrasonography

Abnormal

Identify:
  Choledochal cyst
  Duplication
  Cholelithiasis
  Abscess
  Tumor
  Liver/pancreatic cysts

**Normal (or absent
gallbladder)**

Identify:
  Prolonged
  hyperalimentation (TPN)

Do:
  Radionuclide scan

Treat:
Consider:
  Increase Enteral Feedings
  Discontinue TPN

Ⓗ Biliary atresia

Ⓗ Hepatocellular
disease
Identify:
  α₁-Antitrypsin
  Dubin-Johnson and Rotor syndrome
  Benign recurrent intrahepatic cholestasis
  Defective bile acid synthesis
  Peroxisomal disorders
  Cystic fibrosis
  Galactosemia
  Idiopathic neonatal hepatitis
  Drug/toxic injury

Intrahepatic   Extrahepatic
Consult:
  Surgeon
  Gastroenterologist

Treat:
  Surgery

in the term newborn: A kinder, gentler approach. Pediatrics
  1992; 89:809.
Provisional Committee for Quality Improvement and Subcom-
mittee on Hyperbilirubinemia. Practice parameter: Management of hyperbilirubinemia in the healthy term newborn. Pediatrics 1994; 94:558.

NECROTIZING ENTEROCOLITIS

Susan Niermeyer, M.D.

A. Early recognition of necrotizing enterocolitis (NEC) may limit progression and improve outcome. Most infants (80%) who develop NEC are born prematurely. Age at onset is inversely related to gestational age at birth; thus, NEC presents in the convalescent stage of a preterm infant's course but usually within 2 or 3 days of birth in a term infant. Factors related to the pathogenesis of NEC include intestinal hypoperfusion or hypoxia, abnormal gut motility, cow's milk–based or hypertonic feedings, and bacterial colonization or infection. Significant clinical history includes gastric residuals or vomiting, change in stool pattern (decreased frequency or diarrhea), Hematest or Clinitest positive stools, and nonspecific systemic signs such as temperature instability, glucose instability, lethargy, apnea, and respiratory distress.

B. In the physical examination note any abdominal distention, tenderness, mass, and erythema. Assess perfusion and pulses as well as heart rate and blood pressure (shock); oozing from the umbilical stump or puncture sites suggests disseminated intravascular coagulation (DIC).

C. Evaluation should be directed at detection of sepsis (immature to total neutrophil ratio greater than 1:5, thrombocytopenia, neutropenia). Submit blood and stool cultures for bacterial pathogens (e.g., *Escherichia coli, Klebsiella, Pseudomonas, Salmonella, Clostridium*); electron microscopy of stool detects rotavirus and other viral agents. Obtain an arterial blood gas to detect hypoxemia or metabolic acidosis. Abdominal radiography should include anteroposterior and left lateral decubitus or cross-table lateral views to detect mucosal damage, intramural air (pneumatosis intestinalis), portal venous air, or perforation (pneumoperitoneum).

D. NEC may be indolent or fulminant. Severely ill infants may have microscopic blood in the stool, abdominal distention or tenderness, and localized pneumatosis or ileus pattern. Very severely ill infants may exhibit abdominal wall erythema or a palpable mass; gross GI bleeding, shock, metabolic acidosis and DIC are suggestive of acute perforation; extensive pneumatosis, portal venous air, or pneumoperitoneum are ominous radiographic findings.

TABLE 1 Antibiotic Therapy for Necrotizing Enterocolitis in Infants

Drug	Dosage	Product Availability
Ampicillin	Age ≤7 days Preterm 50–100 mg/kg/day q12h Full term 75–150 mg/kg/day q8–12h Age >7 days 75–150 mg/kg/day q8h	Vial: 125, 250, 500 mg
Gentamicin	Premature newborn Age <7 days: 2.5 mg/kg/dose IV q18h or 3.5 mg/kg/dose IV determined by formula: dosing hours = 50.5–0.76 × gestational age (wk) Term newborn: 2.5 mg/kg/dose q12h Age >7 days: 2.5 mg/kg/dose q8h	IV solution: 10 mg/ml (2 ml) 40 mg/ml (1.5, 2 ml)
Metronidazole	Age 0–4 wk; wt <1200 g 7.5 mg/kg q48h Age <7 days 1200–2000 g: 7.5 mg/kg/day q24h >2000 g: 15 mg/kg/day q12h Age >7 days 1200–2000 g: 15 mg/kg/day q12h >2000 g: 30 mg/kg/day q12h	IV solution: 500 mg/100 ml vial (ready to use isotonic)
Clindamycin	Age <7 days <2000 g: 10 mg/kg/day q12h >2000 g: 15 mg/kg/day q8h Age >7 days <2000 g: 15 mg/kg/day q8h >2000 g: 20 mg/kg/day q8h	Vial: Clindamycin phosphate 150 mg/ml (2, 4, 6 ml) IV solution: 300, 600, 900 mg/ 50 ml

(Continued on page 422)

Newborn with NECROTIZING ENTEROCOLITIS

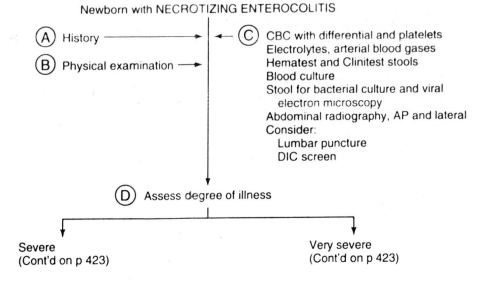

Severe
(Cont'd on p 423)

Very severe
(Cont'd on p 423)

E. Manage severely ill patients by discontinuing feeding, placing an orogastric sump tube to suction, and initiating antibiotic therapy with IV ampicillin and an aminoglycoside (Table 1). Reevaluate radiographic and clinical findings every 6 to 12 hours until condition stabilizes. Treat infants with antibiotics and keep NPO for at least 1 week from the first normal abdominal film. Initiate hyperalimentation promptly by peripheral vein; consider a peripherally inserted central venous catheter after 24 hours of antibiotic therapy. If pneumatosis is present or clinical deterioration occurs, seek surgical consultation.

F. Very severely ill patients should receive immediate surgical consultation and close attention to maintenance of adequate circulating volume and provision of ventilatory assistance prior to respiratory failure. Intestinal capillary leak may deplete circulating fluid volume and protein; DIC and GI hemorrhage may lead to significant blood loss. Maintenance fluids should be provided at 100% to 150% of baseline with additional crystalloid, 5% albumin, and packed red blood cells as indicated by vital signs and urine output. Low-dose dopamine (3 to 5 μg/kg/min) may improve cardiac output and increases mesenteric blood flow. Treat DIC and significant thrombocytopenia with fresh frozen plasma and platelet transfusions. Apnea, respiratory acidosis, and hypoxemia are specific respiratory indicators for assisted ventilation. If intestinal perforation is suspected, add clindamycin or metronidazole to antibiotic coverage (Table 1).

G. Pneumoperitoneum is an absolute indication for surgical exploration. Relative indications include portal venous air, abdominal wall erythema, abdominal mass, persistently dilated intestinal loop, unremitting metabolic acidosis, hyperkalemia or DIC, and rapid clinical deterioration. Paracentesis may be useful to confirm intestinal gangrene.

H. Reintroduce enteral feedings with a diluted elemental formula, and slowly advance volume and strength while tapering parenteral nutrition. Obtain a barium enema 6 to 8 weeks after the episode of NEC to detect stricture formation. Earlier barium enema may be indicated if signs of intestinal obstruction develop or if follow-up after discharge is uncertain.

References

Kanto WP Jr, Hunter JE, Stoll BJ. Recognition and medical management of necrotizing enterocolitis. Clin Perinatol 1994; 21:335.

McClead RE Jr, ed. Neonatal necrotizing enterocolitis: Current concepts and controversies. J Pediatr (suppl) 1990; 117 (1 part 2):S1.

Newborn with NECROTIZING ENTEROCOLITIS

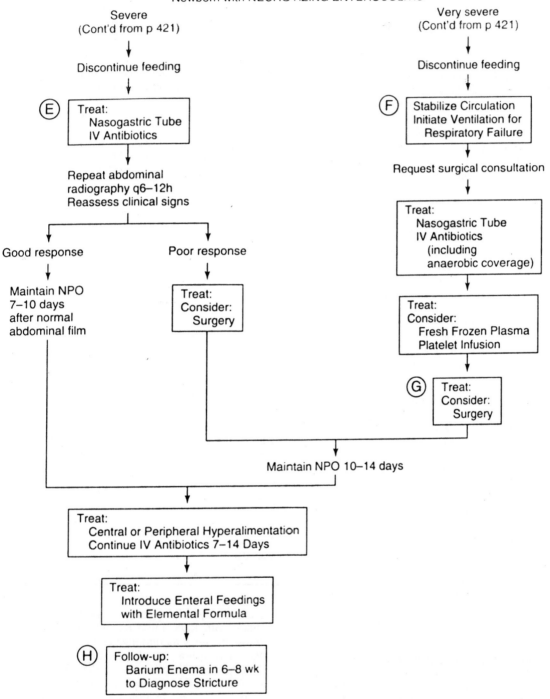

RESPIRATORY DISTRESS SYNDROME

Susan Niermeyer, M.D.

Respiratory distress syndrome (RDS), once called hyaline membrane disease, results from surfactant deficiency, usually in premature infants. RDS should be anticipated in the setting of preterm delivery and/or amniotic fluid indices that indicate pulmonary immaturity. Hormonal therapy using glucocorticoids alone or with thyrotropin-releasing hormone (TRH) can prevent neonatal RDS when administered to the mother at least 24 to 48 hours prior to delivery.

A. In the physical examination focus on accurate assessment of gestational age by defined morphologic and neurologic criteria. Search for evidence of congenital cardiorespiratory malformations (airway obstruction, congenital heart disease). Note the quality of respiratory effort (grunting, flaring, retracting, air entry, adventitial sounds) as well as respiratory rate.

B. The chest radiograph in RDS is characterized by a diffuse reticulogranular, or ground-glass, pattern and hypoexpansion. Near-term infants may have a less-specific hazy infiltrate. The radiographic appearance of RDS cannot be distinguished from that of group B streptococcal (GBS) pneumonia.

C. Include in the differential diagnosis other systemic illnesses with pulmonary manifestations such as congenital heart disease, hypoglycemia or cold stress, and polycythemia. Aspiration syndromes (clear fluid, blood, meconium) even in term infants may lead to acquired surfactant deficiency and RDS.

D. Consider bacterial pneumonia (especially GBS disease) in patients with RDS. Risk factors for infection include maternal fever, amnionitis, and premature rupture of the membranes. Neutropenia or leukocytosis and immature to total leukocyte ratio greater than 0.2 suggest infection. Draw blood cultures; consider urine for bacterial antigen detection and a tracheal aspirate in intubated infants. Initiate antibiotic therapy with ampicillin and an aminoglycoside (Table 1).

E. Worsening occurs over the first 48 to 72 hours in the natural history of RDS; thus, it is important to consider both the postnatal age of the patient and severity of illness in choosing therapeutic interventions. Early initiation of continuous positive airway pressure (CPAP) by nasal prongs or endotracheal tube may stabilize alveoli and prevent atelectasis. A trial of CPAP in the first hours of life is useful if the patient is ventilating adequately but oxygenating poorly in fractional inspired oxygen concentration (Fio_2) of 0.4 to 0.6. Extremely preterm infants and those with severe disease often require intubation during delivery room resuscitation or shortly thereafter. All neonates with RDS who are tachypneic (respiratory rate >60) should be kept NPO with maintenance IV fluids and glucose (80 ml/kg fluids in the first 24 hours; 6 to 9 mg/kg/minute glucose). Institution of total parenteral nutrition by 24 to 48 hours is recommended, especially for preterm infants.

TABLE 1 Drugs Used to Treat Complications in Infants with Respiratory Distress Syndrome

Drug	Dosages

Ampicillin	Age <7 days
	  <2000 g—50 mg/kg/24 hr in 2 divided doses
	  >2000 g—75 mg/kg/24 hr in 3 divided doses
	Age >7 days:
	  <2000 g—75 mg/kg/24 hr in 3 divided doses
	  >2000 g—100 mg/kg/24 hr in 4 divided doses

Gentamicin	Premature newborn
	Age <7 days
	  <1000 g and <28 wk GA—2.5 mg/kg q24h
	  <1500 g and <34 wk GA—2.5 mg/kg q18h
	  >1500 g and >34 wk GA—2.5 mg/kg q12h
	Age >7 days
	  <2000 g—2.5 mg/kg q12h
	  >2000 g—2.5 mg/kg q8h

Indomethacin	Initial 0.2 mg/kg followed by 2 doses of 0.1–0.2 mg/kg q12–24h if age <48 hours at time of first dose; 0.2 mg/kg twice if 2–7 days old at time of first dose; 0.25 mg/kg twice if over 7 days at time of first dose

GA, gestational age.

TABLE 2 Degree of Illness in Respiratory Distress

Moderate	Severe	Very Severe
Adequate Pao_2 in Fio_2 <0.4 and Pco_2 <50 mm Hg and Normal pH	Require Fio_2 >0.4	Require Fio_2 >0.6 and Pco_2 >50 mm Hg and Combined respiratory and metabolic acidosis

F. Monitor arterial oxygen concentration (Pao_2) in every infant with RDS. Pulse oximetry is rapidly available; transcutaneous monitoring can provide information on Pao_2 and carbon dioxide pressure. Consider placing an umbilical artery catheter or radial arterial catheter in infants who require high oxygen, CPAP, or assisted ventilation. Connect arterial lines to pressure transducers for blood pressure monitoring and safety. Monitor glucose, electrolytes, and calcium.

G. Assisted ventilation is usually initiated with pressure-limited, time-cycled intermittent mandatory ventilation (IMV) to achieve good chest wall expansion and normalize arterial blood gases. Synchronous ventilation, high-frequency oscillatory ventilation, and jet ventilation may be indicated under certain circumstances; consult a neonatologist.

H. Consider surfactant replacement therapy in patients with a diagnosis of RDS who require an Fio_2 above 0.4

(Continued on page 426)

Patient with RESPIRATORY DISTRESS SYNDROME

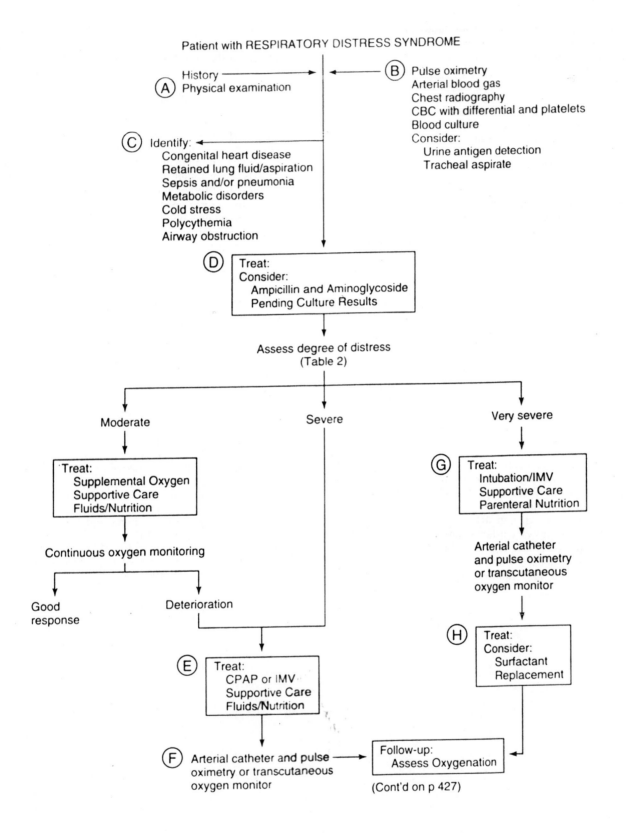

(A) History ——→
    Physical examination

(B) Pulse oximetry
    Arterial blood gas
    Chest radiography
    CBC with differential and platelets
    Blood culture
    Consider:
        Urine antigen detection
        Tracheal aspirate

(C) Identify: ←
    Congenital heart disease
    Retained lung fluid/aspiration
    Sepsis and/or pneumonia
    Metabolic disorders
    Cold stress
    Polycythemia
    Airway obstruction

(D) Treat:
    Consider:
        Ampicillin and Aminoglycoside
        Pending Culture Results

Assess degree of distress
(Table 2)

Moderate

Treat:
    Supplemental Oxygen
    Supportive Care
    Fluids/Nutrition

Continuous oxygen monitoring

Good response

Deterioration

Severe

Very severe

(G) Treat:
    Intubation/IMV
    Supportive Care
    Parenteral Nutrition

Arterial catheter
and pulse oximetry
or transcutaneous
oxygen monitor

(H) Treat:
    Consider:
        Surfactant
        Replacement

(E) Treat:
    CPAP or IMV
    Supportive Care
    Fluids/Nutrition

(F) Arterial catheter and pulse
    oximetry or transcutaneous
    oxygen monitor

Follow-up:
    Assess Oxygenation

(Cont'd on p 427)

TABLE 3 Types of Surfactant Replacement

Natural surfactant preparations
Heterologous
  Bovine surfactant extract
    Calf lung surfactant extract (Infasurf)
    Bovine lung lavage extract
    SF-RI 1 (Alveofact)
  Porcine surfactant extract (Curosurf)
  Modified bovine surfactant extract
    Surfactant TA (Surfacten)
    Beractant (Survanta)
Homologous
  Human amniotic fluid surfactant extract

Synthetic surfactant preparations
Artificial lung expanding compound (ALEC)
Colfosceril palmitate, hexadecanol, typloxapol (Exosurf)

on mechanical ventilation. Neonatology consultation is useful in selecting from an increasing array of natural and synthetic surfactants (Table 3).

I. Acute complications of RDS include pulmonary air leak (pneumothorax and pulmonary interstitial emphysema), pulmonary hemorrhage, and the cardiovascular complications of patent ductus arteriosus (PDA) and persistent pulmonary hypertension. RDS in premature infants is also associated with the chronic complications of retinopathy of prematurity, intracranial hemorrhage and its sequelae, necrotizing enterocolitis, hyperbilirubinemia, and anemia.

J. PDA is common in premature infants weighing less than 1500 g, including those who have received artificial surfactant for RDS. Suspect PDA with a continuous murmur, bounding pulses, diastolic blood pressure less than 26 mm Hg, and active precordium. The chest radiograph shows cardiomegaly with increased pulmonary blood flow and/or pulmonary edema. Color Doppler echocardiography can confirm a left-to-right ductal shunt and demonstrate diastolic runoff from the aorta. Consider indomethacin to promote ductal closure; indomethacin may be contraindicated for a patient with renal failure, thrombocytopenia or other coagulation disorders, or severe hyperbilirubinemia. Surgical ligation of the PDA may be necessary in urgent cases or if medical management is unsuccessful.

K. Persistent pulmonary hypertension in association with RDS most often occurs in near-term or term infants with congenital or acquired surfactant deficiency. Presentation may be immediately after birth or after several days of RDS. Right-to-left shunts through the ductus arteriosus or patent foramen ovale result in refractory hypoxemia. In the presence of PDA, preductal Pao_2 (right radial artery) may be more than 15 to 20 mm Hg higher than postductal Pao_2 (umbilical artery). Echocardiography can confirm right-to-left shunting through the ductus and foramen ovale; the degree of pulmonary hypertension can be estimated by quantitation of a tricuspid regurgitation jet. Initial management includes maintenance of adequate systolic blood pressure and circulating volume, correction of metabolic acidosis, and reversal of hypoxemia. High-frequency oscillatory ventilation (HFOV) and experimental protocols using nitric oxide (NO) offer therapeutic alternatives to extracorporeal membrane oxygenation (ECMO).

References

Kinsella JP, Neish ST, Ivy DD, et al. Clinical responses to prolonged treatment of persistent pulmonary hypertension of the newborn with low doses of inhaled nitric oxide. J Pediatr 1993; 123:103.

Long W. Synthetic surfactant. Semin Perinatol 1993; 17:275.

Moya FR, Gross I. Combined hormonal therapy for the prevention of respiratory distress syndrome and its consequences. Semin Perinatol 1993; 17:267.

Spafford PS, Kendig JW, Maniscalco WM. Use of natural surfactants to prevent and treat respiratory distress syndrome. Semin Perinatol 1993; 17:285.

Patient with RESPIRATORY DISTRESS SYNDROME

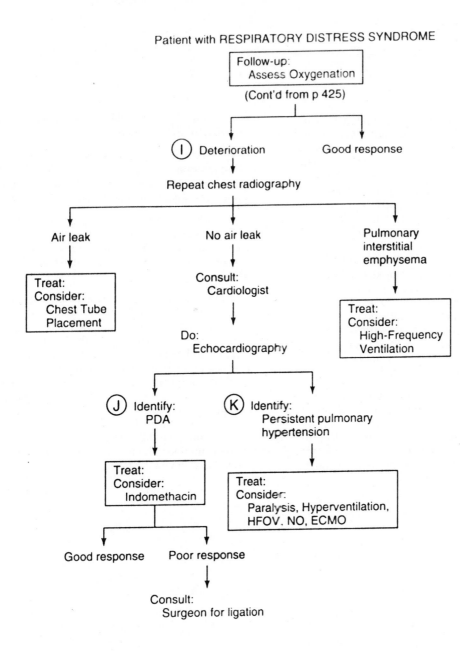

RESUSCITATION

Susan Niermeyer, M.D.

Prompt, skilled evaluation and resuscitation of neonates can restore normal transition and help prevent injury from prenatal or postnatal asphyxia. Effective intervention requires anticipation and preparation to have available trained personnel, proper equipment, supplies, policies, and procedures for resuscitation. Immediate preparation is guided by pregnancy risk factors and intrapartum complications such as prematurity or meconium-stained amniotic fluid. At least one person skilled in neonatal resuscitation should attend each delivery; two persons should be present in high-risk situations, one of them skilled in endotracheal intubation and administration of medications. At every delivery three initial steps in resuscitation should be carried out: (1) prevention of heat loss; (2) opening of the airway; and (3) evaluation of respirations, heart rate (HR), and color. Evaluation, decisions, and actions begin before the 1 minute Apgar score is assigned. While the Apgar score is not the basis for decision making in resuscitation, it is an important objective quantitation of an infant's condition and response to resuscitation.

A. Assess respirations. Provide brief tactile stimulation to an infant who is apneic or gasping. If the rate and depth of respirations do not increase immediately, initiate positive-pressure ventilation (PPV). Continuing to provide tactile stimulation or free-flow oxygen to an infant who is not breathing or whose HR is less than 100 beats per minute (bpm) is of little or no benefit and delays appropriate management.

B. Determine HR. It may be checked by auscultation with a stethoscope or by palpation of umbilical cord pulsations. An HR less than 100 bpm indicates a need for PPV even if the infant has spontaneous respirations.

C. Assess color. Central cyanosis (lips, mucous membranes) reflects hypoxemia; provide free-flow oxygen (100% oxygen at 5 L/min by mask or tubing held to face) to a spontaneously breathing infant whose HR is above 100 bpm.

D. PPV may be given with a resuscitation bag and mask or a bag and endotracheal tube. The bag must deliver 90% to 100% oxygen and be equipped with a pop-off valve and/or pressure gauge. Two or three initial breaths with a prolonged inspiratory time (2 to 3 seconds) and peak pressure of 30 to 40 cm H_2O help open the airways and establish lung volume. Give subsequent ventilations at 40 to 60 breaths per minute at pressures that produce adequate chest wall movement and breath sounds. Perform endotracheal intubation in case of ineffective bag and mask ventilation, prolonged PPV, meconium-stained amniotic fluid in a depressed infant, or suspected diaphragmatic hernia.

(Continued on page 430)

NEONATAL RESUSCITATION IN THE DELIVERY ROOM

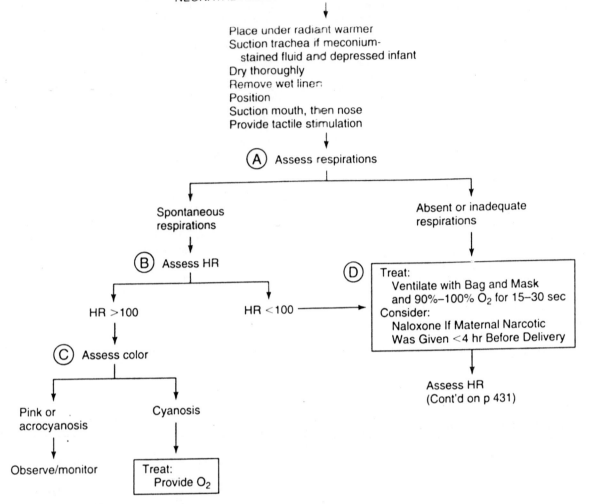

Place under radiant warmer
Suction trachea if meconium-
    stained fluid and depressed infant
Dry thoroughly
Remove wet linen
Position
Suction mouth, then nose
Provide tactile stimulation

(A) Assess respirations

Spontaneous
respirations

Absent or inadequate
respirations

(B) Assess HR

(D) Treat:
    Ventilate with Bag and Mask
    and 90%–100% O_2 for 15–30 sec
Consider:
    Naloxone If Maternal Narcotic
    Was Given <4 hr Before Delivery

HR >100

HR <100

(C) Assess color

Assess HR
(Cont'd on p 431)

Pink or
acrocyanosis

Cyanosis

Observe/monitor

Treat:
    Provide O_2

E. Chest compressions are indicated if after 15 to 30 seconds of PPV with 90% to 100% oxygen the HR remains below 60 bpm or 60 to 80 bpm but not increasing. Apply compression to a depth of ½ to ¾ inch to the lower third of the sternum with the thumbs (hands encircling the chest and supporting the back) or two fingers of one hand (other hand supporting the back). Give compressions in a 3:1 ratio with ventilation to provide 90 compressions and 30 breaths in 1 minute (3 compressions and one pause for ventilation in a 2-second cycle). Check the HR every 30 seconds by counting for 6 seconds and multiplying by 10 to obtain bpm. Discontinue chest compressions when the HR reaches 80 bpm.

F. Most neonates respond to adequate ventilation with 90% to 100% oxygen and chest compressions; however, medication may be necessary to stimulate the heart, increase tissue perfusion, or restore acid-base balance. Give epinephrine if the HR is 0 or below 80 bpm after 30 seconds of PPV with 90% to 100% oxygen and chest compressions. Epinephrine may be given IV or per endotracheal tube (Table 1). If the HR remains below 100 bpm, consider readministration of epinephrine every 3 to 5 minutes as required, volume expander if there is evidence of acute blood loss with signs of hypovolemia or poor response to resuscitative efforts, and sodium bicarbonate in a prolonged arrest

that does not respond to other therapy. Consider dopamine administration if after a prolonged resuscitation the infant has poor peripheral perfusion, thready pulses, and persistent hypotension. Naloxone hydrochloride, a narcotic antagonist, is indicated when there is severe respiratory depression and the mother received a narcotic within 4 hours of delivery.

G. Postresuscitation management includes monitoring of vital signs, perfusion, neurologic status, and urine output. Ongoing ventilatory support and IV fluids are often necessary. A thorough history and physical examination guide further laboratory management and testing. Blood gases, blood glucose, hematocrit, and chest radiography are often informative.

H. Decisions to terminate resuscitation are most often made in the circumstances of extreme prematurity, severe congenital anomalies, and prolonged asphyxia. Prenatal diagnosis facilitates advance discussion with the parents to guide delivery room treatment. In other circumstances the initial approach is aggressive resuscitation; a decision to terminate efforts may become appropriate in the delivery room or later in the intensive care nursery. Dramatic increases in death and severe sequelae occur after 15 minutes or more of resuscitation. Thus, it is probably futile to continue resuscitation longer than 15 minutes in an unresponsive infant.

TABLE 1   Medications for Neonatal Resuscitation

Medication	Concentration to Administer	Preparation	Dosage/Route	Rate/Precautions
Epinephrine	1:10,000	1 ml	0.1–0.3 ml/kg IV or ET	Give rapidly May dilute with normal saline to 1–2 ml if giving ET
Volume expanders	Whole blood 5% albumin-saline Normal saline Ringer's lactate	40 ml	10 ml/kg IV	Give over 5–10 min
Sodium bicarbonate	0.5 mEq/ml (4.2% solution)	20 ml or Two 10-ml prefilled syringes	2 mEq/kg IV	Give slowly, over at least 2 min Give only if infant is being effectively ventilated
Naloxone hydrochloride	0.4 mg/ml or 1 mg/ml	1 ml	0.1 mg/kg IV, ET IM, SC	Give rapidly IV, ET preferred IM, SC acceptable
Dopamine	$6 \times \dfrac{\text{Weight (kg)} \times \text{Desired dose } (\mu g/kg/min)}{\text{Desired fluid (ml/hr)}} =$ mg of dopamine per 100 ml of solution		Begin at 5 µg/kg/min (may increase to 20 µg/kg/min if necessary) IV	Give as a continuous infusion using an infusion pump Monitor heart rate and blood pressure closely Seek consultation

IM, intramuscular; ET, endotracheal; IV, intravenous; SC, subcutaneous.
Modified from *Textbook of Neonatal Resuscitation* © 1987, 1990, 1994 American Heart Association.

NEONATAL RESUSCITATION IN THE DELIVERY ROOM

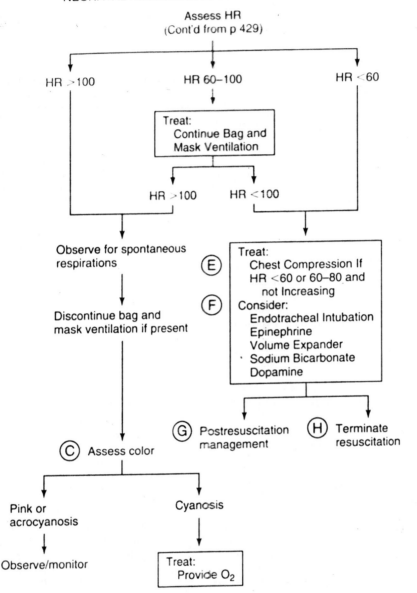

References

Bloom RS, Cropley C, AHA/AAP Neonatal Resuscitation Program Steering Committee. Textbook of Neonatal Resuscitation. Dallas: American Heart Association, 1994.

Burchfield DJ, Berkowitz ID, Berg RA, Goldberg RN. Medications in neonatal resuscitation. Ann Emerg Med 1993; 22:435.

Byrne PJ, Tyebkhan JM, Laing LM. Ethical decision-making and neonatal resuscitation. Seminar Perinatol 1994; 18:36.

Carter BS, Haverkamp AD, Merenstein GB. The definition of acute perinatal asphyxia. Clin Perinatol 1993; 20:287.

Emergency Cardiac Care Committee and Subcommittees, American Heart Association. Guidelines for cardiopulmonary resuscitation and emergency cardiac care. Part VIII. Neonatal resuscitation. JAMA 1992; 268:2276.

SEIZURES

Susan Niermeyer, M.D.

A. In the history inquire about maternal medication and illicit drug use during pregnancy. Note the type of anesthesia used during delivery, abnormalities of fetal monitoring, Apgar score, and resuscitation required at birth (perinatal asphyxia). Determine whether other infants in the family have had seizures.

B. In the physical examination focus on dysmorphic features, evidence of trauma, stigmata of infection, and signs of asphyxia. Evaluate the fontanelle carefully, examine the fundi, and auscultate for cranial bruit. Evaluate alertness, tone, and reflexes between clinical seizures to detect obtundation or coma.

C. Laboratory evaluation should screen for the most common metabolic abnormalities, infection, and exposure to drugs and toxins. Drug screening can be performed on maternal and neonatal urine. Analysis of meconium for drugs and toxins detects exposure in utero.

D. Characterize the clinical seizure activity. Focal clonic seizures, focal tonic seizures (tonic eye deviation or asymmetric tonic posturing), and some myoclonic seizures occur in association with electrical seizure activity. Clinical events without a consistent relationship to electrographic seizures include generalized symmetric tonic posturing, some myoclonic jerking, and most subtle seizures (oral-buccal-lingual movements, random eye movements, nystagmus, and progression movements such as pedaling, stepping, and swimming). Attempt to suppress spontaneous seizures by lightly restraining or repositioning the involved areas of the body. Epileptic motor activity will continue, while jitteriness or tremors will cease with passive flexion. Jitteriness, more common than seizures, occurs frequently in infants with hypocalcemia, hypoglycemia, drug withdrawal, and asphyxia. Attempt to evoke behavior identical to spontaneous clinical seizures. Temporal and spatial summation and eradication of the response characterize reflex response rather than epileptic activity.

TABLE 1 Medications Used in the Treatment of Neonatal Seizures

Medication	Dosage	Preparation
Phenobarbital	Load: 15–20 mg/kg/dose IV, IM Maintenance: 3–5 mg/kg/day q12h IV, IM, PO	Elixir: 20 mg/5 ml Vial: 65 mg/ml
Phenytoin	15 mg/kg/dose IV Maintenance: 3–5 mg/kg/day q12h IV, PO	Susp: 30, 125 mg/5 ml Vial: 50 mg/ml
Lorazepam	0.05–0.1 mg/kg/dose IV	Vial: 2 mg/ml

E. Consider electroencephalogram (EEG) and restriction of anticonvulsant therapy to seizures with a clear epileptic basis. EEG is helpful in establishing cause and prognosis. Seizures with a clear epileptic basis are often associated with focal structural lesions, hemorrhage, and metabolic derangements. Seizures without epileptic cortical discharges are often associated with hypoxic-ischemic encephalopathy. Both epileptic and nonepileptic seizures may occur with infection. Begin anticonvulsant therapy with phenobarbital. If seizures continue with a therapeutic phenobarbital level, add phenytoin as a slow IV loading dose followed by IV maintenance. If seizures persist or interfere with vital functions, consider giving lorazepam (Table 1).

F. Transient hypoglycemia may accompany asphyxia, low birth weight, growth retardation, infant of a diabetic mother, polycythemia, sepsis, cold stress, adrenal hemorrhage, and respiratory distress. Persistent hypoglycemia, much less common, may be due to hyperinsulinism, hormonal deficiency, or defects in carbohydrate, amino acid, or organic acid metabolism. After obtaining a serum glucose, treat Dextrostix values less than 40 by administering 2 ml/kg $D_{10}W$ IV bolus followed by a constant infusion of 6 to 8 mg/kg/minute of glucose.

(Continued on page 434)

Newborn with SEIZURES

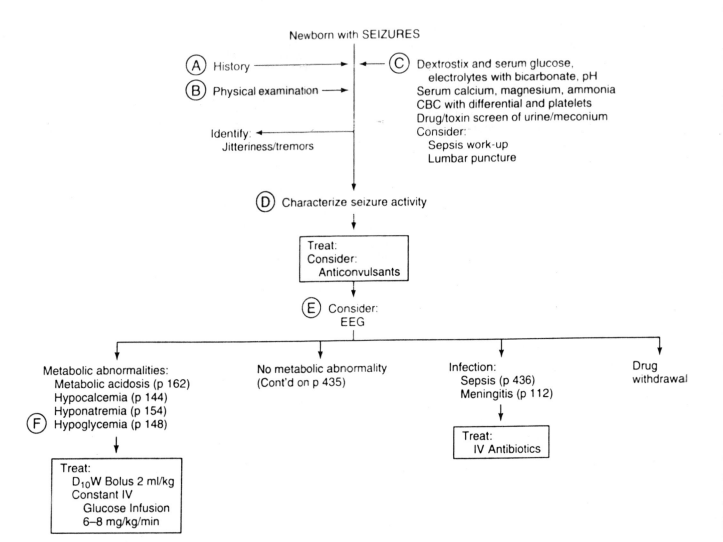

(A) History

(B) Physical examination

(C) Dextrostix and serum glucose,
electrolytes with bicarbonate, pH
Serum calcium, magnesium, ammonia
CBC with differential and platelets
Drug/toxin screen of urine/meconium
Consider:
Sepsis work-up
Lumbar puncture

Identify:
Jitteriness/tremors

(D) Characterize seizure activity

Treat:
Consider:
Anticonvulsants

(E) Consider:
EEG

Metabolic abnormalities:
Metabolic acidosis (p 162)
Hypocalcemia (p 144)
Hyponatremia (p 154)
(F) Hypoglycemia (p 148)

No metabolic abnormality
(Cont'd on p 435)

Infection:
Sepsis (p 436)
Meningitis (p 112)

Drug
withdrawal

Treat:
D₁₀W Bolus 2 ml/kg
Constant IV
Glucose Infusion
6–8 mg/kg/min

Treat:
IV Antibiotics

No metabolic abnormality
(Cont'd on p 435)

G. Perinatal asphyxia is the most frequent cause of neonatal seizures. Intracranial hemorrhage is a common cause of seizures in preterm infants less than 32 weeks gestation. Intracranial hemorrhage commonly occurs in the periventricular or intraventricular region in prematures; in term infants bleeding is more common in the subarachnoid or subdural space. Developmental defects and tumors are less common causes of neonatal seizures.

H. If seizures of unknown origin persist despite therapeutic levels of anticonvulsants, consider a trial of pyridoxine. Paroxysmal electrical activity on EEG ceases after IV injection of pyridoxine in cases of pyridoxine deficiency.

I. The prognosis of infants with neonatal seizures relates most directly to the underlying cause. Perinatal asphyxia and intraventricular hemorrhage frequently result in permanent sequelae, as do intracranial infections, significant and prolonged hypoglycemia, and early-onset hypoglycemia. The EEG and clinical examination at 1 week are helpful in predicting outcome: infants with a normal EEG and neurologic examination usually have a favorable outcome, while an abnormal EEG and neurologic examination are worrisome.

References

Mizrahi EM. Consensus and controversy in the clinical management of neonatal seizures. Clin Perinatol 1989; 16:485.
Novotny EJ Jr. Neonatal seizures. Semin Perinatol 1993; 17:351.
Seashore MR, Rinaldo P. Metabolic disease of the neonate and young infant. Semin Perinatol 1993; 17:318.
Volpe JJ. Neurology of the newborn. Philadelphia: Saunders, 1994.

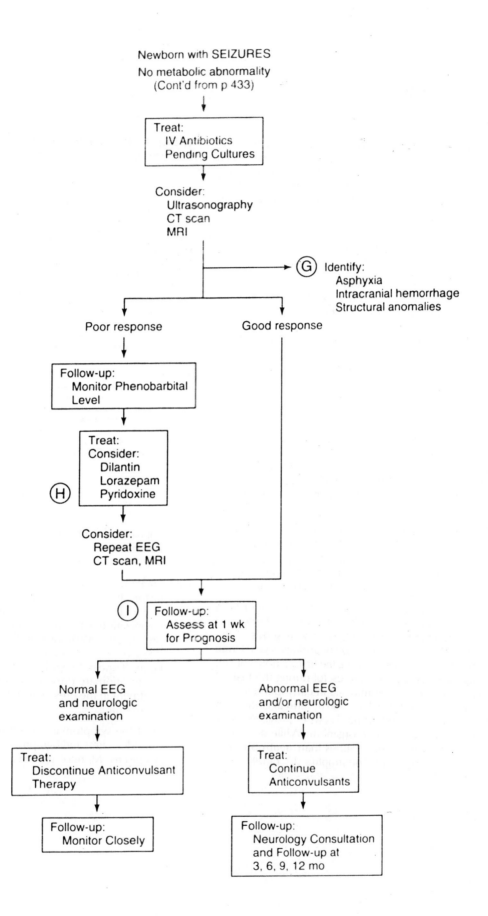

Newborn with SEIZURES
No metabolic abnormality
(Cont'd from p 433)

Treat:
IV Antibiotics
Pending Cultures

Consider:
Ultrasonography
CT scan
MRI

(G) Identify:
Asphyxia
Intracranial hemorrhage
Structural anomalies

Poor response

Good response

Follow-up:
Monitor Phenobarbital
Level

Treat:
Consider:
Dilantin
(H) Lorazepam
Pyridoxine

Consider:
Repeat EEG
CT scan, MRI

(I) Follow-up:
Assess at 1 wk
for Prognosis

Normal EEG
and neurologic
examination

Abnormal EEG
and/or neurologic
examination

Treat:
Discontinue Anticonvulsant
Therapy

Treat:
Continue
Anticonvulsants

Follow-up:
Monitor Closely

Follow-up:
Neurology Consultation
and Follow-up at
3, 6, 9, 12 mo

SEPSIS

Susan Niermeyer, M.D.

Perinatally acquired bacterial sepsis often presents with subtle or nonspecific signs but may progress rapidly to death. In such a condition, with high mortality, low incidence, and relatively benign treatment, clinical practice dictates therapy for infants at risk on the basis of historical factors and diagnostic tests as well as those who are symptomatic.

ETIOLOGY

Neonatal sepsis is most commonly caused by group B streptococcus (GBS) and *Escherichia coli,* followed by *Klebsiella, Enterobacter, Staphylococcus aureus,* group D streptococci, *Haemophilus influenzae, Pseudomonas,* and others. While this chapter focuses on perinatally acquired bacterial infection, congenital infection (bacterial and viral), perinatally acquired nonbacterial infection (e.g., herpes, enterovirus, *Mycoplasma/Ureaplasma*), and nosocomial infection (bacterial, viral, yeast) are other important causes of illness in the neonate.

A. The perinatal history provides important early information to assess the risk of sepsis in a newborn infant. Note risk factors (Table 1). Suspect chorioamnionitis with maternal fever above 100.4° F (38° C), uterine tenderness, purulent or foul-smelling amniotic fluid, or fetal tachycardia.

B. In the physical examination note nonspecific signs such as lethargy, hypotonia, fever or hypothermia, respiratory distress (tachypnea, cyanosis, grunting, apnea), glucose instability, feeding intolerance, poor perfusion or shock, petechiae or purpura, and unexplained jaundice.

C. Obtain a blood culture by sterile venipuncture or from a newly placed sterile umbilical catheter. Perform a lumbar puncture in neonates in whom sepsis is the primary diagnosis or who exhibit neurologic signs. Urine cultures have a low yield during the first 72 hours of life. Tracheal aspirate cultures are useful during the first 12 hours of life; Gram stain may aid in early identification of bacteria. GBS antigen detection by latex agglutination (LA) on concentrated urine likewise provides early specific identification of an organism. While neutropenia is a better predictor of sepsis than neutrophilia, a ratio of immature to total neutrophils (I/T ratio) $>1:5$

TABLE 1 Risk Factors for Neonatal Sepsis

Condition	Incidence	
	Proven Sepsis	Proven & Highly Suspected Sepsis*
PROM >18–24 hr	1%	1%–2%
Maternal + GBS	0.5%–1%	1%–2%
PROM and + GBS	4%–6%	7%–11%
+ GBS and maternal fever	3%–5%	6%–10%
PROM and chorioamnionitis	3%–8%	6%–10%
PROM or + GBS and preterm	4%–6%	7%–11%
PROM and 5 min Apgar <6	3%–4%	6%–10%
Male sex	Risk ↑ 4-fold	Risk ↑ 4-fold

PROM, prolonged rupture of membranes; GBS, group B streptococcus.
*Highly suspected sepsis includes cases in which cultures were negative, but the clinical presentation was highly consistent with bacterial infection such as pneumonia.
Adapted from Gerdes JS. Clinicopathologic approach to the diagnosis of neonatal sepsis. Clin Perinatol 1991; 18:361.

improves the predictive value. Toxic granulation and vacuolization of neutrophils and thrombocytopenia are useful but not definitive.

D. Treat the asymptomatic infant after evaluation of the risk factors. If maternal colonization with GBS is present with one additional risk factor, begin treatment. If maternal colonization with GBS and no additional risk factors are present and WBC/differential and urine GBS-LA are negative, a term infant may be observed closely for 48 hours. If one or two risk factors other than GBS maternal colonization are present, carry out screening. Consider treatment in the presence of three risk factors regardless of screening.

E. Treat the symptomatic infant regardless of risk factors. Consider chest radiography in infants with respiratory symptoms. Monitor glucose, oxygenation, blood pres-

(Continued on page 438)

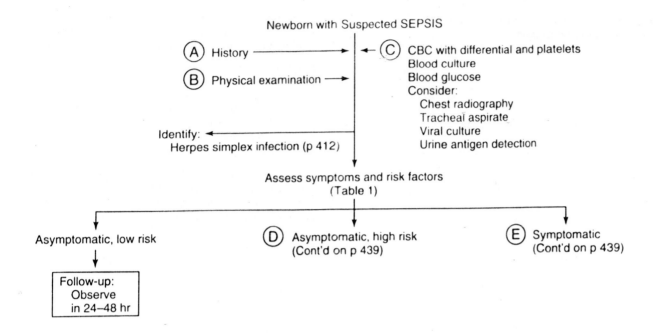

Newborn with Suspected SEPSIS

Ⓐ History ──────────▶ ◀── Ⓒ CBC with differential and platelets
                                Blood culture
Ⓑ Physical examination ──▶   Blood glucose
                                Consider:
                                   Chest radiography
                                   Tracheal aspirate
Identify: ◀─────────────   Viral culture
   Herpes simplex infection (p 412)   Urine antigen detection

Assess symptoms and risk factors
(Table 1)

Asymptomatic, low risk   Ⓓ Asymptomatic, high risk   Ⓔ Symptomatic
                               (Cont'd on p 439)   (Cont'd on p 439)

┌─────────────┐
│ Follow-up: │
│ Observe   │
│ in 24–48 hr│
└─────────────┘

TABLE 2 Medications Used in the Treatment of Neonatal Sepsis

Drug	Dosage	Product Availability

Ampicillin	Sepsis:
	  < 7 days
	    Preterm 50–100 mg/kg/day q12h
	    Full term 100–150 mg/kg/day q12h
	  > 7 days
	    100–150 mg/kg/day q8h
	Meningitis:
	  < 7 days
	    Preterm 100 mg/kg/day q12h
	    Full term 150–200 mg/kg/day q8–12h
	  > 7 days: 200–300 mg/kg/day q6–8h
		Vials: 125, 250, 500 mg

Gentamicin	Premature newborn
	  < 7 days
	    2.5 mg/kg/dose IV q18–24h or 3.5 mg/kg/dose IV determined by formula: dosing hours = 50.5 − 0.76 × gestational age (wk)
	Term newborn
	  2.5 mg/kg/dose q12h
		IV solution: 10 mg/ml (2 ml), 40 mg/ml (1.5, 2 ml)

Cefotaxime	≤ 7 days:
	  50 mg/kg/dose IV q12h
	> 7 days:
	  50 mg/kg/dose IV q8h
		Vials: 1, 2 g

Immunoglobulin, Intravenous	Premature newborn
	  500 mg/day
	Term newborn
	  750 mg/day
	  Graded, slow infusion
		Vials: 2.5, 5 g Reconstitute to 5% solution

sure, renal function, electrolytes, and coagulation. Consider viral cultures and serology if congenital infection or viral infection is possible.

F. Begin antibiotic therapy with IV or IM ampicillin and an aminoglycoside (Table 2). Continue appropriate antibiotic treatment on the basis of culture results. Consider 7 to 10 days of therapy for positive GBS-LA. Treat positive blood culture for 10 to 14 days and meningitis for 14 to 21 days. If cultures are negative, discontinue antibiotics after 48 to 72 hours.

G. Stabilize acutely ill infants with intubation, volume and pressor support, and coagulation factors as indicated. Treat seizures. IV immunoglobulin may be useful in certain circumstances associated with neutropenia. Granulocyte transfusions and cytokines continue under investigation.

References

Committee on Infectious Diseases and Committee on Fetus and Newborn, American Academy of Pediatrics. Guidelines for prevention of group B streptococcal (GBS) infection by chemoprophylaxis. Pediatrics 1992; 90:775.

Gerdes JS. Clinicopathologic approach to the diagnosis of neonatal sepsis. Clin Perinatol 1991; 18:361.

Gibbs RS, McDuffic RS Jr, McNabb F, et al. Neonatal group B streptococcal sepsis during 2 years of a universal screening program. Obstet Gynecol 1994; 84:496.

Klein JO, Marcy SM. Bacterial sepsis and meningitis. In: Remington JS, Klein JO, eds. Infectious diseases of the fetus and newborn infant. 3rd ed. Philadelphia: Saunders, 1990:601.

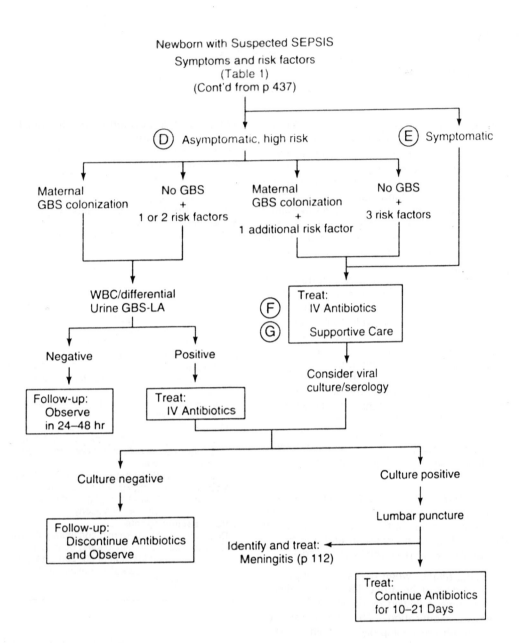

Newborn with Suspected SEPSIS
Symptoms and risk factors
(Table 1)
(Cont'd from p 437)

(D) Asymptomatic, high risk

(E) Symptomatic

Maternal GBS colonization

No GBS + 1 or 2 risk factors

Maternal GBS colonization + 1 additional risk factor

No GBS + 3 risk factors

WBC/differential
Urine GBS-LA

(F)
(G)
Treat:
IV Antibiotics

Supportive Care

Negative

Positive

Follow-up:
Observe
in 24–48 hr

Treat:
IV Antibiotics

Consider viral
culture/serology

Culture negative

Culture positive

Follow-up:
Discontinue Antibiotics
and Observe

Lumbar puncture

Identify and treat: ◄
Meningitis (p 112)

Treat:
Continue Antibiotics
for 10–21 Days

TETANUS

Susan Niermeyer, M.D.

Tetanus is a major cause of neonatal mortality in the developing world; even in industrialized countries continued awareness is vital when dealing with migrant workers, immigrants from developing countries, and other patients with limited access to health care and inadequate immunization. Mortality in neonatal tetanus ranges from 12% to 90%, depending on severity and medical facilities available. Neonatal tetanus results from the toxin tetanospasmin, elaborated by the anaerobic bacterium *Clostridium tetani,* which most frequently enters through the umbilical stump. Unhygienic birth conditions (lack of hand washing, use of unsterile implement to cut the cord) and certain traditional practices (dressing the cord with dung, yam flour, Shea butter, plant or industrial oils, herbs or plant juices; neonatal surgical procedures such as circumcision, uvulectomy, and ear piercing) predispose to contamination of susceptible tissue. Absence of protective levels of tetanus-specific IgG may result from absent or inadequate maternal immunization (administration late in pregnancy, insufficient antibody response, defective tetanus toxoid preparation). Even with protective maternal immunity, cord levels of tetanus-specific antibody may be nonprotective when mothers have high circulating levels of IgG (chronic parasites) or impaired placental transfer, as in placental malaria. As many as a third of neonatal tetanus cases occur in infants born to mothers of another affected child.

A. In the history determine the incubation period, time of onset (appearance of symptoms to first generalized spasm), and immunization history of the mother. Short incubation period, rapid progression, and absence of any passive antibody are poor prognostic factors.

B. Suspect neonatal tetanus when typical signs appear in the first 3 to 10 days of life: irritability, early weakness and failure to nurse, followed by rigidity and spasms. In the physical examination note hypothermia or hyperthermia; both are poor prognostic signs. Tachycardia, hypotension, or hypertension suggests autonomic involvement. Trismus (masseter rigidity), risus sardonicus (increased tone of the orbicularis oris), and abdominal rigidity reflect general muscle stiffness. General spasms triggered by tactile, visual, or auditory stimuli resemble decorticate posturing with flexion of the arms and extension of the legs in an opisthotonic posture. Airway obstruction during spasms may result in transient cyanosis or lethal apnea. Examine the umbilicus for signs of omphalitis or fasciitis and seek other possible entrance sites.

C. Culturing of the umbilicus or wounds for *C. tetani* is not useful in diagnosis. Cultures are commonly negative even when organisms are present; presence of organisms does not always result in disease if the toxin-producing plasmid is absent or immunity is adequate. Laboratory evaluation should, however, include cultures of blood, urine, and cerebrospinal fluid (CSF) for other bacterial infections, most commonly due to

TABLE 1 Drugs Used in Treatment of Neonatal Tetanus

Passive immunization
HTIG 500–6000 U IM (optimum therapeutic dose has not been established)
IV immunoglobulin (dose not established for this indication)
Equine ATS 3000 IU IM in 2 divided doses

Active immunization
Diphtheria-tetanus-pertussis vaccine 0.5 ml IM (to age 7 yr)
Diphtheria-tetanus vaccine 0.5 ml IM (age 7 yr–adult)

Antibiotics
Penicillin G 100,000 U/kg/24 hr IV in 4–6 divided doses for 10–14 days
Procaine penicillin 50,000 U/kg/day IM q24h to complete 10–14 days
Ampicillin 100 mg/kg/24 hr IM or IV in 4 divided doses
Gentamicin 7.5 mg/kg/24 hr IM or IV in 3 divided doses
Metronidazole 30 mg/kg/24 hr IV in 2 divided doses

Sedatives, muscle relaxants
Diazepam 0.2–0.8 mg/kg/24 hr PO in 3 or 4 divided doses up to 2.5–5 mg PO t.i.d.-q.i.d. for maintenance muscle relaxation
0.25 mg/kg/dose IV q15min for 2–3 doses for emergent control of spasms
Midazolam 0.1–0.2 mg/kg IV loading dose followed by continuous infusion of 2 µg/kg/min (titrate 0.4–6 µg/kg/min to achieve desired effect) for conscious sedation during mechanical ventilation
Phenobarbital 6–10 mg/kg/24 hr PO in 3–4 divided doses
Vecuronium 0.1 mg/kg IV for intubation
Pancuronium 0.03–0.1 mg/kg IV q30–60min p.r.n. movement during mechanical ventilationy

Cardiovascular agents
Dopamine 5–20 µg/kg/min continuous IV infusion
Esmolol 500 µg/kg/min loading dose IV over 1 min, followed by continuous infusion of 50–200 µg/kg/min
Labetalol 50–100 µg/kg/hr continuous IV infusion (not approved for infants)

coliforms and *Staphylococcus aureus,* which complicate more than a third of cases. Evaluate electrolytes and serum bicarbonate for signs of dehydration or unexpected acidosis, which might suggest an alternative diagnosis, inborn error of metabolism. Obtain serum creatinine and BUN to evaluate renal function.

D. Stabilize the infant immediately by assuring an adequate airway and controlling muscle spasm and rigidity. Administer a benzodiazepine and titrate the dose to produce sedation and minimize reflex spasms (Table 1). If airway compromise results, perform endotracheal intubation, using a short-acting neuromuscular blocking agent. Insert a soft, small-diameter nasogastric feeding tube. Transfer the patient to a quiet, darkened area and group further interventions to minimize stimulation. Administer human tetanus immunoglobulin (HTIG); as an alternative, consider IV pooled immunoglobulin or equine antitetanus serum (ATS) if other preparations are not available. Begin crystalline penicillin or ampicillin

(Continued on page 442)

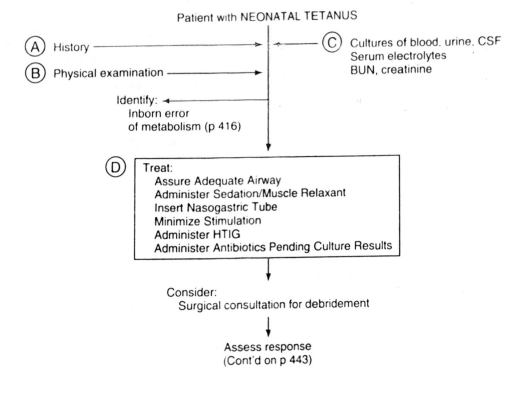

Patient with NEONATAL TETANUS

(A) History

(B) Physical examination

(C) Cultures of blood, urine, CSF
Serum electrolytes
BUN, creatinine

Identify:
Inborn error
of metabolism (p 416)

(D) Treat:
Assure Adequate Airway
Administer Sedation/Muscle Relaxant
Insert Nasogastric Tube
Minimize Stimulation
Administer HTIG
Administer Antibiotics Pending Culture Results

Consider:
Surgical consultation for debridement

Assess response
(Cont'd on p 443)

and an aminoglycoside. Metronidazole treatment to eradicate *C. tetani* has been correlated with better outcome in adult patients. Debride any significant necrotic tissue.

E. If benzodiazepines do not adequately control spasms, intubate and institute long-term neuromuscular blockade; continue benzodiazepines for sedation. Consider tracheostomy to decrease reflex stimulation from airway irritation and minimize airway compromise from persistent spasms. If small bolus feedings or continuous drip feedings are not tolerated in volumes sufficient to meet the high fluid and caloric needs, place a central catheter for parenteral nutrition. Treat sympathetic hyperactivity with esmolol or labetalol. Correct hypotension with volume expansion and dopamine or norepinephrine. Sustained bradycardia may reflect hypoxia or myocardial damage.

F. Chronic management in the intermediate phase may extend 2 to 3 weeks and depends on continuous observation and meticulous nursing care. Family members can be trained in observation and airway clearance. After initial control of spasms is achieved, administer benzodiazepines by nasogastric tube. Decrease the dose of benzodiazepines if apnea occurs. Phenobarbital may be used as an adjunct in sedation. If neuromuscular junction blockade has been initiated, discontinue daily to assess the physical examination and decrease the likelihood of excessive accumulation of the blocking agent. Apply gentle splinting to maintain neutral position of hands and feet. Monitor growth and electrolyte balance.

G. In the convalescent phase focus on rehabilitation and active immunization. Maintain benzodiazepines until any neuromuscular blockade has been discontinued and spasms have subsided. Taper oral benzodiazepines over 14 to 21 days. Begin physical therapy as indicated for contractures and weakness. Assure close developmental follow-up, as cognitive delays are common among survivors. Administer a dose of diphtheria-pertussis-tetanus vaccine to the infant prior to discharge and continue for a series of three doses. Administer adult diphtheria-tetanus vaccine to mother if previously unimmunized.

References

Anlar B, Yalaz K, Dizmen R. Long-term prognosis after neonatal tetanus. Dev Med Child Neurol 1989; 31:76.

Antia-Obong OE, Ekanem EE, Udo JJ, Utsalo SJ. Septicaemia among neonates with tetanus. J Trop Pediatr 1992; 38:173.

Bleck TP. *Clostridium tetani.* In: Mandell GL, Bennett JE, Dolin R, eds. Principles and practice of infectious diseases. 4th ed. New York: Churchill-Livingstone, 1995:2173.

Einterz EM, Bates ME. Caring for neonatal tetanus patients in a rural primary care setting in Nigeria: A review of 237 cases. J Trop Pediatr 1991; 37:179.

Kumar S, Malecki JM. A case of neonatal tetanus. South Med J 1991; 84:396.

Okuonghae HO, Airede AI. Neonatal tetanus: Incidence and improved outcome with diazepam. Dev Med Child Neurol 1992; 34:448.

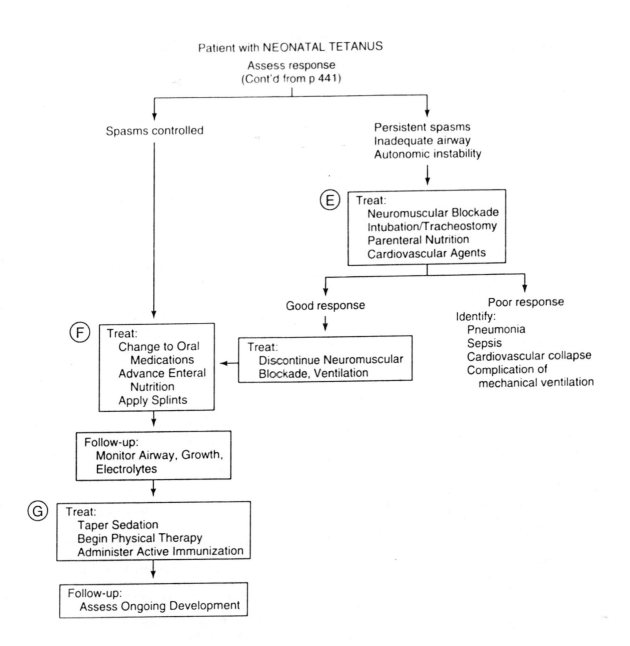

Patient with NEONATAL TETANUS
Assess response
(Cont'd from p 441)

Spasms controlled

Persistent spasms
Inadequate airway
Autonomic instability

(E) Treat:
  Neuromuscular Blockade
  Intubation/Tracheostomy
  Parenteral Nutrition
  Cardiovascular Agents

Good response

Poor response
Identify:
  Pneumonia
  Sepsis
  Cardiovascular collapse
  Complication of
    mechanical ventilation

(F) Treat:
  Change to Oral
    Medications
  Advance Enteral
    Nutrition
  Apply Splints

Treat:
  Discontinue Neuromuscular
    Blockade, Ventilation

Follow-up:
  Monitor Airway, Growth,
  Electrolytes

(G) Treat:
  Taper Sedation
  Begin Physical Therapy
  Administer Active Immunization

Follow-up:
  Assess Ongoing Development

THROMBOCYTOPENIA IN THE NEWBORN

Peter A. Lane, M.D.
Rachelle Nuss, M.D.

A. In the history ask about any maternal illnesses that suggest maternal autoimmune thrombocytopenia (idiopathic thrombocytopenic purpura [ITP], systemic lupus erythematosus [SLE]). Inquire about drug use, hypertension, and preeclampsia during pregnancy. Document a history of rubella immunization, the maternal rubella titer, a serologic test for syphilis, and a maternal red cell antibody screen. Consider risk factors for bacterial infection such as prematurity, prolonged rupture of membranes, maternal amnionitis, or fetal distress during labor. Note any family history of bleeding disorders and assess risk for HIV.

B. In the physical examination note any growth retardation, rash, jaundice, or hepatosplenomegaly (congenital infection, severe hemolysis), congenital anomalies (trisomy syndromes, congenital rubella, thrombocytopenia with absent radii, Fanconi anemia), or a cavernous hemangioma. Examine the placenta to detect a placental chorangioma.

C. Perform a CBC with differential and a platelet count; review the peripheral blood smear. Anemia (hemolysis, infection, congenital leukemia, or osteopetrosis), polycythemia, extreme leukocytosis (congenital leukemia, Down syndrome), or neutropenia (infection) may all be clues to the cause of the thrombocytopenia. The peripheral smear may suggest infection or disseminated intravascular coagulation (DIC) (red cell fragmentation), extramedullary hematopoiesis (extreme nucleated erythrocytosis), or Wiskott-Aldrich syndrome (small platelet size in a boy). Any platelet count less than 150,000 is abnormal, and an explanation should be sought.

D. Any infant with clinical bleeding other than skin petechiae or with other signs of systemic illness (lethargy, irritability, poor feeding, temperature instability) is considered symptomatic.

E. Perform a coagulation screen (prothrombin time [PT], partial thromboplastin time [PTT], fibrinogen) to determine whether a diffuse coagulopathy is present. Symptomatic infants with thrombocytopenia are commonly septic. Evaluate infants with thrombocytopenia and CNS symptoms for intracranial hemorrhage with a CT scan or ultrasonographic examination of the head. Bloody stools or abdominal distention suggests necrotizing enterocolitis (NEC).

F. Infants with clinical bleeding secondary to thrombocytopenia should be given 10 ml/kg platelet concentrate. This should stop the bleeding and produce a marked rise in the platelet count. An inadequate response suggests either rapid platelet consumption (DIC, NEC) or antiplatelet antibodies (isoimmune or maternal autoimmune). Bleeding in an infant with isoimmune thrombocytopenia may require a platelet transfusion from the mother. Bleeding in an infant whose mother has autoimmune thrombocytopenia may require exchange transfusion and/or steroids prior to transfusion with random-donor platelets. IV immunoglobulin may be effective in either isoimmune or autoimmune thrombocytopenia. Thrombocytopenic infants without clinical bleeding may be observed and not transfused.

G. Perform a platelet count on the mother and review her history for any clues to autoimmune disease. Neonatal thrombocytopenia secondary to maternal autoimmune disease may occur despite a normal platelet count in the mother.

References

Andrew M, Kelton J. Neonatal thrombocytopenia. Clin Perinatol 1984; 11:359.

Bussell J, Kaplan C, McFarland J, et al. Recommendations for the evaluation and treatment of neonatal autoimmune and alloimmune thrombocytopenia. Thromb Haemost 1991; 65:631.

Gill FM. Thrombocytopenia in the newborn. Semin Perinatol 1983; 7:201.

Hathaway WE, Bonnar J. Hemostatic disorders of the pregnant woman and newborn infant. New York: Elsevier, 1987:115.

Naiman JL. Disorders of platelets. In: Oski FA, Naiman JL, eds. Hematologic problems in the newborn. 3rd ed. Philadelphia: Saunders, 1982:175.

Samuels P, Bussell J, Braitman L, et al. Estimation of the risk of thrombocytopenia in the offspring of pregnant women with presumed immune thrombocytopenic purpura. N Engl J Med 1990; 323:229.

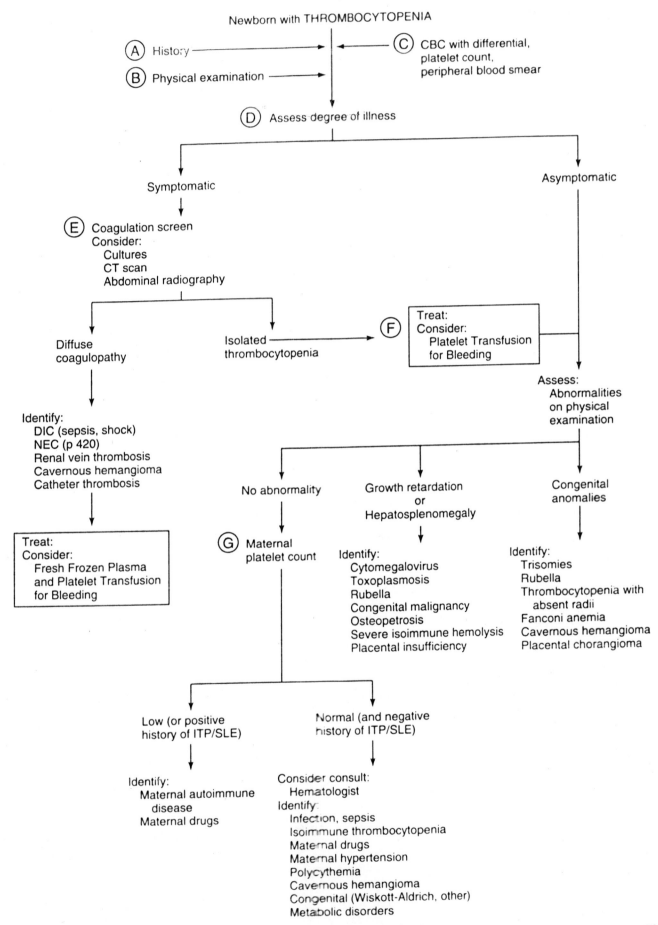

Newborn with THROMBOCYTOPENIA

(A) History

(B) Physical examination

(C) CBC with differential,
platelet count,
peripheral blood smear

(D) Assess degree of illness

Symptomatic

Asymptomatic

(E) Coagulation screen
Consider:
Cultures
CT scan
Abdominal radiography

Diffuse
coagulopathy

Isolated
thrombocytopenia

(F) Treat:
Consider:
Platelet Transfusion
for Bleeding

Identify:
DIC (sepsis, shock)
NEC (p 420)
Renal vein thrombosis
Cavernous hemangioma
Catheter thrombosis

Treat:
Consider:
Fresh Frozen Plasma
and Platelet Transfusion
for Bleeding

Assess:
Abnormalities
on physical
examination

No abnormality

Growth retardation
or
Hepatosplenomegaly

Congenital
anomalies

(G) Maternal
platelet count

Identify:
Cytomegalovirus
Toxoplasmosis
Rubella
Congenital malignancy
Osteopetrosis
Severe isoimmune hemolysis
Placental insufficiency

Identify:
Trisomies
Rubella
Thrombocytopenia with
absent radii
Fanconi anemia
Cavernous hemangioma
Placental chorangioma

Low (or positive
history of ITP/SLE)

Normal (and negative
history of ITP/SLE)

Identify:
Maternal autoimmune
disease
Maternal drugs

Consider consult:
Hematologist
Identify:
Infection, sepsis
Isoimmune thrombocytopenia
Maternal drugs
Maternal hypertension
Polycythemia
Cavernous hemangioma
Congenital (Wiskott-Aldrich, other)
Metabolic disorders

NEUROLOGIC DISORDERS

EVALUATION OF A NEUROLOGIC DISORDER

Patricia H. Ellison, M.D.
Stephen Berman, M.D.

In almost all cases a child with a neurologic disorder has symptoms that are confirmed by signs in the examination. Occasionally the picture is unclear and the clinician must localize the lesion in an organized way.

A. In the history start with the brain. Ask about injury. In the infant first obtain the history of developmental milestones: what that child can do and when he or she learned to do it. Ask whether the child has lost any skills. What are they and when were they lost? If a parent says the child does not remember anything, ask for examples. If the parent says the child sleeps all the time, ask about the history of bedtime, when the child usually awakens, whether there are any naps, and how long they are. School data may be very helpful for both rate of progress and any loss of skills. Compare report cards, achievement test scores, and teacher evaluations. Most schools release these with proper authorization. Try to obtain the school information before your evaluation. Ask about irritability, lethargy, or rapid change of mood. Consider the cranial nerves. Ask about vision, especially evidence of loss of vision. A mother can tell you about an infant who used to pick up small items and no longer does so. A child can often describe changes in the vision. This helps to diagnose optic glioma or craniopharyngioma impinging on the optic pathways or visual compromise from increased intracranial pressure. Ask about and look for head tilt. Ask the child whether he or she ever sees double. Be especially careful to ask about and examine for other cranial nerves when a facial nerve palsy has been identified. Ask about changes in hearing and any problems with swallowing, choking, sputtering, or aspirating food or liquid into the trachea. Next comes the spinal cord. Ask about neck or back pain and injury: car accidents, slips, and falls. Ask about repetitive tasks: lifting smaller children, carrying a heavy backpack, helping with moving. Ask about sports, gymnastics, wrestling, football, any sensory loss, bowel and bladder control. For the neuromuscular junction, ask about family history of myasthenia. Ask at what time of day the child is weak; myasthenia often worsens during the day. For the peripheral nerves ask about trauma, weakness, sensory loss, numbness, and tingling. Ask about high arched feet in the child and in the parents. For the muscles ask which are weak or which parts of the body the child is not using well. Ask for examples and about the use of stairs. Ask about family history of loss of walking ability or wheelchair use.

B. In the physical examination inspect the skin: neurocutaneous disorders are among the most common causes of brain problems. Look for adenoma sebaceum, shagreen patches, café-au-lait or depigmented spots, ecchymoses, and other evidence of trauma. Examine the fundi. Look also for chorioretinitis, neurophakomatous lesions, and retinal hemorrhages. Examine the cranial nerves (Table 1). If the child is too young to do

TABLE 1 Cranial Nerve Testing

Nerve	Testing Age	Comments
I (smell)	About 4 yr	Head injury, coup contra coup, some frontal tumors
II (vision)	From birth	*Decrease* Optic nerve tumor in infancy; craniopharyngioma in childhood; increased ICP (hydrocephalus); degenerative (neuronal ceroid lipofuscinosis)
III, IV, VI	Some from birth	Eye does not move fully; VI: ICP, tumor in brain stem; III: herniation; IV: often frontal trauma (e.g., fall off tricycle) Child reports double vision, may tilt head; try to determine field of diplopia Brain stem glioma, herpes or other brain stem infection
V	About 4 yr	Touch three sensory divisions, palpate masseter while child bites
VII	From birth	Traumatic, facial nerve palsy; congenital, Moebius; acquired, Bell palsy; brain stem glioma (requires others)
VIII	From birth Early hearing test	Audiologic testing, brain stem auditory evoked response
IX	From birth	Acquired: document loss of gag; diagnosis of brain stem tumor requires other cranial nerve dysfunction
XI	From birth	Fasciculations, Werdnig-Hoffman; to one side: brain stem tumor (vs. infection)

ICP, intracranial pressure.

finger to nose, entice him or her to reach for an object, checking for ataxia. Ages 4 and up can do finger to nose, rapid alternating motion, and finger to thumb opposition. Check handedness: present object to each side of an infant to examine hand use (early handedness, i.e., under 12 months, is an important clue to hemiplegia). Tap reflexes: biceps, triceps, brachioradialis, patella, and ankle. If cognitive function is the concern, do a sufficient number of drawing items for age to be reliable,

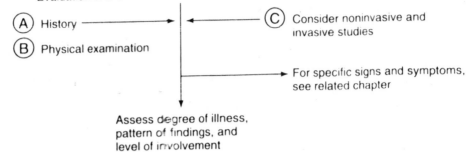

Evaluation of a Child with a NEUROLOGIC DISORDER

(A) History

(B) Physical examination

(C) Consider noninvasive and invasive studies

For specific signs and symptoms, see related chapter

Assess degree of illness, pattern of findings, and level of involvement
(Cont'd on p 451)

use age-appropriate reading paragraphs and obtain school records, and do some age-appropriate math problems.

Many nonneurologists shy away from the cranial nerves. However, they are a map of the brain with so little individual variation that mastery of the basics often yields the correct diagnosis. When you have identified dysfunction in one cranial nerve, always look for dysfunctions in others. That will help you localize the lesion. The cranial nerves traverse the brain, and dysfunction cannot always be localized, especially when only one cranial nerve is involved. With two or more dysfunctional cranial nerves, the brain stem is the most likely location. It is easy to teach parents some simple guidelines so they can report to you when a new cranial nerve becomes dysfunctional. Parents can report failure of the eyes to move in all directions, onset of diplopia or head tilt, asymmetric smile or cry, repetitive cough, sputter, or choke with eating and protrusion of the tongue to one side. Parental help increases the probability of making the right diagnosis. With localization to the brain stem, an MRI is the best imaging test because of its capacity to show small things. The possibilities in children are usually brain stem glioma and infection. There is a rare possibility of multiple sclerosis (MS) in adolescents.

For the spinal cord palpate along the vertebral column, watching for evidence of pain. Either depressed or brisk patella reflexes can result from trouble in the spinal cord. Ease of walking on toes and difficulty in walking on heels may help. A sensory level is helpful but seldom happens. Asymmetric arch of feet, tendency to toe walk, or clonus might help place the lesion in the spinal cord. Auscultation of distended bladder or palpable hard feces in colon can be clues to this also. Diagnosis of spinal cord problems is facilitated by MRI that shows displacement of disk material, extradural and intradural tumor, infections, and a variety of congenital abnormalities. For imaging of a portion of the spinal column, especially lumbar, CT scanning is quick and usually relatively cheap. Imaging of the entire spine seldom is necessary; when it is, choose MRI over CT scan to avoid the radiation. If myelography is considered, seek neurologic or neurosurgical consultation. Consider the anterior horn cell, the target of polio infections. The clinical symptoms of polio are usually asymmetric. Guillain-Barré, which originates beyond

the anterior horn cell, tends to have fairly symmetric findings. Get electromyography–nerve conduction velocity (EMG-NCV) testing. Always consider Werdnig-Hoffman syndrome in infancy and Kugelberg-Weylander disease in older children.

Consider the neuromuscular junction. Most infants with botulism are sick enough to be hospitalized. An acutely weak infant with depressed reflexes who is still sucking well may be confusing. Consider botulism toxin assays. Myasthenia gravis may be even more confusing because it can appear at various ages and in various ways. For an edrophonium (Tensilon) test you need a sign obvious enough to reveal improvement. For some signs, you also need a cooperative child. Often the weakness is most prominent during late afternoon or early evening, so the test must be done then. Drooping eyelids, weak hand grasp, and inability to get up from the floor without using hands are useful signs. If the edrophonium increases muscle strength objectively, consider EMG-NCV.

For the peripheral nerves remember their two basic functions: motor and sensory. Signs and symptoms tend to be distal first, so focus on hands and feet. Test hand strength by asking child to spread all fingers and not let you push them together. Then check strength of index finger to thumb opposition, then little finger to thumb opposition, then all fingers flexed (slip your fingers under them and try to pull up). Then have child extend hand and you try to push it back. Throughout this keep telling the child to be strong. Test the ulnar, median, and radial nerves by light touch to back of hand, little finger, thumb, and middle finger. Touch each hand and ask whether it can be felt on each hand and if it feels the same on both hands. If all have decreased sensation, use light touch from fingertips up the arm looking for the glove of glove-stocking distribution. Ask the child to tell you when he or she feels it better. Do three or four different routes. If you find glove-stocking on hands, be sure to do the feet, and vice versa. Test the feet first by asking the child to stand on tiptoes, then on heels with the toes up. You can add to this. Tell the child to turn the foot out and not let you push it in, then turn it in and not let you push it out. Then test sensation as with hands. If you detect neither sensory loss nor weakness, it is generally not peripheral neuropathy yet. There may be irritation of the nerve as manifested by numbness, tingling, or burning. Or it may not be in the nerve but in the muscle, which tends to be proximal. EMG-NCV may help to distinguish proximal from distal and anterior horn cell from neuromuscular function from peripheral nerve. Consider toxins and heavy metals: lead, arsenic, mercury. Consider juvenile diabetes, which does not start with neuropathy, but over the years most diabetics get peripheral neuropathy.

Nerve disorders start peripherally; muscle disorders start proximally. This usually helps except with the overall weakness of muscle disorders such as some congenital myopathies. Test upper body strength. Ask child to flex arms and be strong while you try to pull against arm (biceps). Ask child to extend arm; you push, trying to flex arm (triceps). Ask child to get up from a chair without using hands or arms, get up from the floor without using hands or arms, and step up with each foot on a small stepstool. Look at calves (gastrocnemius), especially of 3 to 5 year old boys, for the enlargement of Duchenne disease. Test toe and heel walking; heel walking usually deteriorates first.

If you have obtained a careful history and physical examination, and the signs, symptoms, and testing do not fit a well-recognized configuration, consider conversion hysteria. Pseudoseizures, vision loss, and limb paralysis are all well known to pediatric neurologists.

C. Start with noninvasive testing. In most cases CT scan is sufficient. For hypomyelination, brain tumor within brain tissue, temporal lobe lesions, such as mesial temporal sclerosis, and multiple sclerosis, and for some spinal cord lesions, MRI is necessary. Consider infection or systemic disease such as *Mycoplasma*, lupus, *Borrelia*, and Epstein-Barr virus (EBV). A high sedimentation rate is a nonspecific indication of infection. In most situations, except acute illness, lumbar puncture is done last. Then consider special studies such as TB, oligoclonal bands for MS, possibly *Cryptococcus* in addition to cells, protein, and glucose.

For seizure-like episodes order EEG. Rather than do this twice, order sleep deprivation the first time to enhance any seizure activity. **EEG** is a helpful tool when done well and read by a knowledgeable clinician. But an EEG full of movement artifact is of little use. The technicians must know how to work with children. Sedation is usually not used. The child must fall asleep for some of the recording. Photic stimulation should be used for absence seizures. Usually sleep deprivation before the test encourages sleep and increases the chance of capturing a spike-wave discharge. The EEG must be read by a person well trained in babies' and children's EEGs. This is generally not available at every hospital or clinic. Use the following categories of outcome: (1) conspicuously abnormal: spike-wave discharge, repetitive slow waves, very low voltage, well-defined asymmetries; (2) mildly abnormal such as paroxysms or runs of θ-waves or excess β-waves, usually not diagnostic of anything; and (3) normal.

EMG-NCV is an unpleasant test. Have good reason to order it and know that the person who does it is experienced in interpretation of children's EMG-NCV. **Muscle biopsy** is invasive. Consultation with a neurologist who has special expertise in muscle is essential. The biopsy must be done well, the specimen treated well, and an experienced clinician or pathologist must read it. One reason to seek neurologic consultation at this point is to assure that all parts of the system will function well. This is not available at every hospital or clinic.

CT scanning requires less time than **MRI**, but the child must not move or the artifact will obscure the results. MRI takes longer, it often requires heavier sedation, and the patient cannot always be seen throughout the test. In emergencies the test should be done as needed. When there is more leeway, often it is better to choose CT or wait months or even 1 to 2 years until the test can be done well.

Few institutions have any reason to do **brain biopsy**. It requires extremely skillful pathologists, electron microscopists, and neurologists. That combination exists in few places.

In most cases all test results are normal and often the child is normal. The parent says, "We still do not know what caused the seizures." I tell them that is the best neurologic diagnosis. Other times the child is clearly dysfunctional, a thoughtful basic work-up has been done without finding a cause, and then another group of selective tests were done and maybe another with still no cause. Often it is time then to address the community programming, preservation of the family if possible, and maintenance of the primary caretaker.

D. In most difficult medical situations there remains hope for improvement if not a cure. Small heads with large ventricles still rarely need a shunt. Small brains with early-closing sutures rarely need major reconstructive surgery. Surgical treatment of seizures for brains that do not work well in other respects may be questioned. Second or third brain biopsies (or even the first) generally offer no change in function. At some point a good clinician has to say, this is about what we are able to do well.

References

Barkovich AJ. Pediatric neuroimaging. 2nd ed. New York: Raven, 1995.

Diebler C, Dulac O. Pediatric neurology and neuroradiology: Cerebral and cranial diseases. New York: Springer-Verlag, 1987.

Faerber EN, ed. CNS magnetic resonance imaging in infants and children. New York: Cambridge, 1995.

Jones HR, Bolton, CF, Harper CM. Pediatric clinical electromyography. Philadelphia: Lippincott-Raven, 1995.

Orlow SJ. When to suspect a neurocutaneous disorder. Contemp Pediatr 1995; 12:59.

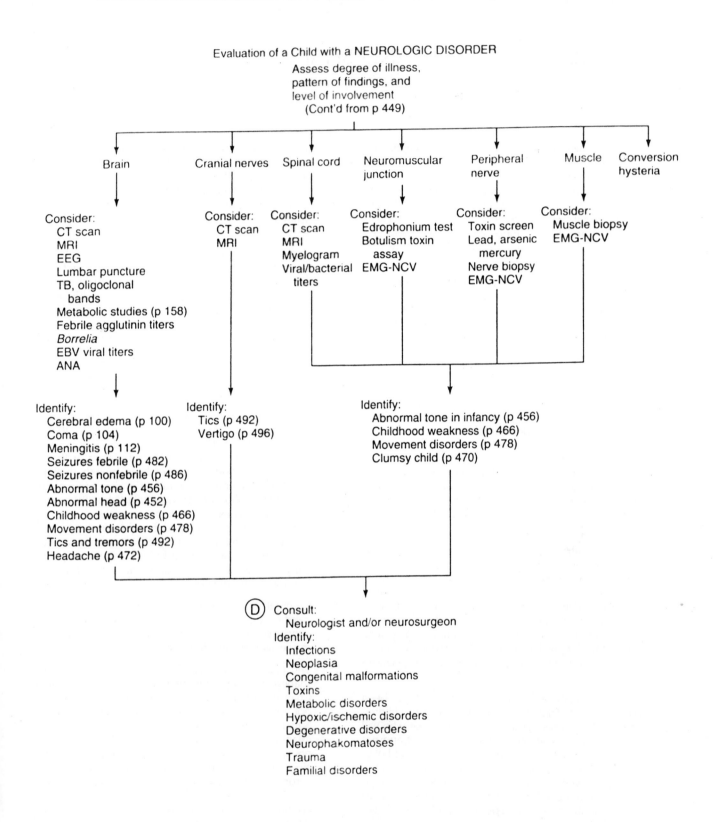

Evaluation of a Child with a NEUROLOGIC DISORDER

Assess degree of illness,
pattern of findings, and
level of involvement
(Cont'd from p 449)

Brain

Consider:
CT scan
MRI
EEG
Lumbar puncture
TB, oligoclonal
bands
Metabolic studies (p 158)
Febrile agglutinin titers
Borrelia
EBV viral titers
ANA

Identify:
Cerebral edema (p 100)
Coma (p 104)
Meningitis (p 112)
Seizures febrile (p 482)
Seizures nonfebrile (p 486)
Abnormal tone (p 456)
Abnormal head (p 452)
Childhood weakness (p 466)
Movement disorders (p 478)
Tics and tremors (p 492)
Headache (p 472)

Cranial nerves

Consider:
CT scan
MRI

Identify:
Tics (p 492)
Vertigo (p 496)

Spinal cord

Consider:
CT scan
MRI
Myelogram
Viral/bacterial
titers

Neuromuscular junction

Consider:
Edrophonium test
Botulism toxin
assay
EMG-NCV

Peripheral nerve

Consider:
Toxin screen
Lead, arsenic
mercury
Nerve biopsy
EMG-NCV

Muscle

Consider:
Muscle biopsy
EMG-NCV

Conversion hysteria

Identify:
Abnormal tone in infancy (p 456)
Childhood weakness (p 466)
Movement disorders (p 478)
Clumsy child (p 470)

Ⓓ Consult:
Neurologist and/or neurosurgeon
Identify:
Infections
Neoplasia
Congenital malformations
Toxins
Metabolic disorders
Hypoxic/ischemic disorders
Degenerative disorders
Neurophakomatoses
Trauma
Familial disorders

ABNORMAL HEAD: SIZE AND SHAPE

Patricia H. Ellison, M.D. ⁻

Abnormal head sizes are either too small (microcephaly) or too large (macrocephaly). The latter may be due to a large brain (megalencephaly). Usually there is a progressive change in head size of two or more percentiles on a grid marked 1st, 10th, 25th, 50th, 75th, 90th, and 99th percentiles. Abnormal brain function is most highly associated with heads that are three or more standard deviations (SD) from the mean (50th percentile) (under 1st or more than 99th percentile).

A. In the history ask about relatives with a large or small head. Families often relate this to the purchase of hats or caps. Measure the parents' heads. Ask about birthmarks on the child, siblings, and parents. Review the birthing history for prematurity, hypoxic-ischemic encephalopathy, and subarachnoid hemorrhage.

B. Inspection of the head and measurement of the occipital frontal circumference should be a part of every physical examination. Most of these abnormalities are first noted by the child's physician. Inspect the skin on the entire body for depigmented spots, café-au-lait lesions, and other phakomatous lesions. Examine the fundi and eyegrounds for retinal hemorrhages, abnormal fundi, chorioretinitis, and phakomatous lesions. Evaluate the legs for tonicity. Abnormal head shape is often best seen by sighting from the top down, which is easily done with the infant supine on the examining table.

C. Consider brain imaging. In young infants with an open fontanelle cerebral ultrasound is quick, easy, and less expensive than other radiologic studies. In most situations when the fontanelle is closed, CT without contrast is sufficient. Ventricle size shows well, subdural effusions are usually identifiable, and tumors and arteriovenous malformations (AVM) are rare in infants. In general reserve MRI for possible degenerative diseases of gray or white matter and for the few children whose diagnosis is puzzling.

D. In macrocephaly, if brain imaging has not yet been done, order it. That should quickly separate children who require neurosurgical referral from those who will be followed. Two situations are less clear-cut and not uncommon: (1) An infant who has excessive fluid over the brain surfaces may have some hypotonia but is developing well cognitively. This is generally a benign condition that needs monthly follow-up. (2) A child has macrocephaly, some mild to perhaps moderate enlargement of ventricles, and some school problems. The hope has always been that a shunt would improve the

schoolwork. However, few data support that. A conservative approach is to repeat MRI in 6 to 12 months. This will show any change in ventricle size as well as any fluid in the tissue near the ventricles. Without such change and without evidence of loss of cognitive function, shunting may complicate or worsen neurologic problems.

E. Children with a large brain (megalencephaly) often function normally. A large head in a child whose relatives with large heads function normally needs no further diagnostic testing. However, some children with megalencephaly are developmentally delayed. Some deteriorate progressively from specific neurodegenerative diseases. Refer to a pediatric neurologist. Others progress developmentally but slowly. Consider TORCH (toxoplasmosis, rubella, cytomegalovirus [CMV], and herpes) titers. Follow the child monthly for 3 to 6 months, then at regular intervals.

F. Small head also runs in families whose members with small heads function normally. However, small heads, especially three SD below the mean (about or below the 1st percentile), have a high correlation with poor cognitive function. Failure of head growth shown by serial head circumference identifies slow brain growth. Imaging may show enlarged ventricles, but this is usually hydrocephalus ex vacuo (large ventricles due to atrophied or poorly developed brain tissue). It is not a pressure phenomenon; it does not require a shunt. Sutures may close early and the fontanelle may shrink early. No amount of neurosurgic intervention will improve brain function.

G. Cerebral imaging may give clues to a cause such as calcification of CMV, toxoplasmosis infection, or dysgenesis of parts of the brain. Many of such children are in special programs from young ages.

H. The major types of craniosynostoses (abnormal head shapes) are readily identified by inspection (Figs. 1 to 3). Changes in head shape from mild craniosynostosis do not appear to modify brain function. Dolichocephaly (sagittal suture, narrow head) is common in premature infants. In extreme cases the sagittal suture can be opened surgically, largely for cosmetic purposes. Plagiocephaly (one coronal suture) and acrocephaly (both coronal sutures) also cause abnormal shape. In severe acrocephaly vision can be affected because of the position of the eyes. Trigonocephaly (metopic suture) is released largely for cosmetic purposes. Early fusion of all sutures for reasons other than poor brain growth is rare.

(Continued on page 455)

Patient with an ABNORMAL HEAD

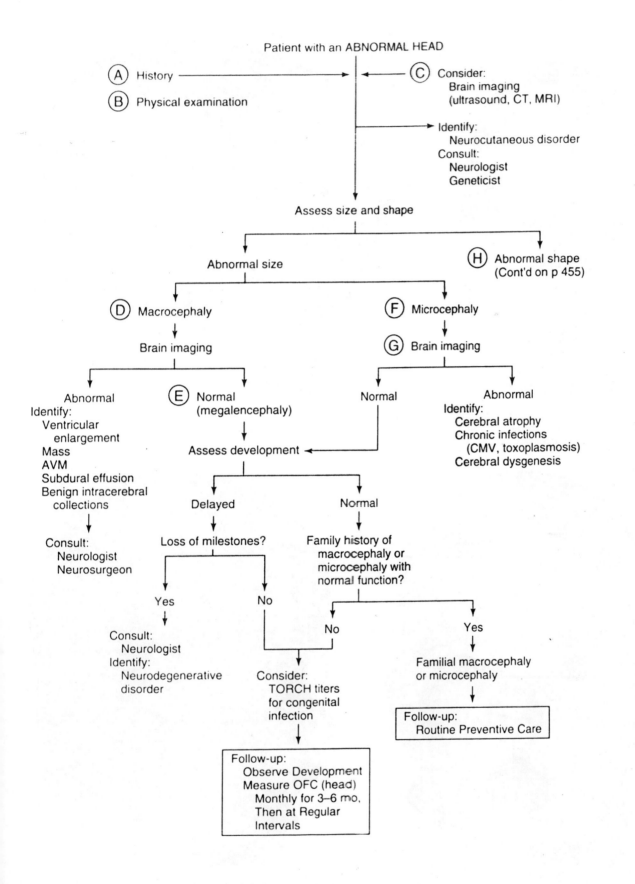

Abnormal shape
(Cont'd on p 455)

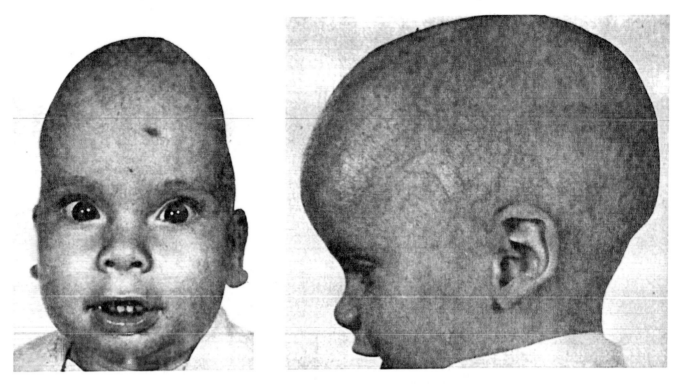

Figure 1 Craniosynostosis. Premature fusion of the sagittal suture. The vault of the skull is narrow transversely and elongated in the anteroposterior diameter. (From Till K. Paediatric neurosurgery for paediatricians. London: Blackwell Scientific, 1975.)

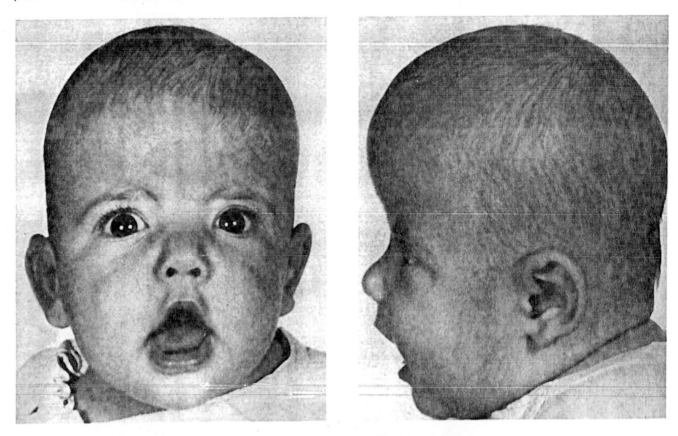

Figure 2 A 3 month old baby with premature fusion of the coronal sutures. There is poor formation of the frontal bones with a reduction in the anteroposterior diameter of the skull and a conpensatory broadening in the transverse diameter. (From Till K. Paediatric neurosurgery for paediatricians. London: Blackwell Scientific, 1975.)

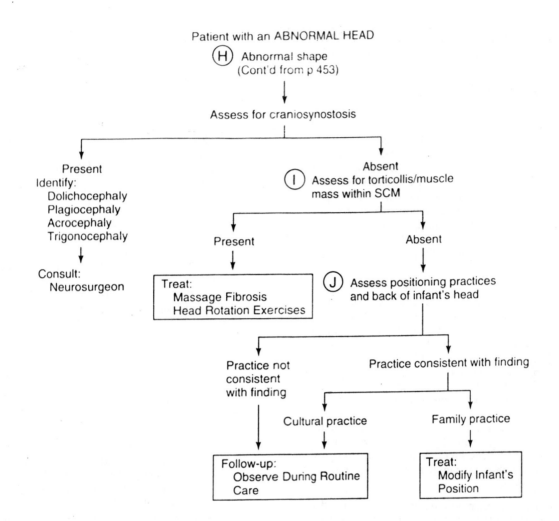

Patient with an ABNORMAL HEAD

(H) Abnormal shape
(Cont'd from p 453)

↓

Assess for craniosynostosis

Present
Identify:
Dolichocephaly
Plagiocephaly
Acrocephaly
Trigonocephaly

↓

Consult:
Neurosurgeon

Absent
(I) Assess for torticollis/muscle mass within SCM

Present

Treat:
Massage Fibrosis
Head Rotation Exercises

Absent

(J) Assess positioning practices and back of infant's head

Practice not consistent with finding

Practice consistent with finding

Cultural practice

Family practice

Follow-up:
Observe During Routine Care

Treat:
Modify Infant's Position

I. A few infants with secondary fibrosis have stretched or torn a sternocleidomastoid (SCM) muscle during delivery. Such an infant sits with the head turned, sleeps with the head turned, and often cries if you try to turn the head in the opposite direction. Ask the mother to sit and to hold the infant on the back between her legs with the infant's legs toward her. The infant's head then easily drops back at the mother's knees and you can palpate the SCM muscles. Treatment consists of massage of the abnormal SCM muscle and deliberate turning of the head by the mother several times a day to stretch the muscle.

J. Head shape may be abnormal because an infant habitually lies in the same position. In some cultures the infant is positioned to flatten the back of the head because the resultant head shape is valued. Some families do this without realizing the consequence and without trying to achieve a certain head shape. Abnormal head shapes from habitual assumption of the same position do not change brain functions. Some infants who are slow of motor development flatten the part of the head placed against the mattress because they cannot turn their head well. For the latter two groups, modify the sleeping position.

Reference

Aicardi J. Hydrocephalus and nontraumatic pericerebral collections. In: Aicardi J, ed. Diseases of the nervous system in childhood. London: Mac-Keith Press, 1992:291.

ABNORMAL TONE IN INFANCY

Patricia H. Ellison, M.D.
Stephen Berman, M.D.

Abnormal tone is common in children who graduate from neonatal intensive care units (NICUs), particularly those who were born prematurely, were depressed at birth, or had neonatal seizures. Perform a neurologic assessment when the parents or grandparents express concern about development delay, chiefly in failure to achieve motor milestones such as rolling over, sitting, crawling, standing, or when the developmental screening indicates delay in motor milestones. Then a neurologic assessment is mandatory.

A. In the history ask about the pregnancy, labor, delivery, and whether the mother saw the delivery or saw the baby shortly thereafter. Ask whether the baby needed any special help after delivery and what that was. Ask how long the baby was hospitalized. If more than 24 to 48 hours, ask why. Ask whether the baby was treated with a breathing machine (ventilator) or had seizures as a newborn. Ask whether there is family history of children with delayed motor or cognitive development. Ask the parents at what age they learned to walk and about any clumsiness in parents or near relatives. Ask whether any extended family members were confined to a wheelchair or unable to walk and at what age. Ask whether any relatives died as infants or children and of what. Ask whether any family members had muscle or nerve disorders.

B. On physical examination measure and chart head size and percentile. Palpate the suture lines for sprung sutures. Examine fundi for increased intracranial pressure. Examine the skin for depigmentation and café-au-lait lesions. Identify syndromes (e.g., Down, Prader-Willi). Most infants treated by pediatricians and family practitioners are neurologically normal, making it difficult to learn the signs of neurologic abnormality and their changes across time. This is easier when the neurologic assessment method builds these changes into the scoring system, enabling the physician to examine the infant, record the findings systematically, and score the infant appropriately for gestational age. Newborns now are hospitalized only briefly, reducing observation by experienced nursing staff. The physician may not be aware of an infant's signs of neurologic problems. Thus the assessments at 2 weeks and 2 months of age are increasingly important in the identification of neurologic problems.

Neoneuro & Up (Fig. 1): These areas are assessed: irritability and apathy as noted by caretaker, primitive reflexes, French angles, head control, neck and trunk tone, neurologic irritability or apathy, alertness, and responsiveness. This assessment is designed for neurologic evaluation of infants from 38 weeks gestation to 16 weeks of age. Ask the caretaker about the first four items and observe for the last four. Items are the following:

1. How often must the caretaker awaken the infant to feed?

2. How many feedings are given between 6 PM and 6 AM?
3. Describe how easy or difficult it is to care for the infant.
4. How long does the infant cry before you can console him or her?
5. Posture. Observe both arms and legs of the infant lying quietly for strong flexion, semiflexion, flexion, or extension.
6. Observe for decorticate (legs extended, arms flexed), decerebrate (legs and arms extended), or opisthotonic (neck hyperextended) postures.
7. Hands open/closed. Observe the hands for clenching (closed too tightly), clenched under stress (closed too tightly when crying or during the neurologic evaluation), closed, sometimes closed, and open positions.
8. Palmar grasp. Place your index finger in the palm of the hand approaching from the ulnar side and observe the flexion of the fingers and arm.
9. Plantar grasp. Place your thumb on the balls of the foot and observe the flexion of the toes.
10. Asymmetric tonic neck reflex. With the infant supine, turn the head from side to side. Observe for the fencing position—extension of the arm in front of the infant's face and flexion of the arm at the back of the head.
11. Scarf sign. Grasp the upper arm near the elbow and move the arm across the chest until resistance. Measure the angle between a line dropped from the armpit and the upper arm.
12. Popliteal angle. Grasp the lower leg near the knee and extend the leg until resistance. Measure the angle at the knee.
13. Heel to ear. Keep the infant's buttocks on the table. Grasp the upper leg and flex the legs at the hip until resistance. Measure the angle between the leg and the trunk.
14. Knee reflex. Relax the leg by some knee flexion, then tap below the patella and observe the quality of the reflex.
15. Ankle clonus. Grasp one foot and quickly flex it, counting any spontaneous beats.
16–17. Pull to sit. Grasp both wrists and pull the infant slowly to sitting position. Score arm flexion and head lag separately.
18. Held sit. Hold the infant upright, supporting each shoulder, noting the amount of time the head remains upright. If the infant has head control for more than 10 seconds, support the infant on the trunk and observe the number of the lumbar vertebra from which the back is bent.
19. Posterior neck. Support the infant at the shoulders, moving the trunk forward until the head drops forward. Count the seconds until the infant

(Continued on page 460)

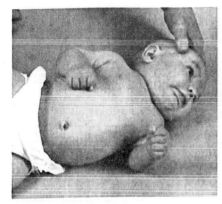

HANDS CLENCHED
Abnormal
Clenched with stress maneuver
Age 2½ mo

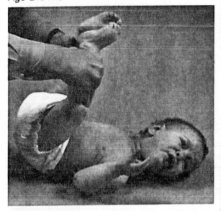

HEEL TO EAR
Abnormal
Hypertonic
Age 7–9 mo

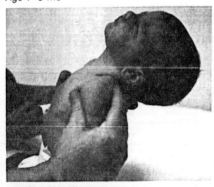

ANTERIOR NECK
Normal
Neonate

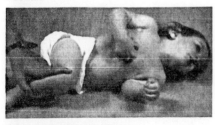

BODY DEROTATIVE
Abnormal
Age 10–12 mo

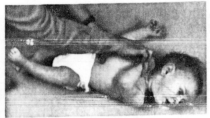

SCARF SIGN
Abnormal
Hypertonic
Age 7–9 mo

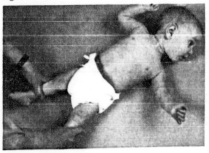

LEG ABDUCTION
Abnormal
Hypertonic
Age 7–9 mo

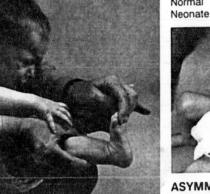

DORSIFLEXION OF FOOT
Abnormal
Hypertonic
Age 4 mo

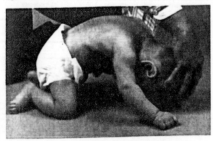

TONIC LABYRINTHINE PRONE
Abnormal
Age 7 mo

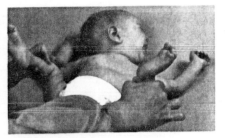

POPLITEAL ANGLE
Abnormal
Hypertonic
Age 7–9 mo

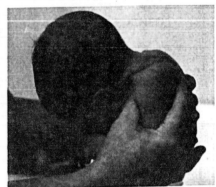

POSTERIOR NECK
Normal
Neonate

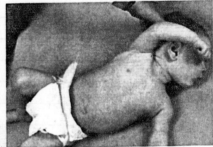

**ASYMMETRIC TONIC
NECK REFLEX**
Abnormal
Age 5 mo

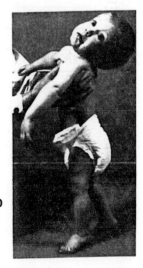

**WEIGHT BEARING AND
POSITIVE SUPPORT
REACTION**
Abnormal
Age 10–12 mo

Name _____
Date _____

Date of birth _____
Gestational age at birth _____

Corrected gestational age _____
Sex _____

Item	Description						
1. CARETAKER MUST AWAKEN TO FEED	a) rarely	b) sometimes	c) often				
2. NUMBER OF FEEDINGS BETWEEN 6 PM - 6 AM	a) none	b) 1	c) 2	d) 3	e) 4	f) 5	g) 6 or more
3. EASY OF CARING FOR	a) too easy	b) easy	c) not so easy	d) difficult			
4. HOW LONG CRIES BEFORE CONSOLED?	a) 1-3 min	b) 4-7 min	c) 8-12 min	d) 13-18 min	e) 19-24 min	f) 25 or more min	
5. POSTURE	Upper limbs a) extended / Lower limbs a) extended	b) semi-flexed or flexed / b) semi-flexed or flexed	c) strongly flexed / c) strongly flexed				
6. POSTURING	a) decorticate	b) decerebrate	c) opisthotonic	d) none of these			
7. HANDS OPEN/CLOSED	a) clenched	b) clenched with stress maneuver	c) closed	d) sometimes closed	e) open		
8. PALMAR GRASP	a) absent	b) weak flexion	c) medium flexion	d) strong flexion spread to	e) very strong lifts off bed		
9. PLANTAR GRASP	a) absent or weak	b) medium to strong	c) very strong				
10. ASYMMETRICAL TONIC NECK REFLEX	a) persistent or spontaneous	b) present, not persistent	c) absent				
11. SCARF SIGN	a) > 85°	b) 60° to 85°	c) 45° to 60°	d) 15° to 45°	e) 0° to 15°		
12. POPLITEAL ANGLE	a) >180°	b) 150° to 180°	c) 130° to 150°	d) 110° to 130°	e) 90° to 110°	f) < 90°	
13. HEEL TO EAR	a) < 10°	b) 10° to 40°	c) 40° to 60°	d) 60° to 90°	e) 90° to 100°	f) ≥ 100°	
14. KNEE REFLEX	a) absent	b) 1 + to 2 +	c) brisk	d) very brisk			
15. ANKLE CLONUS	a) > 2 beats	b) 1-2 beats	c) absent				
16. PULL TO SIT	Arm Flexion - angle at elbow / Head Lag	a) > 170°	b) 140° to 170°	c) 110° to 140°	d) 70° to 110°	e) < 70°	
17.		a)	b)	c)	d)	e)	f)
18. HELD SIT	a) head stays forward or backward	b) head up < 3 sec	c) head up 3-10 sec	d) head up > 10 sec	e) bends from L3		
19. POSTERIOR NECK	a) no attempt to raise head	b) tries but cannot raise head	c) head upright by 30 sec, drops head	d) head upright by 30 sec, maintained	e) examiner cannot extend head		
20. ANTERIOR NECK	a) no attempt to raise head	b) tries but cannot raise head	c) head upright by 30 sec, drops head	d) head upright by 30 sec, maintained	e) examiner cannot flex head		
21. AUDITORY	a) no reaction or startle	b) brightens or stills	c) shifts eyes	d) shifts and turns	e) prolonged head turning		
22. VISUAL	a) no focus or following	b) focuses	c) follows 30° horizontally	d) follows 30°-60° horizontally	e) also follows vertically	f) follows past midline	g) follows full circle
23. ALERT	a) 0-4 sec.	b) 5-10 sec	c) 11-30 sec	d) 31-60 sec	e) > 60 sec.	f) regards hand or object in hand	
24. VENTRAL SUSPENSION	a)	b)	c)	d)			
25. ALL FOURS/PRONE	a) no head turning	b) turns head side to side	c) lifts head 45° drops	d) lifts head 45° holds	e) head up 90° drops	f) head up 90° holds	
26. MORO	a) absent or minimal	b) partial	c) full	d) exaggerated - immediate brisk response			
27. SUCK	a) no attempt	b) weak	c) strong irregular	d) strong regular	e) jaw clenched		
28. TREMOR	a) all states	b) only in states 5, 6	c) also in state 4	d) only in sleep or after moro	e) none		
29. RESPONSIVENESS	a) no smile	b) smiles to self	c) smiles responsively	d) gets excited anticipation of food	e) breathes heavily gets excited		
30. VOCALIZATION	a) none	b) small noises	c) talks back some way	d) chuckles	e) squeals, laughs outloud		
31. ATTENDS TO EXAMINER	a) no stimulus needed	b) with mild stimuli	c) moderate stimuli	d) really have to stimulate	e) does not attend		
32. ATTENDS DURING EXAM	a) does not attend	b) with stimulus only	c) some	d) recurrently	e) most of exam		

ASK CARETAKER (items 1–4)

Figure 1   Neoneuro & Up.

458

Scoring-Use corrected gestational age   Factors

0-48 Hrs
Severely abnormal = < 95
Moderately abnormal = 95 - 119
Mildly abnormal = 120 - 139
Normal = 140 up

48 Hrs. - 16 weeks
Severely abnormal = < 100
Moderately abnormal = 100 - 124
Mildly abnormal = 125 - 144
Normal = 145 up

★ Abnormal auditory or visual requires hearing or vision testing. May be secondary to brain dysfunction

Assymmetry	38-39	0-4 weeks	4.1-8 weeks	8.1-12 weeks	12.1-16 weeks	1	2	3	4	5	6
			a=5, b=3, c=1								
		d,e=5 / c,f=3 / a,b,g=1	c,d=5 / b,e=3 / a,f,g=1	b,c=5 / a,d=3 / e,f,g=1							
			b=5, c=3, a,d=1								
		a=5 / b=3 / c,f=1		b,c=5 / a,d=3 / e,f=1	c,d=5 / b,e=3 / a,f=1						
R d = levels ≥1 L		arms b=5 / c=3 / a,d=1	legs b=5 / c=3 / a,d=1	Sum: divide by 2							
			d=5, a,b,c=1								
R f = levels ≥2 L		c,d=5 / a,b,e,f=1		d,e=5 / c=3 / a,b,f=1	e=5 / d=3 / a,b,c,f=1						
R f = levels ≥2 L			b,c=5 / a,d=3 / e,f=1	c,d=5 / b=3 / a,e,f=1	b,c=5 / a,d=3 / e,f=1						
R d = levels ≥1 L			b=5, a,c,d=1								
R d = levels ≥1 L			b,c=5 / a,d=1		c=5 / b=3 / a,d=1						
R f = levels ≥2 L			d,e=5 / c=3 / a,b,f=1		c,d=5 / b,e=3 / a,f=1						
R g = levels ≥2 L			d,e=5 / c,f=3 / a,b,g=1		c,d=5 / b,e=3 / a,f,g=1						
R g = levels ≥2 L			d,e=5 / c,f=3 / a,b,g=1		d=5 / c,e=3 / a,b,f,g=1						
R e = levels ≥2 L			b=5, a,c=3, d=1								
R d = levels ≥1 L			c=5, b=3, a,d=1								
R f = levels ≥2 L		b,c=5 / a=3 / d,e,f=1		c=5 / b=3 / a,d,e,f=1							
		b,c=5 / a,d,f=1		c=5 / b,d=3 / a,e,f=1	d=5 / c,e=3 / a,b,f=1						
		b,c=5 / a,d,e=1	c,d=5 / b,e=3 / a=1	d,e=5 / c=3 / a,b=1	e=5 / c,d=3 / a,b=1						
		c=5 / b,d=3 / a,e=1	c,d=5 / b=3 / a,e=1	d=5 / c=3 / a,b,e=1							
		c=5 / b,d=3 / a,e=1	c,d=5 / b=3 / a,e=1	d=5 / c=3 / a,b,e=1							
★ if assymmetry, consider hearing test		b-e=5 / a=1	c-e=5 / b=3 / a=1	d,e=5 / c=3 / a,b=1							★
	b-g=5 / a=1	c-g=5 / b=3 / a=1	d-g=5 / c=3 / a,b=1	f,g=5 / d=3 / a,c=1	g=5 / f=3 / a,e=1						★
		b-f=5 / a=1		c,f=5 / b=3 / a=1 d,f=5 / c=3 / a,b=1	f=5 / e=3 / a,d=1						
		b,c=5 / a,d=1	c,d=5 / b=3 / =1	d=5 / c=3 / a,b=1							
		a,b=5	b,c=5 / a=1	c,f=5 / b=3 / a=1	d,f=5 / c=3 / a,b=1						
R e = levels ≥2 L		c=5 / b=3 / a,d,e=1	b,c=5 / a=3 / d,e=1	a,b=5 / c=3 / d,e=1							
		d=5 / b,c=3 / a,e=1		d=5 / c=3 / a,b,e=1							
		d,e=5 / b,c=3 / a=1	e=5 / c,d=3 / a,b=1	e=5 / d=3 / a,b,c=1							
		a,b=5	b,e=5 / a=1	c,e=5 / b=3 / a=1	d,e=5 / c=3 / a,b=1						
		a,b=5	b,e=5 / a=1	c,e=5 / b=3 / a=1	d,e=5 / c=3 / a,b=1						
		a-c=5 / d=3 / e=1	a,b=5 / c=3 / d,e=1	a=5 / b=3 / c,e=1							
		b-e=5 / a=1	c-e=5 / b=3 / a=1	d,e=5 / c=3 / a,b=1	e=5 / d=3 / a,c=1						
					FACTOR SCORES						

TOTAL SCORE [   ]

returns the head to upright position, noting also ability to maintain the head upright.

20. Anterior neck. Support the infant at the shoulders, moving the trunk backward until the head drops back. Count the seconds until the infant returns the head to upright position, noting also ability to maintain the head upright.

21. Auditory. Ask the caretaker to call the infant's name from each side, holding the infant so the head can be easily turned. Or use a rattle held 6 to 10 inches from each ear.

22. Visual. Use a black and white bull's-eye about 12 inches from the face for horizontal and vertical tracking, tracking well past midline, and following in a full circle.

23. Alert. Use voice or tongue clucking, holding the infant's face about 12 inches from your face. Note that the infant is focusing and count the seconds until the infant averts his/her gaze.

24. Ventral suspension. Support the infant in the air under the abdomen, noting the body position.

25. All fours/prone. Place the infant abdomen down on a firm surface and observe head and arm position.

26. Moro. Place one hand behind the infant's head and support the infant's back with the other, then drop the infant 10 to 20 cm. Observe the hand and arm movements.

27. Suck. Wash your hands, place your finger in the infant's mouth with finger pad toward the palate, and note sucking response.

28. Tremor. Note presence or absence of tremor and state in which it occurs.

29. Responsiveness. Talk to or cluck tongue at the baby, trying to engage the baby, and ask the caretaker about the response to seeing bottle or breast.

30. Vocalization. Talk to or cluck tongue at the infant and note the vocal response.

31. Assess the amount of stimulus needed to get the infant's attention.

32. Assess the infant's attention to you throughout the evaluation.

Infanib (Fig. 2): Assessment of primitive reflexes, trunk control, vestibular function, legs, and French angles designed for the neurologic evaluation of infants ages 4 to 15 months. Items are the following:

1. Hands closed/open. See Neoneuro & Up, item 7.
2. Scarf sign. See Neoneuro & Up, item 11.
3. Heel to ear. See Neoneuro & Up, item 13.
4. Popliteal angle. See Neoneuro & Up, item 12.
5. Leg abduction. Grasp the lower legs and move them apart until resistance. Measure the angle between the legs.
6. Dorsiflexion of the foot. Grasp the foot and flex it until resistance. Measure the angle between the foot and leg.
7. Foot grasp. Place thumb on balls of foot. Observe curling of toes.
8. Tonic labyrinthine supine. Place hand between the infant's shoulder blades and rub the skin. Observe shoulder retraction, extension of arms, legs, and trunk.

9. Asymmetric tonic neck. See Neoneuro & Up, item 10.
10. Pull to sit. See Neoneuro & Up, items 16 and 17. Here they are scored as one with preference given to head lag.
11. Body derotative. With the infant supine, grasp the lower legs near the feet and rotate them to start the roll from back to prone. Observe infant's ability to continue the roll.
12. Body rotative. The infant spontaneously rolls from back to front, then pulls to standing.
13. All fours. See Neoneuro & Up, item 25.
14. Tonic labyrinthine prone. Support the abdomen with one hand and raise the infant to crawling position, then flex the head with your other hand. Observe shoulder protraction and flexion of arms, legs, and hips.
15. Sitting position. Place the infant in sitting position, supporting the trunk. Observe truncal flexion and extension and the lumbar vertebra at which flexion occurs.
16. Sideways parachute. Support the infant in sitting position, then tip the infant to each side, noting extension of hand for support.
17. Backward parachute. Support the trunk, then gently and firmly thrust backward, observing posturing of arms.
18. Weight bearing. Support infant under the arms in standing position. Observe amount of weight bearing and body position.
19. Positive support reaction. Lift the infant under arms to standing position and return the feet to surface. Observe the position of the feet.
20. Forward parachute. Grasp infant at the trunk, support in midair, then thrust infant head first toward a surface. Observe the reaction and placement of the arms.

Scoring. Circle the appropriate description of each item during and immediately after the examination. Circle any notable differences between one side and the other in the asymmetry column of Neoneuro & Up. Then go to a quiet place to do the formal scoring, placing the points within the black enclosed space for each item. Total the items for factor (subscale) and total score. The degree of normality or abnormality is determined from the ranges of scores on the scoring form (see Figs. 1 and 2).

C. For the occasional infant who was not sick at birth and did not have brain imaging studies, consider a CT scan. Identify mass, cyst, tumor, malformation, dysgenesis, cerebral atrophy, and enlarged ventricles. Consult neurologist or neurosurgeon as appropriate. Obtain occupational and physical therapy services.

D. Identifiable congenital syndromes associated with hypotonia include trisomy 21, congenital hypothyroidism, Ehlers-Danlos syndrome, Prader-Willi syndrome, Laurence-Moon-Biedl syndrome, and congenital brain anomalies (hydrocephalus, Dandy-Walker cyst, Arnold-Chiari syndrome).

E. Hypotonia is more common than hypertonia in both premature and term babies who were sick as newborns. Some hypotonia in infants less than 4 to 6 months will

(Continued on page 464)

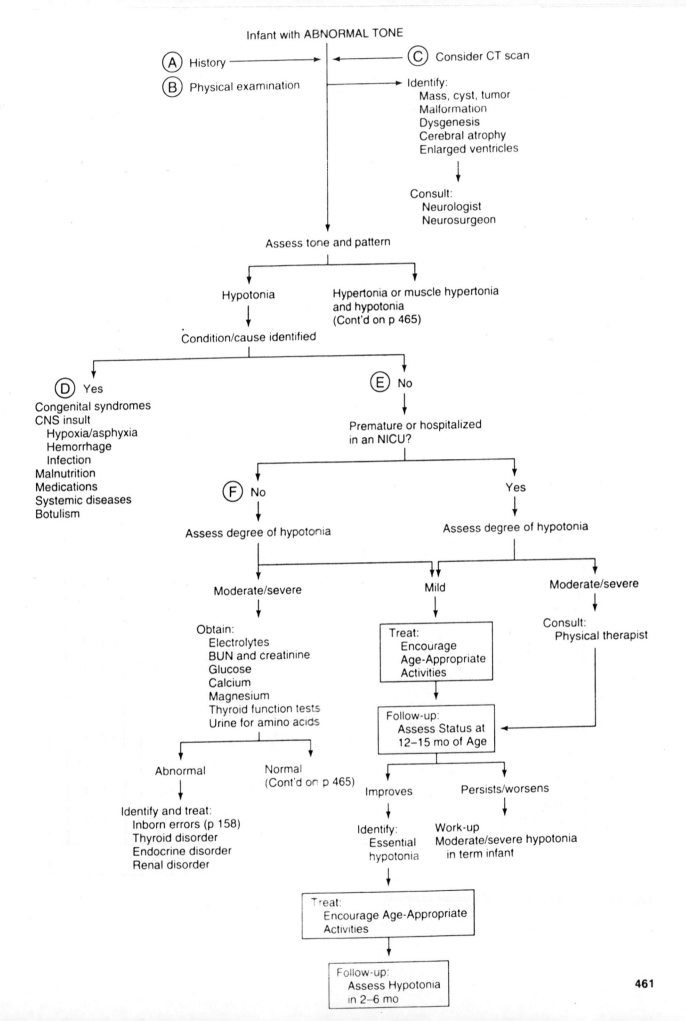

Infant with ABNORMAL TONE

(A) History ——————→←—— (C) Consider CT scan

(B) Physical examination

Identify:
    Mass, cyst, tumor
    Malformation
    Dysgenesis
    Cerebral atrophy
    Enlarged ventricles

Consult:
    Neurologist
    Neurosurgeon

Assess tone and pattern

Hypotonia

Hypertonia or muscle hypertonia
and hypotonia
(Cont'd on p 465)

Condition/cause identified

(D) Yes

Congenital syndromes
CNS insult
    Hypoxia/asphyxia
    Hemorrhage
    Infection
Malnutrition
Medications
Systemic diseases
Botulism

(E) No

Premature or hospitalized
in an NICU?

(F) No

Assess degree of hypotonia

Yes

Assess degree of hypotonia

Moderate/severe

Obtain:
    Electrolytes
    BUN and creatinine
    Glucose
    Calcium
    Magnesium
    Thyroid function tests
    Urine for amino acids

Mild

Treat:
    Encourage
    Age-Appropriate
    Activities

Moderate/severe

Consult:
    Physical therapist

Follow-up:
    Assess Status at
    12–15 mo of Age

Abnormal

Normal
(Cont'd on p 465)

Identify and treat:
    Inborn errors (p 158)
    Thyroid disorder
    Endocrine disorder
    Renal disorder

Improves

Identify:
    Essential
    hypotonia

Persists/worsens

Work-up
Moderate/severe hypotonia
in term infant

Treat:
    Encourage Age-Appropriate
    Activities

Follow-up:
    Assess Hypotonia
    in 2–6 mo

461

INFANIB

Date of Exam _____

Corrected Gestational Age _____

CIRCLE ONE

NAME _____

ITEM	START SCORE	MAJOR CHANGE														
1	Birth		**SUPINE** Hands closed/open	Clenched	Clenched with stress maneuver	Closed	Sometimes closed	Open								
2	Birth		Scarf sign	Less Than #1	0° to 15° — 1	15° to 45° — 2	45° to 60° — 3	60° to 85° — 4	Past #4						
3	Birth		Heel to ear	Over 100°	90° to 100°	60° to 90°	40° to 60°	10° to 40°	Under 10°						
4	Birth		Popliteal angle	Under 80°	80° to 90°	90° to 110°	110° to 150°	150° to 170°	Over 170°						
5	Birth		Leg abduction	Under 40°	40° to 70°	70° to 100°	100° to 130°	130° to 150°	Over 150°						
6	Birth		Dorsiflexion of foot	0° to 10°	10° to 40°	40° to 70°	70° to 80°	80° to 90°							
7	Birth	9 mos	Foot grasp		No Grasp	Barely Grasp	Average grasp	Excessive grasp or grasp with stress maneuver							
8	Birth	6 mos	Tonic labyrinthine supine	Absent		Some shoulder retraction or some extension of trunk or legs		Shoulder retraction and full leg extension or flexed arms and legs							
9	Birth	6 mos	Asymmetric tonic neck reflex	Absent		Postures in, can move out		Persistent or spontaneous							
10	Birth		Pull to sitting	Head extended Arms extended	Head up Arms ext.	Head flexed Arms ext.	Head flexed Arms flexed								
11	4 mos.		Body derotative	Present to both sides	Slow or mildly asymmetrical	Absent or markedly asymmetrical									
12	9 mos		Body rotative	Present to both sides	Slow or mildly asymmetrical	Absent or markedly asymmetrical									
13	Birth		**PRONE** All fours	Lifts Head	Head up 45°	Forearms only	Head up 90°	Bears weight on extended arms	Assumes all fours unsteadily	Assumes all fours well	Stands up through Plantigrade					
14	Birth	9 mos	Tonic labyrinthine prone	Absent		With Head Flexion — Some shoulder protraction or some flexion of legs		Shoulder protraction and arms, hips, or legs under trunk							
15	Birth		**SITTING** Sitting position			L3	L5								
16	6 mos.		Sideways parachute	Present in both arms	Slow or mildly asymmetrical	Absent or markedly asymmetrical									
17	9 mos		Backwards parachute	Present in both arms	Slow or mildly asymmetrical	Absent or markedly asymmetrical									
18	Birth		**STANDING** Weight bearing	Primitive reflex	No weight bearing	Poor weight bearing Breaks at knees	Unequal weight bearing								
19	3 mos.		Positive support reaction	Feet flat	5 to 30 sec. on toes then drop to feet flat	> 30 sec. on toes									
20	7 mos.		**SUSPENDED** Forward parachute	Present	Slow or mildly asymmetrical	Absent or markedly asymmetrical									

FACTOR SCORES

TOTAL SCORE

Figure 2   Infanib (Infant neurologic international battery).

Overall Normal = 5. Mildly abnormal = 3
Markedly abnormal = 1

Comments

Corrected gestational age

ITEM	0-9	1-1.9	2-2.9	3-3.9	4-4.9	5-5.9	6-6.9	7-7.9	8-8.9	9-18 months	Comments
											matches age = 5
1	Closed		Sometimes closed	Open				At any age, clenched or clenched with stress maneuver = 1			One stage delay = 3 / Two stage delay = 1 / One closed, one open = 1
2	0 - 15°			15 - 45°			45 - 60°			60 - 85°	5 = Picture matches age / 3 = One stage away ← or → / 1 = Two stages away ← or →
3	100 - 90°			90 - 60°			60 - 40°			40 - 10°	As above except definite asymmetry = 1
4	80 - 90°			90 - 110°			110 - 150°			150 - 170°	
5	40 - 70°			70 - 100°			100 - 130°			130 - 150°	As for # 2 & 3
6	0-10° = 1 / 10-40° = 3	40-80° = 5 / 80-90° = 3		0-10° = 1	10 - 40° = 3		40 - 70° = 5		70 - 80° = 3	80 - 90° = 1	Definite asymmetry = 1
7	Excessive grasp or grasp with stress maneuver = 1 , Other = 5							Absent = 5	Barely Grasp = 3	Grasp = 1	Definite asymmetry = 1
8	Shoulder retraction and full leg extension or flexed arms and legs = 1, Other = 5							Absent = 5	Some = 3	Full = 1	
9	Persistent or spontaneous = 1, Other = 5					Absent = 5	Postures in Can move out = 3		Persistent = 1		
10						Full = 5 / Partial head lag or not using arms = 3 / Complete head lag and not using arms = 1					Picture matches age = 5 / One stage delay = 3 / Two stage delay = 1 / 0-4 months head flexion and arm flexion = 1
11				Present to both sides = 5		Slow or mildly asymmetrical = 3		Absent or markedly asymmetrical = 1			
12								Present = 5 / Slow or mildly asymmetrical = 3 / Absent or markedly asymmetrical = 1			
13	Lifts Head	Head up 45°	Forearms only	Head up 90°	Bears weight on extended forearms	All fours unsteadily	All fours well		Plantigrade		Picture matches age = 5 / One stage delay = 3 / Two stage delay = 1
14	Shoulder protraction, arms, hips or legs under trunk = 1, other = 5							Absent = 5	Some = 3	Full = 1	
15				L3 →	L5 →						Picture matches age = 5 / One stage delay = 3 / Two stage delay = 1 / 0-5 months L5 break and head extension = 1
16						Present in both arms = 5	Slow or mildly asymmetrical = 3		Absent or markedly asymmetrical = 1		
17									As Above		
18	Primitive Reflex	No Weight-bearing	Poor weight bearing Breaks at knee			Unequal weight bearing					Picture matches age = 5 / One stage delay = 3 / Two stage delay = 1 / Persistent weight-bearing (> 60 sec) at 2.5 - 5 months = 1
19				Maintains weight feet flat = 5	5 - 30 sec on toes then drop to feet flat = 3				> 30 sec on toes = 1		
20							Present = 5	Slow or mildly asymmetrical = 3	Absent or markedly asym = 1		

Degree of normality/abnormality based on total score

Less than 4 months	4 to 8 months	8 months or more
Abnormal ≤ 48	Abnormal ≤ 54	Abnormal ≤ 68
Transient 49 - 65	Transient 55-71	Transient 69-82
Normal ≥ 66	Normal ≥ 72	Normal ≥ 83

Category of abnormality

If abnormal, choose a category

Spastic Tetraparesis/Dyskinesia   Spastic Hemiparesis   Spastic Diplegia   Hypotonia later change to hypertonia. After 6 months much of the hypotonia and even mild mixed hypotonia with hypertonia lessens with time, especially in those with milder hypotonia (transient neurologic abnormality of infancy).

F. Assess the degree of hypotonia in infants who were premature or hospitalized in an NICU. With mild hypotonia observation and follow-up are generally sufficient. The hypotonia should improve some by 12 to 15 months and throughout the preschool years. For moderate to severe hypotonia in infants not hospitalized in the NICU, obtain electrolytes, BUN, creatinine, glucose, calcium, magnesium, thyroid panel, and urine for amino and organic acids. This will identify inborn errors of metabolism, thyroid disorders, and other endocrine and renal disorders. When moderate to severe hypotonia persists at 12 to 15 months of age, especially among infants who are developing well cognitively, obtain a creatine phosphokinase (CPK) and electromyography–nerve conduction velocity (EMG-NCV).

G. For those with increasing hypotonia and absent or depressed reflexes, obtain a CPK and EMG-NCV. A motor unit consists of the anterior horn cell, its axon, and the muscle fibers it innervates. In myopathic disorders individual muscle fibers are lost and EMG demonstrates small motor unit potentials. In neuropathic disorders involving the anterior horn cell or peripheral nerves, the motor units have increased size and motor unit potentials. Nerve conduction studies assess the function of peripheral motor and sensory nerves. A relatively normal NCV associated with decreased amplitude suggests axonal pathology related to metabolic disorders. A markedly decreased NCV associated with asynchronous evoked potentials suggests demyelinization caused by Guillain-Barré syndrome, inflammatory polyneuropathy, or leukodystrophy. The muscle biopsy, besides separating myopathic from neuropathic disorders, may help in characterizing the specific type of myopathy. For elevated CPK consult a neurologist for muscle biopsy and identification of myopathic changes.

H. Most myopathic disorders are diagnosed and treated by the special pediatric neuromuscular clinic funded by the Muscular Dystrophy Association. Muscular dystrophies include Duchenne, Emery-Dreifuss, and other congenital dystrophies. Myotonic disorders include myotonic dystrophy, myotonia congenita, and paramyotonia congenita. Congenital myopathies are central core disease, nemaline (rod), myotubular, and fiber-type disproportion. Metabolic myopathies include storage and mitochondrial disorders (carnitine deficiency syndromes). Myotonic dystrophy, the most common infantile genetic myopathy, in early infancy causes poor feeding and respiratory distress secondary to diaphragmatic and intercostal weakness. Because electrical myotonia is not present at birth and muscle biopsy findings are nonspecific, the diagnosis is suggested by electrical myotonia in the mother. Prenatal diagnosis and carrier detection can be made by measuring apolipoprotein C-II. Surviving infants can eventually stand and walk independently but have a high incidence of mental retardation and speech difficulties. See also weakness (p 466) for discussion of neuropathic, myopathic, and myoneural junction disorders.

I. For progressive hypertonia in children who are not graduates of the NICU and progressive hypotonia in children with normal CPK and EMG-NCV, refer to a neurologist. Some of these infants have degenerative neurologic disorders, most of which still are not treatable. Diagnosis is important largely for genetic counseling, parental support, and education about the anticipated outcome.

References

Dubowitz V. The floppy infant. In: Dubowitz V. Clinics in developmental medicine. 2nd ed. London: Spastics International, 1980.

Ellison PH. The Infanib: A reliable method for the neuromotor assessment of infants. Tucson: Therapy Skill Builders, 1994.

Ellison PH. The neurologic examination of the newborn and infant. In: David RB, ed. Pediatric neurology for clinicians. 2nd ed. Norwalk, CT: Appleton & Lange, 1996.

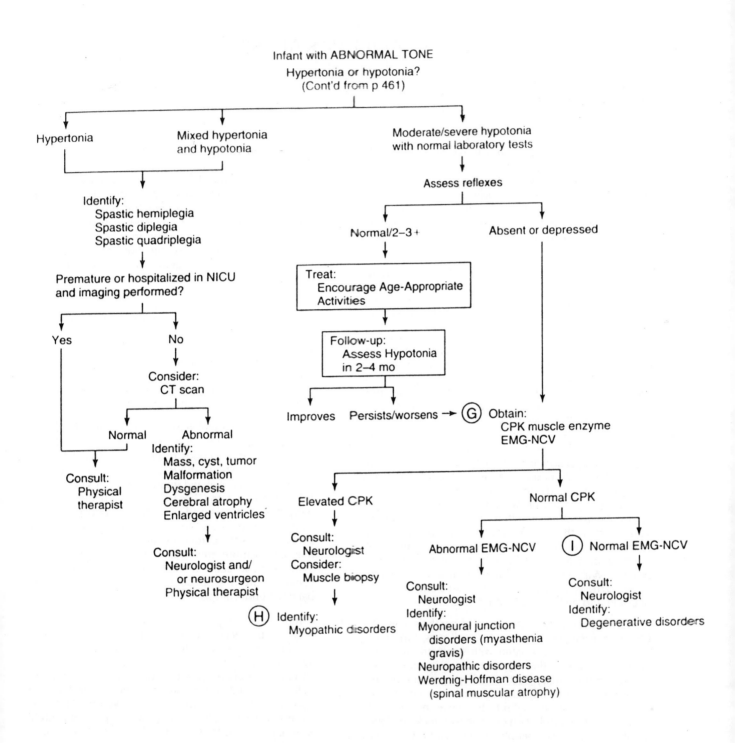

Infant with ABNORMAL TONE
Hypertonia or hypotonia?
(Cont'd from p 461)

Hypertonia

Mixed hypertonia and hypotonia

Identify:
Spastic hemiplegia
Spastic diplegia
Spastic quadriplegia

Premature or hospitalized in NICU and imaging performed?

Yes

No

Consider:
CT scan

Normal

Abnormal
Identify:
Mass, cyst, tumor
Malformation
Dysgenesis
Cerebral atrophy
Enlarged ventricles

Consult:
Physical
therapist

Consult:
Neurologist and/
or neurosurgeon
Physical therapist

Moderate/severe hypotonia with normal laboratory tests

Assess reflexes

Normal/2–3 +

Absent or depressed

Treat:
Encourage Age-Appropriate
Activities

Follow-up:
Assess Hypotonia
in 2–4 mo

Improves

Persists/worsens → (G) Obtain:
CPK muscle enzyme
EMG-NCV

Elevated CPK

Normal CPK

Consult:
Neurologist
Consider:
Muscle biopsy

Abnormal EMG-NCV

(I) Normal EMG-NCV

(H) Identify:
Myopathic disorders

Consult:
Neurologist
Identify:
Myoneural junction
disorders (myasthenia
gravis)
Neuropathic disorders
Werdnig-Hoffman disease
(spinal muscular atrophy)

Consult:
Neurologist
Identify:
Degenerative disorders

CHILDHOOD WEAKNESS AND PARALYSIS

Patricia H. Ellison, M.D.
Stephen Berman, M.D.

Because most children move so much, weakness is usually readily recognized by the parents when its onset is acute. It is more difficult to judge when there is pain. More subtle weakness that does not prevent movement of arms or legs, especially when present from birth or gradual in onset, may also be harder for parents to identify. Paralysis is identified by absence of movement and decreased or absent deep tendon reflexes.

A. In the history ask in which limb the weakness started and when. Ask what the child cannot do. Ask whether the weakness is getting better, getting worse, or staying the same. If it is getting worse, ask how it is getting worse—what abilities the child has lost.

B. In the physical examination use the reflex hammer to seek asymmetric or depressed reflexes. If an arm is weak, check the leg carefully. In hemiplegia the arm is more involved than the leg. Check both proximal and distal strength. Ask the child to spread his or her fingers and not let you push them together (see p 448). Ask the child to remove socks and shoes, walk on heels, and walk on toes. Check proximal strength of arms by asking child to hold up arm and be strong. Ask child to get up from a chair without using hands, get up from the floor without using hands. In a toddler observe stoop and recover (place a toy or two on the floor). Inspect the calves. Asymmetries are often more subtle. On extension of arms with eyes closed tell the child you are going to tap the arms. Tap several times looking for displacement of one arm or failure to return to the same position. Watch for some elbow flexion of one arm. On heel and toe walking watch for decreased arm swing on one side and awkward use of one leg.

C. Assess involvement. Acute onset of paralysis suggests CNS hemorrhage or trauma. A spinal mass, tumor, or infarction may be associated with symmetric involvement, loss of anal reflex, rectal or urinary incontinence, and recurrent urinary tract infections. Asymmetric involvement is most likely due to anterior horn cell, nerve root lesions, or lesions distal to the nerve root. Loss of sensation in the distribution of a nerve or stocking-glove distribution suggests a peripheral neuropathy. Consider conversion reaction when paralysis or weakness occurs in a nonanatomic pattern and the patient is capable of withdrawal movements to appropriate stimuli.

D. Neurotoxins that prevent the release of acetylcholine at the nerve endings are produced by ticks, diphtheria, and *Clostridium botulinum*. Removal of the tick brings rapid relief of symptoms. Botulism causes blurred vision, loss of accommodation, diplopia, and constipation in association with weakness or paralysis of the extremities. Consider *Corynebacterium diphtheriae* in the inadequately immunized child with a history of severe exudative pharyngitis and myocarditis. Guillain-Barré syndrome often causes symmetric progressive motor weakness and areflexia. Cranial nerve involvement and signs of autonomic dysfunction may be present. Cerebrospinal fluid (CSF) examination reveals elevated protein levels in association with absent or slight pleocytosis (< 10 WBCs/mm^3). Symptoms generally progress for the first 4 weeks, then plateau for 2 to 4 weeks prior to recovery. Transverse myelitis is a parainfectious process resulting in inflammation and infarction of the spinal cord. Suspect this entity if you find acute flaccid paralysis of lower extremities, sensory loss to pain and temperature, and rectal and bladder incontinence. No specific therapy is available. Suspect poliomyelitis in the patient with asymmetric involvement, CSF pleocytosis, and signs of meningeal irritation.

E. If reflexes are depressed or absent on one side, a brain CT scan will identify most tumors, acute hemorrhages (e.g., from arteriovenous malformation [AVMs]), brain abscess, and cysts of various worms and amoebae (most common with travel and immigration). In sick children MRI is preferable to CT scan because it better identifies early brain abscess and early herpes encephalitis. In acute stroke you may see little on CT scan. Even in old stroke such as the chronic hemiplegias of infancy, there may be no more abnormality than a mild ventricular asymmetry. In acute hemiplegia in a child with congenital heart disease be sure to look for subacute bacterial endocarditis.

F. If reflexes are depressed or absent bilaterally, even if only in the legs, obtain electromyelography-nerve conduction velocity (EMG-NCV), especially if there is evidence of progression within the acute episode. An EMG-NCV identifies most anterior horn cell disease: radicular, neural, and myoneural junction; and muscle disorders. While the weakness of Werdnig-Hoffman syndrome is generally not acute, it may present acutely with pneumonia. With abnormal EMG-NCV, consult a neurologist.

G. With normal reflexes, obtain potassium and creatine phosphokinase (CPK) levels. If both are normal, order the urine porphyrins. Suspect acute intermittent porphyria when abdominal pains and altered mental function are associated with porphyrins in the urine. Periodic paralysis, an autosomal dominant familial disorder, can be associated with hypokalemia.

(Continued on page 468)

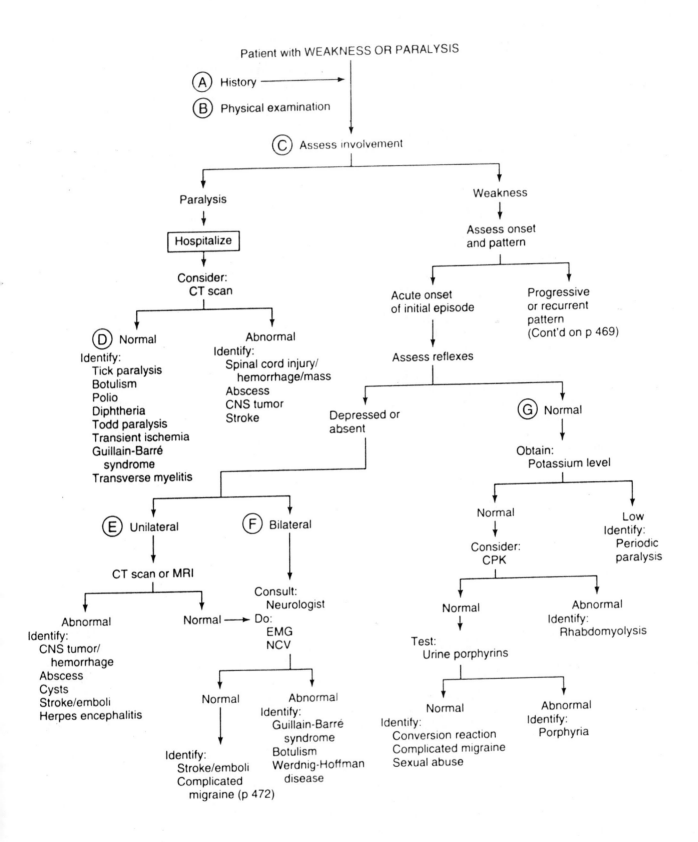

Patient with WEAKNESS OR PARALYSIS

(A) History

(B) Physical examination

(C) Assess involvement

Paralysis

Hospitalize

Consider:
CT scan

(D) Normal
Identify:
  Tick paralysis
  Botulism
  Polio
  Diphtheria
  Todd paralysis
  Transient ischemia
  Guillain-Barré
    syndrome
  Transverse myelitis

Abnormal
Identify:
  Spinal cord injury/
    hemorrhage/mass
  Abscess
  CNS tumor
  Stroke

(E) Unilateral

CT scan or MRI

Abnormal
Identify:
  CNS tumor/
    hemorrhage
  Abscess
  Cysts
  Stroke/emboli
  Herpes encephalitis

Normal →

Identify:
  Stroke/emboli
  Complicated
    migraine (p 472)

(F) Bilateral

Consult:
  Neurologist
Do:
  EMG
  NCV

Normal

Abnormal
Identify:
  Guillain-Barré
    syndrome
  Botulism
  Werdnig-Hoffman
    disease

Weakness

Assess onset
and pattern

Acute onset
of initial episode

Assess reflexes

Depressed or
absent

Progressive
or recurrent
pattern
(Cont'd on p 469)

(G) Normal

Obtain:
  Potassium level

Normal

Consider:
  CPK

Normal

Test:
  Urine porphyrins

Normal
Identify:
  Conversion reaction
  Complicated migraine
  Sexual abuse

Abnormal
Identify:
  Porphyria

Abnormal
Identify:
  Rhabdomyolysis

Low
Identify:
  Periodic
    paralysis

H. With recurrent episodes, write a laboratory slip for the family to obtain the blood and urine tests during the next episode. If all tests are normal, consider conversion hysteria, either separately from or as a manifestation of sexual abuse. Consider also complicated migraine.

I. For weakness greater in the legs, obtain a CPK. With a normal CPK, consider a CT scan. That will identify hydrocephalus, some masses, and some neurodegenerative diseases. MRI better identifies the white matter diseases.

J. In a boy 4 to 5 years of age an elevated CPK usually indicates Duchenne muscular dystrophy. In older boys the diagnosis may be Becker muscular dystrophy. Obtain an EMG-NCV to confirm. Some other myopathies may be identified.

K. If the CT scan is normal, obtain an EMG-NCV. This will enable you to separate peripheral neuropathy (very uncommon in children) from myopathic disorders from conditions such as Charcot-Marie-Tooth. While Charcot-Marie-Tooth is categorized as a hereditary motor sensory neuropathy, some patients have spinal cord or even cerebellar involvement. Charcot-Marie-Tooth is often recognized by pes cavus and the wasted lower leg muscles. The myopathies may require a muscle biopsy for precise diagnosis, since many are named by unique features of the cellular contents. Consult a neurologist with expertise in children's muscle disease before biopsy to make certain the biopsy is done well, handled well, and read well. Proper diagnosis separates progressive from nonprogressive disorders. Many of these disorders are diagnosed and treated through clinics funded by the Muscular Dystrophy Association. Support groups for families, knowledge about maintenance of function as long as possible, and resources for purchase of proper equipment are all available. Anterior horn cell disease can appear in an intermediate form between 6 months and 2 years and in a juvenile after 2 years of age. Suspect leukodystrophy when signs of both upper and lower motor neuron disease are present.

L. If the condition is no greater in the legs, consider an edrophonium (Tensilon) test. Myasthenia gravis results from failure of neuromuscular transmission caused by antibodies against acetylcholine receptors. The administration of edrophonium produces improvement in patients with myasthenia. Remember that the test requires a measurable weakness—drooping eyelids, weak hand grasp—something you can test reasonably objectively before and after the drug. If the weakness worsens near the end of the day, have the test done then.

References

Evans OB. Manual of child neurology. New York: Churchill Livingstone, 1981.

Patterson MC, Gomez MR. Muscle disease in children: A practical approach. Pediatr Rev 1990; 12:73.

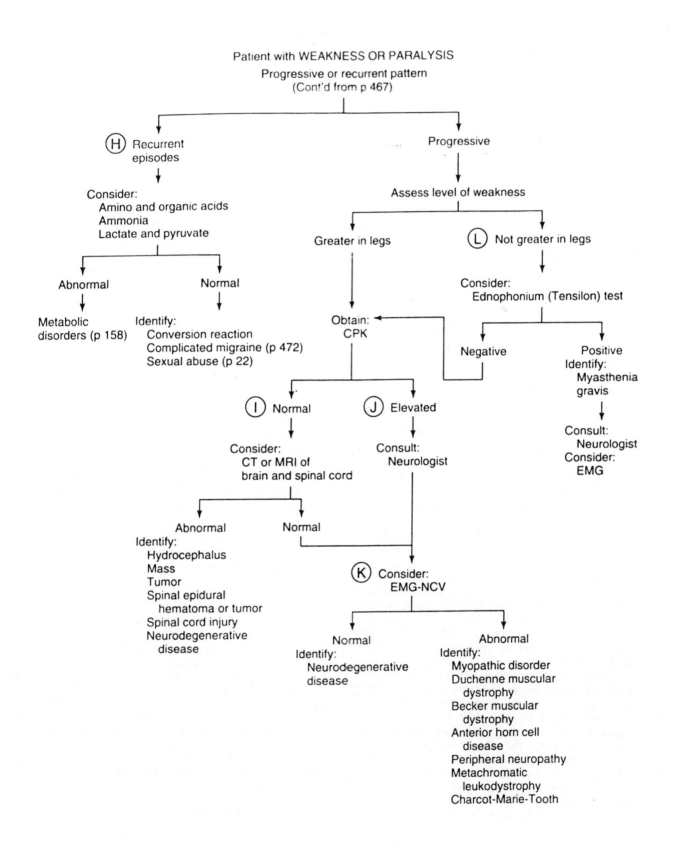

Patient with WEAKNESS OR PARALYSIS
Progressive or recurrent pattern
(Cont'd from p 467)

(H) Recurrent episodes

Consider:
Amino and organic acids
Ammonia
Lactate and pyruvate

Abnormal

Metabolic disorders (p 158)

Normal

Identify:
Conversion reaction
Complicated migraine (p 472)
Sexual abuse (p 22)

Progressive

Assess level of weakness

Greater in legs

(L) Not greater in legs

Consider:
Ednophonium (Tensilon) test

Obtain: CPK

Negative

Positive
Identify:
Myasthenia gravis

Consult:
Neurologist
Consider:
EMG

(I) Normal

(J) Elevated

Consider:
CT or MRI of brain and spinal cord

Consult:
Neurologist

Abnormal
Identify:
Hydrocephalus
Mass
Tumor
Spinal epidural hematoma or tumor
Spinal cord injury
Neurodegenerative disease

Normal

(K) Consider:
EMG-NCV

Normal
Identify:
Neurodegenerative disease

Abnormal
Identify:
Myopathic disorder
Duchenne muscular dystrophy
Becker muscular dystrophy
Anterior horn cell disease
Peripheral neuropathy
Metachromatic leukodystrophy
Charcot-Marie-Tooth

CLUMSY CHILD

Patricia H. Ellison, M.D.

DEFINITION

Clumsiness is poor speed and dexterity in motor tasks. Parents may call a child clumsy for a variety of neurologic disorders. It is best to make a careful assessment before deciding this is just another clumsy child.

A. Observe the child throughout the history. Have age-appropriate blocks or puzzles available. Ask what the parent means by clumsiness. Ask whether the child has always been clumsy. Was the child floppy or hypotonic as an infant? Is the clumsiness in arms, legs, or both? Is it getting better, getting worse, or staying the same? Is anyone else in the family clumsy—siblings, parents, grandparents, aunts and uncles, cousins? How old were other family members when thought to be clumsy? Did they get better, worse, or stay the same? Did any family member end up in a wheelchair? Why? How old was this child when he or she learned to walk? What can the child do and not do now: running, ascending and descending stairs, skipping, hopping, drawing, writing? Ask why the parents are seeking medical consultation now.

B. In the physical examination be alert for movement disorders. For infants and young children hold an object on either side and verbally offer it to the child. Watch for ataxia or dyskinesia when reaching. For children old enough to do the finger to nose of cerebellar testing (about age 4 years), observe for ataxia, tremor, or chorea on the cerebellar testing (finger-to-nose, rapid alternating movement, and thumb to second digit repetitive opposition). Have the child extend both arms and close eyes. Observe for chorea. If you think you see some ataxia in the arms, try big toe to your finger, looking for ataxia in the feet. Observe movements such as stoops and recovers, very helpful in children not old enough to walk on tiptoe or do tandem gait. Put some toys on the floor near the child to encourage this. Look for wide-based gait persisting after 3 months of walking independently. Test tandem gait forward and backward, walking on tiptoes and heels, jumping, skipping, and hopping with age norms (Motor subscale of McCarthy). Search for other clues: the skin markers of neurocutaneous disorders; thin, long face and nasal speech of myotonia; the enlarged head of the gastrocnemius of Duchenne muscular dystrophy. If fine motor skills are a concern, have the child do some age-appropriate pencil and paper and grooved pegboard tasks. For school-age children these should include printing and writing name in cursive when age-appropriate, drawing a sufficient number of items to be reliable, and grooved pegboard (see Bloch Peterson, et al. and Rapin, et al. for a detailed description of pegboard activities). For younger children use inch-cube blocks.

C. At this point other neurologic conditions are ruled out, and the patient is defined as a clumsy child. Some children are sufficiently clumsy to merit adaptive physical therapy (PT) or occupational therapy (OT) through school programs. For school-age children suggest that the parents help the child develop skills that do not depend on fine coordination. Ages 6 to 12 years are key to self-mastery. These children should not always be asked to do what they simply cannot do. Some suggestions: swimming, hiking, fishing. Try to find out strengths or interests of the parents that might successfully unfold in the child.

D. Reevaluate the child in 6 months. Your detailed and quantified notes from the previous examination should enable you to judge progress, plateau, or worsening clumsiness. For those who improve, inquire about the techniques being used and encourage those that are emotionally and physically appropriate. For those on a plateau, inquire again about family resources for developing skills the child can master.

E. Children who are deteriorating need further diagnostic work-up. Neurodegenerative diseases, such as metachromatic leukodystrophy, adrenoleukodystrophy, or neuronal ceroid lipofuscinosis, are high on this list. Neurologic consultation is appropriate.

References

Bloch Petersen M, Ellison P, Sharpsteen D. A review of neuromotor tests and the construction of a scored neuromotor examination of four-year-olds. Acta Paediatr Scand 1994; 83(Suppl 401).

Deuel RK. Disorders of motor execution II: Higher-order motor deficits. In: David RB, ed. Pediatric neurology for the clinician. Norfolk, CT: Appleton & Lange, 1992:486.

McCarthy D. McCarthy scale of children's abilities. New York: Psychological Corp., 1972.

Rapin I, Tourk LM, Costa LD. Evaluation of the Purdue pegboard as a screening test for brain damage. Dev Med Child Neurol 1966; 8:45.

Taft LT, Barowsky EI. Clumsy child. Pediatr Rev 1989; 10:247.

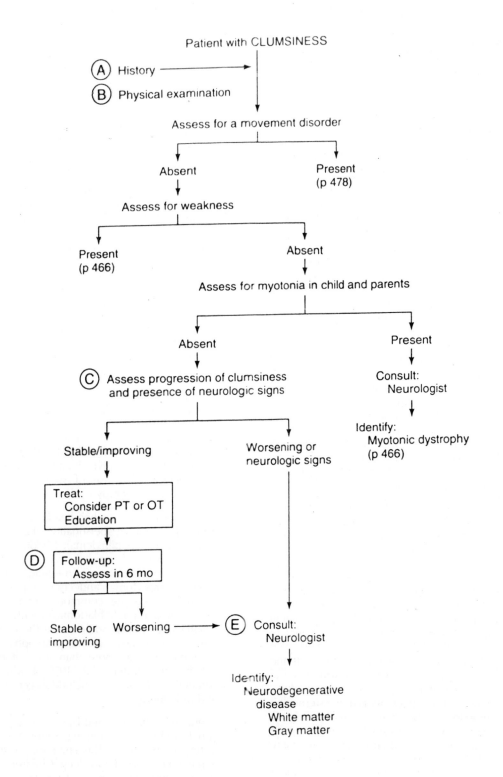

Patient with CLUMSINESS

(A) History

(B) Physical examination

Assess for a movement disorder

Absent → Assess for weakness

Present (p 478)

Present (p 466)

Absent → Assess for myotonia in child and parents

Absent

(C) Assess progression of clumsiness and presence of neurologic signs

Present → Consult: Neurologist → Identify: Myotonic dystrophy (p 466)

Stable/improving

Worsening or neurologic signs

Treat: Consider PT or OT Education

(D) Follow-up: Assess in 6 mo

Stable or improving

Worsening → (E) Consult: Neurologist → Identify: Neurodegenerative disease White matter Gray matter

HEADACHE

Patricia H. Ellison, M.D.
Stephen Berman, M.D.

Headaches occur frequently in children and are a common reason for neurologic consultation. The vast majority are easily treated.

A. In the history ask about family history of migraines, sick headaches, or headaches that sent the relative to bed; not all familial migraines are called such by family members. Ask about and be wary of recurrent morning vomiting, a possible sign of increased intracranial pressure (ICP). Ask about injury to the head or neck, specifically car accidents, slips, or falls. Ask about activities that use the trapezius muscles: backpacks with heavy books or gear or caring for very young children (common in early-teen-aged girls from families with new babies). Ask the child about the quality of the headache; even very young children understand throbbing or pounding. Ask about warning symptoms of headache: flashing lights or other visual symptoms, tingling in an arm, vertigo. Ask where the headache starts and where it goes (this often gives clues to headaches triggered by cervical muscle spasm). Ask what treatment has been tried and how well it works. Ask what works for relatives with bad headaches. Ask about the frequency of the headache and where the child usually is when it starts. Ask what the child does when a headache occurs at home and at school.

B. The neurologic examination is key to the diagnosis of increased ICP. Examine the fundi, measure the head circumference, tap the skull (listening for the sound of ICP), palpate the coronal sutures for widening, and look for increased tone in the legs or inability to use the legs well. Check blood pressure for the rare case of hypertension. Examine the teeth for obvious cavities; check the pharynx and sinuses for infection. Assess cervical and suboccipital muscle tone. Muscle palpation can be a big help in the diagnosis and treatment of headache. First ask the child to put chin on chest, then put head back as far as possible, then rotate to left and right, leading with the chin. Children with cervical muscle spasm have better range of motion than adults. Palpate the right and left attachments of the sternocleidomastoid muscles to the sternum. If there is no evidence of pain, move your fingers 1 to 2 inches up the muscle and squeeze gently, again observing for pain. Squeeze gently between thumb and fingers the upper part of the trapezius that runs from neck to shoulder bilaterally and observe for pain. Palpate the trapezius from the upper edge to well below and around the shoulder blade, seeking knots of muscle in spasm. If you are not certain that the mass is a knot of muscle, push gently, which will be painful if it is muscle. Palpate firmly the suboccipital muscle attachments, starting at the mastoid and working along to the midposterior base of the skull. Palpate the upper attachments of the trapezius to the cervical vertebrae about midway on each side of the neck. Keep talking to the child while your fingers are

at work, observing for pain. If you are not certain but have reason to consider this a problem, do the palpation again after you complete the rest of the examination.

C. Consider CT scan. The parents may be extremely anxious, even in families with strong histories of migraine, about possible brain tumor. Appropriate work-up includes attention to this concern. Early use of a CT scan to rule out a brain tumor may be the best approach. A noncontrast CT scan is an excellent screen. It shows fresh hemorrhages, the size of the ventricles, and some tumors, especially some cerebellar tumors and some arteriovenous malformations (AVMs). Some headaches cannot be treated well until the CT scan is done. At the conclusion of history, physical, and CT scans, you will have ruled out most serious causes of headache plus a variety of other causes. Two types of headache usually remain: (1) vascular (migraine) and (2) muscle tension.

D. Pseudotumor cerebri or benign intracranial hypertension can cause headache, visual disturbances (double vision and visual obscurations), papilledema, and retinal hemorrhage in a well-appearing patient. The cause is usually unknown, but most patients respond to removal of risk factors (excessive vitamin A intake, some antibiotic therapy, and use of steroid medications) and acetazolamide therapy.

E. Suspect brain tumor when headache is associated with neurologic deficit, personality change, or signs of increased ICP (papilledema). Childhood brain tumors have varying peak ages of occurrence. In infancy the most common tumors are medulloblastoma, ependymoma, astrocytoma, and choroid plexus tumors. In preadolescence the common tumors are cerebellar astrocytoma, medulloblastoma, ependymoma, and craniopharyngioma. In adolescence the common tumors are cerebellar astrocytoma, craniopharyngioma, and medulloblastoma. More than 50% of the childhood tumors are infratentorial, 40% of which are in the cerebellum. Treatments include surgery, chemotherapy, and radiotherapy.

F. Migraine is characterized by aura (e.g., flashing lights) and throbbing or pounding. Often there is a family history of migraine. The child may seek a quiet or darkened room and may sleep. Children of any age can get migraines. They may last for days, especially from junior high on. Cervical muscle spasm can trigger vascular headaches, so it is best to palpate the cervical musculature for either vascular or muscle tension headache. Treatment is based on frequency and severity of headache and age of the child.

G. Treat acute sporadic mild headaches with acetaminophen or ibuprofen, ice packs, and sleep. Caffeine may help moderate headaches; an easily ingested source is Coca-Cola Classic with high-dose acetaminophen or

(Continued on page 474)

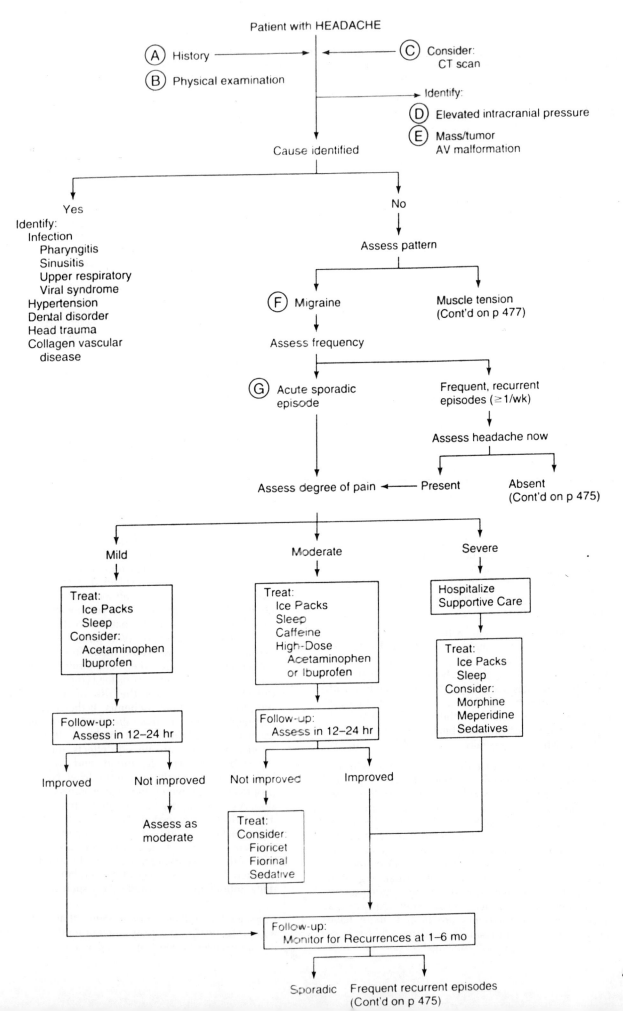

Patient with HEADACHE

(A) History

(B) Physical examination

(C) Consider: CT scan

Identify:

(D) Elevated intracranial pressure

(E) Mass/tumor AV malformation

Cause identified

Yes

Identify:
  Infection
    Pharyngitis
    Sinusitis
    Upper respiratory
    Viral syndrome
  Hypertension
  Dental disorder
  Head trauma
  Collagen vascular
    disease

No

Assess pattern

(F) Migraine

Muscle tension
(Cont'd on p 477)

Assess frequency

(G) Acute sporadic episode

Frequent, recurrent episodes (≥1/wk)

Assess headache now

Assess degree of pain ← Present

Absent
(Cont'd on p 475)

Mild

Treat:
  Ice Packs
  Sleep
Consider:
  Acetaminophen
  Ibuprofen

Follow-up:
  Assess in 12–24 hr

Improved   Not improved

                  Assess as
                  moderate

Moderate

Treat:
  Ice Packs
  Sleep
  Caffeine
  High-Dose
    Acetaminophen
    or Ibuprofen

Follow-up:
  Assess in 12–24 hr

Not improved   Improved

Treat:
  Consider:
    Fioricet
    Fiorinal
    Sedative

Severe

Hospitalize
Supportive Care

Treat:
  Ice Packs
  Sleep
Consider:
  Morphine
  Meperidine
  Sedatives

Follow-up:
  Monitor for Recurrences at 1–6 mo

Sporadic   Frequent recurrent episodes
            (Cont'd on p 475)

TABLE 1 Drugs Used for the Treatment of Migraine in Children and Adolescents

Drugs	Dosage	Product Availability	Comments
Analgesics			
Acetaminophen	8–10 mg/kg q4h Max 5 doses/day	Tabs: 160, 325, 500, 650 mg Chewables: 80 mg	Liver toxicity with overdose or overuse
Ibuprofen	4–10 mg/kg q6–8h	Susp: 100 mg/5 ml Tabs: 200, 300, 400, 600, 800 mg	Take with food or milk to decrease stomach irritation
Butalbitol, aspirin, caffeine (Fiorinal)	Max 4 doses/day	Tabs: Butalbital 50 mg, aspirin 325 mg, caffeine 40 mg	Contraindicated in porphyria; safety and effectiveness not established under age 12
Butalbitol, acetaminophen, caffeine (Fioricet)	Max 4 doses/day	Tabs: Butalbital 50 mg, acetaminophen 325 mg, caffeine 40 mg	Dependency possible with daily use
Vasoconstrictors			
Ergotamine (Ergomar, Ergostat)	½ tablet at onset of episode, then ½ tablet q30min p.r.n. to max 1½ tablet	Tabs: 2 mg ergotamine Sublingual: 2 mg Inhaler: 9 mg/ml Suppository: 2 mg ergotamine	If use of ergotamine exceeds 1.2 mg/day, switch to daily use of Bellergal-S
Ergotamine with caffeine (Cafergot)	1 tablet at onset of episode, then 1 tablet q30min p.r.n. to max 3 tablets	Tabs: 1 mg ergotamine, 100 mg caffeine	Do not use with arm or leg symptoms or speech disturbance
Isometheptene (Midrin)	1 capsule at onset of episode, then 1 capsule qh p.r.n. to max 3 capsules	Caps: Isometheptene (vasoconstrictor) 65 mg, dichloralphenazone (sedative) 100 mg, acetaminophen 325 mg	Contraindicated in renal disease, hypertension, hepatic disease, or with MAO inhibitors

Continued on page 476

ibuprofen plus ice packs and sleep. If this does not help, consider aspirin with butalbital and caffeine (Fioricet, Fiorinal) or a sedative (Table 1). Occasionally a child has such a severe headache that hospitalization is appropriate for additional treatments of morphine, meperidine, and a sedative.

H. For children under 10 years with headaches more than once a week, the first choice is daily cyproheptadine; start with 4 mg at bedtime. In 2 or 3 days add a second 4 mg in the morning. Some children need a midday dose. This drug has been a boon to young children with migraine, and it has few side effects. If that does not work, try a slow start of phenobarbital. For both cyproheptadine and phenobarbital, slow starts decrease sedation, which is generally unacceptable to parents.

I. In children 10 years or older the headache is much more like adult migraine, and many children approach adult size, making it possible to use some drugs that come in fairly large doses (e.g., ergotamine with belladonna, or Bellergal-S). If the headache is occasional, try ergotamine with caffeine (Cafergot) at the start of the headache. Usually the child must carry the drug or go to the nurse's office. Alternatives include a good dose of acetaminophen or ibuprofen (e.g., 400 mg) with a regular Coca-Cola for caffeine, or isometheptene. If headache occurs more than once a week, preventive medicines are best. If there have already been days of headache and the child is over 80 to 90 lb., start with Bellergal-S, one tablet at bedtime for a couple of days, then 1 tablet b.i.d. Bellergal-S works as quickly as anything, has less ergotamine per week than repetitive use of Cafergot, and quells the nausea. Explain that there are about five types of preventive treatments for migraine, each chemically different. It is not yet possible to take a blood test and match the patient to the medication, so use therapeutic trials. With patience, it is usually possible to find a workable medication. Do not use vasoconstrictive drugs (i.e., ergotamine, isometheptene) in children with arm or leg symptoms or speech disturbance because of the risk of a stroke. Such symptoms imply brain ischemia. If the headaches are common but not a crisis (already days of headache), try 10 mg amitriptyline at bedtime. If that is not enough and there are no side effects, increase to 20 mg at bedtime. The dry mouth and constipation of higher doses are rarely seen at this level. Next consider propranalol but remember that it can cause depression. A careful history may identify some children who are at risk for depression. For a couple days give 40 mg at night, then add another 40 mg in the morning; this is usually enough. It is contraindicated in children with asthma. Cyproheptadine can be tried in older children but is less successful. Another possibility is daily antiinflammatory medication such as naproxen.

J. Consider biofeedback sooner rather than later as an adjunct to therapy. For those who master the techniques it is an excellent approach to migraine from a lifetime

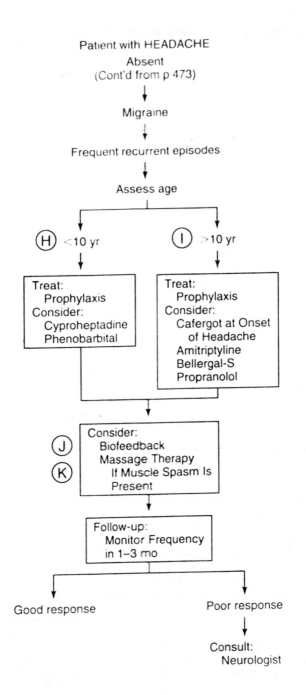

Patient with HEADACHE
Absent
(Cont'd from p 473)

Migraine

Frequent recurrent episodes

Assess age

(H) <10 yr   (I) >10 yr

Treat:
  Prophylaxis
Consider:
  Cyproheptadine
  Phenobarbital

Treat:
  Prophylaxis
Consider:
  Cafergot at Onset
    of Headache
  Amitriptyline
  Bellergal-S
  Propranolol

(J)
(K) Consider:
  Biofeedback
  Massage Therapy
    If Muscle Spasm Is
    Present

Follow-up:
  Monitor Frequency
    in 1–3 mo

Good response   Poor response

Consult:
  Neurologist

viewpoint. Children with migraine tend to be more conscientious than other children. These days that often means saying no to drugs. Both children and parents are often open to treatments without drugs or decrease in the use of drugs. Many children do well in the summer or vacation times with little medication.

K. For cervical muscle spasm consider a certified massage therapist. Sessions of half an hour are enough. Ask if the parent can observe a session so the parent can massage the child at home. Some physical therapists have trained in massage, but most have not. In my experience massage therapists have been most successful in release of muscle spasm of the trapezius and neighboring muscles. Tell the parents and child to have the child avoid neck flexion. Get a book stand so that reading is at eye level when sitting. Older children should take breaks from studying, do stretch exercises, or take hot showers aimed at the neck. Heat helps chronic muscle spasm. Teach the child to lower the eyes rather than flexing the neck while taking notes at school or using a computer. Advise avoidance of heavy backpacks or book bags and repetitive lifting of heavy things.

TABLE 1 Drugs Used for the Treatment of Migraine in Children and Adolescents *Continued*

Drugs	Dosage	Product Availability	Comments
Prophylaxis			
Ergotamine, phenobarbital, belladonna (Bellergal-S)	Start 1 tab h.s.; increase to 1 tab b.i.d.	Tabs: 0.6 mg ergotamine, 40 mg phenobarbital, 0.2 mg belladonna	May interact with β-blockers or propranolol Belladonna and tricyclics may give increased anticholinergic effects Bellergal-S tends to give more rapid relief than tricyclics
Amitriptyline hydrochloride (Elavil)	Start 1 tab h.s.; 25–30 mg usually sufficient	Tabs: 10–25 mg	Advise patient that it may take 2–3 wk to work
Cyproheptadine (Periactin)	Start 1 dose h.s.; 0.2–0.4 mg/kg/day b.i.d. or t.i.d. PO	Syrup: 2 mg/5 ml Tabs: 4 mg	Start slowly because of sedation
Propranolol (Inderal)	20–40 mg/dose PO t.i.d. or q.i.d.	Tabs: 10, 20, 40, 60, 80, 90 mg	Can cause depression; contraindicated in asthma
Narcotics			
Morphine	0.1–0.2 mg/kg q4h SC	Injection: 2, 4, 8, 10, 15 mg/ml	Do not use with arm or leg symptoms or speech disturbance
Meperidine	1–2 mg/kg q4h PO	Tabs: 50, 100 mg Syrup: 50 mg/5 ml	
Sedatives			
Chloral hydrate	30 mg/kg q6h	Caps: 250, 500 mg Syrup: 250, 500 mg/5 ml	
Diazepam	0.1–0.2 mg/kg q6h PO	Tabs: 2, 5, 10 mg	

L. Treat acute sporadic muscle tension headaches with ibuprofen, acetaminophen, or isometheptene. For frequent recurrent headaches, assess cervical muscle spasm. Also palpate the scalp, looking for tender places at suture lines; some of these headaches are in the scalp muscles. Use comb or brush to stimulate these muscles four or five times a day. Use heat on the scalp. Order massage therapy for cervical and scalp muscle spasm (in general, scalp muscle spasm follows cervical muscle spasm).

M. Use amitriptyline 10 mg at bedtime for prophylaxis. If it is unsuccessful, a limited course of several weeks to 3 months of Bellergal-S may work. Biofeedback can also be very helpful.

N. Try to keep children with headache in school. Arrange with the school nurse so medication can be taken in school if needed. Usually twice a day is sufficient. A brief time in the nurse's room lying down with a cold cloth on the forehead is fine (maximum about 15 minutes). Do not automatically allow the child to be picked up from school for headache, since that can quickly escalate the headaches.

References

Igaraski M, May WN, Golden GS. Pharmacologic treatment of childhood migraine. J Pediatr 1992; 120:653.

Maytal J, Bienkowski RS, Patel M, Eviatar L. The value of brain imaging in children with headaches. Pediatrics 1995; 96:413.

Olness K, MacDonald JT, Uden DL. Comparison of self-hypnosis and propranolol in the treatment of juvenile classic migraine. Pediatrics 1987; 79:593.

Rothner AD. Migraine headaches. In: Swaiman KF, ed. Pediatric neurology: Principles and practice. 2nd ed. St. Louis: Mosby, 1994:865.

Shinnar S, D'Souza B. Migraine in children and adolescents. Pediatr Rev 1982; 3:257.

Singer HS, Rowe S. Chronic recurrent headache in children and adolescents. Pediatr Ann 1992; 21:369.

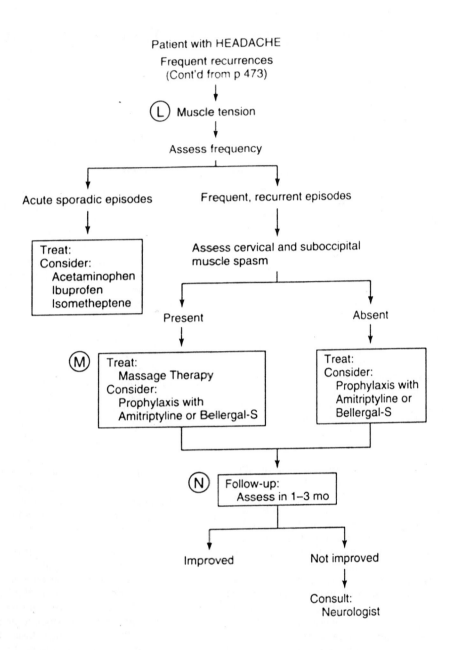

Patient with HEADACHE
Frequent recurrences
(Cont'd from p 473)

Ⓛ Muscle tension

Assess frequency

Acute sporadic episodes

Treat:
Consider:
  Acetaminophen
  Ibuprofen
  Isometheptene

Frequent, recurrent episodes

Assess cervical and suboccipital
muscle spasm

Present

Absent

Ⓜ Treat:
  Massage Therapy
Consider:
  Prophylaxis with
  Amitriptyline or Bellergal-S

Treat:
Consider:
  Prophylaxis with
  Amitriptyline or
  Bellergal-S

Ⓝ Follow-up:
  Assess in 1–3 mo

Improved

Not improved

Consult:
  Neurologist

MOVEMENT DISORDERS (ATAXIA, DYSTONIA, CHOREA)

Patricia H. Ellison, M.D.
Stephen Berman, M.D.

DEFINITIONS

Ataxia, dystonia, and chorea are types of abnormal movements. **Ataxia** is uncoordinated motor function, especially with voluntary movement. **Dystonia** is abnormal muscle tone associated with slow, sometimes writhing movement. In the more extreme forms there is distortion of the body. **Chorea** is twitching resulting from involuntary muscle contractions. Parents rarely use a precise neurologic term unless another family member or acquaintance has had such a diagnosis.

A. In the history ask when the movement was first observed. What is it like? Is it getting better, getting worse, or staying the same? Is it acute, recurrent, or chronic? Does anyone else in the extended family have abnormal movements? Were they ever confined to a wheelchair, unable to walk, or confined to a long-term care institution, including mental institutions? Could the child have access to medicines of other family members or a babysitter? Does the parent know what these medicines are? Ask about trauma, including head trauma.

B. As a part of the physical and neurologic examination, check the skin carefully for depigmented areas, café-au-lait lesions, and other indicators of neurocutaneous disorders. Examine for ecchymoses, other evidence of trauma, and telangiectasia in conjunctiva, earlobes, and chest. Check the ears for infection, which is sometimes a cause of acute ataxia. Examine the fundi for papilledema. Do eye tracking several times rapidly from side to side, trying to elicit vertigo. Observe throughout for the axial and limb movements of dystonia. This may also be brought out with heel and toe walking. Test for ataxia in several ways: finger to nose, eyes closed; finger to nose, eyes open; thumb to second digit opposition; rapid alternating motion of hands bilaterally. Check the feet: each big toe to your finger in three different directions. Ask the child to extend arms, close eyes, stick out tongue, then observe the fingers for choreiform movements. Ask the child to squeeze the index finger of your hand, assessing for milkmaid hand movements. Look for a wide-based gait associated with ataxia.

C. Based on the examination results, identify the abnormal movement as ataxia, dystonia, or chorea (tremors are discussed on p 492).

D. Acute ataxia is more common in children old enough to walk but below school age than in older children. The three most common causes are toxin ingestion, sequela of infection, and brain tumor. Obtain a toxicology screen and treat appropriately. If the toxin screen is negative, consider a CT scan, which will show posterior fossa problems but not the brain stem. If that is negative and the history is compatible, the diagnosis probably is postinfectious ataxia.

E. While there is no specific treatment for postinfectious ataxia, about a third of patients improve spontaneously. Follow weekly. About a third of postinfectious ataxias take several weeks to recover and another third may take months; some of these become chronic. Consider a course of oral steroids after 2 to 4 weeks. Always recheck the eye movements with vertical and horizontal tracking, looking for opsoclonus. Also check for myoclonus, presenting with brief limb or head jerks.

F. If opsoclonus and myoclonus are present, perform lumbar puncture and obtain cerebrospinal fluid protein, glucose, and cells. This unusual condition can be caused by encephalitis but is a hallmark of neuroblastoma. Order imaging studies to identify a site for neuroblastoma. Consult a neurologist.

G. When ataxia is chronic, recurrent, or progressive, obtain a CT scan for identification of posterior fossa tumor, cerebellar dysgenesis, arteriovenous (AV) malformation, stroke, and hydrocephalus. If it is normal, obtain serum IgA and ammonia levels during an ataxic period and urine for amino and organic acids. The IgA identifies those with ataxia-telangiectasia often before telangiectasia develops. (Even carriers of ataxia telangiectasia are at increased risk for some cancers.) The serum ammonia and urine for amino acids and organic acids generally identify the rare inborn errors of metabolism (see p 158). If those studies are normal and the child is school age, the most common diagnosis is Freidrich ataxia. Both cardiology and neurologic consultations are appropriate. The remaining undiagnosed ataxic conditions

(Continued on page 480)

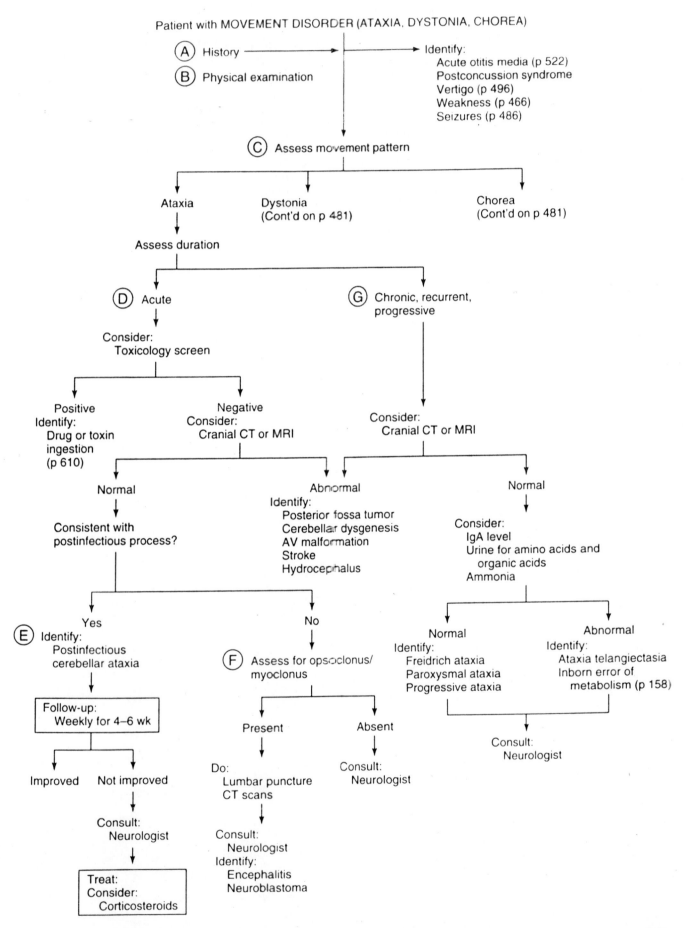

Patient with MOVEMENT DISORDER (ATAXIA, DYSTONIA, CHOREA)

(A) History ——————→ Identify:
Acute otitis media (p 522)
Postconcussion syndrome
(B) Physical examination
Vertigo (p 496)
Weakness (p 466)
Seizures (p 486)

(C) Assess movement pattern

Ataxia | Dystonia (Cont'd on p 481) | Chorea (Cont'd on p 481)

Assess duration

(D) Acute | (G) Chronic, recurrent, progressive

Consider:
Toxicology screen

Positive
Identify:
Drug or toxin
ingestion
(p 610)

Negative
Consider:
Cranial CT or MRI

Consider:
Cranial CT or MRI

Normal

Consistent with
postinfectious process?

Abnormal
Identify:
Posterior fossa tumor
Cerebellar dysgenesis
AV malformation
Stroke
Hydrocephalus

Normal

Consider:
IgA level
Urine for amino acids and
organic acids
Ammonia

Yes
(E) Identify:
Postinfectious
cerebellar ataxia

No

(F) Assess for opsoclonus/
myoclonus

Normal
Identify:
Freidrich ataxia
Paroxysmal ataxia
Progressive ataxia

Abnormal
Identify:
Ataxia telangiectasia
Inborn error of
metabolism (p 158)

Follow-up:
Weekly for 4–6 wk

Present

Absent

Improved   Not improved

Do:
Lumbar puncture
CT scans

Consult:
Neurologist

Consult:
Neurologist

Consult:
Neurologist

Consult:
Neurologist
Identify:
Encephalitis
Neuroblastoma

Treat:
Consider:
Corticosteroids

479

are very uncommon and generally familial. Consult a neurologist.

H. Some drugs cause dystonia. Some cerebral palsies have dystonic qualities, although most of those resulting from kernicterus have disappeared. The remaining dystonias tend to be familial and infrequent.

I. Acute onset of chorea associated with uncontrollable facial grimaces is most probably Sydenham chorea (St. Vitus dance). Obtain an antistreptolysin (ASO) titer to document streptococcal infection. Other uncommon causes are familial: Wilson disease, which most commonly presents with liver disease in children; Huntington chorea, which may have more stiffness than chorea in children; and benign familial chorea.

References

Chun RWM, Shapiro SM. Movement disorders. In: David RB, ed. Pediatric neurology for the clinician. Norwalk, CT: Appleton & Lange, 1992:229.

Franz DN. Tremor in childhood. Pediatr Ann 1993; 22:60.

Kastan M. Ataxia telangiectasia: Broad implications for a rare disorder. N Engl J Med 1995; 333:662.

Klawans HL, Brandabur MM. Chorea in childhood. Pediatr Ann 1993; 22:41.

MacDonald GP. Ataxia of childhood. In: Berg BO, ed. Child neurology: A clinical manual. Philadelphia: Lippincott, 1994:287.

Pranzatelli MR. Miscellaneous movement disorders of childhood. Pediatr Ann 1993; 22:65.

Stacy M, Jankovic J. Childhood dystonia. Pediatr Ann 1993; 22:53.

Patient with MOVEMENT DISORDER (ATAXIA, DYSTONIA, CHOREA)
Assess movement pattern
(Cont'd from p 479)

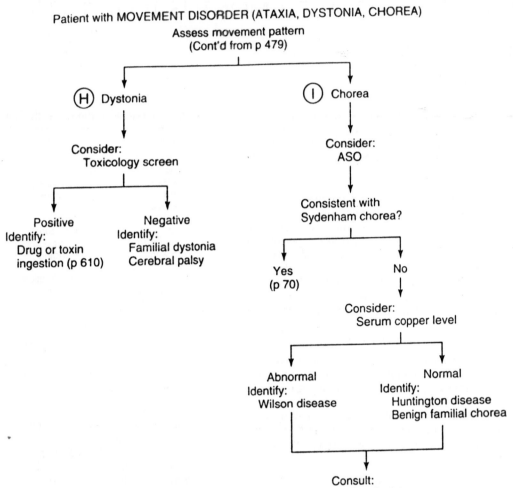

SEIZURES: FEBRILE (AGE 3 MONTHS TO 6 YEARS)

Patricia H. Ellison, M.D.
Stephen Berman, M.D.

Febrile seizures are the most common neurologic disorder treated by pediatricians and family physicians. Febrile seizures with no identifiable cause occur in 4% of children. The clinical approach addresses the diagnosis and management of both the fever and the seizure.

A. The initial seizure frightens most parents. Immediate, appropriate telephone communication can often prevent the 911 call and emergency room service; neither of which is necessary for a simple febrile seizure, yet both of which are necessary for status epilepticus. For the ongoing event, ask the parent whether the tonic-clonic (seizure) movement is still present. Ask whether it involved one side or both sides. Ask about the degree of sickness of the child, the general intellectual and motor function of the child, and family history of seizures, including febrile seizures.

B. In the physical examination identify the source of fever. In children under 18 months the symptoms and signs of meningitis are not specific. Thus, considering meningitis remains key (missed meningitis not only may be devastating but remains a continual source of malpractice litigation). Other common sites of infection include ears, urinary tract, lungs, and less commonly GI tract and blood.

C. Febrile seizures are simple or complex. On presentation the simple seizure is brief (tonic-clonic activity <20 minutes but usually much shorter). The child is normal, and there is often a family history of outgrown febrile seizures. The complex seizure is long (>20 minutes); it may be focal and may have focal findings; two or more episodes of seizures may occur with the same febrile event; and the child may be abnormal. Subsequent EEG information is also helpful for classification: the child with a simple seizure must have a normal EEG (best done about 2 weeks later).

TABLE 1 Degree of Illness with Febrile Seizures

Mild/Moderate	Severe	Very Severe
No serious bacterial infection and Benign febrile seizure or Complex seizure in child with history of febrile seizures or known underlying neurologic disorder	Two or more seizures during the same episode or Focal seizure or Focal finding or Seizure duration >20 min or Serious bacterial infection	Status epilepticus or Shock or Respiratory failure or Severe hypoxia

Spike-wave abnormalities on the EEG place the seizure in the complex category.

D. It is important to impress on the parent that a brief seizure does not harm the child. Even children with repetitive simple seizures have been shown to have intelligence equal to that of their siblings. Tell the parent to look at the clock at the beginning of tonic-clonic movement. If the movement ends in 5 to 10 minutes and the child does not appear ill, there is no need to seek emergency medical treatment. If the movement is still going on at 10 minutes, the parent should get the child to the nearest emergency facility so that the seizures can be stopped with anticonvulsants. For the next seizure, request that the parent place the child so he or she will sustain no injury, loosen any constricting clothing, and tip the child to one side so that secretions can drip from the mouth and call the physician. Phone the family in 24 to 48 hours for follow-up.

(Continued on page 484)

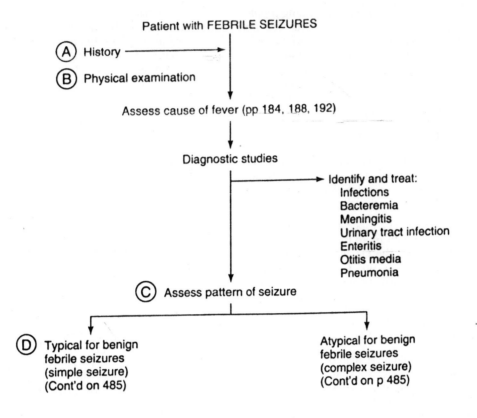

Patient with FEBRILE SEIZURES

(A) History

(B) Physical examination

Assess cause of fever (pp 184, 188, 192)

Diagnostic studies

Identify and treat:
Infections
Bacteremia
Meningitis
Urinary tract infection
Enteritis
Otitis media
Pneumonia

(C) Assess pattern of seizure

(D) Typical for benign
febrile seizures
(simple seizure)
(Cont'd on 485)

Atypical for benign
febrile seizures
(complex seizure)
(Cont'd on p 485)

E. There is no hard and fast rule about providing prophylactic treatment for recurrent simple febrile seizures. Note the amount of parental anxiety. Consider prophylaxis for more than three to five febrile seizures a year, especially when febrile viral infections are common. Phenobarbital is effective. Another approach when the parent is considered very responsible is treatment for each seizure with rectal diazepam or lorazapam.

F. For a generalized seizure consider lumbar puncture and additional laboratory tests: ammonia, toxin screen, electrolytes, glucose, BUN, creatinine, calcium. The frequency of both bacterial and viral meningitis and encephalitis is higher in complex than simple febrile seizures (9% and 3% respectively).

G. Consider obtaining an EEG, especially with preexisting neurologic disease or with more than one marker of a complex febrile seizure. The EEG can be done several days or weeks after the seizure. General slowing may reflect an acute diffuse process such as encephalitis, a longstanding alteration, or a postictal state. A spike-wave discharge pattern is considered epileptogenic. Treat with anticonvulsants if the EEG has spike-wave activity or if the child has multiple seizures.

H. For a focal seizure obtain a CT scan or MRI (preferably the latter if the child is sick), looking for early identification of herpes encephalitis as well as abscess, mass, arteriovenous (AV) malformation, hematoma, or stroke. With normal imaging studies, obtain an EEG. A focal slowing suggests an acute focal abnormality such as encephalitis, infarction, tumor, or a postictal state. Children with complex seizures, except those with an acute infectious brain condition, often have underlying seizure disorders triggered by fever. See p 486 for recommendations about anticonvulsant therapy.

References

Annegers JF, Hauser WA, Shirts SB, et al. Factors prognostic of unprovoked seizures after febrile convulsions. N Engl J Med 1987; 316:493.

Autret E, Billard C, Bertrand P, et al. Double-blind, randomized trial of diazepam versus placebo for prevention of recurrence of febrile seizures. J Pediatr 1990; 117:490.

Chamberlain JM, Gorman RL. Occult bacteremia in children with simple febrile seizures. Am J Dis Child 1988; 142:1073.

Freeman JM. What have we learned from febrile seizures? Pediatr Ann 1992; 21:355.

Joffe A, McCormick M, De Angelis C. Which children with febrile seizures need lumbar puncture? Am J Dis Child 1983; 137:1153.

Knudsen FU. Effective short-term diazepam prophylaxis in febrile convulsions. J Pediatr 1985; 160:487.

National Institutes of Health Consensus Statement. Febrile seizures. Pediatrics 1980; 66:1009.

Offringa M, Bossuyt PMM, Lubsen J, et al. Risk factors for seizure recurrence in children with febrile seizures: A pooled analysis of individual patient data from five studies. J Pediatr 1994; 124:574.

Patient with FEBRILE SEIZURES

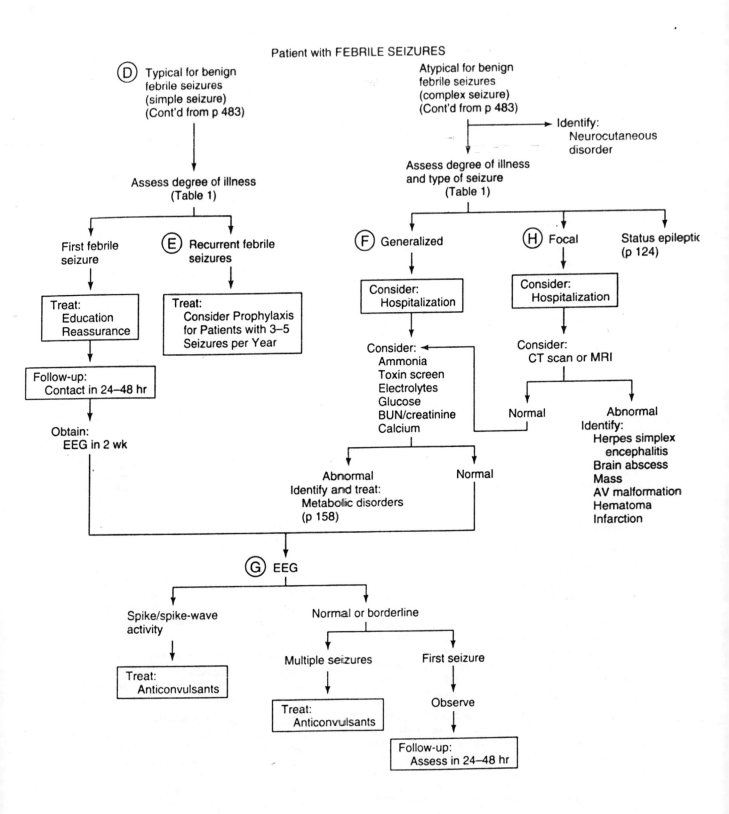

SEIZURES: NONFEBRILE

Patricia H. Ellison, M.D.
Stephen Berman, M.D.

Pediatricians should be able to treat most seizure disorders of infancy, childhood, and adolescence. The guidelines are straightforward although occasionally a child has seizures that are quite difficult to control. Most difficult seizures occur in children with other neurologic conditions, usually developmental and/or motor delay. A physician seldom witnesses a seizure unless the child has a positive response to hyperventilation in the office, or the physician gets to the emergency department before status is stopped, the child has so many seizures almost anyone can see them, or it is a pseudoseizure. Therefore, the physician must rely on the parent or another reliable observer for details of the event. Most seizures fall into one of four clinical types: (1) absence: eye blinking, staring, and/or mental absence; (2) generalized seizure; (3) focal seizure; many start with eye deviation to one side, jerking on one side of the body at least initially; and (4) brief jerks, including flexion or extension body jerks (myoclonus). Myoclonus is the most difficult to recognize as a seizure from the parent's description. This may delay the diagnosis. From the history you should be able to categorize the clinical type of seizure, then proceed to the correct algorithms for diagnostic tests and treatment.

A. In the history ask what was seen and when it happened. What time of day or night did it happen? How long did the movement part of the seizure last? (Postictal lethargy or sleeping is not included in length of seizure.) Was there any triggering event such as head trauma, sleep deprivation, or failure to eat for many hours? Many adolescents and college students are sleep deprived. Did the child have a sore tongue or urinate? Is there any family history of seizures? If so, what is the relationship of that person to this child? How old was the relative when the seizures started? Is the relative still being treated? Does the relative have any other neurologic problems? Does the child or either parent have any birthmarks? Has the child had meningitis or moderate to severe head trauma? Ask about the birthing history, birth weight, length of neonatal hospitalization, and any treatment with a ventilator. Did the child have neonatal seizures?

B. The most common diagnosis made from the physical examination in childhood seizures is a neurocutaneous disorder. Look carefully at the skin and eyes, including fundi. Measure and graph the head size. Do a careful neurologic examination. Look for evidence of trauma from abuse: bruises, retinal hemorrhages, signs of increased intracranial pressure. For an absence seizure, ask the child to hyperventilate. Make certain the parent can see the child's face. Demonstrate hyperventilation and breathe with the child, offering encouragement ("good job, keep going"). You may pause for dry mouth or to catch your breath, but the child must go on. Three minutes can seem a very long time; watch the clock. Often a seizure will occur. If so, the discussion with parent is easier and treatment is straightforward. Children with classical petit mal tend to have a seizure with hyperventilation; those with temporal lobe seizures do not.

C. In a generalized seizure the patient is on the floor, unconscious, stiffening, then jerking. Try to find out whether jerks were one-sided or bilateral; one-sided implies focal seizures. Obtain an EEG about 2 weeks after the seizure. An abnormal EEG is defined as spike or spike-wave activity. Mildly abnormal EEGs are lumped with normal EEGs here. Waiting 2 weeks for the EEG decreases the frequency of mildly abnormal EEGs.

D. With an initial seizure plus an abnormal EEG or two or more seizures or a normal EEG in an abnormal child, consider further diagnostic work-up, including CT scan, glucose, electrolytes, BUN, creatinine, calcium, toxicology screen, metabolic studies, and stool for *Shigella*. Of these tests the most important to the parents is the CT scan because of worry about brain tumor. The diagnostic yield from normal children is very small. Parents and adolescent patients often become upset if the seizures remain without a cause identified. An appropriate response to this is "I'm sorry. I can't provide a diagnosis, that's good news. The outcome is generally better when we can't find the cause." Any child who is losing motor and/or intellectual skills generally requires a more comprehensive work-up to make a diagnosis. Some children with long recurrent generalized seizures lose intellectual function with time. Drops of 10 to 20 or more IQ points are not uncommon, even though there is no diagnosed neurodegenerative disorder.

E. Start treatment with carbamazepine, valproic acid, phenytoin, or phenobarbital (Table 1). Usually carbamazepine is the first choice, but if there is a lot of spike-wave activity on the EEG, valproic acid may be more effective.

F. In a normal child with a normal EEG (i.e., an EEG without spike-wave activity 2 weeks later) and *only one* seizure, treatment usually can be postponed until a second event occurs.

G. A focal seizure generally tells the neurologist to be more careful. Consider MRI, as the patient may have a focal brain process ranging from tumor to herpes encephalitis. If the child is sick and has a focal seizure, consider herpes encephalitis. The MRI shows early changes well. If the child is not sick and there are no focal findings, you can wait for a second seizure before treating with anticonvulsants. With neurologic signs or two or more seizures, obtain an MRI to identify mass, arteriovenous (AV) malformation, infarction, or hematoma. Even with an MRI, most children have normal studies; the second most frequent finding is an area of sclerosis in the temporal lobe. Treat with carbamazepine or valproic acid.

H. Often the parent sees and describes repetitive brief jerks (myoclonus), but the description is not enough

(Continued on page 488)

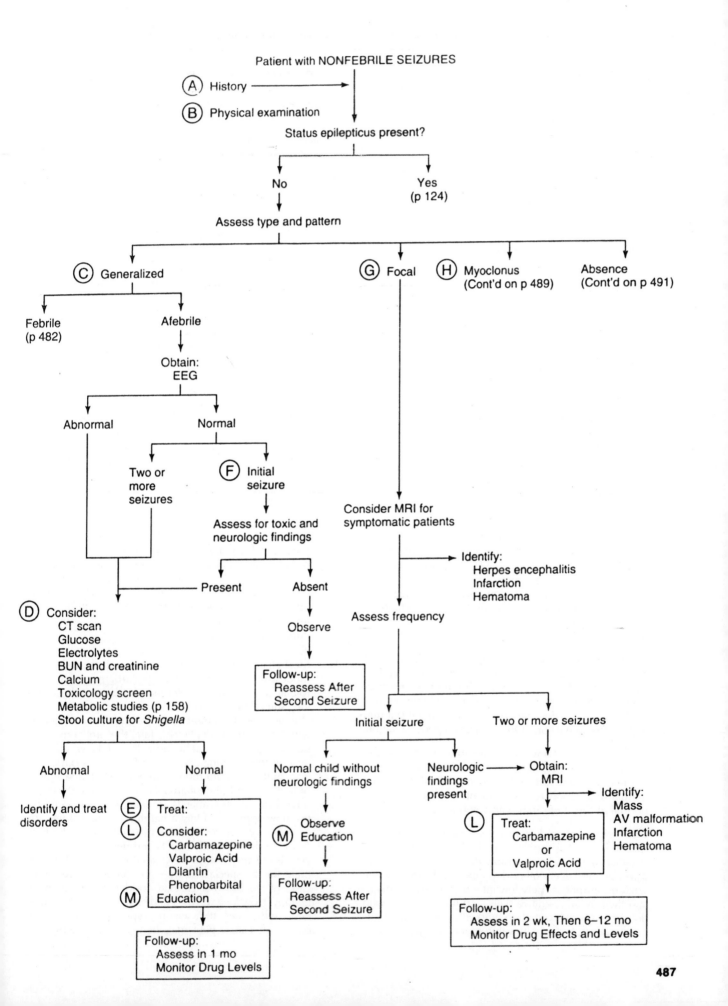

Patient with NONFEBRILE SEIZURES

(A) History

(B) Physical examination

Status epilepticus present?

No   Yes (p 124)

Assess type and pattern

(C) Generalized   (G) Focal   (H) Myoclonus (Cont'd on p 489)   Absence (Cont'd on p 491)

Febrile (p 482)   Afebrile

Obtain: EEG

Abnormal   Normal

Two or more seizures   (F) Initial seizure

Assess for toxic and neurologic findings

Consider MRI for symptomatic patients

Present   Absent

Identify:
Herpes encephalitis
Infarction
Hematoma

(D) Consider:
CT scan
Glucose
Electrolytes
BUN and creatinine
Calcium
Toxicology screen
Metabolic studies (p 158)
Stool culture for *Shigella*

Observe

Assess frequency

Follow-up:
Reassess After
Second Seizure

Abnormal   Normal

Initial seizure   Two or more seizures

Identify and treat disorders

(E)
(L) Treat:

Consider:
Carbamazepine
Valproic Acid
Dilantin
Phenobarbital
(M) Education

Normal child without neurologic findings   Neurologic findings present → Obtain: MRI

(M) Observe
Education

Identify:
Mass
AV malformation
Infarction
Hematoma

(L) Treat:
Carbamazepine
or
Valproic Acid

Follow-up:
Reassess After
Second Seizure

Follow-up:
Assess in 1 mo
Monitor Drug Levels

Follow-up:
Assess in 2 wk, Then 6–12 mo
Monitor Drug Effects and Levels

487

TABLE 1 Drugs Used in the Treatment of Seizures in Children and Adolescents

Drug	Dosage	Therapeutic Blood Level	Comments	Products	Monitor
Carbamazepine (Tegretol)	15–25 mg/kg/day b.i.d., t.i.d.	5–12 μg/ml	Start slowly: 1 tab h.s.; in 3–4 days add second tab; often requires upper end of therapeutic range	Chew: 100 mg Tab: 200 mg	CBC and platelets q2wk for 2 mo, then q6mo
Phenytoin (Dilantin)	< 1 yr: 5–10 mg/kg/day > 1 yr: 5 mg/kg/day	10–20 μg/ml	Some younger children need b.i.d., t.i.d. dose; with older children use h.s. dose	Chew: 50 mg Caps: 30, 100 mg	CBC yearly
Phenobarbital	< 1 yr: 4–11 mg/kg/day 1–12 yr: 3–7 mg/kg/day > 12 yr: 1–2.5 mg/kg/day	10–40 μg/ml	Start slowly	Syrup: 20 mg/5 ml Tabs: 15, 30, 60, 100 mg	None
Valproic acid (Depakene, Depakote)	15–60 mg/kg/day b.i.d.	60–100 μg/ml; to 150 μg for difficult seizures	Effective for spike wave on EEG	Liquid: 250 mg/5 ml Caps: 125, 250, 500 mg	CBC q6mo Liver function and ammonia tests in 2 wk, then 1 mo, then q6mo
Ethosuximide (Zarontin)	20–40 mg/kg/day	40–100 μg/ml	Does not control generalized seizures	Liquid: 250 mg/5 ml Caps: 250 mg	CBC yearly
Primidone (Mysoline)	10–25 mg/kg/day	4–12 μg/ml	Start slowly	Liquid: 250 mg/5 ml Tabs: 50, 250 mg	None
ACTH nonsynthetic	60 IU/day IM; if seizures still present after 2 wk, increase 10 IU/wk to 80 IU/day; change to q.o.d. in 2–3 wk		Treat for at least 1 mo after seizures stop	Vials: 25, 40 USP units	Weekly blood pressure; electrolytes q1–2wk
Clonazepam (Clonodine)	Start 0.01–0.02 mg/kg/day t.i.d.; maintenance 0.1–0.2 mg/kg/day	0.02–0.08 μg/ml	Start slowly	Tab: 0.5, 1, 2 mg	None

to tip off the physician to myoclonus in young infants and older children. Get an EEG. In most cases the spike-wave discharge shows up and provides the diagnosis. High-amplitude slow waves and exaggerated spike-wave discharges may be seen in infants; a spike-wave pattern typical of myoclonus may be seen in older children.

I. Treat juvenile myoclonic epilepsy with valproic acid. Treatment of a child with myoclonus and normal EEG can be delayed until signs and symptoms become more clear-cut. If the myoclonus continues, obtain another EEG. Myoclonus does not localize to the brain but may include the spinal cord. Obtain neurologic consultation.

J. An infant does not always have an abnormal or typically hypsarrhythmic EEG at the start of infantile spasms, yet it is mandatory to initiate treatment, since the resultant mental retardation is less frequent in those who were normal at the start. Start with valproic acid.

K. Especially in normal infants, the diagnosis of infantile spasms with a hypsarrhythmic EEG requires immediate initiation of steroids, preferably IM ACTH daily for 2 to 3 weeks, then every other day, tapering the dose as the seizures disappear. Very few infants with spasms maintain their initial cognitive skills, and most of those who do were initially normal. In markedly abnormal infants some specialists start with valproic acid (be careful; liver

toxicity is highest in the very young) or clonazepam; sedation and drooling are common side effects. Side effects of IM ACTH tend to be few, especially if the daily course is limited to 2 or 3 weeks, then switched to every other day. Improvement in the EEG pattern is not necessarily associated with maintenance, much less improvement, in cognition.

L. Most children with seizures can be well treated with a modest armamentarium of drugs: carbamazepine, valproic acid, phenytoin (preference for boys), ethosuximide, sometimes primidone, sometimes phenobarbital (Tables 2 and 3). In most cases (perhaps in most patients without status epilepticus) start the anticonvulsant slowly, e.g., one dose at bedtime. In 3 or 4 days add one dose in the morning and in another 3 to 4 days, one dose in the early afternoon if needed. Carbamazepine, primidone, and phenobarbital "snow" patients at full dose. Side effects (Table 2) are markedly decreased by the slow approach. Only a handful of good drugs are available for seizures; it is wiser to increase medication slowly to decrease side effects and defuse parental anger. There are several new anticonvulsants. Reserve them for the specialists. They are needed in very few cases of childhood seizures. Consider the duration of therapy. How long will the child have to take medicine? First, remember the seizure types that are often outgrown: classic petit mal, benign central temporal

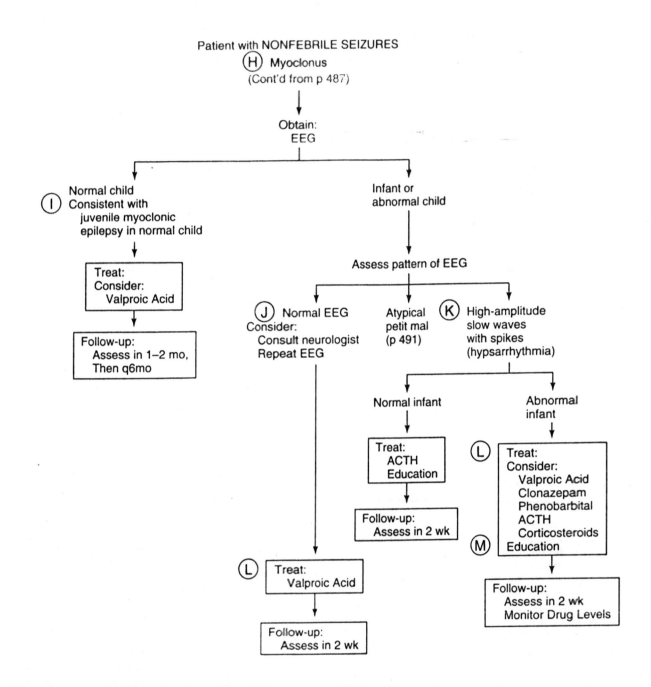

Patient with NONFEBRILE SEIZURES
(H) Myoclonus
(Cont'd from p 487)

Obtain:
EEG

(I) Normal child
Consistent with
juvenile myoclonic
epilepsy in normal child

Treat:
Consider:
Valproic Acid

Follow-up:
Assess in 1–2 mo,
Then q6mo

Infant or
abnormal child

Assess pattern of EEG

(J) Normal EEG
Consider:
Consult neurologist
Repeat EEG

Atypical
petit mal
(p 491)

(K) High-amplitude
slow waves
with spikes
(hypsarrhythmia)

Normal infant

Treat:
ACTH
Education

Follow-up:
Assess in 2 wk

Abnormal
infant

(L) Treat:
Consider:
Valproic Acid
Clonazepam
Phenobarbital
ACTH
Corticosteroids
(M) Education

Follow-up:
Assess in 2 wk
Monitor Drug Levels

(L) Treat:
Valproic Acid

Follow-up:
Assess in 2 wk

lobe epilepsy, and some generalized seizure disorders. There are studies about the withdrawal of anticonvulsants after 4 years of treatment, but most parents get itchy long before that. For normal children some consider discontinuing therapy after 2 years on medication without a seizure. Remember that abnormal children, children with an underlying disorder (e.g., one of the neurocutaneous disorders), and children with recurrent spike or spike-wave activity on the EEG tend to seize readily. Pick a good time of the year, often summer. Tell the parents the drug level will usually drop below the therapeutic level with a decrease of one pill a day, so seizures may occur. Most recurrent seizures occur within 6 months of withdrawing therapy, with less likelihood of a recurrence as the months pass. However, the biologic tail is long, and some patients may have recurrent seizures during the next several years. Patients who

are in late adolescence may discontinue anticonvulsants on their own at some time. Some are successful; some are not. Explain that it is better to taper anticonvulsants than to stop abruptly.

M. Seizures cause great anxiety in parents. Emphasize the importance of having the child lead a normal life, including riding a bicycle, sleeping alone, and learning to drive a car (assuming the seizures are totally controlled). A person with a seizure disorder should not go swimming alone (nor should anyone else) and should not play competitive sports conducive to head injuries (e.g., football, lacrosse). Touch football is allowed. Many parents are worried that the child has a brain tumor, and it is difficult to alleviate that anxiety without an imaging study. Ask the parents if they have any other questions; encourage them to call if they

TABLE 2 Side Effects of Drugs Used to Treat Seizures

Drug	Comments	Idiosyncratic Reactions	Drug Interactions
Carbamazepine	Start too fast: drowsiness Dose too high: double vision, rare drowsiness	Allergy, usually rash (2%) Granulocytopenia (1%) usually appears early	Erythromycin increases level Lessens effectiveness of birth control
Valproic acid	Occasional behavior change Decreased appetite, especially with mild ammonia elevations Tremor	Alopecia, thrombocytopenia, pancreatitis Liver failure: most frequent in young children; in older children, usually associated with use of additional anti-convulsants	Increases phenobarbital and primidone levels
Phenytoin	Levels too high: lethargy, nystagmus, ataxia When blood level is 5–9, add only small amount more (easy to reach toxic level at that range of dose/response curve)	Allergy, usually rash Gingival hyperplasia (40%); encourage tooth brushing and gum stimulation Hypertrichosis (5%) Facial skeletal remodeling across years Rare aplastic anemia Some anemia, leukopenia, lymphadenopathy	
Phenobarbital	Start too fast: drowsiness Very young children: hyperactivity (30%) Dose too high: lethargy, ataxia Possible decreased cognitive impairment	Allergy, usually rash First choice if liver disease or early pregnancy	
Ethosuximide	Headaches and stomach upset in early weeks, months (generally can continue use)	Allergy, usually rash Rare: drug-induced lupus leukopenia, pancytopenia	
ACTH	Cushingoid obesity frequent	Growth retardation, mood change, skin eruption including acne Hypertension, electrolyte disturbances, susceptibility to infections, osteoporosis	
Clonazepam	Start slowly	Depression, sedation, drooling	

do. Tell the parents what to do in the event of seizures. Turn the child to the side so any secretions slide out of the mouth. Make certain nothing constricts breathing or hurts the child. Look at a clock at the start. Minutes may seem like hours. If jerking stops in 5 to 10 minutes, all is well. The child may be poorly responsive for several hours or may sleep. If jerking lasts more than 10 minutes, head for the nearest emergency room to get the seizure stopped (often with IV benzodiazepam). When the family calls, order a drug level. (The most common reason for a seizure while on anticonvulsants is a less than therapeutic blood level because of noncompliance, forgetfulness, or insufficient dose.) Carbamazepine often works best near the top of the therapeutic range. Valproic acid can often be pushed above 100 (some say to 150). You may have to add a second drug.

N. Absence seizures manifest as repetitive blinking, staring, and/or mental absence. In a typical presentation the parent or school teacher wonders whether the child may be having seizures. Occasionally a child can recognize gaps in time. More often the child is noted to stare, fail to respond to voice, or progress poorly in school. Obtain an EEG.

O. Classic petit mal: 3 cycles per second (cps) pattern. The child is almost always normal. Treat with ethosuximide or valproic acid. Start a young child without generalized seizures with ethosuximide, an effective drug with few side effects. It does not control generalized seizures. Explain to the parents that some children with classic petit mal get generalized seizures. If so, the drug must be changed to valproic acid. Use school performance and parental observation as end points for adequate seizure control. This type of seizure is often outgrown.

P. Benign central temporal spike (Rolandic, Sylvian) is good news. The seizures are usually easily controlled and eventually outgrown. Start with carbamazepine.

Q. Other EEG patterns may be either normal or the great gray of EEG, perhaps with a little φ-activity here or there; nothing very specific, nothing diagnostic. Often this is interpreted as mildly abnormal. Seizures that originate from the temporal lobe may show no abnormality or only mild changes in EEG. The temporal lobe originations are usually deep in the brain: discharges do not register well on scalp electrodes. Sleep deprivation increases the chance of showing some seizure discharge. So do nasopharyngeal electrodes, which are unpleasant. If the events sound like absence seizures witnessed on several occasions, a trial course of medication may settle it. Try carbamazepine, valproic acid, primidone, or (for boys only) phenytoin. Get the dose well into the therapeutic range. Use clinical observation and school performance to assess effectiveness.

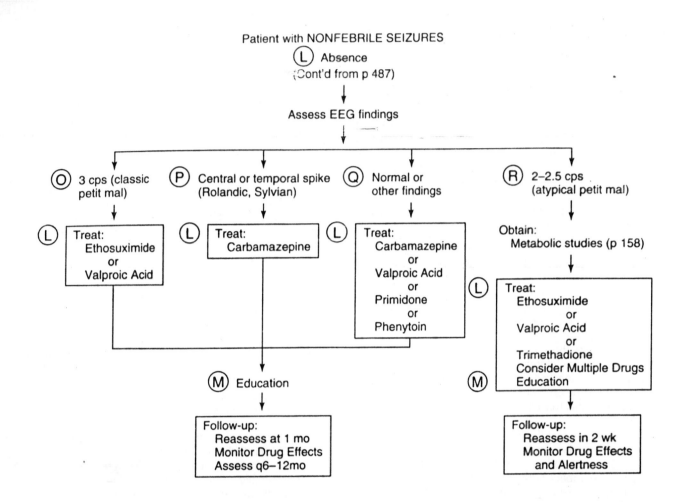

Patient with NONFEBRILE SEIZURES

(L) Absence
(Cont'd from p 487)

↓

Assess EEG findings

(O) 3 cps (classic petit mal)

(L) Treat:
Ethosuximide
or
Valproic Acid

(P) Central or temporal spike (Rolandic, Sylvian)

(L) Treat:
Carbamazepine

(Q) Normal or other findings

(L) Treat:
Carbamazepine
or
Valproic Acid
or
Primidone
or
Phenytoin

(M) Education

Follow-up:
Reassess at 1 mo
Monitor Drug Effects
Assess q6–12mo

(R) 2–2.5 cps (atypical petit mal)

Obtain:
Metabolic studies (p 158)

(L) Treat:
Ethosuximide
or
Valproic Acid
or
Trimethadione
Consider Multiple Drugs
Education

(M) Follow-up:
Reassess in 2 wk
Monitor Drug Effects
and Alertness

TABLE 3   Interactions between Anticonvulsants

Original Drug	Added Drug	Effect on Original Drug Level
Carbamazepine	Phenobarbital	Decrease
	Phenytoin	Decrease
	Primidone	Decrease
Phenobarbital	Carbamazepine	No change
	Methsuxamide	Increase
	Phenytoin	Increase
	Valproate	Increase
Phenytoin	Carbamazepine	Increase
	Methsuxamide	Increase
	Phenobarbital	No change
	Primidone	No change
	Valproate	Decrease
Primidone	Carbamazepine	Increase phenobarbital
	Phenytoin	Increase phenobarbital
	Valproate	Increase primidone
Valproate	Carbamazepine	Decrease
	Phenobarbital	Decrease
	Phenytoin	Decrease
	Primidone	Decrease

From Browne TR. Clinical pharmacology of antiepileptic drug administration. In: Penny JK, ed. Epilepsy: Diagnosis and management and quality of life. New York: Raven, 1986:26; with permission.

R. A 2 to 2.5 cps is atypical, not classic, petit mal. It is usually seen in abnormal children. The seizures are more difficult to control with medications. Often the child has more than one type of seizure, which may change over time. Start with one solid baseline drug such as valproic acid. Push the drug to the upper limits. If seizures continue, add a second drug. A spike-wave drug, such as trimethadione, ethosuximide, or valproic acid, may help some of the small seizures for a time. Push the second drug to the top of the therapeutic range. This may eliminate most of the seizures. When breakthrough occurs, check the drug levels. If there is room to increase one of the drugs, do so. If both are at the top of the range, rotate one drug. Add one new drug, building it to the top of the range, and then over 3 to 4 weeks remove one of the old drugs. Some pediatric neurologists try for total seizure control in these children. That is often associated with multiple drug use and sedation. Some parents will tolerate some seizures to achieve alertness. There is no indication that this approach is any less valid than the total control approach.

References

Aicardi J. Epilepsy and other seizure disorders. In: Aicardi J, ed. Diseases of the nervous system in childhood. London: Mac-Keith Press 1992:911.

Pranzatelli MR. Myoclonic disorders. Pediatr Ann 1993; 22:33.

TICS AND TREMORS

Patricia H. Ellison, M.D.

Tics range from the common garden variety to full-blown Tourette syndrome with multiple types of tics, guttural noises, and obscenities. Since the establishment of the Tourette's Foundation and increased publicity about tics, more children have been referred for diagnosis and treatment of tic disorders. The tics of early childhood used to be considered benign, and parents were counseled to ignore them. This deemphasis usually led to the lessening or disappearance of the tics. Now there is more concern that early childhood tics will turn into Tourette syndrome. Anxiety of parents and child may increase their frequency and severity.

Tremors are most common in neonates and infants. The quality of movement distinguishes them from other hand and foot movements. Tremors are equal in amplitude, while the movement in clonic seizures has a downbeat quality. In neonates and infants the concern usually is that they may be seizures. Tremor in children is rare but often of great concern to the parent or teacher. The tremor may be viewed as a forerunner of some ominous neurologic condition. Usually it is a benign essential tremor, and an elderly relative also has it.

A. In the history seat the child within your full view so that you can observe any tics or tremors. Take your time with the history to allow time for observation. Ask about family members with tics or neurotic or obsessive-compulsive behavior. Often you can identify a relative with a similar tic disorder. Ask about use of methylphenidate (Ritalin), which may trigger tics. In newborns and young infants with tremor ask about associated irritability. The presenting complaint may be tremor, but the major problem may be repetitive crying at a volume or range that irritates the caretaker or interrupts sleep. In an older child ask when the tremor occurs. If when drinking, drawing, or writing, it is an action tremor. If the child sits with hands resting on the chair arms or in lap and has no tremor, the child does not have tremor at rest. Give the child a pencil and paper and continue history taking and observing.

B. In the physical examination continue your observation. Perform cerebellar testing: extend the child's arms and ask the child to close the eyes. Try to elicit tremor during action (which defines action tremor) by having the child put a finger of each hand on the nose. Rarely are there jerky or dystonic movements. If you observe dystonia, see p 478.

C. Decide whether to treat with medication or to observe. In the past there was only one drug, haloperidol. Now several medications, all of which change some neurotransmitters, are available. Key reasons to treat are disruption in the classroom (e.g., noises so loud they can be heard down the hall), public humiliation, embarrassment, and the child's *(not the parents')* inability to cope with it. Some children with tics cope with teasing fairly well; others do not. Middle school or junior high is a particularly devastating time. If the tics are common and obvious, this is an excellent time to initiate treatment. There are four medications to try in this order: clonidine, haloperidol, pimozide, and paroxetin. Start them at low doses, as they may cause undesirable side effects (Table 1). Warn parents about the dramatic haloperidol crisis, which can be treated quickly and successfully with diphenhydramine. If nothing works, consider a diagnosis of pseudotics.

D. At follow-up determine how well the child is responding, especially a child with Tourette syndrome. Ask the parent to keep a calendar, scoring each day (0, good day, few tics; 1, some tics; 2, more tics; 3, bad day, many tics). The calendar should be brought to follow-up.

(Continued on page 494)

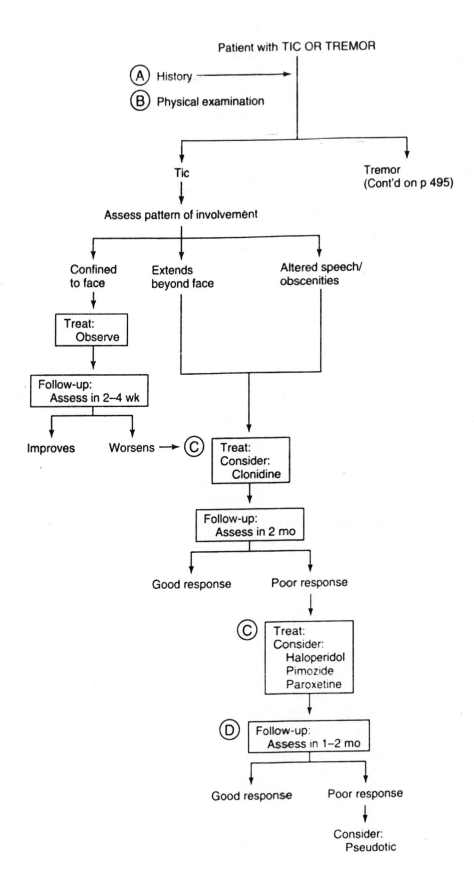

Patient with TIC OR TREMOR

(A) History
(B) Physical examination

Tic

Tremor
(Cont'd on p 495)

Assess pattern of involvement

Confined
to face

Extends
beyond face

Altered speech/
obscenities

Treat:
  Observe

Follow-up:
  Assess in 2–4 wk

Improves

Worsens → (C)

Treat:
Consider:
  Clonidine

Follow-up:
  Assess in 2 mo

Good response

Poor response

(C) Treat:
Consider:
  Haloperidol
  Pimozide
  Paroxetine

(D) Follow-up:
  Assess in 1–2 mo

Good response

Poor response

Consider:
  Pseudotic

TABLE 1 Drug Therapy for Tics and Tremors

Drug	Dosage	Side Effects	Tablets
Clonidine	Start 0.05 mg/day Increase to 0.1–0.3 mg/day	Dry mouth, sedation, hypotension	0.1, 0.2, 0.3 mg
Haloperidol	Start 0.25–0.5 mg/day Increase to 3–5 mg/day	Haloperidol crisis: treat with diphenhydramine; sedation, fatigue, tardive dyskinesia, may lower seizure threshold	0.5, 1, 2, 5 mg
Pimozide	Start 1 mg/day Increase to 5–10 mg/day	Contraindicated if congenital long QT syndrome or cardiac arrhythmia (obtain baseline ECG) Tardive dyskinesia, sedation	2 mg
Paroxetine	Start 10 mg/day in AM Increase to max 20 mg if child > 100 lb	Sedation, insomnia, nausea	20 mg scored
Propranolol	< 100 lb: Start 10 mg t.i.d. Increase to 20 mg t.i.d. > 100 lb: Start 20 mg t.i.d. Increase to 40 mg t.i.d. Target times when control of tremor is important	Contraindicated in asthma Hypotension Hypoglycemia, especially when not eating well Depression	10, 20, 40, 60, 80 mg Available in long-acting tab

E. In young infants the effect of prolonged, repetitive irritability is much worse than that of tremor. The excessive irritability may originate from the CNS. Repeat the neurologic evaluation, including tone, posture, and alertness, at follow-up.

F. Total control of action tremor (benign essential tremor) may not be possible. Target the medication (propranolol) for school hours. Propranolol is contraindicated in asthma. The other risk is hypoglycemia, particularly if the child is not eating well or is vomiting. Some patients choose to use propranolol only when performing, e.g., during piano recitals.

References

Chun RWM, Shapiro SM. Benign familial tremors and tics. In: David RB, ed. Pediatric neurology for the clinician. Norwalk, CT: Appleton & Lange, 1992:239.

Franz DN. Tremor in childhood. Pediatr Ann 1993; 22:60.

Singer HS. Tic disorders. Pediatr Ann 1993; 22:22.

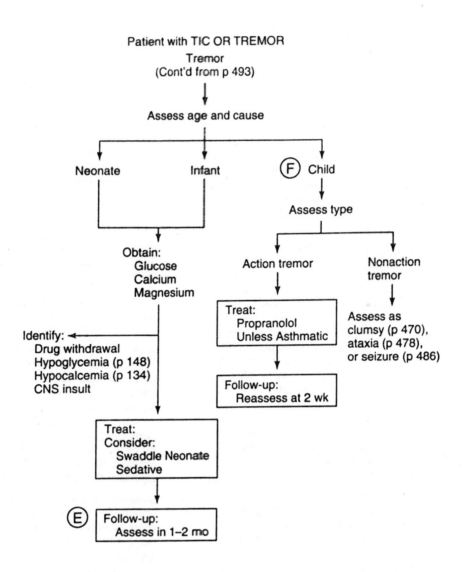

Patient with TIC OR TREMOR

Tremor
(Cont'd from p 493)

↓

Assess age and cause

Neonate   **Infant**   Ⓕ Child

↓

Assess type

Obtain:
 Glucose
 Calcium
 Magnesium

Action tremor   Nonaction
                   tremor

Identify: ◄―――
 Drug withdrawal
 Hypoglycemia (p 148)
 Hypocalcemia (p 134)
 CNS insult

Treat:
 Propranolol
 Unless Asthmatic

Assess as
clumsy (p 470),
ataxia (p 478),
or seizure (p 486)

Follow-up:
 Reassess at 2 wk

Treat:
Consider:
 Swaddle Neonate
 Sedative

Ⓔ Follow-up:
 Assess in 1–2 mo

VERTIGO

Patricia H. Ellison, M.D.

DEFINITION

Vertigo is the sensation of moving around in space or the sensation that objects, the room, or the horizon is moving around you. With moderate to severe vertigo, the child may have difficulty maintaining balance. Rarely do parents use the word vertigo, and it may be difficult to tell what is happening from their description.

A. In the history ask the parents what they observed. If the child passed out, likely diagnoses include breath holding, syncope, and possibly seizure. Preferentially sitting or lying down may indicate vertigo. Some children with benign paroxysmal vertigo steady themselves by briefly touching a wall or furniture. A worsening condition when the child is riding in a car may indicate vertigo. However, vertigo does not usually accompany motion sickness. Ask about the likelihood of toxic ingestion. Ask about any indication or report of headache after the episode. Basilar artery migraine often starts with an aura of vertigo or other posterior brain symptoms. Ask about birth marks, ear infections, and injury to head or neck. Identify nonvertiginous dizziness, syncope, hyperventilation, and anxiety or panic attacks. These are most common in adolescent girls.

B. During the examination of cranial nerves, do horizontal tracking of eyes several times. This may elicit either nystagmus or vertigo. Test hearing, checking for additional evidence of dysfunction of cranial nerve VIII. Examine skin and fundi for neurocutaneous lesions. Palpate the sternocleidomastoid muscles, especially at the mastoid attachment, trapezius, and suboccipital muscles. Assess cerebellar functions with several tests looking for mild dysfunction. Assess Romberg and tandem gait. Ask the child to hop on each foot, seeking signs of incoordination, which may indicate demyelinating disease, especially in adolescence. Examine the ears and identify and treat otitis media and/or cholesteatoma.

C. Identify and treat postvertiginous migraine. If it is not among the symptoms, obtain a toxic screen. If that is negative, consider acute labyrinthitis. Treat the vertigo with meclizine, starting with one 12.5 mg tablet at bedtime, increasing to 1 tablet t.i.d.

D. In recurrent vertigo ask both parent and child about headache following vertigo, which identifies basilar artery migraine. If there is no evidence of such headache and no skin lesions of neurocutaneous disorders and the child is under 10 years, consider benign paroxysmal vertigo. In adolescents, particularly in girls, obtain an MRI of the brain to identify demyelinating disease (multiple sclerosis). If that is normal, consider benign paroxysmal vertigo, which also occurs in adolescents.

E. In chronic or progressive vertigo identify neurocutaneous disorders. All of them carry an increased risk of a variety of brain tumors, including acoustic neuromas. Obtain a CT scan of the brain. In children without neurophakomatous skin lesions, palpate the cervical neck muscles (see p 470) with special attention to the sternocleidomastoid attachment at the mastoid. Cervical vertigo may be associated with this muscle spasm. It generally disappears as the muscle spasm is released, especially through massage therapy.

F. Sometimes it is not possible to find the immediate cause of vertigo. Continued observation, instruction to parents about identifying additional cranial nerve abnormalities (see p 448), and the use of meclizine for symptoms are appropriate.

Reference

Eviatar L. Vertigo. In: Swaiman KF, ed. Pediatric neurology. Principles and practice. 2nd ed. St. Louis: Mosby, 1994:297.

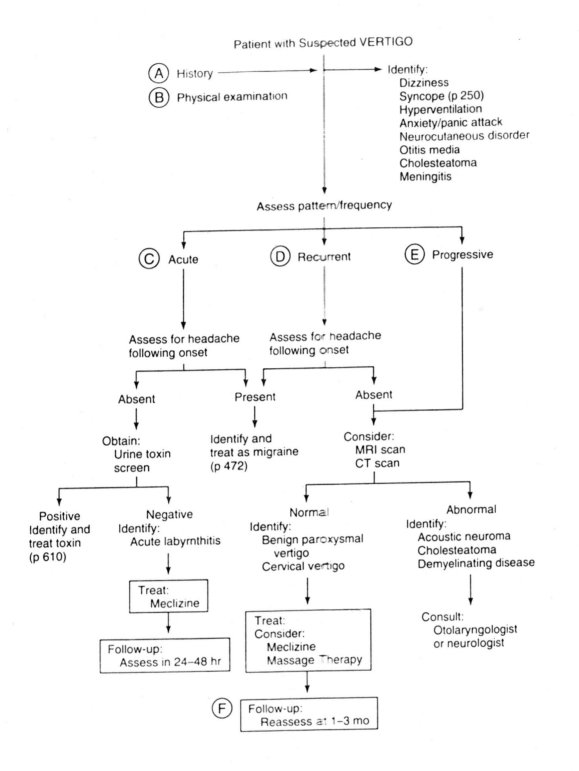

Patient with Suspected VERTIGO

(A) History ⟶ Identify:
　　　　　　　　　　　　　Dizziness
(B) Physical examination 　　Syncope (p 250)
　　　　　　　　　　　　　Hyperventilation
　　　　　　　　　　　　　Anxiety/panic attack
　　　　　　　　　　　　　Neurocutaneous disorder
　　　　　　　　　　　　　Otitis media
　　　　　　　　　　　　　Cholesteatoma
　　　　　　　　　　　　　Meningitis

Assess pattern/frequency

(C) Acute　　　(D) Recurrent　　　(E) Progressive

Assess for headache　　Assess for headache
following onset　　　　following onset

Absent　　　Present　　　Absent

Obtain:　　　Identify and　　　Consider:
Urine toxin　treat as migraine　MRI scan
screen　　　(p 472)　　　　　CT scan

Positive　　　Negative　　　Normal　　　　　Abnormal
Identify and　Identify:　　　Identify:　　　　Identify:
treat toxin　Acute labyrnthitis　Benign paroxysmal　Acoustic neuroma
(p 610)　　　　　　　　　vertigo　　　　Cholesteatoma
　　　　　　　　　　　　Cervical vertigo　Demyelinating disease

Treat:　　　　　　　Treat:　　　　　　Consult:
Meclizine　　　　　Consider:　　　　　Otolaryngologist
　　　　　　　　　Meclizine　　　　　or neurologist
Follow-up:　　　　Massage Therapy
Assess in 24–48 hr

(F) Follow-up:
Reassess at 1–3 mo

497

OPHTHALMOLOGIC DISORDERS

Evaluation of Poor Vision
Conjunctivitis/Red, Painful Eyes
Orbital Cellulitis or Abscess

Periorbital (Preseptal) Cellulitis
Strabismus (Eye Muscle Imbalance)

EVALUATION OF POOR VISION

Robert D. Gross, M.D.
Joel N. Leffler, M.D.

A. Obtain a careful history, including prenatal, perinatal, and postnatal development, as well as a family history of general developmental problems, systemic abnor- malities, seizures, and medication usage. If possible, determine the time of onset of vision loss to differentiate congenital from acquired causes.

TABLE 1 Vision Screening Guidelines for Children Ages 3 to 5 Years

Function	Recommended Tests	Referral Criteria	Comments

Distance visual acuity	Snellen letters
	Snellen numbers
	Tumbling E
	HOTV
	Picture tests
	  Allen figures
	  LH test
		Fewer than 4 of 6 correct on 20 ft line with either eye tested at 10 ft monocularly (i.e., < 10/20 or 20/40)
		or
		Two-line difference between eyes, even within the passing range (i.e., 10/12.5 and 10/20 or 20/25 and 20/40)
			Tests are listed in decreasing order of cognitive difficulty. The highest test that the child is capable of performing should be used. In general, the Tumbling E or HOTV test should be used for ages 3–5 yr.
			Testing distance of 10 ft is recommended for all visual acuity tests.
			A line of figures is preferred to single figures.
			The nontested eye should be covered by an occluder held by the examiner or by an adhesive occluder patch applied to the eye. The examiner must ensure that it is not possible to peek with the nontested eye.

Ocular alignment	Unilateral cover test at 10 ft (3 m) or Random dot E stereotest at 40 cm (630 secs of arc)	Any eye movement Fewer than 4 of 6 correct	

From American Academy of Pediatrics Section on Ophthalmology. Vision screening guidelines. Pediatrics, July 1995.

TABLE 2 Vision Screening Guidelines for Children Ages 6 Years and Older

Function	Recommended Tests	Referral Criteria	Comments

Distance visual acuity	Snellen letters
	Snellen numbers
	Tumbling E
	HOTV
	Picture tests
	  Allen figures
	  LH test
		Fewer than 4 of 6 correct on 15 ft line with either eye tested at 10 ft monocularly (i.e., < 10/15 of 20/30)
		or
		Two-line difference between eyes, even within the passing range (i.e., 10/10 and 10/15 or 20/20 and 20/30)
			Tests are listed in decreasing order of cognitive difficulty. The highest test that child is capable of performing should be used. In general, Snellen letters or numbers should be used for ages 6 yr or older.
			Testing distance of 10 ft is recommended for all visual acuity tests.
			A line of figures is preferred to single figures.
			The nontested eye should be covered by an occluder held by the examiner or by an adhesive occluder patch applied to the eye. The examiner must ensure that it is not possible to peek with the nontested eye.

Ocular alignment	Unilateral cover test at 3 m or Random dot E stereotest at 40 cm (630 secs of arc)	Any eye movement Fewer than 4 of 6 correct	

From American Academy of Pediatrics Section on Ophthalmology. Vision screening guidelines. Pediatrics, July 1995.

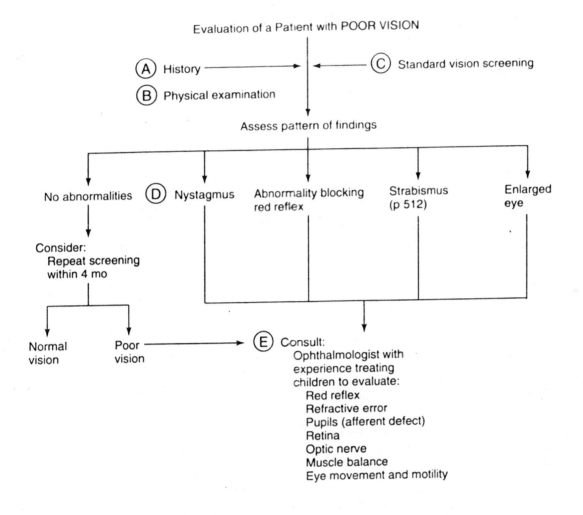

Evaluation of a Patient with POOR VISION

(A) History   (C) Standard vision screening

(B) Physical examination

Assess pattern of findings

- No abnormalities
- (D) Nystagmus
- Abnormality blocking red reflex
- Strabismus (p 512)
- Enlarged eye

No abnormalities →
Consider:
Repeat screening within 4 mo

→ Normal vision
→ Poor vision → (E) Consult:
Ophthalmologist with experience treating children to evaluate:
Red reflex
Refractive error
Pupils (afferent defect)
Retina
Optic nerve
Muscle balance
Eye movement and motility

B. Examine the patient to assess visual acuity, ocular motility, and muscle balance. Infants who are at least 3 to 4 months old will follow a fixation target such as a toy. A sign of poor vision in one eye is objection to covering the other eye. Children older than 2 years may have more traditional vision testing. The corneal light reflex (Hirschberg) test can be used to test for an eye muscle imbalance (see p 512). Examine the external eye to rule out microphthalmia, coloboma, aniridia, cataract, and glaucoma (enlarged eye, corneal clouding). Use the direct ophthalmoscope set at zero and held 12 to 18 inches from the eye to assess the red reflex of each eye. Inequality, obstruction, or absence of the red reflex may occur in a variety of conditions. Ophthalmoscopy is an excellent screening device for detecting media opacities, strabismus, and unequal refractive errors. The important differential diagnosis of an absent red reflex (leukocoria) includes cataract, retinoblastoma, retinopathy of prematurity, and congenital glaucoma.

C. Newborns should be screened for risk factors that may cause visual problems, and all children should have their visual status evaluated regularly. All pediatricians should be familiar with the screening guidelines of the American Academy of Pediatrics (Tables 1 and 2).

D. Nystagmus, a sign of reduced vision, is often associated with abnormalities of the anterior visual pathways. Infants and children with nystagmus, media opacities, poor vision or fixation, or strabismus should be referred to an ophthalmologist with experience treating children.

E. Many infant and pediatric eye problems, such as high refractive errors, asymmetric refractive errors (anisometropia), media opacities (cataract, corneal clouding, retinal or vitreous hemorrhage), and retinal and optic nerve problems, can impair vision and visual development, and they require early detection and referral to an ophthalmologist with experience treating children for optimal treatment.

References

Isenberg S. The eye in infancy. 2nd ed. St. Louis: Mosby, 1994.
Taylor D. Pediatric ophthalmology. Boston: Blackwell Scientific Publications, 1990.

CONJUNCTIVITIS/RED, PAINFUL EYES

Stephen Berman, M.D.
Robert D. Gross, M.D.

Conjunctivitis, an inflammation of the conjunctiva, can be caused by bacterial and viral infections, allergy, irritation, and trauma. In the neonate infectious conjunctivitis is most often caused by *Chlamydia*. *Neisseria gonorrhoeae*, a less common agent, can cause very severe disease. Chemical conjunctivitis following eye prophylaxis is common. Beyond the neonatal period, bacterial infection accounts for 50% to 80% and adenovirus 20% to 30% of cases. Nontypable *Haemophilus influenzae* is the most common bacterium followed by *Streptococcus pneumoniae*. *N. gonorrhoeae* and *Neisseria meningitidis* infections are rare, but these organisms cause severe disease. In the United States *Chlamydia*, the most common cause of conjunctivitis in neonates, occasionally causes infection in older children and adolescents. However, *Chlamydia trachoma* is endemic in certain areas of the world, where it is an important cause of infection and blindness. The roles of *Staphylococcus aureus*, α-hemolytic streptococci, and anaerobes are unclear because these organisms have similar rates of isolation from conjunctivae in control and infected patients. Additional viral agents associated with conjunctivitis include herpes simplex, adenovirus, and enteroviruses.

A. In the history evaluate the severity of the inflammation by asking about the amount of exudate, the degree of swelling, pain, and the effect on vision. Ask about the onset and duration of the inflammation, pattern of symptoms, and prior episodes. Note associated symptoms, including fever, rash, cough, rhinorrhea, nasal congestion, malodorous breath, headache, vomiting, and malaise. Severe headache, protracted vomiting, seizures, focal neurologic signs, or an altered mental status suggests CNS involvement. Identify precipitating factors or predisposing conditions such as trauma, insect bites, exposure to allergens, and sinusitis.

B. In the physical examination note the degree of conjunctival injection, periorbital swelling, purulent discharge, evidence of trauma or local infection, and degree of tenderness. Periorbital swelling associated with mucopurulent rhinorrhea, facial tenderness, and malodorous breath suggests periorbital cellulitis secondary to sinusitis. Ophthalmoplegia, proptosis, edema of the eyeball (chemosis), and abnormal visual acuity suggest orbital cellulitis. Erythroderma with fever suggests infection or toxin (toxic shock, staphylococcal

scarlet fever, leptospirosis) or Kawasaki disease. Carefully examine the tympanic membranes because of the frequent association with nontypable *H. influenzae* acute otitis media (conjunctivitis-otitis syndrome).

C. Hordeolum (stye) of the eyelid is caused by a staphylococcal infection of a hair follicle or sebaceous gland. A chalazion is a granulomatous inflammation of the meibomian glands. Treat with warm compresses for 20 minutes q.i.d. until no longer red and tender. If pointing, express the discharge. Consider topical antibiotics when response is not prompt.

D. Herpes simplex keratitis usually presents with marked irritation and eye pain. Herpetic-like lesions at the eyelid margins or around the lips or unilateral disease suggests herpes simplex infection. Fluorescein examination reveals branching dendritic etchings on the anterior part of the cornea. Symptoms may be exacerbated by the use of topical or systemic corticosteroids. Refer these patients to the ophthalmologist for confirmation and treatment with 0.5% idoxiuridine ophthalmic ointment or vidarabine or acyclovir. Reduce the patient's level of eye discomfort by instilling a cycloplegic and patching the eye.

E. Fluorescein examination of patients with phlyctenular keratoconjunctivitis reveals nodules near the limbus with surrounding hyperemia. The lesions indicate a hypersensitivity reaction. Treat this disorder with topical steroids. Apply a PPD (purified protein derivative test) to rule out tuberculosis. Hypertrophy of the dorsal conjunctiva with elevated grayish areas near the limbus is consistent with vernal conjunctivitis. Manage mild cases with topical steroids and refer more severe cases to the ophthalmologist.

F. Adenovirus is the cause of approximately 20% to 30% of cases of conjunctivitis. Also called pharyngoconjunctival fever, it is often associated with a nonpurulent discharge, fever, and pharyngitis, and it frequently occurs in epidemics. Enteroviral infections also cause conjunctivitis. Acute hemorrhagic conjunctivitis caused by enterovirus or adenovirus manifests as eyelid swelling, nonpurulent discharge, and bulbar conjunctival hemorrhages.

(Continued on page 504)

Patient with CONJUNCTIVITIS/RED, PAINFUL EYES

(A) History ⟶ Identify:
Periorbital cellulitis (p 510)
(B) Physical examination ⟶ Orbital cellulitis (p 508)
Red eyes, red skin (p 210)

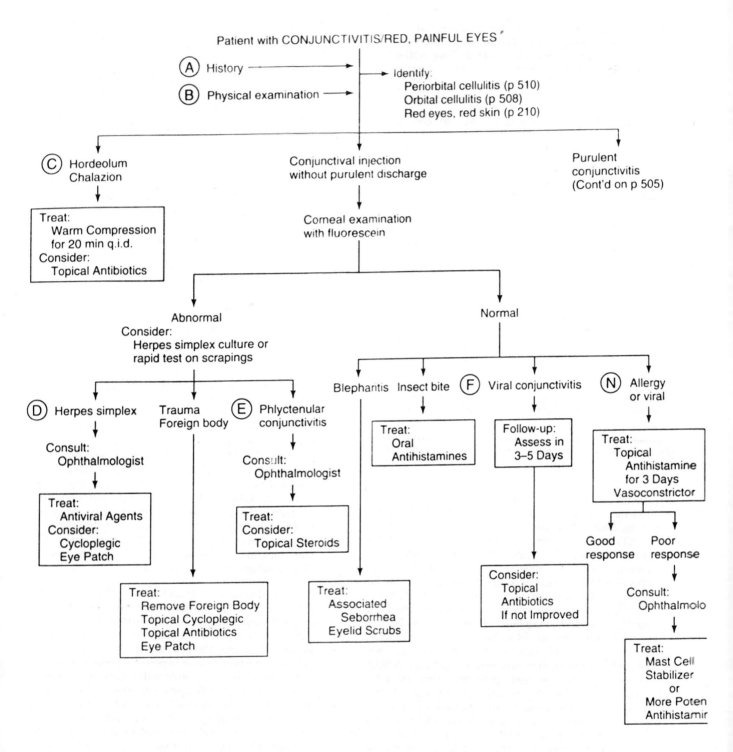

(C) Hordeolum
Chalazion

Treat:
Warm Compression
for 20 min q.i.d.
Consider:
Topical Antibiotics

Conjunctival injection
without purulent discharge

Corneal examination
with fluorescein

Purulent
conjunctivitis
(Cont'd on p 505)

Abnormal
Consider:
Herpes simplex culture or
rapid test on scrapings

Normal

(D) Herpes simplex   Trauma   (E) Phlyctenular
                      Foreign body   conjunctivitis

Consult: Consult:
Ophthalmologist   Ophthalmologist

Treat: Treat:
Antiviral Agents   Consider:
Consider: Topical Steroids
Cycloplegic
Eye Patch

Treat:
Remove Foreign Body
Topical Cycloplegic
Topical Antibiotics
Eye Patch

Blepharitis   Insect bite   (F) Viral conjunctivitis   (N) Allergy
                                                                or viral

              Treat: Follow-up: Treat:
              Oral   Assess in   Topical
              Antihistamines 3–5 Days   Antihistamine
                                                          for 3 Days
                                                          Vasoconstrictor

Treat:
Associated
Seborrhea
Eyelid Scrubs

Consider:
Topical
Antibiotics
If not Improved

Good   Poor
response   response

Consult:
Ophthalmolo

Treat:
Mast Cell
Stabilizer
or
More Poten
Antihistamir

503

TABLE 1 Antibiotics Used in the Treatment of Gonococcal Ophthalmia Neonatorum, Dacryocystitis, and Bilateral Conjunctivitis

Drug	Dosage	Product Availability
IV route		
Penicillin G	25,000 U/kg/dose q12h	Vials: 600,000; 900,000; 1.2 million U
Cefotaxime	50 mg/kg/dose IV q8h	Vials: 0.5, 1, 2 g
Gentamicin	2.5 mg/kg/dose q12h	Vials: 20, 80 mg
Oral route		
Erythromycin	10 mg/kg/dose q.i.d.	Liquid: 200, 400 mg/ 5 ml Chewables: 200 mg Tabs, caps: 250, 500 mg
TMP-SMX*	5 mg/kg (TMP)/ dose b.i.d. or 0.5 ml/kg/dose b.i.d.	Liquid: 40 mg/5 ml Tabs: 80, 160 mg
Topical route		
Sodium sulfaceta-mide	Apply q.i.d.	Ointment or solution 10%
Gentamicin sulfate	Apply q.i.d.	Ointment or solution 0.3%
Erythromycin	Apply q.i.d.	Ointment 0.5%
Tobramycin sulfate	Apply q.i.d.	Ointment or 0.3% solution

*All dosages and products express trimethoprim component. Ratio of T to S, 1:5.

G. Allergic conjunctivitis may cause considerable itching, mucous discharge, tearing, and conjunctival hyperemia. Allergic conjunctivitis associated with sinusitis or rhinitis or other systemic allergies may be effectively treated by systemic treatment of the associated condition. If allergic conjunctivitis is isolated or is unresponsive to treatment of systemic allergies, it may be managed by prudent use of topical antihistamine-vasoconstrictor combinations such as those containing naphazoline and antazoline. Preservative-free Tears is recommended for use in children for minor irritation, burning, or mild itching, and the naphazoline-antazoline combination may relieve significant itching. These drops may be used up to three times daily for 3 consecutive days. If symptoms are not relieved after 3 days, refer the child to an ophthalmologist experienced in the care of children for consideration of a more potent topical antihistamine preparation or a mast cell stabilizer. It is important to adhere to the three times a day and 3 day maximum treatment

period for naphazoline-antazoline preparations due to the significant potential for rebound hyperemia following long-term use.

H. The use of silver nitrate as prophylaxis against ophthalmic gonorrhea produces an excoriation of the superficial conjunctival layer and mild purulent discharge. The discharge appears within 24 hours of prophylaxis and resolves within 3 days.

I. *Chlamydia* conjunctivitis develops in 20% to 44% of infants born vaginally to infected mothers. The incubation period varies from 5 to 15 days. Infants with *Chlamydia* conjunctivitis may become nasopharyngeal carriers and subsequently develop pneumonia. Treatment with oral erythromycin (Table 1) decreases the risk of relapse or reinfection of conjunctiva, eradicates the carrier state, and prevents *Chlamydia pneumonia*. Erythromycin prophylaxis has a minimal failure rate of 7% to 20%. Consider the need to treat parents and contacts of parents.

J. In the treatment of nonspecific purulent conjunctivitis, administer antibiotics with attention to safety and effectiveness. With conjunctival irritation in purulent nonspecific conjunctivitis, any topical eye drop may cause great discomfort. By contrast, ophthalmic ointments are generally painless upon administration and remain in the conjunctival sac longer. Consider alternatives to sodium sulfacetamide for routine use in children because of its high level of discomfort, general ineffectiveness as an antibiotic, and potential for sensitization, including the risk of ocular Stevens-Johnson syndrome. Neomycin-containing antibiotics, while more comfortable and more effective than sulfacetamide, have a sensitivity rate as high as 10%. Gentamicin and tobramycin are both highly effective, although gentamicin may be a bit more irritating to the conjunctiva. Erythromycin is a very safe and comfortable antibiotic. Erythromycin ointment should be used with systemic treatment when chlamydial infection is suspected.

K. *N. gonorrhoeae* is a gram-negative diplococcus that may cross an intact cornea, leading to perforation and loss of the eye. Suspect *N. gonorrhoeae* with infection during the first 2 days of life; confirm by appropriate smear and culture. The clinical signs of gonorrheal conjunctival infection include hyperemic boggy conjunctiva with large amounts of purulent discharge. Treat with IV ceftriaxone or IM or IV penicillin. Irrigate the purulent discharge from the conjunctival sac with sterile saline or topical antibiotic drops. Consider admitting to the hospital any infant whose eyes may be damaged by the infection. Consult an ophthalmologist experienced in the care of infants and small children.

(Continued on page 506)

Patient with CONJUNCTIVITIS/RED, PAINFUL EYES
Purulent conjunctivitis
(Cont'd from p 503)

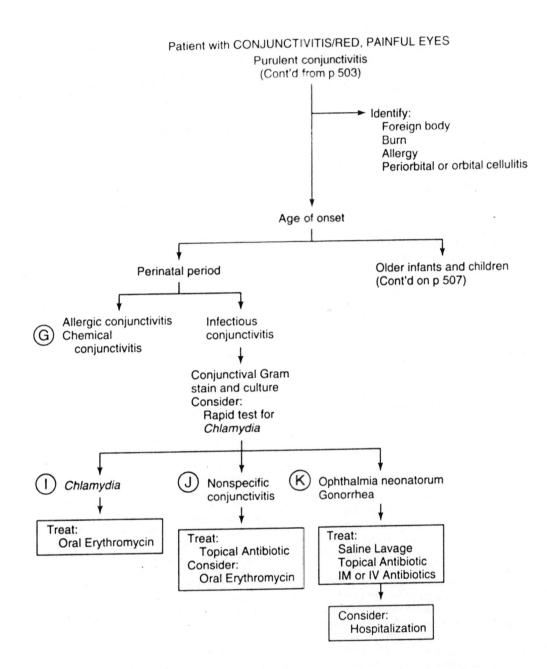

L. Dacryocystitis, an infection of the lacrimal sac, may present with purulent discharge associated with swelling and erythema under and associated with the medial canthus of the affected eye. Although dacryocystitis is rare in typical dacryostenosis or nasolacrimal duct obstruction, it is common in association with lacrimal sac mucocele, in which there is both nasolacrimal duct obstruction and obstruction proximal to the lacrimal sac. Most commonly seen in the perinatal period, lacrimal sac mucocele is treated by massage. If massage is unsuccessful, a lacrimal probe in the office may be required to decompress the lacrimal sac. Dacryocystitis associated with significant swelling and erythema, particularly in cases associated with overlying induration, should be treated as periorbital cellulitis (see p 510) unless proved otherwise. Consult an ophthalmologist experienced in the treatment of infants.

M. Dacryostenosis (narrowing of the nasolacrimal duct) or nasolacrimal duct obstruction commonly results in secondary bacterial infection of the lacrimal sac. Nasolacrimal duct obstruction is apparent in at least 6% of newborn infants. Signs of it may not occur at birth but may become apparent within the first 4 to 6 months of life as tear production increases. Differentiation between purulent conjunctivitis and an infected lacrimal drainage system is made by observing purulent discharge despite a white, quiet conjunctiva on the affected side. Patients with conjunctivitis typically demonstrate significant hyperemia and other abnormalities of the conjunctiva. Diagnosis of an infected lacrimal drainage system is further confirmed by massage of the tear sac, which may express additional discharge via the puncta.

N. The treatment of an infected lacrimal drainage system and prophylaxis for infections in lacrimal drainage obstruction free of infection is massage of the lacrimal sac each morning upon awakening and each night at bedtime. When the lacrimal drainage system is normal, only clear tears should emanate from the puncta upon massage. If mucus or pus emanates, infection is present. Massage should then be increased to four or five times daily. If after a day or so the amount of discharge continues unabated, apply erythromycin ophthalmic ointment to the conjunctival sac after massage and removal of the discharge. Continue the antibiotic ointment after each massage for 2 or 3 days until no further pus or mucus emanates. Gradually reduce the frequency of the massages until they are back to baseline, each morning and each evening. Teach parents that the massage keeps the lacrimal drainage system free of infection. If the ointment is used without the massage, the discharge may not improve. When parents complain that the infection has become resistant to the erythromycin, ineffective massage is usually the cause. Infants whose nasolacrimal duct obstruction persists beyond 12 months of age may be candidates for a nasolacrimal probe and irrigation by an ophthalmologist experienced in the care of infants and small children. The usual site of obstruction is the valve of Hasner, a one-way valve at the nasal end of the nasolacrimal duct. Nasolacrimal probes are successful in almost all patients on the first attempt.

References

Black-Payne C, Bocchini JA, Cedotal C. Failure of erythromycin ointment for postnatal ocular prophylaxis of chlamydial conjunctivitis. Pediatr Infect Dis J 1989; 8:491.

Bodor FF, Marchant CD, Shurin PA, et al. Bacterial etiology of conjunctivitis: Otitis media syndrome. Pediatrics 1985; 76:26.

Gigliotti F. Acute conjunctivitis. Pediatr Rev 1995; 16:203.

Gigliotti F. Acute conjunctivitis of childhood. Pediatr Ann 1993; 22:353.

Gigliotti F, Hendley JO, Morgan J. Efficacy of topical antibiotic therapy in acute conjunctivitis in children. J Pediatr 1984; 104:623.

Hammerschlag MR. Neonatal conjunctivitis. Pediatr Ann 1993; 22:346.

Heggie AD, Jaffe AC, Stuart LA, et al. Topical sulfacetamide vs. oral erythromycin for neonatal chlamydial conjunctivitis. Am J Dis Child 1985; 139:564.

Kushner BJ. Congenital nasolacrimal system obstruction. Arch Ophthalmology 1982; 100:597.

Laga M, Naamara W, Brunham RC, et al. Single dose therapy of gonococcal ophthalmia neonatorum with ceftriaxone. N Engl J Med 1986; 315:1382.

Lohn JA. Treatment of conjunctivitis in infants and children. Pediatr Ann 1993; 22:359.

Lohr JA, Austin RD, Grosman M, et al. Comparison of three topical antimicrobials for acute bacterial conjunctivitis. Pediatr Infect Dis J 1988; 7:626.

Wagner RS. The differential diagnosis of the red eye. Contemp Pediatr 1991; 8:26.

Weiss AH. Chronic conjunctivitis in infants and children. Pediatr Ann 1993; 22:366.

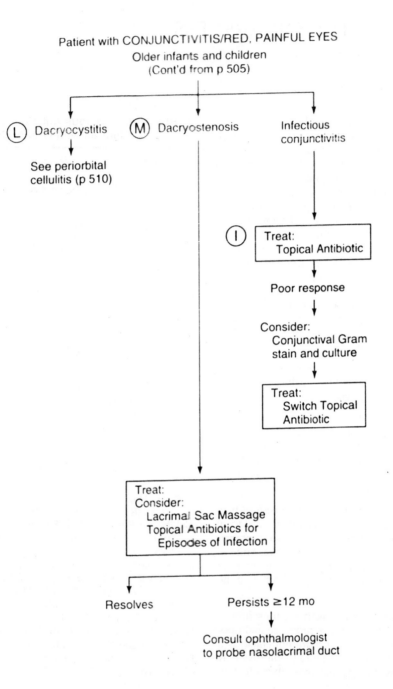

Patient with CONJUNCTIVITIS/RED, PAINFUL EYES
Older infants and children
(Cont'd from p 505)

(L) Dacryocystitis

(M) Dacryostenosis

Infectious conjunctivitis

See periorbital
cellulitis (p 510)

(I) Treat:
Topical Antibiotic

Poor response

Consider:
Conjunctival Gram
stain and culture

Treat:
Switch Topical
Antibiotic

Treat:
Consider:
Lacrimal Sac Massage
Topical Antibiotics for
Episodes of Infection

Resolves

Persists ≥12 mo

Consult ophthalmologist
to probe nasolacrimal duct

ORBITAL CELLULITIS OR ABSCESS

Stephen Berman, M.D.

The orbital septum, a reflection of orbital bone periosteum, separates the superficial soft tissues surrounding the eye (eyelid and periorbital areas) from the deeper areas within the orbit. Orbital infection is internal to this septum, whereas periorbital infection is superficial (preseptal). The risk of CNS complications (meningitis and cavernous sinus thrombosis) is increased because the posterior orbit has a direct connection with the dura through the orbital fissures and foramina and the valveless ophthalmic venous system communicates directly with the cavernous sinus. Orbital infections are usually caused by *Haemophilus influenzae, Streptococcus pneumoniae, Staphylococcus aureus, Streptococcus pyogenes,* or anaerobes. Suspect *S. aureus* or *S. pyogenes* when the infection appears related to local superficial infection (impetigo) or trauma. *H. influenzae* is the most common pathogen in immunized children under 5 years of age without a history of trauma or superficial infection.

A. Orbital involvement is characterized by periorbital swelling, loss of vision, edema of the eyeball (chemosis), proptosis, and ophthalmoplegia.

B. Children with suspected orbital infection should have a CT scan to determine the presence and extent of an abscess that requires surgical drainage. Perform a lumbar puncture, because the risk of meningitis in children with orbital infection is high, regardless of the presence of meningeal signs.

C. Altered mental status, severe headache, persistent high fever, persistent vomiting, seizures, paralysis, and focal neurologic signs suggest a CNS complication (meningitis, cavernous sinus thrombosis, brain abscess). Sudden loss of vision associated with pus in the anterior chamber of the eye (hypopyon) results from septic emboli in the posterior ciliary arteries.

D. Begin initial IV antibiotic therapy with a semi-synthetic penicillin (nafcillin) and a third-generation cephalosporin (cefotaxime or ceftriaxone). Chloramphenicol is a reasonable alternative (Table 1). Failure to improve may indicate a need to cover a possible anaerobic infection

TABLE 1 Intravenous Antibiotics for Hospitalized Children with Orbital Cellulitis or Abscess

Antibiotic	Dosage	Product Availability
Cefotaxime (Claforan)	50 mg/kg/dose q8h	Vials: 0.5, 1, 2 g
Ceftriaxone (Rocephin)	50 mg/kg/dose q12–24h	Vials: 0.25, 0.5, 1 g
Chloramphenicol	25 mg/kg/dose q6h	Vials: 1 g
Nafcillin	25 mg/kg/dose q6h	Vials: 0.5, 1, 2 g
Clindamycin (Cleocin)	10 mg/kg/dose q6–8h	Ampules: 0.15, 0.3, 0.6 g
Vancomycin	10 mg/kg/dose q6h	Ampules: 500 mg/10 ml

with clindamycin or a possible resistant *S. pneumoniae* infection with clindamycin or vancomycin and/or obtain studies to identify a CNS complication. Treat improving orbital infections for 10 to 21 days IV and then consider continuing therapy orally to complete a 4 to 6 week course.

References

Gellady AM, Shulman ST, Ayoub EM. Periorbital and orbital cellulitis in children. Pediatrics 1978; 61:272.

Goldberg F, Berne AS, Oski FA. Differentiation of orbital cellulitis from preseptal cellulitis by computed tomography. Pediatrics 1978; 62:1000.

Gomez-Barreto J, Nahmias AJ. Hypopyon and orbital cellulitis associated with *Haemophilus influenzae* type B meningitis. Am J Dis Child 1977; 131:215.

Israele V, Nelson JD. Periorbital and orbital cellulitis. Pediatr Infect Dis J 1987; 6:404.

Londer L, Nelson DL. Orbital cellulitis due to *Haemophilus influenzae.* Arch Ophthalmol 1974; 91:89.

Powell KR. Orbital and periorbital cellulitis. Pediatr Rev 1995; 16:163.

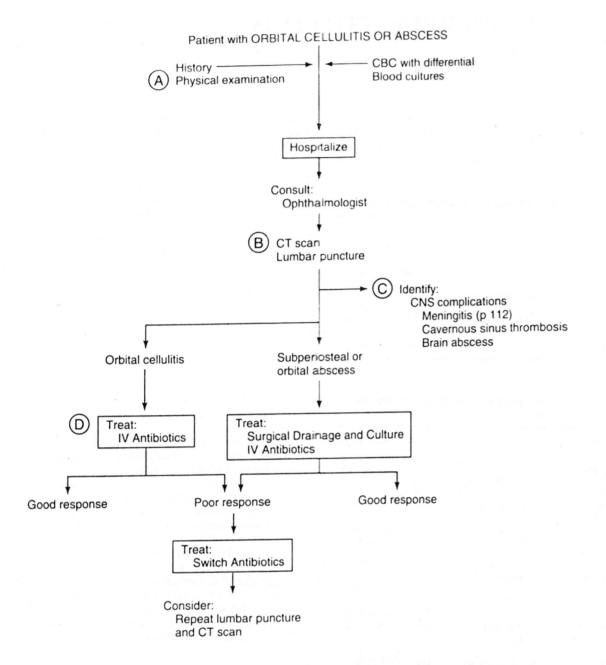

Patient with ORBITAL CELLULITIS OR ABSCESS

History ──────────→   ←────── CBC with differential
(A) Physical examination   Blood cultures

Hospitalize

Consult:
Ophthalmologist

(B) CT scan
Lumbar puncture

(C) Identify:
CNS complications
Meningitis (p 112)
Cavernous sinus thrombosis
Brain abscess

Orbital cellulitis   Subperiosteal or
                            orbital abscess

(D) Treat: Treat:
IV Antibiotics   Surgical Drainage and Culture
                        IV Antibiotics

Good response   Poor response   Good response

Treat:
Switch Antibiotics

Consider:
Repeat lumbar puncture
and CT scan

PERIORBITAL (PRESEPTAL) CELLULITIS

Stephen Berman, M.D.

The swelling and redness of the eyelids in periorbital cellulitis can be caused by reactive preseptal edema or cellulitis. Preseptal edema is often associated with sinusitis. Cellulitis can be related to local trauma, local infection (conjunctivitis or impetigo), or bacteremia. *Haemophilus influenzae* and *Streptococcus pneumoniae* are the most frequent pathogens in patients under 5 years of age, followed by *Streptococcus pyogenes* and *Staphylococcus aureus*. The incidence of *S. pyogenes* and *S. aureus* infections increases in association with local skin infection and trauma and in children older than 5 years of age. Bacteremia with *H. influenzae* occurs in one third of the immunized children with periorbital cellulitis unrelated to local trauma or infection.

A. Treat moderately ill patients in the outpatient setting with IM or oral antibiotics. Use IM ceftriaxone or oral amoxicillin/clavulanate, erythromycin/sulfamethoxazole, TMP-SMX, clarithromycin, or a third-generation cephalosporin to cover *H. influenzae* and gram-positive organisms (Table 2). Daily follow-up is indicated, and failure to respond in 12 to 24 hours requires hospitalization for IV therapy.

B. Admit severely and very severely ill children to the hospital and consider a diagnostic work-up (blood cultures, lumbar puncture, urine culture) to diagnose associated meningitis or sepsis. Obtain sinus films when paranasal sinusitis is suspected. Obtain a CT scan to exclude orbital cellulitis when ophthalmoplegia, proptosis, loss of vision or edema of the eyeball is noted. Severe headaches, meningeal or focal neurologic findings, and seizures are additional indications for a CT scan to identify brain abscess or cavernous sinus thrombosis. Treat periorbital cellulitis in patients younger than 5 years of age without local infection or trauma with IV cefotaxime or ceftriaxone initially, pending culture results. When staphylococcal disease is suspected in this age group, consider adding nafcillin to the cephalosporin. In older children in whom the cellulitis is related to a local trauma or a skin infection, a semi-synthetic penicillin (nafcillin) may be used alone. Vancomycin is an alternative for children with penicillin allergy or with a resistant *S. aureus* infection. Use clindamycin or vancomycin for highly resistant *S. pneumoniae*.

TABLE 1 Degree of Illness in Periorbital Cellulitis

Moderate	Severe	Very Severe
Temperature < 38.5° C without associated systemic symptoms	Temperature ≥ 38.5° C or Systemic symptoms or Severe pain or headache	Altered mental status or signs of meningitis or Focal neurologic signs or seizures or Signs of shock

TABLE 2 Antibiotic Therapy for Periorbital Cellulitis in Children

Drug	Dosage	Product Availability
Oral Antibiotics		
TMP-SMX (Bactrim, Septra)	5 mg T/kg/dose b.i.d. or 0.5 ml/ kg/dose b.i.d.	Liquid: 40 mg T/ 5 ml Tabs: 80, 160 mg T:S = 1:5
Erythromycin-sulfisoxazole (Pediazole)	10 mg E/kg/ dose q.i.d.	Liquid: 200 E mg, 600 S mg/5 ml
Amoxicillin-clavulanate (Augmentin)	10–15 mg/kg/ dose t.i.d.	Liquid: 125, 250 mg/5 ml, Chewables: 125, 250 mg Tabs: 250, 500 mg
Cefaclor (Ceclor)	10 mg/kg/dose q.i.d.	Liquid: 125, 250 mg/5 ml, Caps: 250, 500 mg
Cefixime (Suprax)	8 mg/kg/day as single dose or divided b.i.d.	Liquid:100 mg/5 ml Tabs: 200, 400 mg
Clarithromycin (Biaxin)	7.5 mg/kg/dose b.i.d.	Liquid: 125, 250 mg/5 ml Tabs: 250, 500 mg
IV Antibiotics for Hospitalized Patients		
Cefotaxime (Claforan)	50 mg/kg/dose q8h	Vials: 0.5, 1, 2 g
Ceftriaxone (Rocephin)	50 mg/kg/dose q12–24h	Vials: 0.25, 0.5, 1 g
Chloramphenicol	25 mg/kg/ dose q6h	Vials: 1 g
Nafcillin	25 mg/kg dose q6h	Vials: 0.5, 1, 2 g
Clindamycin (Cleocin)	10 mg/kg/ dose q6–8h	Ampules: 0.15, 0.3, 0.6 g
Vancomycin (Vancocin)	10 mg/kg dose q6h	Vials: 0.5, 1 g

T, trimethoprim component; E, erythromycin component.

References

Israele V, Nelson JD. Periorbital and orbital cellulitis. Pediatr Infect Dis J 1987; 6:404.

Malinow I, Powell KR. Periorbital cellulitis. Pediatr Ann 1993; 22:241.

Powell KR. Orbital and periorbital cellulitis. Pediatr Rev 1995; 16:163.

Powell K, Kaplan SB, Hall CB, et al. Periorbital cellulitis: Clinical and laboratory findings in 146 episodes, including tear countercurrent immunoelectrophoresis in 89 episodes. Am J Dis Child 1988; 142:853.

Sankrithi VM, Lipuma JJ. Clinically inapparent meningitis complicating periorbital cellulitis. Pediatr Emerg Care 1991; 7:28.

Teele DW. Management of the child with red and swollen eye. Pediatr Infect Dis J 1983; 2:258.

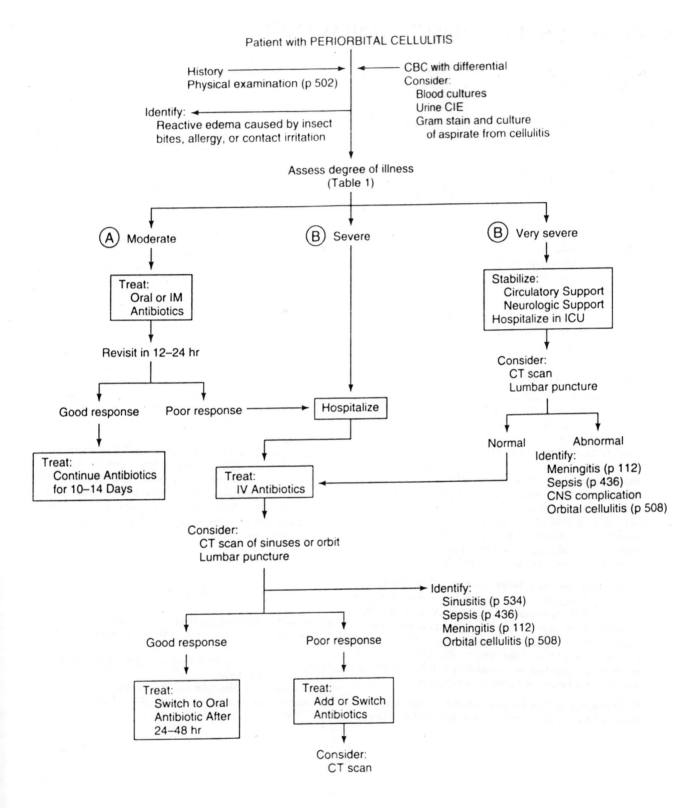

Patient with PERIORBITAL CELLULITIS

History ⟶
Physical examination (p 502)

⟵ CBC with differential
Consider:
  Blood cultures
  Urine CIE
  Gram stain and culture
    of aspirate from cellulitis

Identify: ⟵
Reactive edema caused by insect
bites, allergy, or contact irritation

Assess degree of illness
(Table 1)

(A) Moderate

(B) Severe

(B) Very severe

Treat:
Oral or IM
Antibiotics

Revisit in 12–24 hr

Good response   Poor response ⟶ Hospitalize

Stabilize:
  Circulatory Support
  Neurologic Support
Hospitalize in ICU

Consider:
CT scan
Lumbar puncture

Normal   Abnormal

Treat:
  Continue Antibiotics
  for 10–14 Days

Treat:
  IV Antibiotics

Identify:
  Meningitis (p 112)
  Sepsis (p 436)
  CNS complication
  Orbital cellulitis (p 508)

Consider:
  CT scan of sinuses or orbit
  Lumbar puncture

Identify:
  Sinusitis (p 534)
  Sepsis (p 436)
  Meningitis (p 112)
  Orbital cellulitis (p 508)

Good response   Poor response

Treat:
  Switch to Oral
  Antibiotic After
  24–48 hr

Treat:
  Add or Switch
  Antibiotics

Consider:
  CT scan

STRABISMUS (EYE MUSCLE IMBALANCE)

Robert D. Gross, M.D.
Joel N. Leffler, M.D.

DEFINITION

Strabismus, eyes looking in different directions, occurs in approximately 5% of the population. Children with strabismus may be symptomatic but unaware of blurred vision or diplopia. The cosmetic stigma of misaligned eye may cause psychological problems.

A. Obtain a careful history, including a family history of strabismus, amblyopia, farsightedness, patching therapy, glasses, and eye muscle surgery. Infantile or childhood strabismus may be associated with neurologic or neuromuscular disease or may result from visual deprivation (cataract) or other problems (e.g., coloboma, retinoblastoma, optic nerve hypoplasia). Strabismus may accompany cerebral palsy, hydrocephalus, and prematurity associated with intraventricular hemorrhage or regressed retinopathy.

B. Vision screening or assessment is essential for the detection of conditions, such as strabismus, that can interfere with vision (see Tables 1 and 2 on p 500). Assess ocular alignment (muscle balance) at the same time, using a penlight to evaluate the light reflection from the cornea, the so-called corneal light reflex. The light reflections should appear symmetrically on both corneas in relation to the pupil. Asymmetry of the corneal light reflex may indicate an eye muscle imbalance. The cover test may also be used to identify an eye muscle imbalance (vision screening guidelines). Equal vision does not exclude strabismus. Reduced or absent stereoscopic vision is a reliable screening test for children older than 3 years.

C. A constant assumed head position (head turn, tilt) commonly suggests an eye muscle imbalance due to a fourth or sixth cranial nerve weakness. A head tilt in the absence of strabismus but in association with other signs, such as tearing, photophobia, and irritability, may indicate a posterior fossa lesion. An MRI scan and neurologic evaluation are mandatory in this situation, as well as for a new-onset cranial nerve palsy.

D. Refer children with reduced or unequal vision, reduced stereoacuity, an abnormal corneal light reflex (Hirschberg) test, or unequal red reflexes as determined by direct ophthalmoscopy to an ophthalmologist experienced in treating children.

E. Treatment of childhood strabismus may involve nonsurgical and/or surgical therapies, depending on the nature and frequency of the deviation, time of onset (infantile versus acquired), and status of vision and depth perception. Glasses may correct significant refractive errors or unequal refractive errors (anisometropia). Amblyopia may also be treated with occlusion therapy or pharmacologic penalization. Infantile esotropia is typically managed with early surgical intervention, usually within the first 2 years of life. Children who have proper eye alignment by 2 years of age have the best chance of developing binocular vision. Acquired esotropia may be due to a paretic muscle (e.g., sixth nerve palsy) or more commonly, accommodative influences (significant hyperopia or increased accommodative convergence). Accommodative esotropia is usually treated with glasses; bifocals may be required to control the esotropia at near range. Exotropia may also develop in infancy but is usually acquired and intermittent. Treatment may be nonsurgical (glasses; patching) if the exodeviation is relatively infrequent and vision and stereoacuity are not compromised. If conservative measures fail to control the deviation or significant frequency and/or disruption of stereoacuity develops, surgery should be considered.

References

American Academy of Ophthalmology. Pediatric ophthalmology and strabismus. Section 6. AAO Basic and Clinical Science Course, 1995–96.

Taylor D. Pediatric ophthalmology. Boston: Blackwell Scientific Publications, 1990.

von Noorden GK. Binocular vision and ocular motility: Theory and management of strabismus. 4th ed. St. Louis: Mosby, 1990.

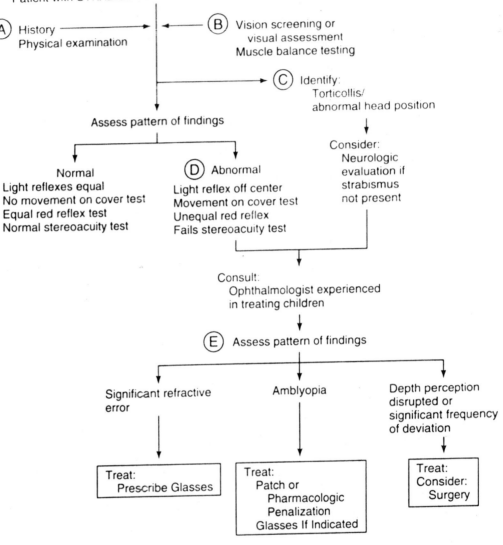

Patient with STRABISMUS/EYE MUSCLE IMBALANCE

(A) History
Physical examination

(B) Vision screening or
visual assessment
Muscle balance testing

(C) Identify:
Torticollis/
abnormal head position

Consider:
Neurologic
evaluation if
strabismus
not present

Assess pattern of findings

Normal
Light reflexes equal
No movement on cover test
Equal red reflex test
Normal stereoacuity test

(D) Abnormal
Light reflex off center
Movement on cover test
Unequal red reflex
Fails stereoacuity test

Consult:
Ophthalmologist experienced
in treating children

(E) Assess pattern of findings

Significant refractive
error

Amblyopia

Depth perception
disrupted or
significant frequency
of deviation

Treat:
Prescribe Glasses

Treat:
Patch or
Pharmacologic
Penalization
Glasses If Indicated

Treat:
Consider:
Surgery

OTOLARYNGOLOGIC DISORDERS

Mastoiditis
Neck Mass/Cervical Adenitis
Otitis Media
Parotid Swelling/Parotitis

Rhinitis—Chronic
Sinusitis
Snoring/Adenoidal Hypertrophy
Sore Throat/Pharyngitis/Tonsillitis

MASTOIDITIS

Stephen Berman, M.D.

Mastoiditis, an infection of the mastoid antrum and air cells, is an infrequent complication of acute otitis media. Prior to routine antibiotic treatment of acute otitis, mastoiditis was common. Signs of mastoiditis are postauricular pain, swelling, and erythema. Mastoiditis without postauricular swelling can occur. Mastoiditis is unusual before age 2 years but can cause swelling superior to the ear, with the pinna pushed down rather than out. The most common agents are *Streptococcus pneumoniae, Staphylococcus aureus, Streptococcus pyogenes, Haemophilus influenzae,* and anaerobes. Other agents reported less frequently include *Moraxella catarrhalis, Pseudomonas aeruginosa,* gram-negative enterics, and *Mycobacterium tuberculosis.*

A. In the history ask about earache, ear discharge, and fever. Identify predisposing conditions such as chronic or recurrent otitis media, cystic fibrosis, Kartagener syndrome, and immunodeficiency syndromes. Note signs of CNS complications such as headache, vertigo, vomiting, ataxia, stiff neck, weakness, changes in sensorium, and seizures.

B. In the physical examination note any swelling over the mastoid area with overlying erythema. Examination of the tympanic membrane reveals swelling of the external ear canal and signs of acute otitis media (see p 522). Evaluate the child's mental status and level of activity and identify neurologic signs such as meningeal signs, facial palsy, cranial nerve deficits, focal seizures, and ataxia.

C. Mastoid CT determines subperiosteal abscess with bony destruction, which occurs in approximately 18% of cases. Some otolaryngologists consider the destruction of septal bone (osteitis) in the mastoid air cells (coalescent mastoiditis) an indication for immediate surgery.

D. Assess the degree of illness. Very severely ill children who require immediate surgery appear toxic or have acute suppurative labyrinthitis, facial palsy, coalescent mastoiditis, or a CNS complication. In a simple mastoidectomy the mastoid air cells are removed, and both the inner table of bone over the dura and the middle ear space are left intact.

E. The initial management of uncomplicated, acute mastoiditis includes IV antibiotic therapy (Table 1) and possible surgery. The results of the Gram stain of an initial tympanocentesis may help in selecting antibiotics. Begin treatment with a semisynthetic penicillin effective against *Staphylococcus* (nafcillin) and a third-generation cephalosporin (cefotaxime or ceftriaxone). Consider vancomycin when resistant *S. aureus* or *S. pneumonia* is suspected. Consider coverage for anaerobes with clindamycin when a resistant pathogen has not been isolated and the child fails to respond after 48 hours.

TABLE 1 Antibiotic Therapy for Acute Mastoiditis in Children

Antibiotics	Dosage	Product Availability
Oral Antibiotics		
Amoxicillin with clavulanate (Augmentin)	10–15 mg/kg/ dose t.i.d.	Liquid: 125, 250 mg/5 ml Chewables: 125, 250 mg Tabs: 250, 500 mg
Clindamycin	10 mg/kg/dose t.i.d.	Caps: 75, 150 mg Liquid: 75 mg/5 ml
IV Antibiotics for Hospitalized Patients		
Cefotaxime (Claforan)	50 mg/kg/dose IV q8h	Vials: 0.5, 1.2 g
Ceftriaxone (Rocephin)	50 mg/kg/dose IV q12–24h	Vials: 0.25, 0.5, 1 g
Nafcillin	25 mg/kg/dose IV q6h	Vials: 0.5, 1, 2 g
Clindamycin (Cleocin)	10 mg/kg/dose q6–8h	Ampules: 0.15, 0.3, 0.6 g Caps: 75, 150 mg Liquid: 75 mg/5 ml
Vancomycin (Vancocin)	10–15 mg/kg/ dose q8h	Sol: 1, 10 g Caps: 125, 250 mg

Switch to an oral antibiotic after improvement (usually 2 to 5 days) for a 4 to 6 week course of therapy. When a causative organism has not been identified, consider using amoxicillin with clavulanate.

F. Meningitis complicates approximately 9% of cases of acute mastoiditis. This infection should be suspected when the child has a high fever, stiff neck, severe headache, or other meningeal signs. A lumbar puncture should be performed to diagnose this infection accurately. Brain abscess (2% of cases) may be associated with persistent headache, recurring fever, or changes in sensorium. A CT scan should be performed to identify these cases.

G. Surgery is indicated by the failure to respond to 24 to 48 hours of antibiotic therapy or the development of complications on therapy.

References

Brook I. Aerobic and anaerobic bacteriology of chronic mastoiditis in children. Am J Dis Child 1981; 135:478.

Garcia RDJ, Baker AS, Cunningham MJ, Weber AL. Lateral sinus thrombosis associated with otitis media and mastoiditis in children. Pediatr Infect Dis J 1995; 14:617.

Ginsburg CM, Rudoy R, Nelson JD. Acute mastoiditis in infants and children. Clin Pediatr 1980; 19:549.

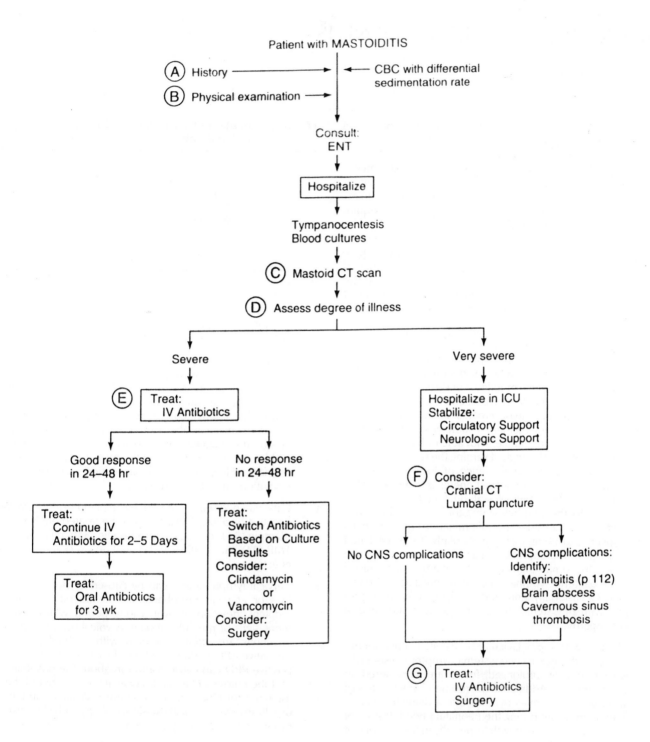

Patient with MASTOIDITIS

(A) History ————————→ ←—— CBC with differential
                                    sedimentation rate
(B) Physical examination ——→

Consult:
ENT

| Hospitalize |

Tympanocentesis
Blood cultures

(C) Mastoid CT scan

(D) Assess degree of illness

Severe   Very severe

(E) | Treat: | | Hospitalize in ICU |
    | IV Antibiotics | | Stabilize: |
                                         | Circulatory Support |
                                         | Neurologic Support |

Good response   No response   (F) Consider:
in 24–48 hr   in 24–48 hr   Cranial CT
                                               Lumbar puncture

| Treat: | | Treat: |
| Continue IV | | Switch Antibiotics | No CNS complications   CNS complications:
| Antibiotics for | | Based on Culture | Identify:
| 2–5 Days | | Results | Meningitis (p 112)
                           | Consider: | Brain abscess
| Treat: | | Clindamycin | Cavernous sinus
| Oral Antibiotics | | or | thrombosis
| for 3 wk | | Vancomycin |
                           | Consider: |
                           | Surgery |

                                                              (G) | Treat: |
                                                                  | IV Antibiotics |
                                                                  | Surgery |

Macadam AM, Rubio T. Tuberculous otomastoiditis in children. Am J Dis Child 1977; 131:152.

Myer CM. The diagnosis and management of mastoiditis. Pediatr Ann 1991; 20:622.

Ogle JW, Laver BA. Acute mastoiditis diagnosis and complications. Am J Dis Child 1986; 140:1138.

Palva T, Virtanen H, Makinen J. Acute and latent mastoiditis in children. J Laryngol Otol 1985; 99:127.

Venezio FR, Naidich TP, Shulman S. Complications of mastoiditis with special emphasis on venous sinus thrombosis. J Pediatr 1982; 101:509.

NECK MASS/CERVICAL ADENITIS

Stephen Berman, M.D.

A. In the history note the duration the mass has been present and determine whether it has been changing in size or character. If painful, determine whether salivation exacerbates the pain (salivary gland enlargement). Record any treatment already undertaken (i.e., antibiotics) and its effect on the size and character of the mass. If the mass is thought to be a lymph node, inquire specifically about previous local infections in the area drained by the node. Note travel and exposure to animals. If there has been exposure to cats, inquire about scratches, papules, or pustules in the area drained by the node (cat-scratch disease). Note any systemic symptoms such as fever, unexplained weight loss, night sweats, irritability, skeletal pain, cough, and wheezing.

B. Perform a complete physical examination. Lymph node enlargement in more than two noncontiguous lymph node regions or of hepatosplenomegaly suggests generalized lymphadenopathy (see p 368). Characterize the mass: note location, mobility, consistency, fluctuation, warmth, erythema, tenderness, and fixation to the skin. Record accurate measurements in two dimensions. Parotid gland enlargement characteristically obscures the angle of the mandible, with at least half of the mass palpable above the angle. Examine the scalp, ears, nose, and oral pharynx for evidence of local infection or neoplasm. Look for sinus tract openings in the skin if the mass is midline (thyroglossal duct cyst; Table 1) or anterior to the sternocleidomastoid muscle (branchial cleft cyst). Consider transillumination of any mass suspected of being cystic, particularly if it is lobulated and lies in the supraclavicular fossa of a young child (cystic hygroma). Signs of acute inflammation suggest acute bacterial lymphadenitis or an infected congenital cyst. Occasionally non-Hodgkin lymphoma may present with persistent tonsillar enlargement and cervical adenopathy.

C. Children with supraclavicular or scalene lymphadenopathy or with unexplained systemic symptoms, especially weight loss or prolonged fever, are considered at significant risk. Additional worrisome characteristics of an undiagnosed mass may include a diameter greater than 3 cm, onset during the neonatal period, history of rapid or progressive growth (especially in the absence of

TABLE 1 Location of Thyroglossal Duct Cysts in 72 Patients

Location	Number
Lingular	0
Submental	2
Suprahyoid	18
Transhyoid	2
Infrahyoid	45
Suprasternal	5

From Ward PH, Strahan RW, Acquarili M, et al. The many faces of cysts of the thyroglossal duct. Trans Am Acad Ophthalmol Otolaryngol 1970; 74:310.

any inflammation), and lack of mobility. Most children with a neck mass fall into the low-risk group.

D. Frequently, clues provided in the history and physical examination allow a presumptive diagnosis. In the absence of severe caries or dental infections (anaerobes), acute unilateral cervical adenitis is most often caused by *Staphylococcus aureus*, *Streptococcus pyogenes*, or an anaerobe. Consider erythromycin, cephalexin, dicloxacillin, or amoxicillin with clavulanate (Table 2). Fluctuant adenitis may require surgical drainage. However, needle aspiration may promote resolution and obviate surgery.

E. Cat-scratch disease, caused by a pleomorphic gram-negative bacillus, *Afipia felis*, can be treated orally with rifampin (87% efficacy), ciprofloxacin (84% efficacy), or TMP-SMX (58% efficacy). IM gentamicin is about 73% effective.

F. Cervical lymphadenitis can be caused by nontuberculous or atypical mycobacteria. The adenitis is often indolent, developing over a long period without systemic signs or much local pain. Atypical mycobacterial infections are often associated with purified protein derivative (PPD) skin reactions less than 10 mm. A positive PPD can cause confusion about the possibility of tuberculosis. Fluctuant cervical nodes should be aspirated for Gram stain and culture. While treatment usually involves surgical excision, therapy with clarithromycin or rifampin may be tried.

(Continued on page 520)

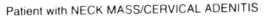

Patient with NECK MASS/CERVICAL ADENITIS

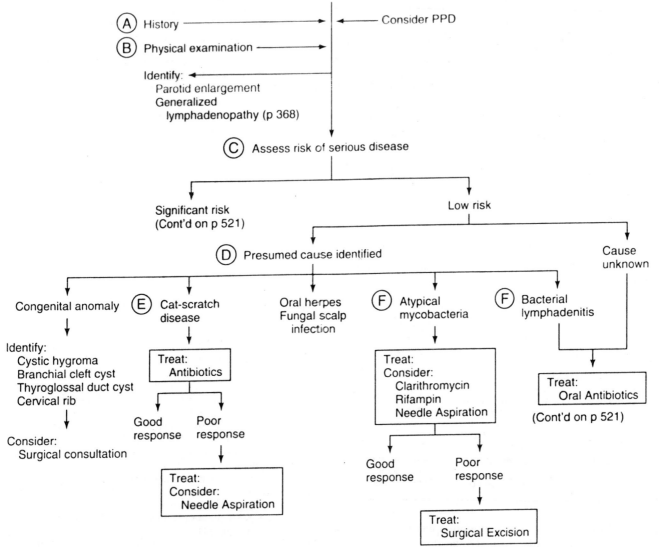

TABLE 2 Antibiotic Coverage for Children with Cervical Adenitis

Antibiotic	Dosage	Product Availability
S. Aureus, S. Pyogenes		
Erythromycin	10 mg/kg/dose q.i.d.	Liquid: 200, 400 mg/5 ml Chewable: 200 mg Tabs, caps: 250, 500 mg
Amoxicillin/ clavulanate	10–15 mg/kg/dose t.i.d.	Liquid: 125, 250 mg/5 ml Chewable: 125, 250 mg Tabs, caps: 250, 500 mg
Dicloxacillin	5–10 mg/kg/dose q.i.d.	Liquid: 62.5 mg/5 ml Caps: 125, 250, 500 mg
Cephalexin	10–20 mg/kg/dose q.i.d.	Liquid: 125, 250 mg/5 ml Caps: 250, 500 mg
Atypical Mycobacteria		
Clarithromycin	7.5 mg/kg/dose b.i.d.	Liquid: 125, 250 mg/5 ml Tabs: 250, 500 mg
Rifampin	5–10 mg/kg/dose q12–24h	Susp: 50 mg/1 ml (extemporaneously prepared) Caps: 150, 300 mg
Cat-scratch Disease		
Rifampin	See above	
Ciprofloxacin	10–15 mg/kg/dose b.i.d. (max 1.5 g/day) (not recommended for children < 18 yr)	Tabs: 250, 500, 750 mg
TMP-SMX	5 mg TMP/kg/dose b.i.d. 0.5 ml/kg/dose b.i.d.	Liquid: 40 mg TMP/5 ml Tabs: 80, 160 mg

G. When there is no apparent presumptive cause of a neck mass in a child determined to be at low risk for serious disease, a 7 to 10 day course of an oral antibiotic is warranted. Consider aspirating an enlarged lymph node, since positive bacterial cultures may be obtained in the absence of inflammation or fluctuance. Run a PPD on young children with unilateral tonsillar or submandibular adenopathy.

H. Perform a PPD, CBC with differential, monospot, and chest radiography. These studies are frequently normal in the face of a lymphoma, so an excisional biopsy is warranted if no cause is apparent, particularly if the mass has continued to enlarge on antibiotics.

I. Obtain an oncology consultation. An excisional biopsy is necessary in most cases. Ultrasonography of the mass may detect cystic components. Gallium avidity suggests infection or neoplasm. Young children, especially those with irritability, fever, skeletal pain, or anemia, should have a urine collection for vanillylmandelic acid (VMA) and catecholamines. The serum lactate dehydrogenase (LDH) is typically elevated in non-Hodgkin lymphoma but is often normal in Hodgkin disease.

References

Friedberg J. Clinical diagnosis of neck lumps: A practical guide. Pediatr Ann 1988; 17:620.

Gorenstein A, Somekh E. Suppurative cervical lymphadenitis: Treatment by needle aspiration. Pediatr Infect Dis J 1994; 7:669.

Hopwood NJ, Kelch RP. Thyroid masses: Approaches to diagnosis and management in childhood and adolescence. Pediatr Rev 1994; 14:481.

Huebner RE, Schein MF, Cauthen GM, et al. Usefulness of skin testing with mycobacterial antigens in children with cervical lymphadenopathy. Pediatr Infect Dis J 1992; 11:450.

Knight PJ, Mulne AF, Vassay LE. When is lymph node biopsy indicated in children with enlarged peripheral nodes? Pediatrics 1982; 69:391.

Knight PJ, Reiner CB. Superficial lumps in children: What, when, and why? Pediatrics 1983; 72:147.

Marcy SM. Cervical adenitis. Pediatr Infect Dis 1985; 4 (Suppl):23.

Margileth AM. Antibiotic therapy for cat-scratch disease: Clinical study of therapeutic outcome in 268 patients and a review of the literature. Pediatr Infect Dis J 1992; 11:474.

Pounds LA. Neck masses of congenital origin. Pediatr Clin North Am 1981; 28:841.

Ridgway D, Wolff LJ, Neerhout RC, et al. Unsuspected non-Hodgkin's lymphoma of the tonsils and adenoids in children. Pediatrics 1987; 79:399.

Spark RP, Fried ML, Bean CK, et al. Nontuberculous mycobacterial adenitis of childhood. Am J Dis Child 1988; 142:106.

Zitelli BJ. Neck masses in children: Adenopathy and malignant disease. Pediatr Clin North Am 1981; 28:813.

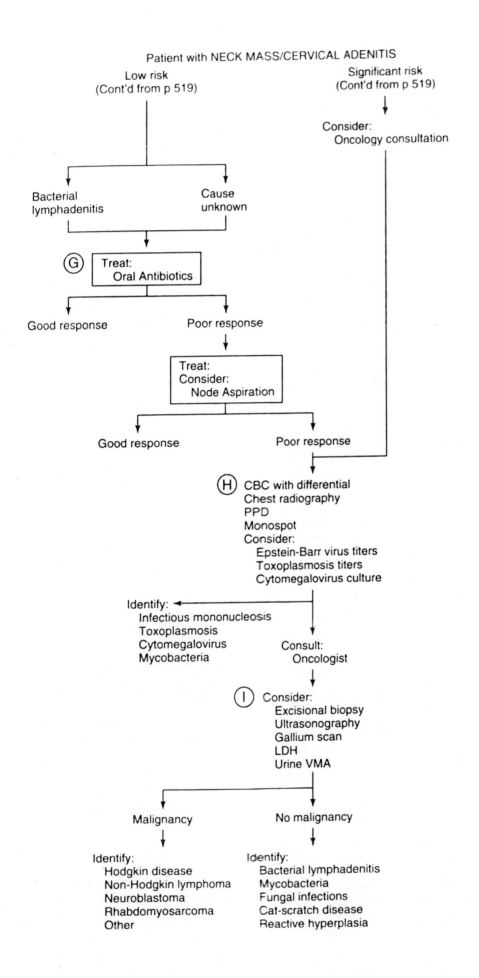

Patient with NECK MASS/CERVICAL ADENITIS

Low risk
(Cont'd from p 519)

Significant risk
(Cont'd from p 519)

Consider:
Oncology consultation

Bacterial
lymphadenitis

Cause
unknown

Ⓖ Treat:
Oral Antibiotics

Good response

Poor response

Treat:
Consider:
Node Aspiration

Good response

Poor response

Ⓗ CBC with differential
Chest radiography
PPD
Monospot
Consider:
Epstein-Barr virus titers
Toxoplasmosis titers
Cytomegalovirus culture

Identify:
Infectious mononucleosis
Toxoplasmosis
Cytomegalovirus
Mycobacteria

Consult:
Oncologist

Ⓘ Consider:
Excisional biopsy
Ultrasonography
Gallium scan
LDH
Urine VMA

Malignancy

No malignancy

Identify:
Hodgkin disease
Non-Hodgkin lymphoma
Neuroblastoma
Rhabdomyosarcoma
Other

Identify:
Bacterial lymphadenitis
Mycobacteria
Fungal infections
Cat-scratch disease
Reactive hyperplasia

521

OTITIS MEDIA

Stephen Berman, M.D.

DEFINITIONS

Acute otitis media (AOM) is an infection of the middle ear space with rapid onset of signs and symptoms of inflammation such as otorrhea, otalgia, fever, irritability, anorexia, vomiting, and/or otoscopic findings of tympanic membrane (TM) inflammation. These findings include decreased mobility of the TM and a bulging contour (recognized by impaired visibility of the ossicular landmarks), yellow and or red color, exudate, or bullae. Approximately one third of AOM cases do not cause fever, pain, or increased irritability. **Otitis media with effusion (OME)** is usually defined by the presence of an asymptomatic middle ear effusion (MEE). Findings that suggest OME include visualization of air fluid levels, serous middle ear fluid, and a translucent TM with diminished mobility. Most cases of OME are residual effusions that remain after treatment of AOM. A residual effusion lasts 6 to 16 weeks after the initial diagnosis of AOM. After 16 weeks the effusion has become persistent. **Unresponsive AOM** is characterized by clinical signs and symptoms associated with otoscopic findings of inflammation that continue beyond 48 hours of therapy. **Recurrent acute otitis media (RAOM)** is three new episodes of AOM within 6 months. **Otitis media with complications** is irreversible damage to the middle ear structures such as retraction pockets, adhesions of the TM to the ossicles, perforations of the TM, ossicular erosion, or cholesteatoma. **AOM with otorrhea**, or draining ears, occurs when the discharge is present less than 6 weeks. In **chronic suppurative otitis media** the discharge persists 6 weeks or longer.

ETIOLOGY

Bacterial pathogens frequently can be isolated from purulent, serous, and mucoid effusions regardless of clinical signs. The most common bacterial pathogens in otitis are *Streptococcus pneumoniae* and *Haemophilus influenzae*. Additional bacterial pathogens include *Moraxella catarrhalis, Streptococcus pyogenes, Staphylococcus aureus,* gram-negative enteric organisms, and anaerobic organisms. The relationship between viral and bacterial infection remains controversial. Since viruses have been isolated as the single agent in only 6% of middle ear aspirates with AOM, it appears that viruses promote bacterial superinfection by impairing eustachian tube function as well as other host immune and nonimmune defenses.

A. In the history ask about earache and discharge, fever, respiratory symptoms, conjunctivitis, irritability, crying, decreased feeding, difficulty sleeping, vomiting, and unsteadiness (ataxia). Inquire about the timing and treatment of the most recent AOM episode and frequency of episodes during the past 6 months. AOM may occur without fever or other symptoms. Ear tugging and other nonspecific symptoms are not reliable predictors of AOM. Identify children with immune disorders, AIDS, cystic fibrosis, or Kartagener syndrome (immotile cilia).

B. Examine the eardrum with pneumatic otoscopy. Signs of AOM are a red or yellow color, bulging contour, and diminished or absent eardrum mobility. Occasionally bullae form between the outer and middle layers of the eardrum (bullous myringitis). Exudate may also be seen on the eardrum. Look for signs of middle ear damage such as tympanosclerosis (chalky white deposits in the eardrum), a retraction pocket, perforation, or cholesteatoma (yellow greasy mass). Evaluate the child's mental status and note signs of meningeal irritation or ataxia. Examine the mastoid area behind the ear for tenderness, swelling, and erythema.

C. Perform a tympanocentesis or myringotomy as part of a diagnostic work-up of a child with suspected sepsis when suppurative labyrinthitis or mastoiditis is identified, in an immunocompromised host, and in an infant less than 6 weeks of age with past neonatal intensive care hospitalization.

D. Treat AOM initially with 10 days of amoxicillin, except in patients who are allergic to penicillin and patients who have received amoxicillin within the past month. In these situations or in areas where β-lactamase–producing pathogens are common, use TMP-SMX or erythromycin-sulfisoxazole (E-S). TMP-SMX is not effective against *S. pyogenes* so should not be used when treating an associated strep throat.

E. The optimal timing of visits after diagnosis and treatment of AOM depends on the child's response to therapy. Children should be reassessed when symptoms continue beyond 48 hours or recur before the next scheduled visit. The timing of a scheduled follow-up visit for asymptomatic children should be 3 to 6 weeks. Follow-up visits for asymptomatic children without risk factors for AOM may be scheduled 6 weeks after initial treatment. Follow-up visits for children with risk factors should be 3 weeks after initial therapy. Risk factors for unresponsive AOM include age under 15 months, a history of RAOM in the child or a sibling, and history of antibiotic treatment of otitis media within the past month.

F. Unresponsive AOM in a child who has been treated initially with amoxicillin can be treated with TMPSMX or E-S and vice versa (Table 1). The sequential administration of these antibiotics provides excellent coverage for most middle ear pathogens. TMP-SMX and E-S cover most β-lactamase–producing organisms resistant to amoxicillin such as *H. influenzae, M. catarrhalis,* and many strains of *S. aureus*. Amoxicillin covers organisms resistant to TMP-SMX such as *S. pyogenes,* group B streptococci, and enterococci. Drug-resistant *S. pneumoniae* may not be covered. However, third-generation cephalosporins and amoxicillin-clavulanate offer mini-

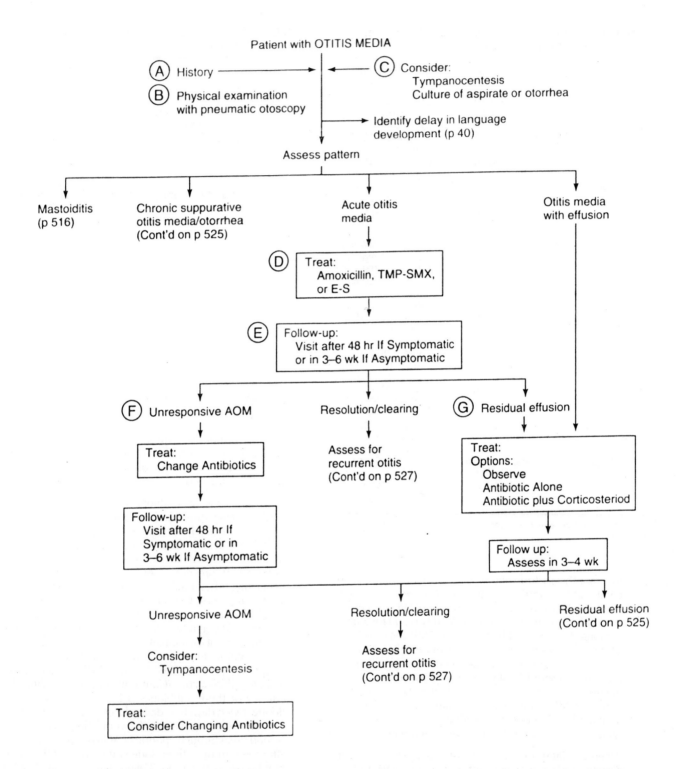

Patient with OTITIS MEDIA

(A) History

(B) Physical examination with pneumatic otoscopy

(C) Consider:
Tympanocentesis
Culture of aspirate or otorrhea

Identify delay in language development (p 40)

Assess pattern

Mastoiditis (p 516)

Chronic suppurative otitis media/otorrhea (Cont'd on p 525)

Acute otitis media

Otitis media with effusion

(D) Treat:
Amoxicillin, TMP-SMX, or E-S

(E) Follow-up:
Visit after 48 hr If Symptomatic or in 3–6 wk If Asymptomatic

(F) Unresponsive AOM

Treat:
Change Antibiotics

Follow-up:
Visit after 48 hr If Symptomatic or in 3–6 wk If Asymptomatic

Unresponsive AOM

Consider:
Tympanocentesis

Treat:
Consider Changing Antibiotics

Resolution/clearing

Assess for recurrent otitis (Cont'd on p 527)

(G) Residual effusion

Treat:
Options:
Observe
Antibiotic Alone
Antibiotic plus Corticosteriod

Follow up:
Assess in 3–4 wk

Resolution/clearing

Assess for recurrent otitis (Cont'd on p 527)

Residual effusion (Cont'd on p 525)

mal advantages in covering these resistant pneumococcal organisms. These more expensive antibiotics are most useful as second-line antibiotics for children who are allergic to either amoxicillin or sulfa-containing antibiotics. When concerned about an associated bacteremia or compliance, treat with an IM injection of ceftriaxone. If unresponsive AOM persists after a second or third course of antibiotics, consider performing a myringotomy or tympanocentesis to isolate the pathogen and determine the most appropriate antibiotic therapy.

G. Approximately 40% of children with AOM who have been treated with a course of antibiotics will have MEE for 3 weeks; about 10% will continue to have the effusion for 6 weeks or longer. Almost 50% of these untreated asymptomatic effusions persist for 3 months, 28% for 6 months, and 5% for 1 year. The main concern when treating otitis media with effusion is the possible negative effects of a conductive hearing impairment produced by the MEE on language development and academic functioning. The management options for otitis media with residual effusion (MEE present 6 weeks

TABLE 1 Antibiotic Therapy for Acute Otitis Media with Effusion in Children

Antibiotic	Dosage	Product Availability
Amoxicillin	10–20 mg/kg/dose t.i.d.	Liquid: 125, 500 mg/5 ml Caps: 250, 500 mg Chewables: 125, 250 mg
Amoxicillin-clavulanate (Augmentin)	10–15 mg/kg/dose t.i.d.	Liquid: 125, 250 mg/5 ml Chewables: 125, 250 mg Tabs: 250, 500 mg
Cefaclor (Ceclor)	10–15 mg/kg/dose t.i.d.	Liquid: 125, 250 mg/5 ml Caps: 250, 500 mg
Cefixime (Suprax)	8 mg/kg/day qd or divided b.i.d.	Liquid: 100 mg/5 ml Tabs: 200, 400 mg
Cefpodoxime proxetil (Vantin)	5 mg/kg/dose b.i.d.	Liquid: 50, 100 mg/5 ml Tabs: 100, 200 mg
Cefprozil (Cefzil)	15 mg/kg/dose b.i.d.	Liquid: 125, 250 mg/5 ml Tabs: 250, 500 mg
Clarithromycin (Biaxin)	7.5 mg/kg/dose b.i.d.	Liquid: 125, 250 mg/5 ml Tabs: 250, 500 mg
Erythromycin-sulfisoxazole (Pediazole)	10 mg E/kg/dose q.i.d.	Liquid: 100 mg (E), 600 mg (S)/5 ml
Loracarbef (Lorabid)	15 mg/kg/dose b.i.d.	Liquid: 100, 200 mg Pulvules: 20, 400 mg
TMP-SMX (Bactrim, Septra)	5 mg T/kg/dose b.i.d. or 0.5 ml/kg b.i.d.	Liquid: 40 (T) mg/5 ml Tabs: 80, 160 mg T:S = 1:5

E, Erythromycin component; S, sulfisoxazole component; T, trimethoprim component.

TABLE 2 Corticosteroid Therapy for Residual Effusions

Corticosteroid	Dosage	Product Availability
Prednisone or prednisolone	0.5 mg/kg/dose b.i.d. Avoid if susceptible to varicella and exposed	Tabs: 5, 10, 20 mg

TABLE 3 Antibiotic Prophylaxis Therapy for Recurrent Otitis Media

Antibiotic	Dosage	Product Availability
Sulfisoxazole (Gantrisin)	75 mg/kg/day qd or b.i.d.	Liquid: 500 mg/5 ml Tabs: 500 mg
Amoxicillin	20 mg/kg/day qd or b.i.d.	Liquid: 125, 500 mg/5 ml Caps: 250, 500 mg Chew: 125, 250 mg

to 4 months) include observation, antibiotics alone, and combination antibiotic and corticosteroid therapy (Table 2). If combination therapy is selected, administer corticosteroid (prednisone 1 mg/kg/day b.i.d.) for 7 days combined with an antibiotic such as TMP-SMX for 14 to 21 days. Children without a history of varicella who have not been immunized and have been exposed to it in the prior month should not receive prednisone because of the risk of disseminated disease. If the patient clears the persistent MEE unilaterally or bilaterally, consider low-dose antibiotic prophylaxis with amoxicillin or sulfisoxazole for 1 to 2 months to prevent recurrence.

H. When a bilateral effusion persists 16 weeks or longer despite medical management, obtain audiology testing to document a bilateral hearing loss (a hearing threshold ≥ 20 dB) and assess the child for any behavioral problems or language delay. The time to place ventilating tubes in a child with a bilateral hearing loss should be individualized at 3 to 6 months, depending on the child's developmental and behavioral status as well as the parents' preference. In the absence of signs of upper airway obstruction, adenoidectomy is a second-line intervention when a child has a complication from the ventilating tubes or requires multiple tube reinsertions. Tonsillectomy in combination with adenoidectomy is no more effective than adenoidectomy alone in treating persistent effusions.

I. The usefulness of antibiotic prophylaxis (Table 3) is unclear, given the rapid emergence of drug-resistant *S. pneumoniae*. Prophlaxis reduces the frequency of AOM episodes by about 1 to 2 episodes a year. While antibiotic prophylaxis is as least as effective as if not better at preventing AOM than surgically placing ventilating tubes, total days with effusion are fewer with ventilating tubes. Consider either continuous antibiotic prophylaxis or intermittent prophylaxis for colds for 1 to 3 months. When intermittent prophylaxis is being used, start the patient on antibiotics if cold symptoms develop, and continue them for 2 weeks or as long as cold symptoms persist. Effective prophylactic antibiotics include sulfisoxazole (Gantrisin) and amoxicillin. The efficacy of these antibiotics is best documented with dosing twice/day, but daily doses may be effective. Consider referring patients for ventilating tubes after a second breakthrough episode of AOM on prophylaxis or after the fifth or sixth episode within 12 months when prophylaxis is not used. Follow patients with RAOM monthly with pneumatic otoscopy, as AOM episodes are often asymptomatic. When clear, obtain audiologic and speech evaluations in these cases, and when appropriate begin a home language intervention program.

(Continued on page 526)

Patient with OTITIS MEDIA

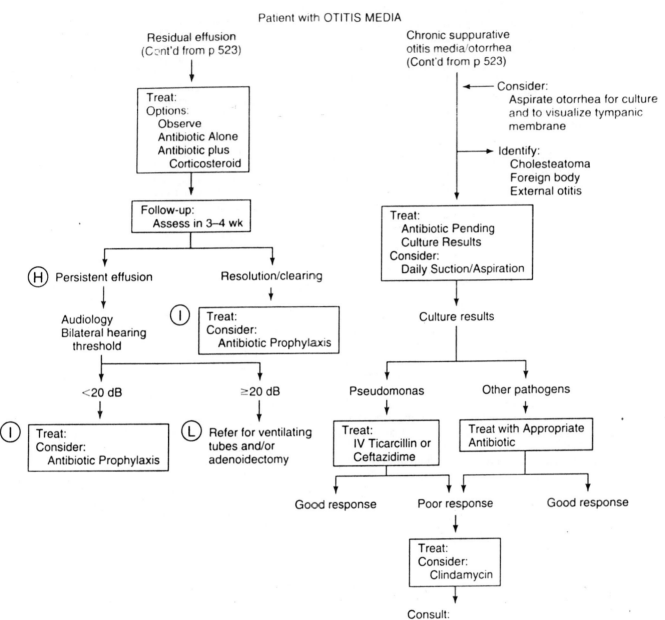

J. Consider immunizing children who have RAOM with influenza vaccine and children older than 2 years with pneumococcal vaccine (Pneumovax). Influenza vaccination during an influenza A epidemic decreases the incidence of AOM. Pneumococcal vaccine reduces AOM episodes in children with a history of RAOM. Clinical trials of the efficacy of newly developed conjugate pneumococcal vaccine to prevent AOM episodes are under way.

K. Chronic suppurative otitis media without cholesteatoma is associated most frequently with *Pseudomonas aeruginosa* infection, followed in frequency by gram-negative enteric pathogens, staphylococci, and *H. influenzae*. The role of anaerobes is unclear. Treat patients with IV ticarcillin or ceftazidime to cover *Pseudomonas* (Table 4). In patients older than 18 ciprofloxacin is an acceptable oral alternative to treat *Pseudomonas.* Consider coverage for anerobes with clindamycin when *Pseudomonas* is not isolated or when other antibiotics fail. Daily suction and debridement may be useful.

L. Refer the following for ventilating tubes: (1) patients with persistent MEE (longer than 4 months despite therapy) and bilateral hearing loss ≥ 20 dB, (2) patients with recurrent AOM who have five or more new episodes within 12 months, and (3) patients with retraction pockets in the eardrum. The benefits of ventilating tubes are improvement in hearing and prevention of recurrent AOM and treatment of permanent damage to middle ear structures. Most ventilating tubes remain in place for 6 to 12 months. Teach parents to avoid getting soapy water in the child's ears. Swimming is acceptable as long as the child does not dive or swim deep underwater.

References

Alho OP, Koivu M, Sorri M. What is an "oqotitis-prone" child? Int J Ped Otorhinolaryngol 1991; 21:201.

Berman S, Nuss R, Roark R, et al. Effectiveness of continuous versus intermittent amoxicillin to prevent episodes of otitis media. Pediatr Infect Dis J 1992; 11:63.

Berman S, Roark R. Factors influencing outcome in children treated with antibiotics for acute otitis media. Pediatr Infect Dis J 1993; 12:20.

Berman S, Roark R, Luckey D. Theoretical cost effectiveness of management options for children with persisting middle ear effusions. Pediatrics 1994; 93:353.

Breiman RF, Butler JC, Tenover FC, et al. Emergence of drug-resistant pneumococcal infections in the United States. JAMA 1994; 271:1831.

Brook I. Management of chronic suppurative otitis media: Superiority of therapy effective against anaerobic bacteria. Pediatr Infect Dis J 1994; 13:188.

Fliss DM, Dagan R, Houri Z, et al. Medical management of chronic suppurative otitis media without choesteatoma in children. J Pediatr 1990; 116:991.

Hathaway TJ, Katz HP, Dershewitz RA, Marx TJ. Acute otitis media: Who needs posttreatment follow-up? Pediatrics 1994; 94:143.

Klein JO. Microbiologic efficacy of antibacterial drugs for acute otitis media. Pediatr Infect Dis J 1993; 12:973.

Nelson CT, Mason EO Jr, Kaplan SL. Activity of oral antibiotics in middle ear and sinus infections caused by penicillin-resistant *Streptococcus pneumoniae:* Implications for treatment. Pediatr Infect Dis J 1994; 13:585.

Rosenfield RM, Post JC. Meta-analysis of antibiotics for the treatment of otitis media with effusion. Arch Otolaryngol Head Neck Surg 1992; 106:378.

Stool SE, Berg AO, Berman S, et al. Otitis media with effusion in young children. Clinical Practice Guideline Number 12. AHCPR Publication No. 94-0622. Rockville, MD: Agency for Health Care Policy and Research, Public Health Service, U.S. Department of Health and Human Services. July 1994.

Williams RL, Chalmers TC, Stange KC, et al. Use of antibiotics in preventing recurrent acute otitis media and in treating otitis media with effusion. JAMA 1993; 270:1344.

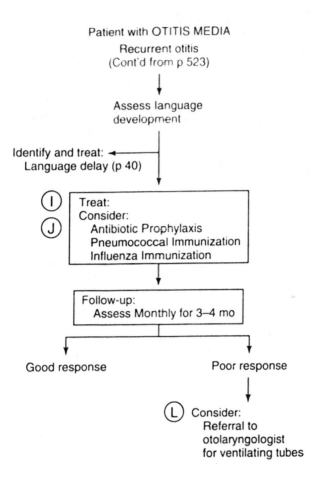

Patient with OTITIS MEDIA
Recurrent otitis
(Cont'd from p 523)

Assess language
development

Identify and treat:
Language delay (p 40)

Ⓘ
Ⓙ
Treat:
Consider:
    Antibiotic Prophylaxis
    Pneumococcal Immunization
    Influenza Immunization

Follow-up:
    Assess Monthly for 3–4 mo

Good response

Poor response

Ⓛ Consider:
    Referral to
    otolaryngologist
    for ventilating tubes

PAROTID SWELLING/PAROTITIS

Stephen Berman, M.D.

Parotid swelling in children is most often caused by mumps virus. Less frequently enterovirus, lymphocytic choriomeningitis virus, HIV, and bacteria can cause parotitis. Noninfectious causes of enlargement include autoimmune disease (Sjögren syndrome), severe weight loss, diabetes, mucoviscidosis, malignancy, cysts, hemangiomas, and stones or strictures in the parotid ducts.

A. In the history ask about the onset, duration, precipitating factors (eating), and frequency of swelling and pain. Enlargement with eating suggests an obstructing lesion (stone or stricture). Nontender progressive enlargement suggests malignancy. Note signs of systemic illness such as fever, rash, weight loss, arthritis, testicular pain or swelling (post-puberty), and alterations in mental status, as well as any underlying conditions, such as diabetes and autoimmune disorders.

B. Perform a careful examination of the parotid gland and Stensen duct. Note whether the swelling is painful or not and generalized or localized. Generalized swelling of the parotid is anterior to the ear and below the mastoid process, with obliteration of the angle of the jaw. Note whether the swelling is hard, firm, fluctuant, or cystic. Inspect the orifice of the Stensen duct and note inflammation and whether the saliva is clear or purulent. Perform a cranial nerve examination and identify facial paralysis (malignancy).

C. Suspect mumps with the first episode of an acute tender swelling. Mumps occurs once and does not produce recurrent disease. The saliva is clear, and the orifice of Stensen duct appears inflamed. Mumps cause fever, headache, anorexia, ear pain, and pain with chewing. Headache may be associated with mild nuchal rigidity, nausea, and vomiting, because meningoencephalitis occurs in 10% of cases. It is not necessary to perform a lumbar puncture to document this complication. Post-pubertal men and boys are at risk for epididymitis or orchitis, but involvement does not cause sterility.

TABLE 1 Drugs Used in the Treatment of Parotid Infection in Children and Adolescents

Drug	Dosage	Product Availability
Erythromycin	10 mg/kg/dose q.i.d.	Liquid: 200, 400 mg/5 ml Chewables: 200 mg Tabs, caps: 250, 500 mg
Amoxicillin clavulanate	10–15 mg/kg/dose t.i.d.	Liquid: 125, 250 mg/5 ml Chewables: 125, 250 mg Tabs: 250, 500 mg
Dicloxacillin	5–10 mg/kg/dose q.i.d.	Liquid: 62.5 mg/5 ml Caps: 125, 250, 500 mg
Cephalexin	10–20 mg/kg/dose q.i.d.	Liquid: 125, 250 mg/5 ml Caps: 250, 500 mg

D. Recurrent parotitis is most often related to repeated bacterial infections with Staphylococcus, Streptococcus pneumoniae, and Streptococcus pyogenes because of a congenital dilation of the salivary gland ductal system (sialectasis). Stones or ductal strictures are additional underlying causes of obstruction and recurrent bacterial infection. Initiate treatment with oral dicloxacillin, cephalexin, erythromycin, or ampicillin with clavulanate (Table 1). Failure to respond may require hospitalization for IV therapy. Sialography identifies stones, strictures, and sialectasis. Refer cases with a ductal stone or stricture to an otolaryngologist for dilation. There is no acceptable treatment of sialectasis other than prompt antibiotic therapy for recurrent infections.

References

Bluestone CD, Stool SE. Pediatric otolaryngology. 3rd ed. Philadelphia: Saunders, 1995.

Cochi SL, Preblud SR, Orenstein WA. Perspectives on the relative resurgence of mumps in the United States. Am J Dis Child 1988; 142:499.

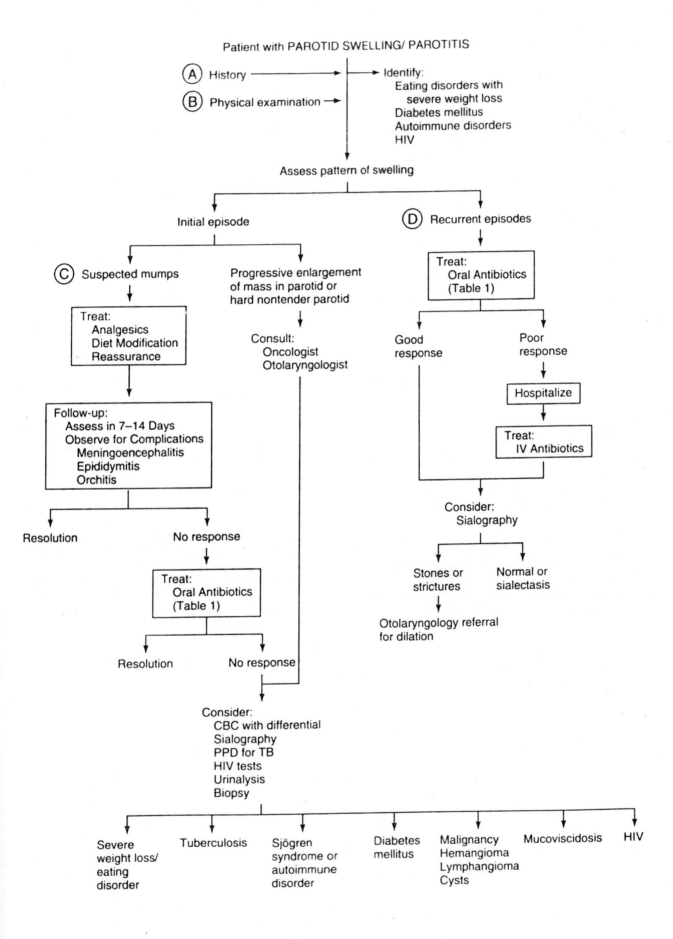

Patient with PAROTID SWELLING/ PAROTITIS

(A) History ⟶ Identify:
⟶ Eating disorders with
    severe weight loss
(B) Physical examination ⟶ Diabetes mellitus
Autoimmune disorders
HIV

Assess pattern of swelling

Initial episode

(D) Recurrent episodes

(C) Suspected mumps

Progressive enlargement
of mass in parotid or
hard nontender parotid

Treat:
  Oral Antibiotics
  (Table 1)

Treat:
  Analgesics
  Diet Modification
  Reassurance

Consult:
  Oncologist
  Otolaryngologist

Good
response

Poor
response

Hospitalize

Follow-up:
  Assess in 7–14 Days
  Observe for Complications
  Meningoencephalitis
  Epididymitis
  Orchitis

Treat:
  IV Antibiotics

Resolution

No response

Consider:
  Sialography

Treat:
  Oral Antibiotics
  (Table 1)

Stones or
strictures

Normal or
sialectasis

Resolution

No response

Otolaryngology referral
for dilation

Consider:
  CBC with differential
  Sialography
  PPD for TB
  HIV tests
  Urinalysis
  Biopsy

Severe
weight loss/
eating
disorder

Tuberculosis

Sjögren
syndrome or
autoimmune
disorder

Diabetes
mellitus

Malignancy
Hemangioma
Lymphangioma
Cysts

Mucoviscidosis

HIV

RHINITIS — CHRONIC

Stephen Berman, M.D.

Chronic rhinitis, an inflammation of the nasal mucosa, is characterized by congestion and increased nasal secretions (rhinorrhea). Causes include alterations in nasal mucosa related to immune-mediated (atopic) conditions, infection, topical decongestants, irritants, polyps, and ciliary defects. Anatomic abnormalities, obstructing masses, and endocrine disorders can also present as chronic rhinitis.

A. In the history determine the onset, severity, type of secretion, and pattern (season and time of day) of rhinitis. Unilateral mucopurulent discharge suggests a foreign body. Note paroxysmal sneezing, nasal itching, burning of the eyes, and the allergic salute. Identify precipitating factors including current medications such as reserpine or β-blockers, overuse of nasal decongestants, pollen exposure, allergens, irritants, and climate changes. Identify atopic conditions such as eczema, asthma, and allergies in the patient or family. Note predisposing endocrine-related conditions such as hypothyroidism, pregnancy, and menstruation.

B. Obtain a nasal smear for eosinophils by having the patient blow the nose into a piece of plastic wrap. Smear the secretion onto a glass slide, stain with Wright stain, and scan the slide for polymorphonuclear leukocytes, bacteria, and eosinophils. If eosinophils constitute more than 5% of the total leukocytes, allergic rhinitis is suggested. Sheets of leukocytes and bacteria suggest infection and sinusitis.

C. Allergic rhinitis results from a type 1 immediate hypersensitivity reaction involving the nasal mucosa. Release of chemical mediators by sensitized mast cells causes vascular dilation and permeability and increased nasal secretions. Symptoms may be seasonal or perennial. Seasonal symptoms are usually related to pollen inhalation, perennial symptoms to dust, mold, dander, or feathers. Clinical manifestations include nasal itching, the allergic salute, a clucking noise caused by using the tongue to scratch the palate, periorbital edema, bluish coloration (allergic shiners), and mouth breathing. Patients often have a history of atopic conditions or problems associated with atopy such as recurrent and/or persistent otitis media, sinusitis, and allergic tension-fatigue syndrome. Whenever possible, recommend limiting or avoiding exposure to known allergens.

D. Perform an environmental survey: review the type of heating system, the bedroom (carpeting, window coverings, mattress, bedding materials, stuffed animals), pets, and exposure to smoke and chemical irritants.

E. Nonallergic rhinitis is divided into groups with and without nasal eosinophilia. Patients without eosinophilia often have vasomotor rhinitis with increased symptoms related to changes in temperature and environmental pollutants. Patients with nonallergic rhinitis with eosinophilia syndrome (NARES) have no history of atopy or identifiable precipitating environmental factors and negative skin tests. This syndrome is less common in children than in adults.

F. Use cromolyn, available in a metered nasal spray, to treat severe allergic rhinitis. In seasonal rhinitis start 1 week prior to the usual onset of symptoms. This drug stabilizes mast cells and prevents allergen-induced release of inflammatory mediators. It has no sedative or stimulant effects. Antihistamines decrease the release of mediators from the mast cell and block the binding of histamine to receptor site. Commonly used classes of

(Continued on page 532)

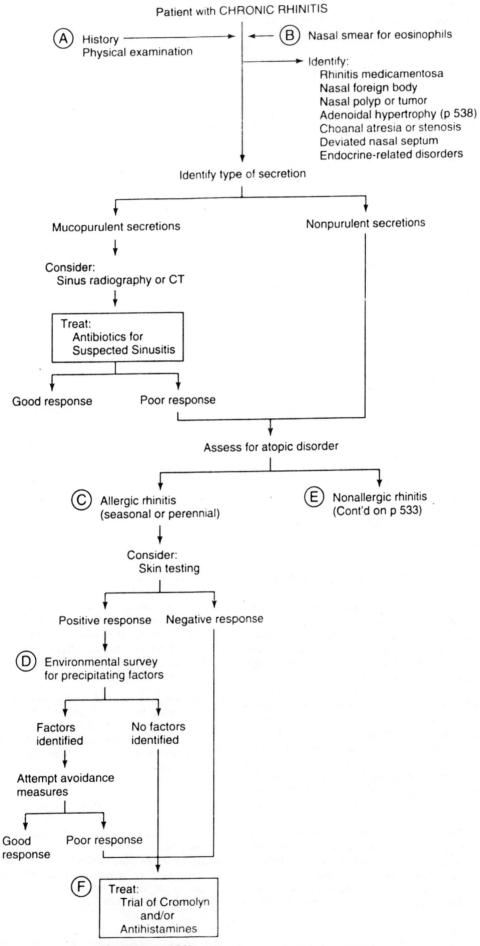

Patient with CHRONIC RHINITIS

(A) History ——————→ ←—— (B) Nasal smear for eosinophils
Physical examination

→ Identify:
Rhinitis medicamentosa
Nasal foreign body
Nasal polyp or tumor
Adenoidal hypertrophy (p 538)
Choanal atresia or stenosis
Deviated nasal septum
Endocrine-related disorders

Identify type of secretion

Mucopurulent secretions   Nonpurulent secretions

Consider:
Sinus radiography or CT

Treat:
Antibiotics for
Suspected Sinusitis

Good response   Poor response

Assess for atopic disorder

(C) Allergic rhinitis   (E) Nonallergic rhinitis
(seasonal or perennial)   (Cont'd on p 533)

Consider:
Skin testing

Positive response   Negative response

(D) Environmental survey
for precipitating factors

Factors   No factors
identified   identified

Attempt avoidance
measures

Good   Poor response
response

(F) Treat:
Trial of Cromolyn
and/or
Antihistamines

(Cont'd on p 533)

TABLE 1 Some Oral Antihistamines for Allergic Rhinitis

Drug	Usual Child Dosage (mg/kg/dose)	Usual Maximum Dosage	Formulations
Alkylamines			
Brompheniramine maleate	0.09 q.i.d.	4 mg q4–6h	4 mg tablets, liquid
Extended release		8–12 mg q8–12h	8 mg, 12 mg tablets
Chlorpheniramine maleate	0.09 q.i.d.	4 mg q4–6h (max 24 mg/day)	4 mg tablets, liquid
Extended release		8–12 mg q8–12h	8 mg, 12 mg tablets, capsules
Dexchlorpheniramine maleate*	0.05 q.i.d.	2 mg q4–6h (max 12 mg/day)	2 mg tablets, liquid
Extended release		4–6 mg q8–10h	4 mg, 6 mg tablets
Triprolidine hydrochloride‡		2.5 mg q4–6h (max 10 mg/day)	2.5 mg tablets, liquid
Ethanolamines			
Carbinoxamine maleate*†	0.2 q.i.d.	4–8 mg q6–8h	4 mg tablets
Clemastine fumarate*		1.34–2.68 mg q12h	
Tavist (Sandoz)			2.68 mg tablets
Tavist-1 (Sandoz)			1.34 mg tablets
Diphenhydramine hydrochloride	1.25 q.i.d.	25–50 mg q4–6h (max 300 mg/day)	25 mg, 50 mg capsules, tablets, liquid
Ethylenediamines			
Pyrilamine maleate	NE	25–50 mg q6–8h (max 200 mg/day)	25 mg tablets
Generic price			
Tripelennamine hydrochloride	1.25 q.i.d.	25–50 mg q4–6h (max 600 mg/day)	25 mg, 50 mg tablets, liquid
PBZ-SR (Geigy)		100 mg q8–12h	100 mg tablets
Phenothiazines			
Promethazine*	0.125 q.i.d.	12.5 mg q12h or 25 mg at bedtime	12.5 mg, 25 mg tablets, liquid
Others			
Azatadine maleate*†	NE	1–2 mg q12h	1 mg tablets
Cyproheptadine hydrochloride*		4 mg q6–8h	4 mg tablets, liquid
Periactin (MSD)	0.06 q.i.d.		
Diphenylpyraline hydrochloride*		5 mg q12h	5 mg spansules
Phenindamine tartrate		25 mg q4–6h (max 150 mg/day)	25 mg tablets
Terfenadine	NE	60 mg q12h	60 mg tablets

*Available only by prescription.
†Extended release formulations available only in combination products.
NE, dosage not established.
Modified from Oral antihistamines. Med Lett 1987;29:753.

antihistamines include alkylamines (chlorpheniramine), ethanolamines (diphenhydramine), ethylenediamines (pyrilamine), and hydroxyzine. Terfenadine and astemizole are nonsedating antihistamines. The most cost-effective initial drug is an alkylamine such as chlorpheniramine. Sustained-release antihistamines are not recommended for children below age 7 years. Large doses are often necessary. Use the lowest dose sufficient to relieve symptoms without producing an unacceptable level of drowsiness. When one drug does not provide relief, switch to a different class. Table 1 lists some oral antihistamines for the treatment of allergic rhinitis. Antihistamines are associated with anticholinergic effects (dry mouth, urinary retention), CNS effects (drowsiness, nervousness, agitation), and GI effects (anorexia, nausea, epigastricpain).Alcohol,barbiturates, and analgesics increase CNS effects.

G. Use an oral decongestant, such as pseudoephedrine, for nonallergic rhinitis and allergic rhinitis when antihistamine therapy is inadequate. Oral sympathomimetics do not cause rebound congestion but are associated with side effects, including headache, tachycardia, excitability, insomnia, tremor, and hyperten-

sion. Advise patients to use nasal decongestants 5 days or less and only when they have complete nasal obstruction secondary to congestion. Overuse of nasal decongestants results in rebound vasocongestion with dry, sore, nasal mucosa (rhinitis medicamentosa). The need for differential titrations of antihistamines and decongestant doses may compromise the benefits of fixed combinations.

H. In resistant cases of allergic rhinitis or rhinitis medicamentosa, try a short course (1 to 3 weeks) of a topical nasal steroid (1 to 2 sprays) such as beclomethasone (Vancenase or Beconase), flunisolide (Nasalide), or fluticasone. Side effects include nasal irritation, epistaxis, and sneezing.

References

Fireman P. Diagnosis of allergic disorders. Pediatr Rev 1995; 16:178.
Fluticasone Propionate Collaborative Pediatric Working Group. Treatment of seasonal allergic rhinitis with once-daily intranasal fluticasone propionate therapy in children. J Pediatr 1994; 125:628.

Patient with CHRONIC RHINITIS

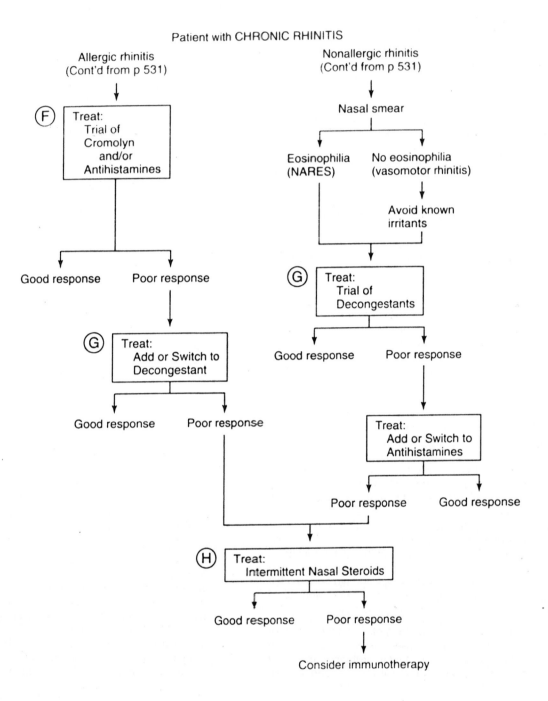

Gentry S. Allergic rhinitis: Always in season. Contemp Pediatr 1991; April:88.

Kaliner M, Eggleston PA, Matthews KP. Rhinitis and asthma. JAMA 1987; 258:2851.

Milgrom H, Bender B. Behavorial side effects of medications used to treat asthma and allergic rhinitis. Pediatr Rev 1995; 16:333.

Miller RE, Paradise JL, Friday GA, et al. The nasal smear for eosinophils: Its value in children with seasonal allergic rhinitis. Am J Dis Child 1982; 136:1009.

Myer CM, Cotton RT. Nasal obstruction in the pediatric patient. Pediatrics 1983; 72:766.

Mygind N, Bisgaard H. Diseases of the nose. In: Bierman CW, Perlman DS, eds. Allergic diseases of infancy, childhood and adolescence. Philadelphia: Saunders, 1988:463.

Rooklin AR, Gawchik SM. Allergic rhinitis—it's that time again! Contemp Pediatr 1994; 11:19.

Shapiro GG. Understanding allergic rhinitis: Differential diagnosis and management. Pediatr Rev 1986; 7:212.

Simons FER. Allergic rhinitis: Recent advances. Pediatr Clin North Am 1988; 35:1053.

Wright AL, Holberg CJ, Martinez FD, et al. Epidemiology of physician-diagnosed allergic rhinitis in childhood. Pediatrics 1994; 94:895.

SINUSITIS

Stephen Berman, M.D.

Sinusitis, inflammation of the paranasal sinuses, occurs in up to 5% of pediatric upper respiratory infections. The ethmoid and maxillary sinuses are most often infected because of anatomic features that impair drainage. The common pathogens responsible for acute infection are *Streptococcus pneumoniae* (25% to 45%), *Haemophilus influenzae* (13% to 30%), and *Morexella catarrhalis* (10% to 15%). Less frequent pathogens include *Streptococcus pyogenes*, *Staphylococcus aureus*, anaerobes, and gram-negative enteric organisms. In 20% to 50% of patients aspirates are sterile or contain non-pathogens. Viruses can be identified in 10% of sinus aspirates, but their pathogenic role is unclear. Anaerobes and mixed anaerobic-aerobic infections are more frequent in chronic sinusitis. Patients with cystic fibrosis and immotile cilia syndrome often have infections with *Pseudomonas aeruginosa* and *S. aureus*. The ethmoid and maxillary sinuses are present at birth and developed by 3 years of age, and the frontal sinuses become pneumatized at 7 to 10 years of age. The valveless ophthalmic venous system allows for free communication among the cavernous sinus, orbit, and paranasal sinuses, and predisposes the patient to a CNS infection.

A. In the history ask about the presence and duration of purulent nasal discharge, daytime cough, malodorous breath, and fever. Persistence of these symptoms for longer than 14 days suggests sinusitis. Ask about other symptoms of sinus infection such as intermittent painless periorbital swelling (often in the morning), discoloration around the eyes, and (in older patients) headache, facial pain or swelling, a sense of fullness, and an altered sense of smell. Identify predisposing conditions such as allergic rhinitis or asthma, recurrent respiratory tract infections, dental infections, anatomic conditions (nasal malformation, nasal trauma, tumors, polyps, foreign bodies, cleft palate), cyanotic congenital heart disease, and barotrauma secondary to swimming and diving.

B. In the physical examination look for tenderness or swelling overlying the sinuses, especially the frontal sinus (Pott puffy tumor), dental problems, including tooth abscess, caries, and apical abscess, and a nasal foreign body. Evaluate the child's mental status and examine for neurologic signs such as focal deficits and meningeal signs. Note signs of periorbital or orbital cellulitis such as periorbital swelling and redness, proptosis, and paralysis of extraocular movements. Listen to the chest for wheezing.

C. Treat acute sinusitis initially with 10 to 14 days of amoxicillin except in patients with penicillin allergy and patients who have received amoxicillin within the preceding month. In these situations and in areas where β-lactamase-producing pathogens are common, use TMP-SMX or erythromycin-sulfisoxazole. TMP-SMX is not effective against *S. pyogenes*, so it should not be used when an associated strep throat is being treated. When symptoms persist beyond 48 hours of therapy, the patient needs to be seen and evaluated for an unresponsive infection or complication. When the infection does not respond, switch antibiotics. If amoxicillin was given initially, change to TMP-SMX or erythromycin-sulfisoxazole. Ampicillin plus clavulanic acid, third generation cephalosporins, and clarithromycin are more expensive alternatives. If erythromycin-sulfisoxazole or TMP-SMX is used initially, consider amoxicillin (Table 2).

D. Treat hospitalized patients with severe illness initially with nafcillin plus a third generation cephalosporin or chloramphenicol. Consider adding clindamycin to cover anaerobes in very severe cases with frontal osteitis or a CNS complication. Admit patients with frontal sinusitis because of the risk of serious complications.

E. Obtain CT sinus studies initially in all hospitalized patients and in children with chronic and/or recurrent infections. The sinus CT can be limited to 4 or 5 transverse cuts when there are no signs of orbital or CNS complications. Patients with moderate disease who have not responded to a course of antibiotic therapy may have sinus radiographic studies. Include the anteroposterior view (Caldwell) for the frontal and ethmoid sinuses, the occipitomental view (Waters) for the maxillary sinuses, and the submentovertex, and

(Contiunued on page 536)

TABLE 1 Degree of Illness in Sinusitis

Moderate	Severe	Very Severe
Nontoxic appearance without signs of facial, periorbital, orbital, or CNS complications	Signs of toxicity or Severe pain or Periorbital or facial cellulitis or Involvement of frontal sinus	Signs of CNS involvement with severe headache, altered mental status, focal neurologic findings, or seizures or Swelling over frontal bone (Pott puffy tumor) or Orbital cellulitis or abscess or Signs of shock

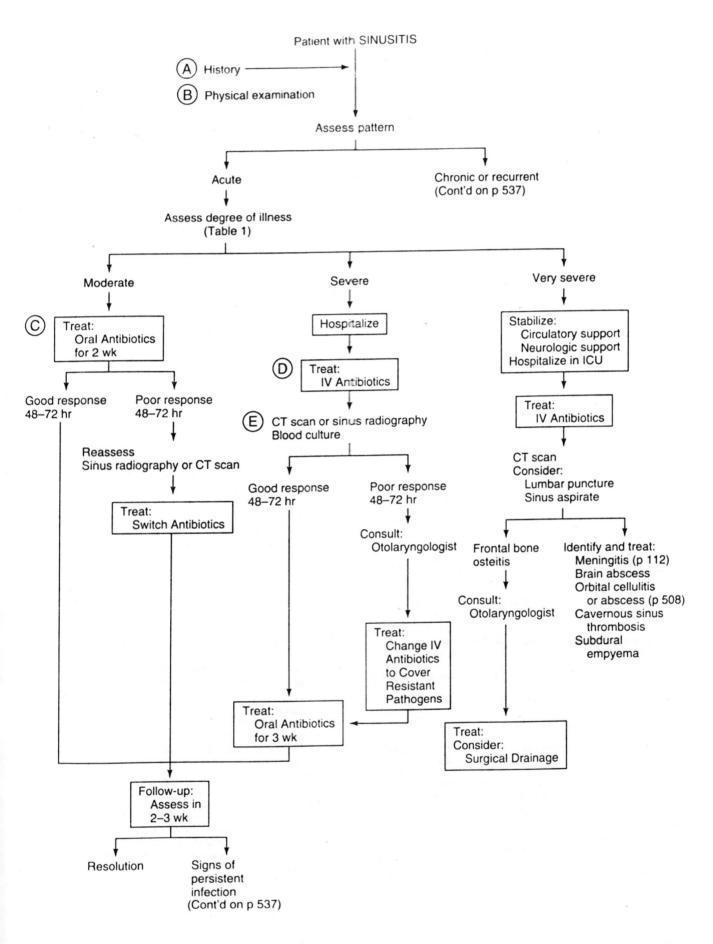

Patient with SINUSITIS

(A) History ──────→

(B) Physical examination

Assess pattern

Acute

Chronic or recurrent
(Cont'd on p 537)

Assess degree of illness
(Table 1)

Moderate

Severe

Very severe

(C) Treat:
Oral Antibiotics
for 2 wk

Hospitalize

Stabilize:
Circulatory support
Neurologic support
Hospitalize in ICU

Good response
48–72 hr

Poor response
48–72 hr

(D) Treat:
IV Antibiotics

Treat:
IV Antibiotics

Reassess
Sinus radiography or CT scan

(E) CT scan or sinus radiography
Blood culture

CT scan
Consider:
Lumbar puncture
Sinus aspirate

Treat:
Switch Antibiotics

Good response
48–72 hr

Poor response
48–72 hr

Frontal bone
osteitis

Identify and treat:
Meningitis (p 112)
Brain abscess
Orbital cellulitis
or abscess (p 508)
Cavernous sinus
thrombosis
Subdural
empyema

Consult:
Otolaryngologist

Consult:
Otolaryngologist

Treat:
Change IV
Antibiotics
to Cover
Resistant
Pathogens

Treat:
Oral Antibiotics
for 3 wk

Treat:
Consider:
Surgical Drainage

Follow-up:
Assess in
2–3 wk

Resolution

Signs of
persistent
infection
(Cont'd on p 537)

TABLE 2 Antibiotic Therapy for Paranasal Sinusitis in Children

Antibiotics	Dosage	Product Availability
Oral Antibiotics		
Amoxicillin	10–15 mg/kg/dose t.i.d.	Liquid: 125, 500 mg/5 ml Caps: 250, 500 mg Chewables: 125, 250 mg
TMP-SMX (Bactrim, Septra)	5 mg T/kg/dose b.i.d. or 0.5 ml/ kg/dose b.i.d.	Liquid: 40 T mg/5 ml Tabs: 80, 160 mg T:S = 1:5
Erythromycin-sulfisoxazole (Pediazole)	10 mg E/kg/dose q.i.d.	Liquid: 200 E mg, 600 S mg/5 ml
Sulfisoxazole (Gantrisin)	30–40 mg/kg/dose q.i.d.	Liquid: 500 mg/5 ml Tabs: 500 mg
Erythromycin	10 mg/kg/dose q.i.d.	Liquid: 200, 400 mg/5 ml Chewable: 200 mg Tabs, caps: 250, 500 mg
Amoxicillin-clavulanate (Augmentin)	10–15 mg/kg/dose t.i.d.	Liquid: 125, 250 mg/5 ml Chewable: 125, 250 mg Tabs: 250, 500 mg
Cefaclor (Ceclor)	10 mg/kg/dose q.i.d.	Liquid: 125, 250 mg/5 ml Caps: 250, 500 mg
Cefixime (Suprax)	8 mg/kg/day as single dose or divided b.i.d.	Liquid: 100 mg/ 5 ml Tabs: 200, 400 mg
Cefpodoxime (Vantin)	5 mg/kg/dose b.i.d.	Susp: 50, 100 mg/ 5 ml Tabs: 100, 200 mg
Loracarbef (Lorabid)	15 mg/kg/dose b.i.d.	Susp: 100, 200 mg/ 5 ml Pulvules: 200, 400 mg
Cefprozil (Cefzil)	15 mg/kg/dose b.i.d.	Susp: 125, 250 mg/ 5 ml Tabs: 250, 500 mg
Clarithromycin (Biaxin)	7.5 mg/kg/dose b.i.d.	Liquid: 125, 250 mg/5 ml Tabs: 250, 500 mg
Intravenous Antibiotics for Hospitalized Patients		
Cefotaxime (Claforan)	50 mg/kg/dose IV q8h	Vials: 0.5, 1, 2 g
Ceftriaxone (Rocephin)	75 mg/kg/dose IV q24h	Vials: 0.25, 0.5, 1 g
Chloramphenicol	10–20 mg/kg/dose q6h	Vials: 1 g
Nafcillin	25 mg/kg/dose IV q6h	Vials: 0.5, 1, 2 g
Clindamycin (Cleocin)	10 mg/kg/dose q6–8h	Ampules: 0.15, 0.3, 0.6 g
Topical Therapy		
Cromolyn 2% nasal solution	1 spray each nostril t.i.d. to q.i.d.	Spray: 0.8 mg/ 0.04 ml
Beclomethasone (Beconase, Vancenase)	2 sprays each nostril b.i.d.	Spray: 50 μg

T, trimethoprim component; E, erythromycin component; S, sulfamethoxazole component.

lateral views for the sphenoid sinus. In young children a Waters view is usually sufficient. Evidence of sinusitis includes the presence of air-fluid levels, complete opacity, and mucosal thickening to greater than 5 mm. Sinus films in children under 1 year of age are often difficult to interpret.

F. The use of topical decongestants and oral decongestants–antihistamine preparations to promote sinus drainage is controversial. Efficacy is unknown, and these drugs may impair ciliary function, reduce blood flow to the mucosa, and reduce diffusion of the antibiotic into the sinuses. Cromolyn and nasal steroids may benefit patients with underlying allergic rhinitis. Nasal lavage with saline delivered by a bulb syringe may be beneficial in recurrent cases.

G. Indications for sinus aspiration or lavage and drainage are CNS complication (intracranial or orbital), frontal bone osteitis, persistence of severe pain despite 48 hours of IV therapy, chronic sinusitis unresponsive to multiple courses of antibiotics, and recurrent episodes of sinusitis.

H. The value of surgical interventions for children with persistent or recurrent sinusitis is unclear. No randomized trials have assessed adenoidectomy. The effectiveness of functional endoscopic sinus surgery for children, while frequently recommended, has not been established. This procedure uses rigid endoscopes to open the osteomeatal complex by removing the uncinate process and widens the maxillary sinus ostia. Revision of the surgery is required in about 7% of cases, and complications include bleeding, damage to the orbital structures, and dural laceration.

References

Dunham ME. New light on sinusitis. Contemp Pediatr 1994; 11:102.

Gwaltney JM, Phillips CD, Miller RD, et al. Computed tomographic study of the common cold. N Engl J Med 1994; 330:25.

Poole MD. Pediatric sinusitis is not a surgical disease. Ear Nose Throat J 1992; 71:622.

Rachelefsky GS, Katz RM, Siegel SC. Chronic sinusitis in the allergic child. Pediatr Clin North Am 1988; 35:1091.

Shapiro GG. Sinusitis in children. J Allergy Clin Immunol 1988; 81:1025.

Simons FER. Allergic rhinitis: Recent advances. Pediatr Clin North Am 1988; 35:1053.

Tinkelman DG, Silk HJ. Clinical and bacteriologic features of chronic sinusitis in children. Am J Dis Child 1989; 143:938.

Wald ER. Acute and chronic sinusitis: Diagnosis and management. Pediatr Rev 1985; 7:150.

Wald ER. Chronic sinusitis in children. J Pediatr 1995; 127:339.

Wald ER, Chiponis D, Ledesma-Medina J. Comparative effectiveness of amoxicillin and amoxicillin-clavulanate potassium in acute paranasal sinus infection in children: A double-blind, placebo-controlled trial. Pediatrics 1986; 77:795.

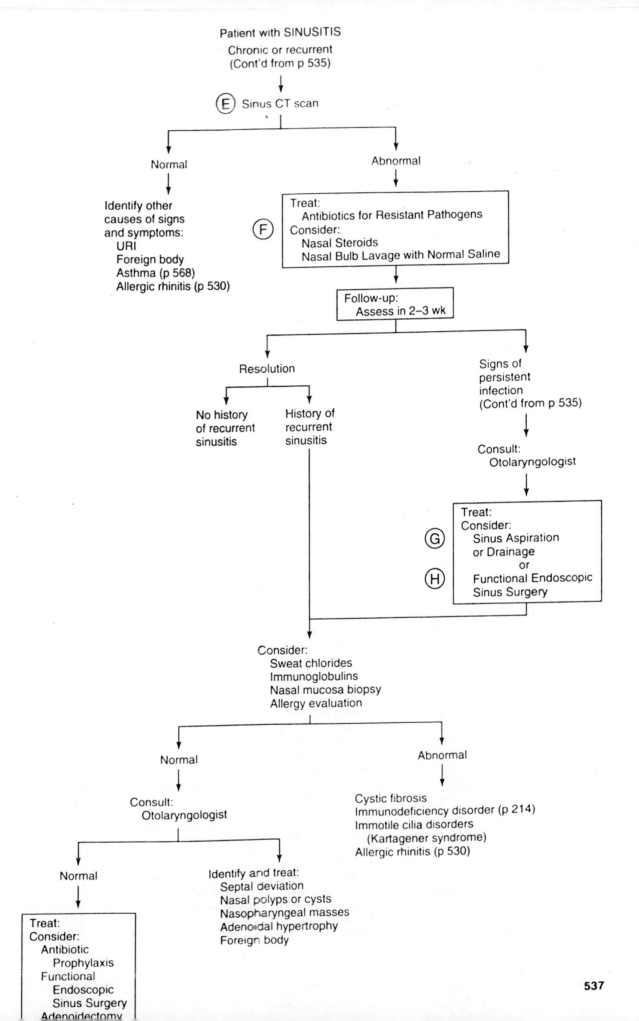

Patient with SINUSITIS
Chronic or recurrent
(Cont'd from p 535)

(E) Sinus CT scan

Normal

Identify other
causes of signs
and symptoms:
    URI
    Foreign body
    Asthma (p 568)
    Allergic rhinitis (p 530)

Abnormal

Treat:
    Antibiotics for Resistant Pathogens
(F) Consider:
    Nasal Steroids
    Nasal Bulb Lavage with Normal Saline

Follow-up:
    Assess in 2–3 wk

Resolution

No history
of recurrent
sinusitis

History of
recurrent
sinusitis

Signs of
persistent
infection
(Cont'd from p 535)

Consult:
    Otolaryngologist

Treat:
Consider:
(G)   Sinus Aspiration
    or Drainage
        or
(H)   Functional Endoscopic
    Sinus Surgery

Consider:
    Sweat chlorides
    Immunoglobulins
    Nasal mucosa biopsy
    Allergy evaluation

Normal

Consult:
    Otolaryngologist

Abnormal

Cystic fibrosis
Immunodeficiency disorder (p 214)
Immotile cilia disorders
    (Kartagener syndrome)
Allergic rhinitis (p 530)

Normal

Identify and treat:
    Septal deviation
    Nasal polyps or cysts
    Nasopharyngeal masses
    Adenoidal hypertrophy
    Foreign body

Treat:
Consider:
    Antibiotic
        Prophylaxis
    Functional
        Endoscopic
        Sinus Surgery
    Adenoidectomy

SNORING/ADENOIDAL HYPERTROPHY

Stephen Berman, M.D.

The adenoids, composed of lymphoid tissue in the nasopharynx, with the palatine and lingual tonsils, constitute the Waldeyer ring. Enlargement of the adenoids with or without infection can obstruct the upper airway, alter normal orofacial growth, and interfere with speech, swallowing, and the eustachian tube. The roles of hypertrophy and chronic infection in the pathogenesis of sinusitis are unclear.

DEFINITIONS

Obstructive apnea consists of periods when airflow stops for longer than 5 seconds. It is associated with respiratory effort, bradycardia, oxygen desaturation, or termination with gasping and agitated arousal. **Hypopnea** is loud snoring during sleep with periods of reduced airflow for 10 seconds or longer associated with oxygen desaturation or arousal.

A. In the history ask about noisy breathing, snoring, mouth breathing, nasal voice, adenoid facies, restless sleep, nasal discharge, bad breath, enuresis, and persistent otitis. When an infant or young child is a restless sleeper, consider alternative reasons such as regular nighttime feedings or play periods. Note neurologic conditions associated with upper airway obstruction such as Down syndrome, cerebral palsy, congenital myopathies, and encephalopathies.

B. In the physical examination note any craniofacial dysostosis, adenoid facies, and dental malocclusion. Listen to the child's speech for a nasal voice. Use pneumatic otoscopy to examine the tympanic membranes. Assess the patient for choanal atresia or stenosis. Note the size of the tonsils. Is the patient obese or neurologically impaired? Perform a careful cardiopulmonary examination for signs of right heart failure or pulmonary hypertension.

C. The initial work-up of a patient varies with findings on history and physical examination. When the severity of any snoring is in doubt, an audiotape during sleep may help. However, it cannot be used to document episodes of hypopnea or obstructive apnea. A lateral neck radiograph or fiberoptic nasopharyngoscopy will assess the relative size of the adenoids. When episodes of hypopnea, obstructive apnea, failure to thrive, or clinical signs of cardiac disease are present, obtain a chest radiograph and ECG initially.

D. Consider treating patients older than 5 years of age who have mild disease or intermittent obstructive symptoms with aqueous nasal beclomethasone 1 spray in each nostril twice daily for 4 to 16 weeks. This treatment appears to reduce adenoidal hypertrophy and nasal airway obstructive symptoms. Immunize children who have not had chickenpox to prevent more serious infection if an exposure occurs while on nasal steroids.

TABLE 1 Degree of Illness in Adenoidal Hypertrophy

Mild	Moderate	Severe
Noisy breathing or Snoring or Restless sleep or Nasal discharge or Mouth breathing	Persistent otitis or Orofacial disorders or Speech disorder or Swallowing disorder or Intermittent respiratory difficulty with colds	Signs of right heart failure (cor pulmonale) or Pulmonary hypertension or ECG changes of right heart strain, hypertrophy or Obstructive sleep apnea, hypopnea or Arterial blood gas with elevated CO_2, chronic hypoxia or Severe failure to thrive
(All are usually intermittent and associated with colds or episodes of rhinitis)		

E. A sleep study polysomnogram records heart rate, oxygen saturation, oronasal airflow, chest wall movement, carbon dioxide, ECG, and EEG. Absent oronasal airflow with the presence of chest wall movement, oxygen desaturation, or bradycardia indicates obstruction sleep apnea.

F. Indications for adenoidectomy with or without tonsillectomy include pulmonary conditions such as chronic hypoxia related to upper airway obstruction, hypopnea, or obstructive sleep apnea; orofacial conditions such as mandibular growth abnormalities, dental malocclusion, and swallowing disorders; speech abnormalities; and persistent middle ear effusion. Children with suspected velopharyngeal insufficiency, such as those with cleft palate, should not have an adenoidectomy unless there is a life-threatening obstruction.

References

Brodsky L. Modern assessment of tonsils and adenoids. Pediatr Clin North Am 1989; 36:1551.

Demain JG, Goetz DW. Pediatric adenoidal hypertrophy and nasal airway obstruction: Reduction with aqueous nasal beclomethasone. Pediatrics 1995; 95:355.

Deutsch ES, Isaacson GC. Tonsils and adenoids: An update. Pediatr Rev 1995; 16:17.

Everett AD, Koch WC, Saulsbury FT. Failure to thrive due to obstructive sleep apnea. Clin Pediatr 1987; 26:90.

Weider DJ, Sateia MJ, West RP. Nocturnal enuresis in children with upper airway obstruction. Otolaryngol Head Neck Surg 1991; 105:427.

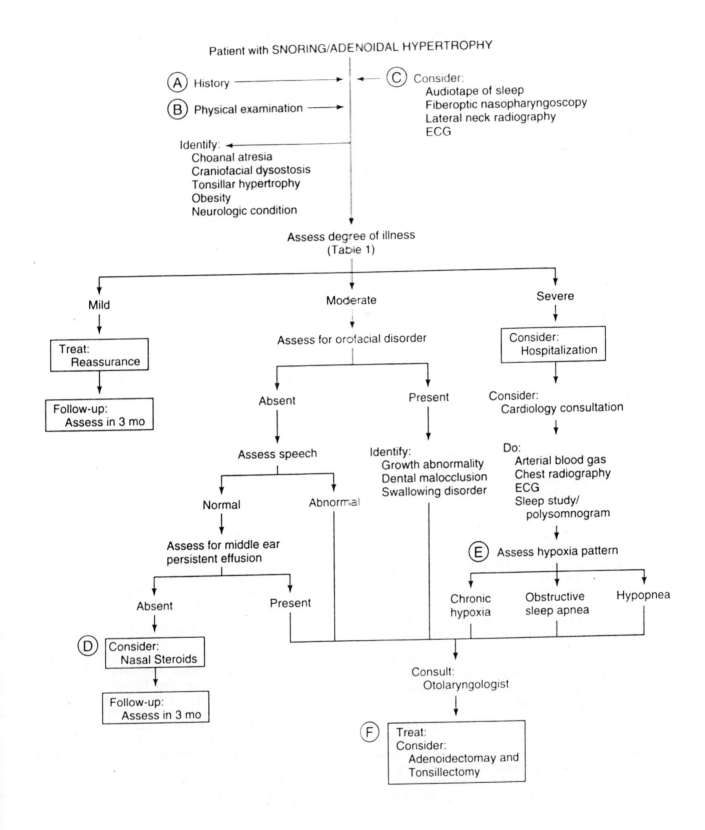

Patient with SNORING/ADENOIDAL HYPERTROPHY

A History

B Physical examination

C Consider:
   Audiotape of sleep
   Fiberoptic nasopharyngoscopy
   Lateral neck radiography
   ECG

Identify:
   Choanal atresia
   Craniofacial dysostosis
   Tonsillar hypertrophy
   Obesity
   Neurologic condition

Assess degree of illness
(Table 1)

Mild

Treat:
Reassurance

Follow-up:
Assess in 3 mo

Moderate

Assess for orofacial disorder

Absent

Assess speech

Normal

Assess for middle ear
persistent effusion

Absent

D Consider:
Nasal Steroids

Follow-up:
Assess in 3 mo

Present

Abnormal

Present

Identify:
   Growth abnormality
   Dental malocclusion
   Swallowing disorder

Severe

Consider:
Hospitalization

Consider:
Cardiology consultation

Do:
   Arterial blood gas
   Chest radiography
   ECG
   Sleep study/
      polysomnogram

E Assess hypoxia pattern

Chronic
hypoxia

Obstructive
sleep apnea

Hypopnea

Consult:
Otolaryngologist

F Treat:
Consider:
   Adenoidectomay and
   Tonsillectomy

SORE THROAT/PHARYNGITIS/TONSILLITIS

Stephen Berman, M.D.

ETIOLOGY

Acute pharyngitis and tonsillitis are caused by bacterial and viral pathogens. Bacterial agents include *Streptococcus pyogenes* (group A β-hemolytic *Streptococcus*), *Mycoplasma pneumoniae*, non–group A β-hemolytic *Streptococcus*, *Neisseria gonorrhoeae*, *Corynebacterium diphtheriae*, and possibly *Chlamydia trachomatis* and anaerobes. Viral agents include influenza viruses, adenovirus, respiratory syncytial virus (RSV), herpes simplex, Epstein-Barr virus (mononucleosis), parainfluenza viruses, and enteroviruses. Common viral syndromes associated with sore throat include herpetic gingivostomatitis, pharyngoconjunctival fever, herpangina, lymphonodular pharyngitis, and hand, foot, and mouth disease.

The goals of diagnosis and treatment of *S. pyogenes* infections are prevention of rheumatic fever and possibly glomerulonephritis, reduction of suppurative sequelae (peritonsillar and retropharyngeal abscess), symptomatic improvement, and interruption of transmission to family members and classmates.

The incidence of acute rheumatic fever (ARF) in the United States has increased since 1985. Treatment begun up to 9 days after the *S. pyogenes* infection prevents rheumatic fever. Adequate treatment requires 10 days of an appropriate oral antibiotic or an adequate dose of long-acting benzathine penicillin. Children under 4 years of age are not usually at risk for ARF.

A. In the history determine the onset, duration, and severity of the sore throat. Note stridor, drooling, inability to swallow, inability to lie down, air hunger, and restlessness. Identify associated symptoms, including fever, rhinorrhea, nasal congestion, cough, earache, fatigue, malaise, vomiting, diarrhea, headache, abdominal pain, and rash. Exposure to a family member with *S. pyogenes* increases the risk of infection. *S. pyogenes* pharyngitis is uncommon in children under 3 years of age and rare in those under 18 months. The clinical presentation in children from 18 to 36 months is nonspecific, and cultures of the nares are often necessary to identify the infection.

B. In the physical examination examine the oropharynx and tonsils and note exudate, petechiae on the palate, peritonsillar swelling with deviation of the uvula, cervical adenitis, or a sandpaper rash suggesting scarlet fever. Identify acute otitis media and mucopurulent rhinorrhea (sinusitis). Note signs of mononucleosis such as lymphadenopathy, hepatosplenomegaly,

TABLE 1   Degree of Illness in Pharyngitis/Tonsillitis

Moderate	Severe	Very Severe
Signs that suggest *S. pyogenes* infection such as tonsillar exudate, petechiae on the palate, cervical adenitis, a scarlatina-type rash, and the absence of URI symptoms	Signs of peritonsillar abscess or cellulitis or Enlarged tonsils that impair swallowing and cause drooling or Systemic toxicity	Signs of upper airway obstruction such as stridor at rest, air hunger, restlessness

URI, upper respiratory infection.

edema of the eyelids, or a rash (frequently associated with ampicillin).

C. Numerous tests, including latex agglutination, enzyme fluorescence, and enzyme immunoassay, are available for rapid detection of *S. pyogenes* antigen. Sensitivity ranges from 62% to 95%, and specificity from 88% to 100%. Advantages of rapid testing and early treatment include increased patient satisfaction, higher treatment rates (especially in clinic settings), reduction in symptomatic discomfort, and possibly decreased transmission. Disadvantages include higher cost, low sensitivity requiring a culture on cases with negative tests, and evidence suggesting that early treatment may compromise the antibody response helpful in preventing relapses and recurrent infections.

D. Treat cases of suspected or proven *S. pyogenes* infection with a 10-day course of oral penicillin V, cephalexin, or an IM injection of benzathine penicillin (Table 2). Use erythromycin for patients with penicillin allergy. Treatment failure after 10 days of penicillin V given three times a day varies from 6% to 23%. Causes of treatment failures are unrecognized carrier states, poor compliance, reinfection with a different strain, inactivation of penicillin by β-lactamase–producing bacteria, and possibly the development of penicillin tolerance by *S. pyogenes* organisms. The small difference between the effectiveness of cephalosporins and penicillin may reflect a difference in eradicating the carrier state rather than treatment failures. Ap-

(Continued on page 542)

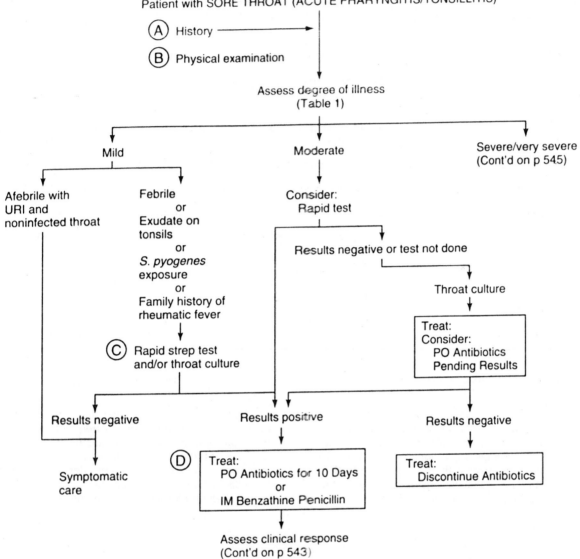

Patient with SORE THROAT (ACUTE PHARYNGITIS/TONSILLITIS)

(A) History ———→

(B) Physical examination

Assess degree of illness
(Table 1)

Mild

Moderate

Severe/very severe
(Cont'd on p 545)

Afebrile with
URI and
noninfected throat

Febrile
or
Exudate on
tonsils
or
S. pyogenes
exposure
or
Family history of
rheumatic fever

(C) Rapid strep test
and/or throat culture

Consider:
Rapid test

Results negative or test not done

Throat culture

Treat:
Consider:
 PO Antibiotics
 Pending Results

Results negative

Results positive

Results negative

Symptomatic
care

(D) Treat:
 PO Antibiotics for 10 Days
 or
 IM Benzathine Penicillin

Treat:
 Discontinue Antibiotics

Assess clinical response
(Cont'd on p 543)

TABLE 2 Antibiotic Therapy for Acute Pharyngitis and Tonsillitis

Antibiotic	Dosage	Product Availability
Oral Antibiotics		
Penicillin V	10–13 mg/kg/dose t.i.d. or max 250 mg t.i.d. × 10 days Prophylaxis: 10 mg/kg/dose b.i.d. or 250 mg b.i.d.	Liquid: 125, 250 mg/5 ml Tabs: 125, 250, 500 mg
Erythromycin Estolate (Ilosone)	10 mg/kg/dose t.i.d. or max 250 mg t.i.d. × 10 days	Liquid: 125, 250 mg/5 ml Chewables: 125, 250 mg Caps: 125, 250 mg
Erythromycin Ethyl succinate	10–13 mg/kg/dose q.i.d. or max 250 mg q.i.d. × 10 days	Liquid: 200, 400 mg/5 ml Chewables: 200 mg Tabs: 400 mg
Amoxicillin and clavulanic acid (Augmentin)	10–13 mg/kg/dose t.i.d. or 250 mg t.i.d. × 10 days	Liquid: 125, 250 mg/5 ml Tabs: 250 mg
Cephalexin monohydrate (Keflex)	10–13 mg/kg/dose t.i.d. or max 250 mg t.i.d. × 10 days	Liquid: 125, 250 mg/5 ml Caps 250, 500 mg
Clindamycin (Cleocin)	5–10 mg/kg/dose t.i.d. or 75 mg t.i.d. × 10 days	Liquid: 75 mg/5 ml Caps: 75, 150 mg
Rifampin (Rifadin, Rimactane)	10 mg/kg/dose q12h b.i.d. × 4 days	Caps: 150, 300 mg
Intramuscular Antibiotics		
Benzathine penicillin	<30 lb 300,000 U 31–60 lb 600,000 U >61–90 lb 900,000 U >90 lb 1,200,000 U	
Intravenous Antibiotics		
Penicillin G sodium	25,000 U/kg q4h	Vials: 5 million U
Clindamycin (Cleocin)	10 mg/kg/dose q8h	Vials: 0.15, 0.3, 0.6 g

proximately 5% of *S. pyogenes* are resistant to erythromycin. TMP-SMX is not an acceptable antibiotic to treat *S. pyogenes.*

E. Document *S. pyogenes* in a symptomatic patient following a course of therapy. If either compliance or the dose of antibiotic therapy is questionable, treat with IM penicillin; otherwise, treat with an antibiotic effective against β-lactamase-producing organisms (Augmentin or a cephalosporin). If this fails to eradicate the orga-

nism, consider a course of clindamycin or benzathine penicillin plus rifampin.

F. Attempt to eradicate the carrier state when the patient or another family member has frequent streptococcal infections or a history of rheumatic fever or glomerulonephritis. If the patient had three or more documented infections within 6 months, consider instituting daily penicillin prophylaxis during the winter strep throat season. Refer for tonsillectomy patients who continue to

(Continued on page 544)

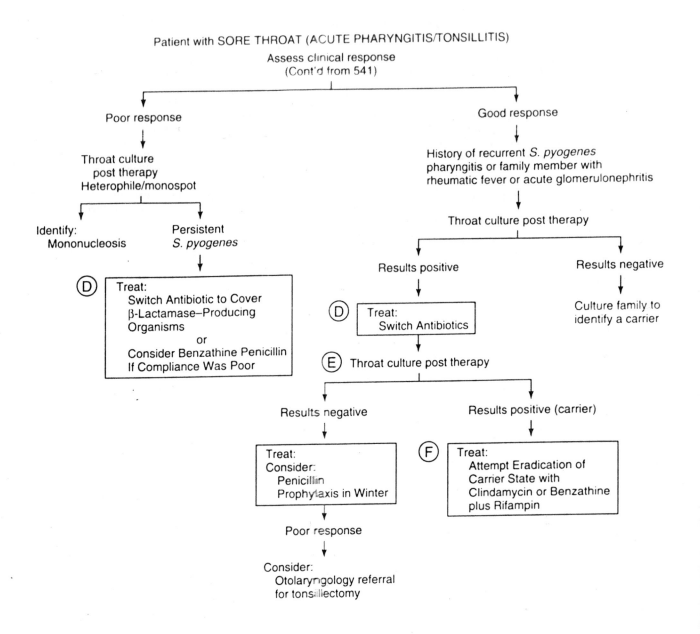

Patient with SORE THROAT (ACUTE PHARYNGITIS/TONSILLITIS)
Assess clinical response
(Cont'd from 541)

Poor response

Throat culture
post therapy
Heterophile/monospot

Identify:
Mononucleosis

Persistent
S. pyogenes

D | Treat:
Switch Antibiotic to Cover
β-Lactamase–Producing
Organisms
or
Consider Benzathine Penicillin
If Compliance Was Poor

Good response

History of recurrent *S. pyogenes*
pharyngitis or family member with
rheumatic fever or acute glomerulonephritis

Throat culture post therapy

Results positive

Results negative

Culture family to
identify a carrier

D | Treat:
Switch Antibiotics

E Throat culture post therapy

Results negative

Results positive (carrier)

Treat:
Consider:
Penicillin
Prophylaxis in Winter

F | Treat:
Attempt Eradication of
Carrier State with
Clindamycin or Benzathine
plus Rifampin

Poor response

Consider:
Otolaryngology referral
for tonsillectomy

have frequent episodes or when persistently enlarged tonsils result in chronic upper airway obstruction.

G. Treat patients hospitalized with tonsillitis or peritonsillar infection with IV benzyl penicillin. Failure to respond in 24 hours is an indication for needle aspiration. Pus indicates an abscess that may need incision and drainage. Consider adding clindamycin for better coverage of β-lactamase–producing anaerobes. Most patients do not need an acute or subsequent tonsillectomy, as the recurrence rate of peritonsillar abscess is low.

References

Denny FW. Tonsillopharyngitis 1994. Pediatr Rev 1994; 15:185.

Deutsch ES, Isaacson GC. Tonsils and adenoids: An update. Pediatr Rev 1995; 16:17.

Durbin WA, Sullivan JL. Epstein-Barr virus infection. Pediatr Rev 1994; 15:63.

Gerber MA, Markowitz M: Streptococcal pharyngitis: Clearing up the controversies. Contemp Pediatr (October) 1992; 9:118.

Levin RM, Grossman M, Jordan C, et al. Group A streptococcal infection in children younger than 3 years of age. Pediatr Infect Dis J 1988; 7:581.

Paradise JL, Bluestone CD, Bachman RZ, et al. Efficacy of tonsillectomy for recurrent throat infection in severely affected children. N Engl J Med 1984; 310:674.

Pichichero ME, Disney FA, Talpey WB. Adverse and beneficial effects of immediate treatment of group A β-hemolytic streptococcal pharyngitis with penicillin. Pediatr Infect Dis J 1987; 6:635.

Shulman ST, Gerber MA, Tanz RR, et al. Streptococcal pharyngitis: The case for penicillin therapy. Pediatr Infect Dis J 1994; 13:1.

Tanz RR, Shulman ST, Barthel MJ, et al. Penicillin plus rifampin eradicates pharyngeal carriage of group A streptococcus. J Pediatr 1985; 106:876.

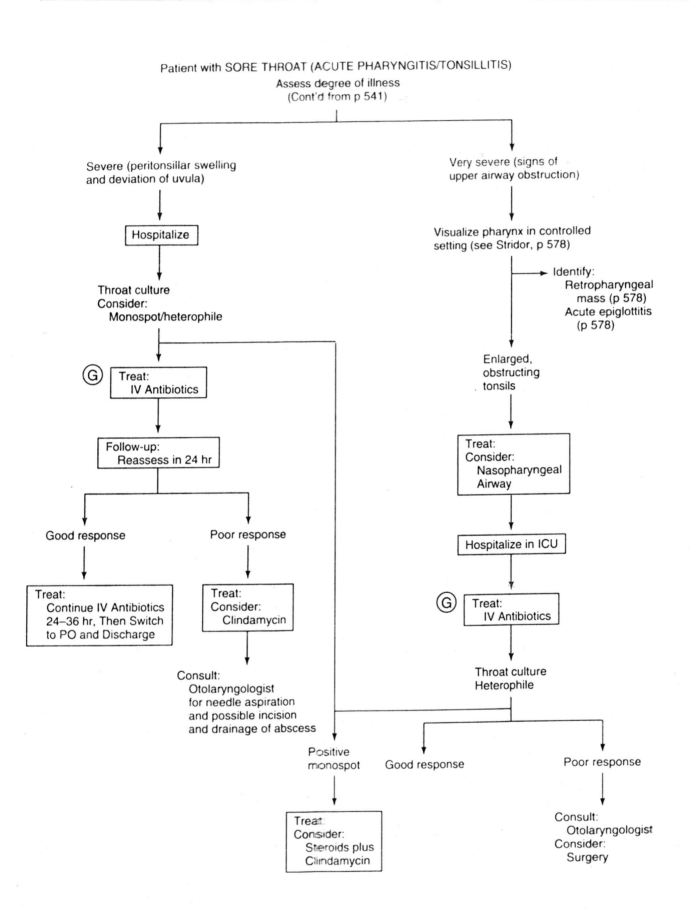

Patient with SORE THROAT (ACUTE PHARYNGITIS/TONSILLITIS)
Assess degree of illness
(Cont'd from p 541)

Severe (peritonsillar swelling and deviation of uvula)

Hospitalize

Throat culture
Consider:
    Monospot/heterophile

(G) Treat:
    IV Antibiotics

Follow-up:
    Reassess in 24 hr

Good response

Poor response

Treat:
    Continue IV Antibiotics
    24–36 hr, Then Switch
    to PO and Discharge

Treat:
Consider:
    Clindamycin

Consult:
    Otolaryngologist
    for needle aspiration
    and possible incision
    and drainage of abscess

Very severe (signs of upper airway obstruction)

Visualize pharynx in controlled setting (see Stridor, p 578)

Identify:
    Retropharyngeal
    mass (p 578)
    Acute epiglottitis
    (p 578)

Enlarged, obstructing tonsils

Treat:
Consider:
    Nasopharyngeal
    Airway

Hospitalize in ICU

(G) Treat:
    IV Antibiotics

Throat culture
Heterophile

Positive monospot

Good response

Poor response

Treat:
Consider:
    Steroids plus
    Clindamycin

Consult:
    Otolaryngologist
Consider:
    Surgery

545

PULMONARY DISORDERS

EVALUATION OF COUGH AND PULMONARY DISORDERS

Stephen Berman, M.D.

A. In the history ask the following: When did the cough begin? How long has the cough been present? Is it difficult for your child to breathe? Is there fast breathing? Wheezing? Is there chest indrawing with breathing? Has your child turned blue or appeared very pale? Did you notice any time when your child stopped breathing? Is your child too weak to feed or play? Has your child had seizures or convulsions? Ask about (1) the presence and duration of upper respiratory symptoms, including runny nose (color), nasal congestion, earache, ear drainage, sore throat, difficulty swallowing, and hoarseness; (2) systemic symptoms, including fever, headache, muscle aches, malaise, vomiting, and diarrhea; (3) current use of medications and allergies to medications; (4) underlying pulmonary cardiac, or immunodeficiency diseases such as reactive airway disease, bronchopulmonary dysplasia, cystic fibrosis, tracheomalacia, HIV infection, and congenital heart disease; and (5) immunization status. Ask about access to a telephone and transportation to the hospital and assess the ability of the family to manage the child at home.

B. During the physical examination count the respirations for 1 minute; look for agitation or restlessness, chest indrawing or retractions, cyanosis, pallor, nasal flaring, drooling, purulent rhinorrhea, and ear discharge; listen for hoarseness, stridor, wheezing, and grunting. With a stethoscope identify signs of (1) bronchiolitis or asthma (wheezing, poor air exchange, prolongation of the expiratory phase of respiration); (2) pneumonia (rales, crepitations, tubular or decreased breath sounds); and (3) cardiac disease such as an irregular heart rate (arrhythmia), abnormal heart sounds, a heart murmur, or a pericardial friction rub. Palpate and percuss the liver because hepatomegaly suggests right heart failure. Use pneumatic otoscopy to assess tympanic membrane color, mobility, and landmarks. Use a tongue blade to examine the pharynx and tonsils for size, exudate, ulcerations, and other lesions.

C. Mild illness has no bacterial upper respiratory tract infections and no findings of lower respiratory involvement (no rales, wheezing, retractions, stridor at rest, cyanosis, or apnea; with good air exchange and a respiratory rate <60/minute in infants <2 months, 50/minute in infants 2 to 12 months, and <40/minute in children over 12 months).

D. Moderate illness includes bacterial upper respiratory infections (acute otitis media, sinusitis, or *Streptococcus pyogenes* pharyngitis); and pneumonia or bronchiolitis without respiratory distress or signs of hypoxia.

E. Severe illness includes signs of respiratory distress such as stridor at rest, respiratory rate greater than 70/minute, marked retractions, cyanosis, grunting respirations, oxygen saturation under 90% to 92% (depending on the altitude) using pulse oximetry, radiographic findings of pleural fluid, abscess, pneumatoceles, or extensive infiltrate. Signs of respiratory distress in wheezing patients include poor response to inhaled bronchodilators with continued wheezing, high respiratory rate, marked retractions, poor air exchange, and oxygen desaturation. Radiographic findings of pleural fluid, abscess, pneumatoceles, or extensive infiltrate indicate severe bacterial disease. Signs of systemic toxicity include mental status changes (inability to feed or drink, lethargy and inability to arouse, disorientation) or dehydration with vascular instability (mottling, poor capillary refill, low blood pressure). Children at high risk for deterioration who need close follow-up not available at home include immunocompromised children, children with sickle cell disease, immunodeficiency disorders (steroid-treated or immunosuppressed children), severe malnutrition, underlying cardiac or pulmonary disease (especially premature infants with bronchopulmonary dysplasia), and premature infants less than 8 weeks of age with documented respiratory syncytial virus infection. Infants and children, early in the course of illness, living in families with little or no means of communication or transportation who are at risk for deterioration should be considered severe.

F. Signs of impending upper airway obstruction that signal very severe illness include stridor at rest with air hunger, restlessness, cyanosis, severe retractions, minimal air exchange, or a clinical presentation suggesting acute epiglottitis (severe sore throat with drooling, sniffing posture, muffled voice, red swollen epiglottis). Very severe illness includes respiratory arrest or signs of impending respiratory failure such as recurrent apnea, cyanosis unresponsive to oxygen (O_2), inability to maintain Pao_2 above 55 torr or O_2 saturation greater than 86% with Fio_2 greater than 80%, and inability to maintain Pco_2 below 50 torr.

References

Acute respiratory infections in children: Case management in small hospitals in developing countries. WHO/ARI/90.5. World Health Organization, Geneva, 1990.

Acute respiratory infections case management charts. World Health Organization Programme for Control of Acute Respiratory Infections, 1990.

Berman S. Epidemiology of acute respiratory infections in children of developing countries. Rev Infect Dis 1991; 13(Suppl 6):S454.

Berman S, Shanks MB, Feiten D, et al. Acute respiratory infections during the first three months of life: Clinical and physiologic predictors of etiology. Pediatr Emerg Care 1990; 6:179.

Simoes EAF, Roark R, Berman S, et al. Respiratory rate: Measurement variability over time and accuracy at different counting periods. Arch Dis Child 1991; 66:1199.

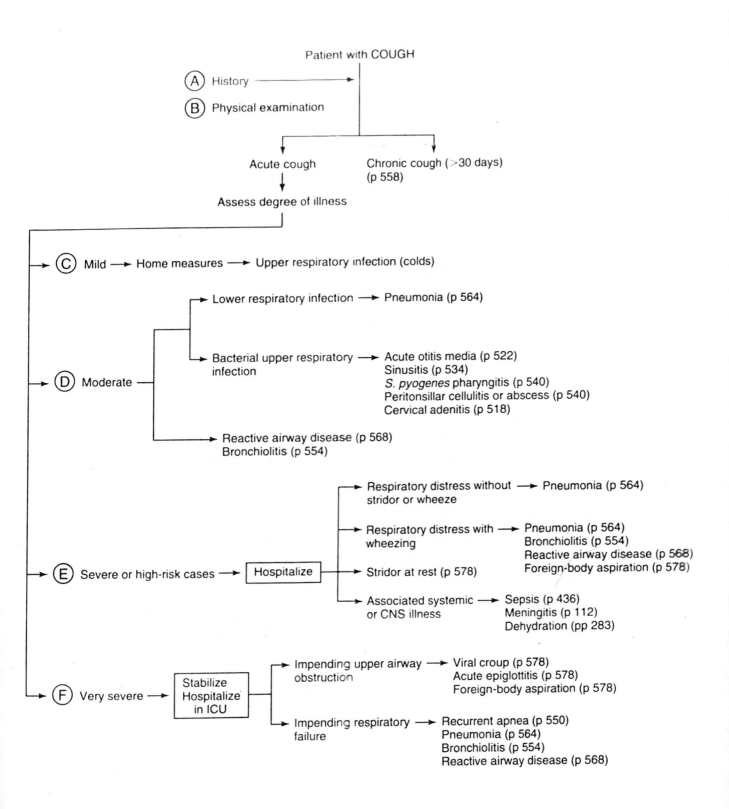

Patient with COUGH

(A) History
(B) Physical examination

Acute cough

Chronic cough (>30 days)
(p 558)

Assess degree of illness

(C) Mild → Home measures → Upper respiratory infection (colds)

(D) Moderate

→ Lower respiratory infection → Pneumonia (p 564)

→ Bacterial upper respiratory infection → Acute otitis media (p 522)
Sinusitis (p 534)
S. pyogenes pharyngitis (p 540)
Peritonsillar cellulitis or abscess (p 540)
Cervical adenitis (p 518)

→ Reactive airway disease (p 568)
Bronchiolitis (p 554)

(E) Severe or high-risk cases → Hospitalize

→ Respiratory distress without stridor or wheeze → Pneumonia (p 564)

→ Respiratory distress with wheezing → Pneumonia (p 564)
Bronchiolitis (p 554)
Reactive airway disease (p 568)
Foreign-body aspiration (p 578)

→ Stridor at rest (p 578)

→ Associated systemic or CNS illness → Sepsis (p 436)
Meningitis (p 112)
Dehydration (pp 283)

(F) Very severe → Stabilize Hospitalize in ICU

→ Impending upper airway obstruction → Viral croup (p 578)
Acute epiglottitis (p 578)
Foreign-body aspiration (p 578)

→ Impending respiratory failure → Recurrent apnea (p 550)
Pneumonia (p 564)
Bronchiolitis (p 554)
Reactive airway disease (p 568)

APNEA AND SUDDEN INFANT DEATH SYNDROME

Stephen Berman, M.D.

DEFINITIONS

Apnea is a failure to breathe spontaneously (exchange air) for 20 seconds or an episode without breathing associated with cyanosis, pallor, bradycardia (< 80 beats per minute), or loss of muscle tone. **Central apnea** (nonobstructive) occurs when inspiratory efforts and airflow are both absent. **Obstructive apnea** is present when inspiratory efforts fail to produce adequate air entry because of airway obstruction. **Periodic breathing** is three episodes of respiratory pauses of 3 seconds or longer within 1 minute separated by not more than 20 seconds of regular breathing. An **apparent life-threatening event (ALTE)** is characterized by apnea with color change, hypotonia, choking, or gagging, in which the observer fears the infant is dying. Resuscitation is often attempted. **Sudden infant death syndrome (SIDS)** is sudden death unexplained by history or a thorough postmortem examination. SIDS is thought to be caused by an alteration in the control of breathing presumed due to a brain stem maturational delay. Having infants sleep on their backs, rather than prone, appears to reduce the frequency of SIDS.

A. In the history determine onset, duration, frequency, pattern (relationship to feeding, crying, sleep), and severity (type of resuscitation required and degree of cyanosis, pallor, or hypotonia) of the apnea. Note symptoms suggestive of seizures such as muscle jerks, eye rolling, tongue thrusting, a postictal state, and frequent recurrences. Suspect breath holding spells if the child is awake and when spells are precipitated by crying, sudden pain, or fear and are associated with stiffening and/or clonus. With breath holding, cyanosis and hypotonia precede any abnormal movements, and there is no postictal state. Identify precipitating factors such as respiratory infection (respiratory syncytial virus [RSV], *Chlamydia*, pertussis), possible drug ingestion, head trauma, and predisposing conditions, including prematurity, heart disease, pulmonary disease (bronchopulmonary dysplasia, asthma), CNS disorders, mucopolysaccharidosis, hypothyroidism, congenital syndromes (Prader-Willi, Pierre Robin), and hematologic diseases causing severe anemia.

B. Perform a thorough examination: rapidly assess vital signs, respiratory status (air entry, respiratory rate, retractions, grunting), signs of shock (pulses, capillary refill, cold, mottled extremities), and neurologic status (mental state, fontanelle, seizures, focal neurologic signs, hypotonia, and fundi). More than 90% of infants with a history of apnea are asymptomatic. Note dysmorphic features or reasons for airway obstruction.

C. A barium swallow identifies gastric reflux, a vascular ring, or tracheoesophageal fistula. The role of gastric reflux as a cause of apnea of infancy is unclear, since gastroesophageal reflux in early infancy is common in children without apnea. Rarely, gastric reflux may result in laryngospasm. Refluxed gastric contents may stimulate upper airway or laryngeal receptors, producing apnea and bradycardia.

D. Diagnoses of upper airway obstruction include macroglossia (mucopolysaccharide syndromes, hypothyroidism), enlarged tonsils and/or adenoids, pharyngeal/retropharyngeal masses, Pierre Robin syndrome, choanal stenosis or atresia, epiglottitis, and supraglottic mass.

(Continued on page 552)

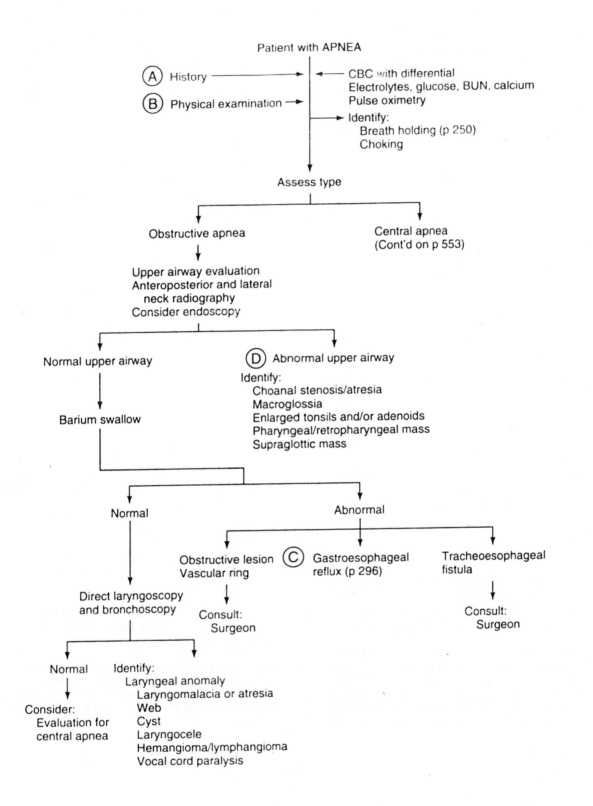

Patient with APNEA

Ⓐ History

Ⓑ Physical examination

CBC with differential
Electrolytes, glucose, BUN, calcium
Pulse oximetry
Identify:
   Breath holding (p 250)
   Choking

Assess type

Obstructive apnea

Central apnea
(Cont'd on p 553)

Upper airway evaluation
Anteroposterior and lateral
   neck radiography
Consider endoscopy

Normal upper airway

Ⓓ Abnormal upper airway
Identify:
   Choanal stenosis/atresia
   Macroglossia
   Enlarged tonsils and/or adenoids
   Pharyngeal/retropharyngeal mass
   Supraglottic mass

Barium swallow

Normal

Abnormal

Direct laryngoscopy
and bronchoscopy

Obstructive lesion
Vascular ring

Ⓒ Gastroesophageal
reflux (p 296)

Tracheoesophageal
fistula

Consult:
   Surgeon

Consult:
   Surgeon

Normal

Consider:
   Evaluation for
   central apnea

Identify:
   Laryngeal anomaly
      Laryngomalacia or atresia
      Web
      Cyst
      Laryngocele
      Hemangioma/lymphangioma
      Vocal cord paralysis

E. Medical evaluation reveals a cause of apnea in only 25% to 50% of cases. The initial laboratory screening tests should include electrolytes, glucose, BUN, calcium, and pulse oximetry. Additional work-up should be guided by the history and physical findings. A sleep study may distinguish obstructive from central apnea as well as assess the extent of hypoxia and degree of obstruction. The most frequent conditions identified in ALTE are GI (gastroesophageal reflux), 12%; seizures, 5%; pneumonia or bronchiolitis, 5%; metabolic disorders (hypocalcemia, hypothyroidism, hypoglycemia), 2%; aseptic meningitis or encephalitis, 1%; cardiac (ventricular septal defect, atrial septal defect, arrhythmias), 1%; anemia, less than 1%. The respiratory pathogens most frequently associated with apnea of infancy are RSV, *Chlamydia*, and pertussis. The risk of infection-induced apnea is highest in infants less than 3 months of age who were born prematurely.

F. The incidence of SIDS in the general population is 1.5 to 2 infant deaths per 1000 live births. Infants are at highest risk at 2 to 4 months of age; 91% of SIDS babies are less than 6 months of age. Prematurity, bronchopulmonary dysplasia, and infants of drug-addicted mothers (especially those addicted to cocaine) are at increased risk. Infants who have had a near-miss SIDS (ALTE requiring vigorous resuscitation) are at high risk for dying (25% to 30%). Siblings of SIDS victims have twice the relative risk of control infants. Pneumograms are not effective in prospective screening. Approximately 80% of SIDS babies have no identifiable risk factors or history of ALTE. Sleeping on the back appears to decrease the risk of SIDS, and exposure to passive smoking may increase the risk. Avoid allowing the infant to sleep on a soft pillow, beanbag, or sheepskin. Consider the possibility of child abuse in recurrent ALTE without an obvious cause.

G. Cardiorespiratory home monitoring is indicated for the following infants at high risk for SIDS: infants with an ALTE requiring mouth-to-mouth, bag resuscitation, or vigorous stimulation; symptomatic preterm infants; siblings of two or more SIDS victims; and infants with predisposing conditions such as central hypoventilation. The routine use of monitoring in infants with a less severe ALTE, those with tracheostomies, and infants of mothers who were opiate or cocaine abusers is controversial. A monitoring program should include a family assessment, anticipatory guidance, parental proficiency in cardiopulmonary resuscitation (CPR), written explanations, demonstration of competence with respect to monitor operation and troubleshooting, and 24 hour availability of support staff and equipment maintenance. Discontinue home monitoring if the infant has not had an ALTE during the preceding 2 to 3 months. Document the infant's ability to handle the stress of immunizations and upper respiratory infections prior to discontinuation.

H. Apnea of prematurity occurs in about 50% of infants less than 32 weeks of gestation. It presents as periodic breathing with apnea and usually resolves when the infant reaches a gestational age of 36 weeks. Theophylline to maintain a blood level of 5 to 10 μg/ml blood level reduces the frequency of episodes. Apnea of prematurity is not an independent risk factor for SIDS.

References

Consensus Statement. National Institutes of Health Consensus Development Conference on Infantile Apnea and Home Monitoring, September 29 to October 1, 1986. Pediatrics 1987; 79:292.

Dunne K, Matthews T. Near-miss sudden infant death syndrome: Clinical findings and management. Pediatrics 1987; 79:889.

Dwyer T, Ponsonby A-L, Blizzard L, et al. The contribution of changes in the prevalence of prone sleeping position to the decline in sudden infant death syndrome in Tasmania. JAMA 1995; 273:783.

Hunt CE, Brouillette RT. Sudden infant death syndrome: 1987 perspective. J Pediatr 1987; 110:669.

Klonoff-Cohen HS, Edelstein SL, Lefkowitz ES, et al. The effect of passive smoking and tobacco exposure through breast milk on sudden infant death syndrome. JAMA 1995; 273:795.

Lewis JM, Ganick DJ. Initial laboratory evaluation of infants with "presumed near-miss" sudden infant death syndrome. Am J Dis Child 1986; 140:484.

McCray PB, Crockett DM, Wagener JS, et al. Hypoxia and hypercapnia in infants with mild laryngomalacia. Am J Dis Child 1988; 142:896.

Oren J, Kelly D, Shannon DC. Identification of a high-risk group for sudden infant death syndrome among infants who were resuscitated for sleep apnea. Pediatrics 1986:495.

Smith RJH, Catlin FI. Congenital anomalies of the larynx. Am J Dis Child 1984; 138:35.

Symposium. Apnea and SIDS: A commonsense approach to the controversies. Contemp Pediatr 1986; August:25.

Taylor JA, Sanderson M. A reexamination of the risk factors for the sudden infant death syndrome. J Pediatr 1995; 126:887.

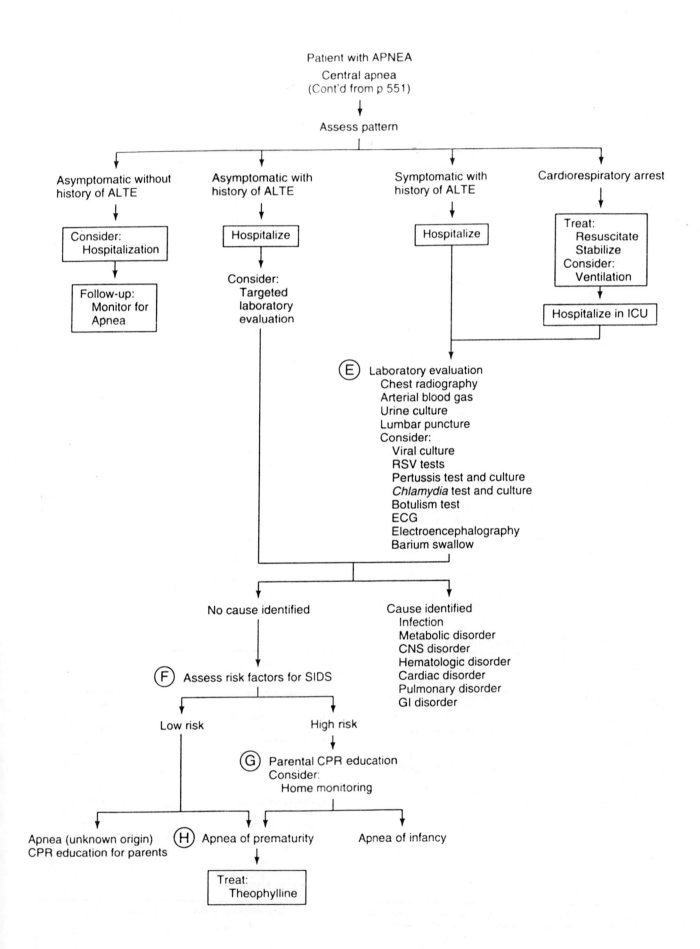

Patient with APNEA

Central apnea
(Cont'd from p 551)

↓

Assess pattern

Asymptomatic without history of ALTE

↓

Consider:
Hospitalization

↓

Follow-up:
Monitor for
Apnea

Asymptomatic with history of ALTE

↓

Hospitalize

↓

Consider:
Targeted
laboratory
evaluation

Symptomatic with history of ALTE

↓

Hospitalize

Cardiorespiratory arrest

↓

Treat:
Resuscitate
Stabilize
Consider:
Ventilation

↓

Hospitalize in ICU

(E) Laboratory evaluation
Chest radiography
Arterial blood gas
Urine culture
Lumbar puncture
Consider:
Viral culture
RSV tests
Pertussis test and culture
Chlamydia test and culture
Botulism test
ECG
Electroencephalography
Barium swallow

No cause identified

Cause identified
Infection
Metabolic disorder
CNS disorder
Hematologic disorder
Cardiac disorder
Pulmonary disorder
GI disorder

(F) Assess risk factors for SIDS

Low risk   **High risk**

↓

(G) Parental CPR education
Consider:
Home monitoring

Apnea (unknown origin)
CPR education for parents

(H) Apnea of prematurity

Apnea of infancy

↓

Treat:
Theophylline

BRONCHIOLITIS

Stephen Berman, M.D.

DEFINITION

Bronchiolitis is a clinical syndrome of infants and young children characterized by wheezing, retractions, and tachypnea. Inflammation of the bronchioles or small airways produces exudate, edema, necrosis, and bronchospasm, which results in air trapping, atelectasis, and ventilation-perfusion mismatch. The most common infectious agent causing bronchiolitis is respiratory syncytial virus (RSV). Other viral pathogens include parainfluenza viruses, influenza viruses, and adenovirus. Chlamydia is a common cause of this syndrome during the first 3 months of life. Rarely, bacterial agents, such as *Haemophilus influenzae* and *Bordetella pertussis*, can cause this clinical syndrome.

A. In the history ask when the cold and cough began. Is there fast breathing? Is it difficult for your child to breathe? Does the chest move in (chest indrawing) when your child breathes? Has your child stopped breathing or turned blue? Is your child too weak to eat or play? Has your child wheezed at other times? Does your child have asthma or heart or lung disease? Was your child born prematurely? Ask about access to a telephone and transportation.

B. In the physical examination look and listen. Count the respirations for 1 minute. In patients with bronchiolitis the respiratory rate correlates well with oxygenation. Respiratory rates above 70/minute indicate a Pao_2 of less than 55 torr. The risk of respiratory failure is also greater at rates over 70/minute. Look for retractions, cyanosis, pallor, and nasal flaring. Listen for grunting, wheezing, hoarseness, stridor, prolonged expiratory phase (the normal inspiration-to-expiration ratio is 2:1), poor air exchange, and rales (may be caused by atelectasis or pneumonia). Note signs of cardiac disease. Using a pneumatic otoscope, note tympanic membrane color, landmarks, and mobility. Acute otitis media is frequently associated with bronchiolitis.

C. Obtain chest films in patients with moderate to severe disease to identify pneumonia and confirm findings of viral bronchiolitis. The radiologic findings of bronchiolitis include hyperexpansion with flattened diaphragm, peribronchial thickening, and patchy atelectasis with or without perihilar infiltrate.

D. Pulse oximetry is a noninvasive technique to determine oxygen saturation. If possible, patients with signs of moderate to severe respiratory distress should be studied. Infants should be monitored before, during, and after feeding. Oxygen saturation below 94% at sea level or 90% at 5000 feet indicates a need for supplemental oxygen therapy.

E. There is no clinical value in obtaining specimens for identifying viral pathogens in children without severe respiratory distress or those not at high risk because of an underlying condition. In severe disease identification of RSV may influence the decision to use ribavirin or hyperimmune globulin. Two rapid viral diagnostic techniques for RSV are widely available: immunofluorescent staining and ELISA (enzyme-linked immunosorbent assay). Both techniques are performed using nasopharyngeal secretions that can be obtained by aspiration with either a Delee tube or small feeding tube attached to a syringe.

F. The many noninfectious causes of airway obstruction and wheezing include asthma, foreign body aspiration, tracheoesophageal fistula, neuromuscular disorders,

TABLE 1 Degree of Illness in Bronchiolitis

Mild	Moderate	Severe	Very Severe
Respiratory rate below thresholds (60 <2 mo, 50 2–12 mo, 40 >12 mo) and Good air exchange and Minimal or no retractions and No signs of dehydration	Respiratory rate elevated over thresholds or Moderate retractions or Prolonged expiratory phase with decreased air exchange	High-risk patients* or Respiratory rate >70/min or Marked retractions or Minimal (poor) air exchange or Grunting respirations or Oxygen saturation <94% at sea level or <90% at 5000 ft or Signs of dehydration or systemic toxicity	Apnea or respiratory arrest or Cyanosis on oxygen or Inability to maintain Pao_2 >50 torr with Fio_2 >80% or Inability to maintain Pco_2 <55 torr or Signs of shock

*High-risk patients are premature infants less than 12 weeks of age (postnatal) and children with congenital heart disease, bronchopulmonary dysplasia, other chronic lung disease, neuromuscular condition, or immunodeficiency disorder.

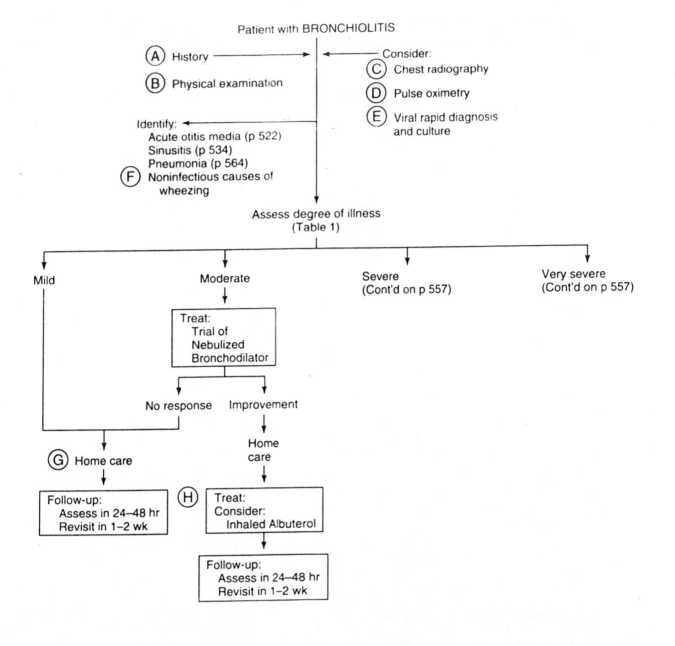

Patient with BRONCHIOLITIS

(A) History

(B) Physical examination

Consider:
(C) Chest radiography
(D) Pulse oximetry
(E) Viral rapid diagnosis and culture

Identify:
Acute otitis media (p 522)
Sinusitis (p 534)
Pneumonia (p 564)
(F) Noninfectious causes of wheezing

Assess degree of illness
(Table 1)

Mild

Moderate

Severe
(Cont'd on p 557)

Very severe
(Cont'd on p 557)

Treat:
Trial of
Nebulized
Bronchodilator

No response   Improvement

Home
care

(G) Home care

Follow-up:
Assess in 24–48 hr
Revisit in 1–2 wk

(H) Treat:
Consider:
Inhaled Albuterol

Follow-up:
Assess in 24–48 hr
Revisit in 1–2 wk

gastroesophageal reflux, structural airway defects (tracheobronchomalacia and bronchial stenosis), and causes of extrinsic compression of the airway such as anomalies of the great vessels and malformation of the lungs (sequestrations, bronchiogenic cysts, and teratomas). Children with chronic lung diseases, such as cystic fibrosis, bronchopulmonary dysplasia, and bronchiectasis, have wheezing without infection. However, these children often have more severe bronchiolitis with infection.

G. Home measures include encouraging the child to drink liquids and eat normally. Discourage the use of antihistamine-decongestant mixtures, especially for infants under 18 months. Educate parents to return if their child develops fast breathing, chest indrawing (retractions), blue color (cyanosis), fever, or becomes too weak to eat.

H. It may be worthwhile to try nebulized albuterol (Table 2). Data assessing the effectiveness of albuterol and other β_2-agonists in treating bronchiolitis are conflicting. It is likely that fewer than half of children with viral bronchiolitis respond to this therapy. It is important to assess each child individually for signs of improvement such as decreased wheezing, less-marked retractions, better air exchange, decreased respiratory rate, increased oxygen saturation, and a more comfortable appearance. Corticosteroids should be reserved for hospitalized children with hypoxia that fails to resolve with oxygen and albuterol nebulizations. Mist tents provide no benefit and impede interaction with and evaluation of the patient. Do not routinely administer antibiotics to children with bronchiolitis. Their use should be reserved for children with signs of systemic toxicity (inability to feed, lethargy, difficulty in arousal) or severe respiratory distress and hypoxia. These children are at risk for mixed

TABLE 2 Albuterol Therapy for Bronchiolitis in Children

Route of Delivery	Dosage	Dosing Intervals	Product Availability
Oral	0.1–0.15 mg/kg/ dose (max 4 mg)	q4–6h	Syrup: 2 mg/ 5 ml Tabs: 2, 4 mg SR tabs: 4 mg
Aerosol		—	
MDI	180 μg/2 puffs	q4–6h	200 puffs/ canister
Nebulized	0.1–0.15 mg/kg/ neb (max 5 mg)	q4–6h	5 mg/1 ml sol 0.83 mg/1 ml sol

viral bacterial infections and need antibiotic treatment to prevent rapid clinical deterioration.

I. Ribavirin is a synthetic nucleoside that limits replication of RSV within the cell. It can be given only by aerosol through a small-particle generator into a mist tent or respirator. Proper filters must be placed on the respirator to prevent plugging and respirator malfunction. Ribavirin therapy is administered 12 to 18 hours a day for 3 to 7 days. Possible indications for use are very severe respiratory distress with impending respiratory failure and high-risk patients with congenital heart disease, bronchopulmonary dysplasia, other chronic lung diseases, neuromuscular conditions, or immunodeficiency disorders. The efficacy of ribavirin in ventilated patients is unclear. Hyperimmune RSV immune globulin has been approved to prevent very severe RSV disease in high-risk patients.

J. Apnea may be a presenting sign of bronchiolitis. It usually occurs early in the course of the infection. Apnea complicates 20% to 25% of cases of RSV bronchiolitis. Infants less than 3 months of age who were born prematurely are at the greatest risk. The mechanism of the disorder is unclear, although it appears to correlate with the degree of hypoxemia. Recurrent or prolonged apnea may present without obvious signs of respiratory distress but still require intubation and assisted ventilation for 24 to 48 hours.

K. Children may be discharged from the hospital when respiratory distress has resolved. Consider discharge on home oxygen when oxygen saturation remains low, but the patient is afebrile, eating well, and appropriately active. A follow-up visit should be scheduled 24 to 48 hours after discharge. Consider a visiting nurse. Parents should be taught to call the physician immediately if signs of respiratory distress (fast breathing or chest indrawing) return.

References

Bruhn FW, Mokrohisky ST, McIntosh K. Apnea associated with respiratory syncytial virus infection in young infants. J Pediatr 1977; 90:777.

Gadomski AM, Aref GH, El Din OB, et al. Oral versus nebulized albuterol in the management of bronchiolitis in Egypt. J Pediatr 1994; 124:131.

Groothius J, Simoes EAF, Hemming VG, et al. Respiratory syncytial virus (RSV) infection in preterm infants and the protective effects of RSV immune globulin (RSVIG). Pediatrics 1995; 95:463.

Hall CB, Powell KR, Schnabel KC, et al. Risk of secondary bacterial infection in infants hospitalized with respiratory syncytial viral infection. J Pediatr 1988; 113:266.

Klassen TP, Rowe PC, Sutcliffe T, et al. Randomized trial of salbutamol in acute bronchiolitis. J Pediatr 1991; 118:807.

Meert KL, Sarnaik AP, Gelmini MJ, Lieh-Lai MW. Aerosolized ribavirin in mechanically ventilated children with respiratory syncytial virus lower respiratory tract disease: A prospective, double-blind, randomized trial. Crit Care Med 1994; 22:566.

Menon K, Sutcliffe T, Klassen TP. A randomized trial comparing the efficacy of epinephrine with salbutamol in the treatment of acute bronchiolitis. J Pediatr 1995; 126:1004.

Sanchez I, De Koster J, Powell RE, et al. Effect of racemic epinephrine and salbutamol on clinical score and pulmonary mechanics in infants with bronchiolitis. J Pediatr 1993; 122:145.

Schuh S, Johnson D, Canny G, et al. Efficacy of adding nebulized ipratropium bromide to nebulized albuterol therapy in acute bronchiolitis. Pediatrics 1992; 90:920.

Shaw KN, Bell LM, Sherman NH. Outpatient assessment of infants with bronchiolitis. Am J Dis Child 1991; 145:151.

Wang EL, Law BJ, Stephens D, et al. Pediatric Investigators Collaborative Network on Infections in Canada (PICNIC) prospective study of risk factors and outcomes in patients hospitalized with respiratory syncytial viral lower respiratory tract infections. J Pediatr 1995; 126:212.

Wang EL, Milner R, Allen U, et al. Bronchodilators for treatment of mild bronchiolitis: A factorial randomised trial. Arch Dis Child 1992; 67:289.

Weiliver RC, Wong DT, Middleton E, et al. Role of parainfluenza virus–specific IgE in pathogenesis of croup and wheezing subsequent to infection. J Pediatr 1982; 101:889.

Wright PE. Bronchiolitis. Pediatr Rev 1986; 7:29.

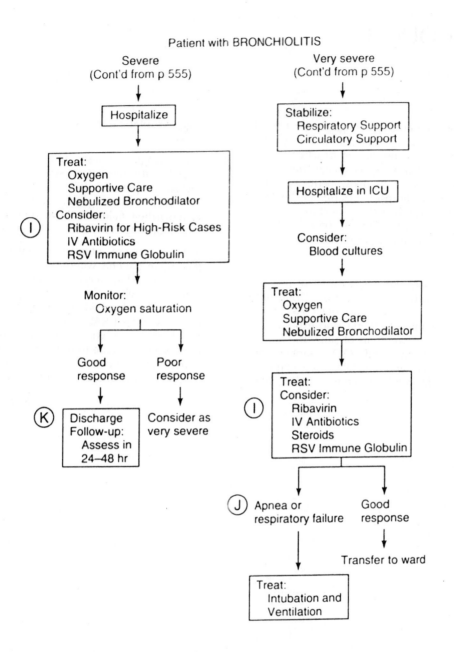

Patient with BRONCHIOLITIS

Severe
(Cont'd from p 555)

↓

Hospitalize

↓

(I) Treat:
Oxygen
Supportive Care
Nebulized Bronchodilator
Consider:
Ribavirin for High-Risk Cases
IV Antibiotics
RSV Immune Globulin

↓

Monitor:
Oxygen saturation

Good response → (K) Discharge Follow-up: Assess in 24–48 hr

Poor response → Consider as very severe

Very severe
(Cont'd from p 555)

↓

Stabilize:
Respiratory Support
Circulatory Support

↓

Hospitalize in ICU

↓

Consider:
Blood cultures

↓

Treat:
Oxygen
Supportive Care
Nebulized Bronchodilator

↓

(I) Treat:
Consider:
Ribavirin
IV Antibiotics
Steroids
RSV Immune Globulin

(J) Apnea or respiratory failure → Treat: Intubation and Ventilation

Good response → Transfer to ward

CHRONIC COUGH

Stephen Berman, M.D.

Children with a history of persistent cough longer than 4 weeks' duration need a thorough evaluation. The type of cough may suggest the cause: productive (reactive airway disease [RAD], infection), brassy (habit cough, tracheitis), barky (croup), paroxysmal (foreign body, pertussis, *Chlamydia, Mycoplasma,* cystic fibrosis), bizarre, or honking (psychogenic). The pattern can be helpful: nocturnal (sinusitis, RAD), early morning (cystic fibrosis, bronchiectasis), exercise-induced (RAD, cystic fibrosis, bronchiectasis), absent during sleep (habit cough).

A. In the history ask about the onset, duration, precipitating factors and pattern of the cough. Distinguish recurrent episodes from continuous cough. Ask about child care, family history of asthma, and exposure to passive smoking. Note symptoms of sinusitis, chronic rhinitis, atopic conditions, and RAD. Examine the upper airway carefully and auscultate the chest to identify wheezing, differential air entry, or rales. Note digital clubbing (chronic hypoxia, cystic fibrosis, heart disease).

B. Rapid diagnostic tests and culture techniques are available for respiratory syncytial virus (RSV), *Chlamydia,* and pertussis. Pertussis cultures should be done on special charcoal agar. Perform a sweat test in patients with diarrhea, failure to thrive, or a history of recurrent respiratory infections (acute otitis, sinusitis, pneumonia).

C. Institute a trial of antiinflammatory and bronchodilator therapy in patients without an upper respiratory tract disorder who have a normal chest film. RAD that causes chronic cough without wheezing is often exercise induced. In older children pre- and postexercise spirometry may suggest RAD. Patients who fail to respond to this therapy and who have associated systemic symptoms, such as failure to thrive, recurrent infections, recurrent fever, stridor, or wheezing, should have a sweat test, sinus films, and/or a barium swallow.

(Continued on page 560)

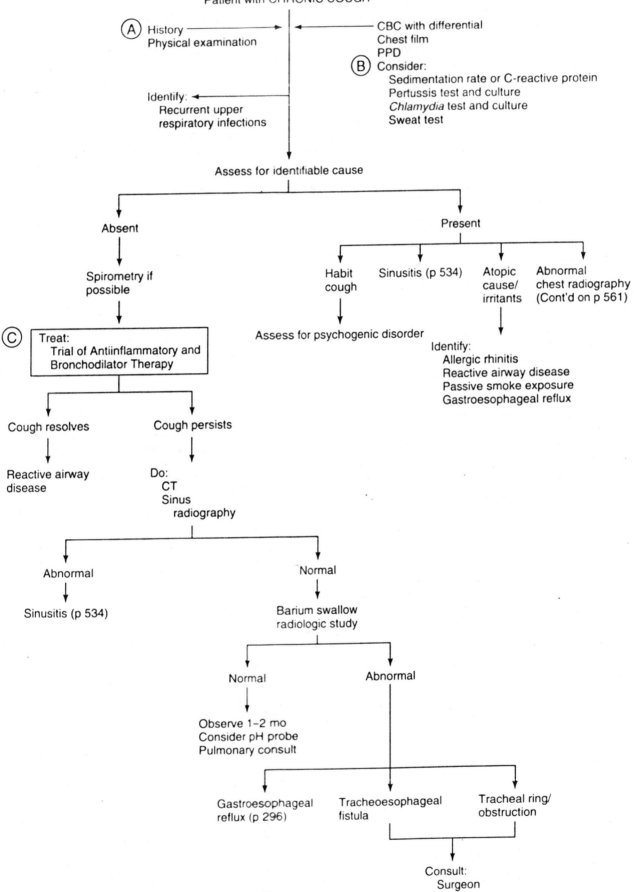

Patient with CHRONIC COUGH

(A) History
Physical examination

CBC with differential
Chest film
PPD
(B) Consider:
  Sedimentation rate or C-reactive protein
  Pertussis test and culture
  Chlamydia test and culture
  Sweat test

Identify:
  Recurrent upper
  respiratory infections

Assess for identifiable cause

Absent

Present

Spirometry if
possible

(C) Treat:
  Trial of Antiinflammatory and
  Bronchodilator Therapy

Cough resolves

Cough persists

Reactive airway
disease

Do:
CT
Sinus
  radiography

Abnormal

Normal

Sinusitis (p 534)

Barium swallow
radiologic study

Normal

Abnormal

Observe 1–2 mo
Consider pH probe
Pulmonary consult

Gastroesophageal
reflux (p 296)

Tracheoesophageal
fistula

Tracheal ring/
obstruction

Consult:
  Surgeon

Habit
cough

Sinusitis (p 534)

Atopic
cause/
irritants

Abnormal
chest radiography
(Cont'd on p 561)

Assess for psychogenic disorder

Identify:
  Allergic rhinitis
  Reactive airway disease
  Passive smoke exposure
  Gastroesophageal reflux

D. Investigate diffuse pulmonary infiltrates for infection with skin tests; rapid diagnostic tests; and cultures for bacterial disease (tuberculosis, pertussis, *Mycoplasma pneumonia,* and *Chlamydia*), fungal disease (*Monilia,* histoplasmosis, coccidioidomycosis), parasitic disease *(Pneumocystis, Echinococcus);* and viral infections (RSV, cytomegalovirus, adenovirus, influenza, parainfluenza). Obtain a pulmonary function consultation to diagnose restrictive lung disease. Consider bronchoalveolar lavage (BAL), brush biopsy, or open-lung biopsy to diagnose noninfectious causes such as hypersensitivity pneumonitis (exposure to organic antigens), pulmonary hemosiderosis, pulmonary alveolar proteinoses, fibrosing alveolitis, and Goodpasture syndrome. Laryngotracheoesophageal cleft is a rare condition that presents with choking and coughing during feedings, repeated aspiration pneumonia, and chronic cough with respiratory distress. Endoscopic diagnosis is difficult but better than radiographic studies.

E. Causes of bronchiectasis include cystic fibrosis, immunodeficiency syndrome, Kartagener syndrome, and chronic infection (pertussis, necrotizing adenovirus, measles).

F. The work-up for mediastinal masses includes a CT scan, possibly tomography, and a surgical consultation for thoracotomy or mediastinoscopy. The most common masses (and their usual location in the mediastinum) are neurogenic tumors (33%, posterior), lymphoma (14%, anterior or middle), teratoma (10%, anterior), thymic lesion (9%, anterior), bronchiogenic cyst (7.5%, middle), angioma (7%, anterior), duplication cyst (7%, posterior), and lymph node infection (4%, middle).

G. Causes of pulmonary mass include pulmonary sequestration, bronchiogenic cysts, eventration of the diaphragm, cystic adenomatoid malformation, lung abscess, massive atelectasis, and tumor. Work up a pulmonary mass with tomography, CT scan, and fluoroscopy. Consider skin tests, bronchoscopy, and angiography.

H. Work up chest radiography findings of tracheal deviation, local infiltrate, or local hyperexpansion with additional studies to diagnose a foreign body, infection, or mass lesion obstructing the airway (intrinsic or extrinsic obstruction). Consider bronchoscopy when a foreign body or obstructing mass is suspected. Manage patients with suspected local infection with a trial of antibiotic therapy combined with postural drainage.

References

Esclamado RM, Richardson MA. Laryngotracheal foreign bodies in children: A comparison with bronchial foreign bodies. Am J Dis Child 1987; 141:259.

McVeagh P, Howman-Giles R, Kemp A. Pulmonary aspiration studies by radionuclide milk scanning and barium swallow roentgenography. Am J Dis Child 1987; 141:917.

Morgan WJ, Taussig LM. The child with persistent cough. Pediatr Rev 1987; 8:249.

Parrillo SJ. Cough variant asthma. Pediatr Emerg Care 1986; 2:97.

Shuper A, Mukamel M, Mimouni M, et al. Psychogenic cough. Arch Dis Child 1983; 58:745.

Wilmott RW. Pursuing the cause of persistent cough. Contemp Pediatr 1987; 4:26.

Wolfson PJ, Schloss MD, Guttman FM, Nguyen L. Laryngotracheoesophageal cleft: An easily missed malformation. Arch Surg 1984; 119:228.

Wood RE, Postma D. Endoscopy of the airway in infants and children. J Pediatr 1988; 112:1.

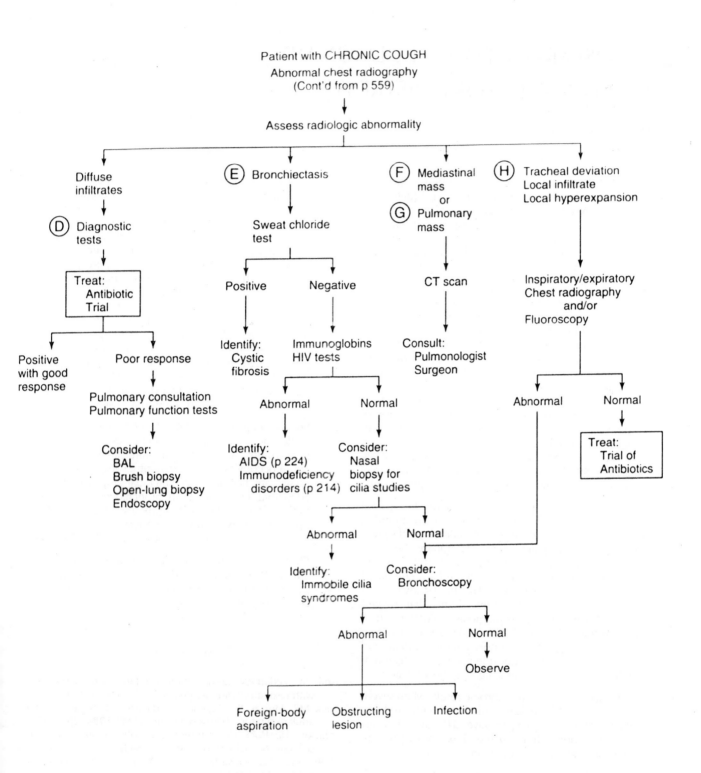

Patient with CHRONIC COUGH
Abnormal chest radiography
(Cont'd from p 559)

↓

Assess radiologic abnormality

Diffuse infiltrates

(D) Diagnostic tests
↓

Treat:
Antibiotic Trial

Positive with good response | Poor response
↓
Pulmonary consultation
Pulmonary function tests
↓
Consider:
BAL
Brush biopsy
Open-lung biopsy
Endoscopy

(E) **Bronchiectasis**
↓
Sweat chloride test

Positive | Negative

Identify: Cystic fibrosis | Immunoglobins HIV tests

Abnormal | Normal

Identify: AIDS (p 224) Immunodeficiency disorders (p 214) | Consider: Nasal biopsy for cilia studies

Abnormal | Normal

Identify: Immobile cilia syndromes | Consider: Bronchoscopy

Abnormal | Normal
↓
Observe

Foreign-body aspiration | Obstructing lesion | Infection

(F) **Mediastinal mass**
or
(G) **Pulmonary mass**
↓
CT scan
↓
Consult:
Pulmonologist
Surgeon

(H) **Tracheal deviation
Local infiltrate
Local hyperexpansion**
↓
Inspiratory/expiratory
Chest radiography
and/or
Fluoroscopy

Abnormal | Normal

Treat:
Trial of Antibiotics

CYANOSIS RELATED TO PULMONARY DISEASE/RESPIRATORY DISTRESS

Stephen Berman, M.D.

Cyanosis related to pulmonary disease can be produced by alveolar hypoventilation, ventilation perfusion inequality, and impairment of oxygen diffusion. Cyanosis is related to the presence of 3 g or more of reduced hemoglobin/100 ml. It is best detected by examining the lips, tongue, and mucous membranes. Peripheral cyanosis related to slow blood flow and large differences in arteriovenous oxygen are often present in the hands, feet, and circumoral areas.

A. Count the respirations for 1 minute. Respiratory rate thresholds are 60/minute in infants less than 2 months old, 50/minute in those 2 to 12 months, and 40/minute in those older than 12 months. Note agitation or restlessness, chest indrawing (retractions), use of accessory muscles, cyanosis, pallor, nasal flaring, and grunting. With a stethoscope listen for wheezing, rales, poor air exchange, tubular breath sounds (suggest consolidation), and prolongation of the expiratory phase of respiration. Note signs of cardiac disease such as an irregular heart rate, gallop, heart murmur, and friction rub. Palpate and percuss the liver (hepatomegaly suggests right heart failure). Absent bowel sounds may suggest ileus, commonly seen with bilateral pneumonia.

B. The arterial blood gas (ABG) measures the partial pressure of dissolved oxygen in blood. The relationship between the ABG and oxygen saturation is displayed in the oxygen dissociation curve. Pulmonary disease is suggested when the administration of 100% oxygen results in a substantial increase in the Pao_2 compared with a gas obtained in room air. The shunt study is useful in identifying fixed right-to-left shunts that suggest cardiac disease or marked pulmonary hypertension. A Pao_2 less than 55 torr on 80% to 100% oxygen or a Pco_2 over 50 torr suggests respiratory failure. Intubate and ventilate these children. Consider the use of sedation or paralysis when the patient is fighting the ventilator.

C. Adult respiratory distress syndrome results when severe damage to the capillary endothelial cells reduces surfactant levels, causing massive atelectasis. Use assisted ventilation with positive end-expiratory pressure to maintain adequate oxygenation.

D. Pulmonary edema results from circulatory overload, decreased oncotic pressure (hypoproteinemia), or capillary damage and leak. Capillary damage can result from a direct pulmonary insult such as a toxic inhalation, near drowning, or a systemic process such as shock, anoxia, or overwhelming sepsis. CNS disorders, such as meningitis, encephalitis, and mass lesions (hematoma, tumor, intracranial hemorrhage), can also produce pulmonary edema. Circulatory overload secondary to renal failure, the syndrome of inappropriate antidiuretic hormone, or water intoxication can cause pulmonary edema. High-altitude pulmonary edema (HAPE) occurs in children and adolescents who live at low altitude and travel above 8500 feet, in residents of high-altitude areas who return home from low altitudes, and in residents of high-altitude areas who develop a viral upper respiratory infection. Clinical signs include dyspnea, cough, periodic breathing, and frothy sputum. Pulmonary edema seen on the x-ray film may be only right-sided with basilar involvement. Manage patients with oxygen and return them to a lower altitude.

E. Space-occupying pulmonary lesions with air leak include pneumothorax, pneumomediastinum, pneumopericardium, and pulmonary interstitial emphysema. Space-occupying lesions without air leaks include diaphragmatic hernia, congenital lobar emphysema, cystic adenomatoid malformation, bronchiogenic cysts, eventration of the diaphragm, lung abscess, and tumor. Work up a pulmonary mass with tomograms and a CT scan. Consider fluoroscopy, bronchoscopy, and angiography.

F. Obstructive lesions of the upper airway include choanal atresia, Pierre Robin syndrome, vocal cord paralysis, stenosis of the trachea, vascular rings, foreign body, and congenital webs and cysts.

References

Anas NG, Perkin RM. Resuscitation and stabilization of the child with respiratory disease. Pediatr Ann 1986; 15:43.

Flick MR, Murray JF. High-dose corticosteroid therapy in the adult respiratory distress syndrome. JAMA 1984; 251:1054.

Johnson TS, Rock PB. Current concepts: Acute mountain sickness. N Engl J Med 1988; 319:841.

Weinberger SE, Schwartzstein RM, Weiss JW. Hypercapnia. N Engl J Med 1989; 321:1223.

Weisman IM, Rinaldo JE, Rogers RM. Current concepts: Positive end-expiratory pressure in adult respiratory failure. N Engl J Med 1982; 307:1381.

Patient with CYANOSIS RELATED TO PULMONARY DISEASE/RESPIRATORY DISTRESS

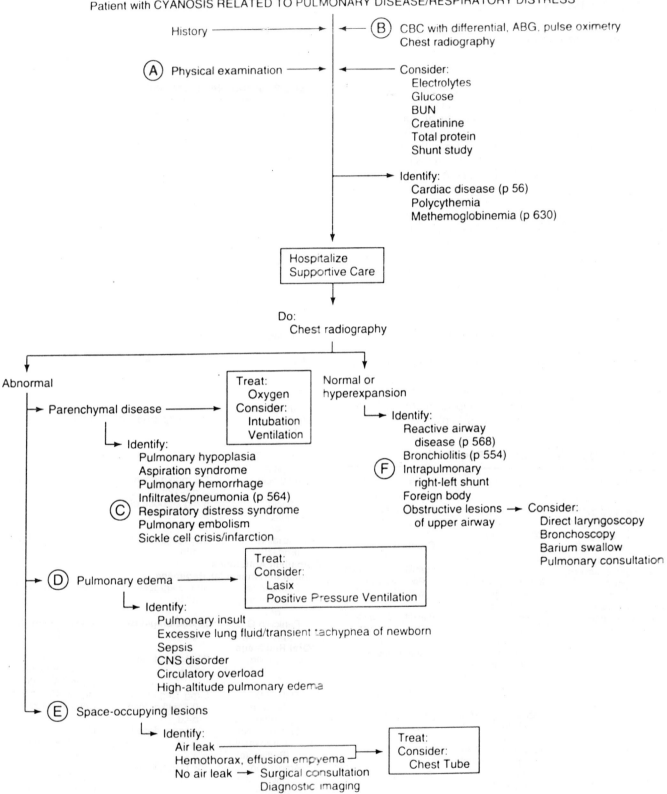

PNEUMONIA

Stephen Berman, M.D.

Pneumonia, or inflammation of the alveoli and/or interstitial space, results from viral and bacterial infections. Viral infections are more common, but bacterial infections are usually more severe. The pathogens that cause most pneumonia in early infancy (younger than 3 months) are respiratory syncytial virus (RSV), *Chlamydia*, group B streptococcus, parainfluenza viruses, and *Bordetella pertussis*. Less common bacterial pathogens in early infancy include *Streptococcus pneumoniae*, *Staphylococcus aureus*, *Haemophilus influenzae*, *Streptococcus pyogenes*, and gram-negative enteric bacteria. Viral respiratory pathogens, especially influenza virus, often infect older children and adolescents. The common bacterial agents in the older group are *Mycoplasma pneumoniae*, *S. pneumoniae*, and *H. influenzae*. Influenza virus infection predisposes to bacterial pneumonia, but the risk of secondary bacterial pneumonia with other viral infections is unclear.

A. In the history ask the following: When did the cough begin? How long has it been present? Is it difficult for your child to breathe? Is there fast breathing? Wheezing? Chest indrawing with breathing? Has your child turned blue or appeared very pale? Did you notice any time when your child may have stopped breathing? Is your child too weak to eat? Too weak to play? Has your child

TABLE 1 Degree of Illness in Pneumonia

Moderate	Severe	Very Severe
RR elevated over thresholds and No O$_2$ desaturation and No signs of severe dehydration and No alterations in mental status	High-risk patient* or RR >70/min or Marked retractions or Minimal (poor) air exchange or Grunting respirations or O$_2$ saturation <94% at sea level or 90% at 5000 ft or Signs of severe dehydration or Radiographic findings of a complicated pneumonia†	Apnea or respiratory arrest or Cyanosis on O$_2$ or Inability to maintain Pao$_2$ >50 torr with Fio$_2$ >80% or Inability to maintain Pco$_2$ <55 torr or Signs of shock

*High-risk patients are premature infants less than 12 weeks of age (postnatal) and children with congenital heart disease, bronchopulmonary dysplasia, other chronic lung disease, or neuromuscular or immunodeficiency disorder. Patients whose family has no phone or car may also be considered high risk.
†Radiographic findings of complicated pneumonia include pleural effusion, abscess, pneumatocoeles, and extensive consolidation.
RR, respiratory rate.

TABLE 2 Antibiotic Treatment of Children with Pneumonia

Antibiotic	Dosage	Product Availability
Cefotaxime (Claforan) or	50 mg/kg/dose IV q8h	Vials: 0.5, 1, 2 g
Ceftriaxone (Rocephin) or	50 mg/kg/dose IV q12h	Vials: 0.25, 0.5, 1 g
Chloramphenicol or	25 mg/kg/dose q6h	Vials: 1 g
Ampicillin plus	50 mg/kg/dose q6h	Vials: 0.25, 0.5, 1, 2, 4 g
Gentamicin	2.5 mg/kg/dose IV q8h	Vials: 20, 80 mg
Suspected S. aureus Add: nafcillin or	25 mg/kg/dose IV q6h	Vials: 0.5, 1, 2 g
Methicillin	50 mg/kg/dose IV q6h	Vials: 1, 4, 6 g
Suspected P. aeruginosa Mezlocillin (Mezlin) or	50 mg/kg/dose q6h	Vials: 1, 2, 3, 4 g
Ticarcillin (Ticar) plus	50 mg/kg/dose q6h	Vials: 1, 3, 6 g
Gentamicin or	2.5 mg/kg/dose q8–12h	Vials: 20, 80 mg
Amikacin (Amikin) or	5 mg/kg/dose q8h	Vials: 0.1, 0.5, 1 g
Ceftazidime (Fortaz)	50 mg/kg/dose IV q8h	Vials: 0.5, 1, 2 g
Outpatient Antibiotics **Initial Intramuscular Regimens** Ceftriaxone (Rocephin) or	50 mg/kg/dose IM q24h	Vials: 0.25, 0.5, 1 g
Penicillin G (procaine)	25,000 U/kg/dose q24h	Vials: 0.3, 0.6, 1, 2, 4 g
Oral Regimens Amoxicillin	20 mg/kg/dose t.i.d.	Liquid: 125, 250 mg/5 ml Caps: 250, 500 mg
TMP-SMX (Bactrim, Septra)	5 mg T/kg or 0.5 ml/kg/dose b.i.d.	Liquid: 40 mg/5 ml Caps: 80, 160 mg
Erythromycin/ sulfisoxazole (Pediazole)	10 mg/kg/dose E q.i.d.	Liquid: 200 mg (E) and 600 mg (S)/5 ml
Amoxicillin/ clavulanate (Augmentin)	10–15 mg/kg/dose t.i.d.	Liquid: 125, 250 mg/5 ml Caps: 250, 500 mg

(Continued on page 566)

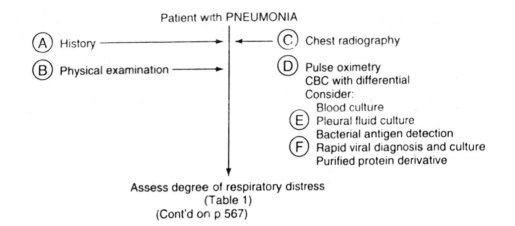

Patient with PNEUMONIA

(A) History ⟶
(B) Physical examination ⟶

(C) Chest radiography ⟵
(D) Pulse oximetry
    CBC with differential
    Consider:
      Blood culture
(E) Pleural fluid culture
    Bacterial antigen detection
(F) Rapid viral diagnosis and culture
    Purified protein derivative

Assess degree of respiratory distress
(Table 1)

(Cont'd on p 567)

had seizures or convulsions? Does your child have a runny nose (color of discharge), nasal congestion, earache, ear drainage, sore throat, difficulty swallowing, or hoarseness? Ask about systematic symptoms, including fever, headache, muscle aches, malaise, vomiting, and diarrhea. Note current use of medications and allergies to medications. Document underlying pulmonary, cardiac, or immunodeficiency diseases such as reactive airway disease, bronchopulmonary dysplasia, cystic fibrosis, tracheomalacia, and congenital heart disease. Ask about immunization status. Evaluate the family situation and note the availability of a telephone and car and the ability of the family to manage the child at home.

B. In the physical examination identify children likely to have pneumonia and assess the severity of illness with respect to oxygen desaturation and bacteremia. Count the respirations for 1 minute. Respiratory rate (RR) thresholds are 60/minute in infants less than 2 months old, 50/minute in infants 2 to 12 months old, and 40/minute in children older than 12 months. Note agitation or restlessness, chest indrawing (retractions), use of accessory muscles, cyanosis, pallor, nasal flaring, and grunting. With a stethoscope listen for wheezing, rales, poor air exchange, tubular breath sounds (suggest consolidation), and prolongation of the expiratory phase of respiration. Note signs of cardiac disease such as an irregular heart rate, gallop, heart murmur, and friction rub. Palpate and percuss the liver (hepatomegaly suggests right heart failure). Absent bowel sounds may suggest ileus, commonly seen with bilateral pneumonia. Mortality is highest when children are both hypoxic and bacteremic. The most useful sign of pneumonia is persistent tachypnea or fast breathing (rates over the thresholds for age). Signs of hypoxia in children with pneumonia are severe chest indrawing (retractions), grunting respirations, central cyanosis, RR above 70 breaths/minute, and altered mental status such as restlessness. Signs that suggest bacteremia are temperature above 39° C (102° F) and altered mental status such as inability to eat normally, decreased activity (lethargy and difficulty arousing), and decreased social interaction. Seizures suggest bacteremia and meningitis.

C. Obtain a chest film in patients with RR over the age-specific threshold, subcostal retractions, altered mental status, signs of toxicity, malnutrition, or other condition associated with immunocompromise. Lobar or segmental infiltrate suggests bacterial infections, while interstitial infiltrate suggests viral infections. Patchy infiltrates (bronchopneumonia) can be caused by either viral or bacterial diseases. In young infants radiographs often do not distinguish viral from chlamydial infection. Abscess and/or pneumatocele formation suggests infection with S. aureus but may also result from infection with S. pneumoniae, H. influenzae, and gram-negative enteric organisms. Pleural fluid suggests bacterial infection and often accompanies infections with M. pneumoniae, S. pneumoniae, and S. aureus but can occur with any bacterial infection.

D. Pulse oximetry is a noninvasive technique used to determine oxygen (O_2) saturation. If possible, patients with pneumonia should be studied. Infants should be monitored before, during, and after feeding. O_2 saturation below 94% at sea level or 90% at 5000 feet indicates a need for supplemental O_2.

E. Blood cultures are positive in 10% to 25% of patients with pneumonia. Cultures are more often positive in patients with fever above 39° C and radiologic evidence of bacterial disease. Patients with pleural fluid should have a diagnostic thoracentesis for culture and fluid analysis. Several bacterial antigen detection tests are available for S. pneumoniae and H. influenzae type B. These can be done on urine or blood, but all lack sensitivity and specificity. Blood culture remains the gold standard for diagnosing bacterial disease.

F. The value of obtaining specimens for identifying viral pathogens in older children with pneumonia is unclear. Results of these studies rarely affect management because identifying a virus does not rule out a mixed bacterial-viral infection. Two rapid viral diagnostic techniques for RSV are widely available: immunofluorescent staining and ELISA. Both techniques are done on nasopharyngeal secretions. The rapid diagnosis of RSV infection helps identify patients who may benefit from early treatment with ribavirin or immune globulin.

TABLE 2 **Antibiotic Treatment of Children with Pneumonia** *Continued*

Antibiotic	Dosage	Product Availability
Cefaclor (Ceclor)	10 mg/kg/dose q.i.d.	Liquid: 125, 250 mg/5 ml Caps: 250, 500 mg
Cefixime (Suprax)	8 mg/kg/dose qd	Liquid: 100 mg/5 ml Tabs: 200, 400 mg
Cefpodoxime proxetil (Vantin)	5 mg/kg/dose b.i.d.	Susp: 50, 100 mg/5 ml Tabs: 100, 200 mg
Cefprozil (Cefzil)	15 mg/kg/dose b.i.d.	Susp: 125, 250 mg/5 ml Tabs: 250, 500 mg
Clarithromycin (Biaxin)	7.5 mg/kg/dose b.i.d.	Liquid: 125, 250 mg/5 ml Tabs: 250, 500 mg

T, trimethoprim component; E, erythromycin component; S, sulfisoxazole component.

G. For outpatient antibiotic therapy of pneumonia in infants under 6 months of age, use erythromycin-sulfisoxazole or TMP-SMX to cover *Chlamydia, S. pneumoniae,* and *H. influenzae.* Treat older patients with amoxicillin, erythromycin-sulfisoxazole, TMP-SMX, a third-generation cephalosporin, clarithromycin, or amoxicillin-clavulanate (Table 2). When *M. pneumoniae* is suspected, use an erythromycin antibiotic. Consider administering one injection of procaine penicillin or ceftriaxone to ensure initial compliance and to avoid vomiting.

H. The aim of the initial management of pneumonia in a child with signs of hypoxia is to correct O_2 desaturation and maintain tissue oxygenation. The initial management of a hypoxic patient should always be O_2 administration. Patients should not be stressed with other procedures or sent to radiology before receiving O_2. There is no benefit to administering albuterol nebulization to patients with pneumonia, and its use without O_2 may cause further desaturation.

I. Base the choice of an initial intravenously administered antibiotic to treat children hospitalized with bacterial pneumonia pending the results of cultures on the patient's age, any underlying condition, radiologic findings, severity of illness, and local antibiotic sensitivity patterns of bacterial pathogens. When pneumonia with *S. aureus* is suspected, use a semisynthetic penicillin (oxacillin or nafcillin) and gentamicin. Resistant *S. aureus* or *S. pneumoniae* may require treatment with vancomycin. Use chloramphenicol or an appropriate cephalosporin (cefotaxime or ceftriaxone) for severe pneumonia associated with meningitis and infections with *H. influenzae.* Use an aminoglycoside antibiotic for possible gram-negative enteric infections. Treat patients with cystic fibrosis for *Pseudomonas* infections. Consider gram-negative enteric organisms and *Pneumocystis* in immunocompromised children at any age. Empyema is associated with many bacterial infections, including *S. pneumoniae, S. aureus, H. influenzae,* group A streptococcus, and gram-negative enteric organisms. If the clinical status deteriorates after 48 to 72 hours of therapy, obtain a repeat chest film to identify air leaks, effusions, empyema, or progression consistent with resistant infection.

J. Ribavirin is a synthetic nucleoside that limits replication of RSV within the cell. It can be given only by aerosol using a small-particle generator in a mist tent or respirator. The respirator must have proper filters to prevent plugging and malfunction. Ribavirin therapy is administered 12 to 18 hours a day for 3 to 7 days. Consider treating patients with documented RSV infection with very severe respiratory distress and high-risk patients with congenital heart disease, bronchopulmonary dysplasia, other chronic lung disease, or neuromuscular or immunodeficiency disorder. However, the efficacy of ribavirin for ventilated patients is unclear. An alternative is RSV hyperimmune globulin, which has been approved to treat or prevent disease in high-risk patients.

K. Children may be discharged from the hospital when their respiratory distress has resolved, and they are afebrile, eating well, and appropriately active. In uncomplicated bacterial pneumonia this usually occurs on the second to fourth day of hospitalization. Consider discharge with home oxygen if mild desaturation persists. Routine repeat chest radiographs are not needed before discharge because resolution of radiographic findings frequently lags clinical improvement. Continue outpatient therapy with oral antibiotics for an additional 7 to 10 days. Schedule a follow-up visit 24 to 48 hours after discharge. Consider a visiting nurse referral. Tell the parents to call immediately if signs of respiratory distress (fast breathing or chest indrawing) or fever return.

References

Block S, Hedrick J, Hammerschlag MR, et al. *Mycoplasma pneumoniae* and *Chlamydia pneumoniae* in pediatric community-acquired pneumonia: Comparative efficacy and safety of clarithromycin vs. erythromycin ethylsuccunate. Pediatr Infect Dis J 1995; 14:471.

Freij BJ, Kusmiesz H, Nelson JD, et al. Parapneumonic effusions and empyema in hospitalized children: A retrospective review of 227 cases. Pediatr Infect Dis J 1984; 3:578.

Margolis PA, Ferkol TW, Marsocci S, et al. Accuracy of the clinical examination in detecting hypoxemia in infants with respiratory illness. J Pediatr 1994; 124:552.

Nohynek H, Eskola J, Kleemola M, et al. Bacterial antibody assays in the diagnosis of acute lower respiratory tract infection in children. Pediatr Infect Dis J 1995; 14:478.

Nohynek H, Valkeila E, Leinonen M, Eskola J. Erythrocyte sedimentation rate, white blood cell count and serum C-reactive protein in assessing etiologic diagnosis of acute lower respiratory infections in children. Pediatr Infect Dis J 1995; 4:484.

Onyango FE, Steinhoff MC, Wafula EM, et al. Hypoxaemia in young Kenyan children with acute lower respiratory infection. BMJ 1993; 306:612.

Programme for the Control of Acute Respiratory Infections. World Health Organization, Geneva. Acute respiratory infections in children: Case management in small hospitals in developing countries. A manual for doctors and other senior health workers. WHO/ARI 90.5, 1991.

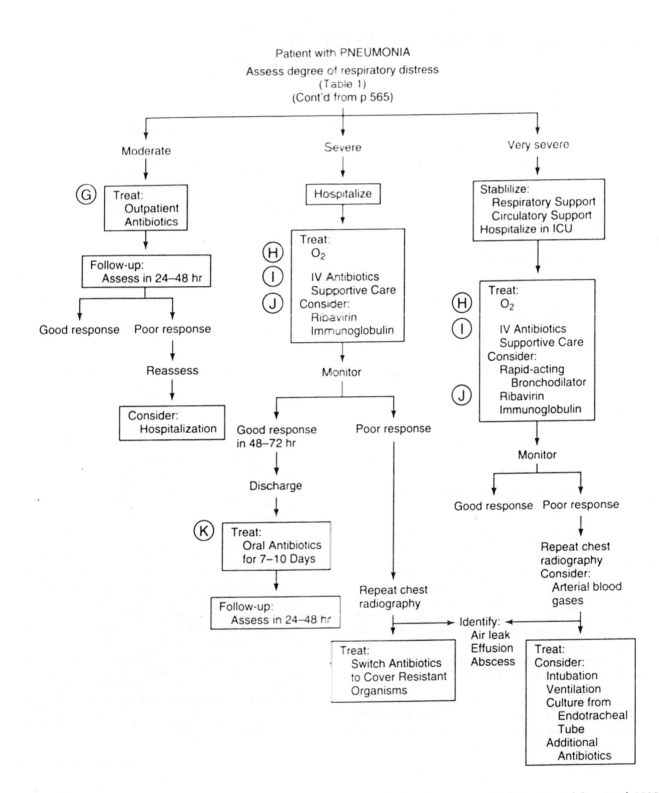

Patient with PNEUMONIA
Assess degree of respiratory distress
(Table 1)
(Cont'd from p 565)

Moderate

(G) Treat:
Outpatient
Antibiotics

Follow-up:
Assess in 24–48 hr

Good response Poor response

Reassess

Consider:
Hospitalization

Severe

Hospitalize

(H) Treat:
O₂
(I) IV Antibiotics
Supportive Care
(J) Consider:
Ribavirin
Immunoglobulin

Monitor

Good response Poor response
in 48–72 hr

Discharge

(K) Treat:
Oral Antibiotics
for 7–10 Days

Follow-up:
Assess in 24–48 hr

Repeat chest
radiography

Treat:
Switch Antibiotics
to Cover Resistant
Organisms

Very severe

Stablilize:
Respiratory Support
Circulatory Support
Hospitalize in ICU

(H) Treat:
O₂
(I) IV Antibiotics
Supportive Care
Consider:
Rapid-acting
Bronchodilator
(J) Ribavirin
Immunoglobulin

Monitor

Good response Poor response

Repeat chest
radiography
Consider:
Arterial blood
gases

Identify:
Air leak
Effusion
Abscess

Treat:
Consider:
Intubation
Ventilation
Culture from
Endotracheal
Tube
Additional
Antibiotics

Programme for the Control of Acute Respiratory Infections. World Health Organization, Geneva. Oxygen therapy for acute respiratory infections in young children in developing countries. WHO/ARI 93.28, 1993.

Regelmann WE. Diagnosing the cause of recurrent and persistent pneumonia in children. Pediatr Ann 1993; 22:561.

Shann F, Barker J, Poore P. Clinical signs that predict death in children with severe pneumonia. Pediatr Infect Dis J 1989; 8:852.

Taylor JA, Del Beccaro M, Done S, Winters W. Establishing clinically relevant standards for tachypnea in febrile children

younger than 2 years. Arch Pediatr Adolesc Med 1995; 149:283.

Turner RB, Lande AE, Chase P, et al. Pneumonia in pediatric outpatients: Cause and clinical manifestations. J Pediatr 1987; 111:194.

Wang EE, Milner RA, Navas L, et al. Observer agreement for respiratory signs in oximetry in infants hospitalized with lower respiratory infections. Am Rev Respir Dis 1992; 145:106.

Welliver RC. Today's approach to pediatric pneumonia and bronchiolitis. J Respir Dis 1991; 12:35.

REACTIVE AIRWAY DISEASE/ASTHMA

Jerrold M. Eichner, M.D.

Asthma is a chronic lung disease with hyperresponsiveness, inflammation, and obstruction of the airway. It is primarily inflammatory rather than bronchospastic. However, some exacerbations of bronchospasm lead to acute episodes of asthma that may be reversible with treatment or spontaneously.

The basics of asthma management include (1) patient and family education to foster a partnership among the patient, family, and physician; (2) environmental measures to control factors that precipitate attacks; (3) comprehensive pharmacologic therapy to prevent and reverse underlying airway inflammation and to relieve bronchospasm; and (4) objective measurement of lung function to assess the severity of asthma and to monitor the course of therapy.

The goals of asthma therapy are to (1) control chronic symptoms (including nighttime symptoms), (2) maintain normal activity (no exercise limitation, no school absences), (3) prevent acute episodes (no emergency room [ER] visits or hospitalizations), (4) maintain normal or nearly normal pulmonary function, (5) maintain normal growth, and (6) avoid adverse affects of medications.

ACUTE ASTHMA

Acute asthma episodes have a variety of infectious, allergic, and nonspecific triggers. The respiratory pathogens most often associated with exacerbations in childhood are rhinovirus, respiratory syncytial virus, influenza virus, parainfluenza virus, and *Mycoplasma pneumoniae*. Acute and chronic sinusitis may trigger asthma in certain individuals. Allergic triggers are usually inhaled, i.e., animal hair and dander, dusts, and so on. Nonspecific triggers include airway irritants, i.e., smoke, air pollution, perfumes, chemicals; weather changes; cold air; vigorous exercise; medications, e.g., salicylates; gastroesophageal reflux; and emotional stress. The threshold for symptoms varies in the same patient diurnally, seasonally, over time, and with combinations of factors. This threshold clearly differs among patients.

A. In the history ask: Has your child been diagnosed as having asthma? Has he or she wheezed before this attack? When? How often? Has he or she been admitted to the hospital with asthma? Bronchitis? Bronchiolitis? Pneumonia? Has he or she ever been in the ICU? On mechanical ventilation? Received steroids? How often? How recently? How long has your child had cough, wheezing, difficulty breathing? Is this a usual episode? What usually triggers an attack? What medicine is he or she taking? Dose? When? What route (inhaler, home nebulizer, oral)? Has your child vomited? Turned blue? Been able to eat and drink? Choked on anything? Had sinusitis? Headache? Bad breath? Facial pain? Fever? Evaluate the family situation; note the availability of a telephone, transportation, and the family's ability to manage the child at home. In the physical examination note signs of respiratory distress, including tachypnea, retractions, dyspnea, nasal flaring, use of accessory muscles, ability to talk, wheezing, prolongation of the expiratory phase, forced expiratory phase, and decreased breath sounds. Signs of severe respiratory distress include markedly decreased or absent breath sounds, cyanosis, and increased pulsus paradoxus (exaggeration of the normal variation of cardiac output with the respiratory cycle). An altered mental status with lethargy, restlessness, disorientation, and air hunger indicates severe hypoxia.

B. Home management of acute asthma requires the family to have appropriate education, the skills to evaluate, and the medication to treat the child. If attempting to treat the child over the phone, ask the questions listed in section A. The family should look for the same physical findings as the physician. If the child is hypoxic or in severe distress, arrange an immediate visit. If not, home treatment should be with an inhaled β_2-agonist, i.e., albuterol by nebulizer or meter dose inhaler (MDI), preferably with a spacer. This may be repeated every 20 minutes for up to an hour. If there is a good response, they should continue with the β_2-agonist every 3 to 4 hours and resume their usual medications. If the response is incomplete, they should continue the β_2-agonist every 2 hours for three doses. Usually at this point it is advisable to begin an oral steroid, i.e., prednisone 1 to 2 mg/kg. If response remains incomplete after the three doses of β_2-agonist or worsens at any time, or if there is a poor response to the initial treatment with β_2-agonist, the child needs to be seen, either in the office or the ER.

(Continued on page 570)

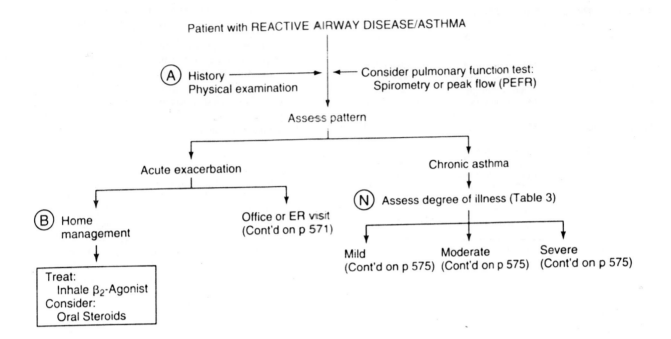

Patient with REACTIVE AIRWAY DISEASE/ASTHMA

Ⓐ History ⟶ ⟵ Consider pulmonary function test:
Physical examination   Spirometry or peak flow (PEFR)

Assess pattern

Acute exacerbation

Chronic asthma

Ⓝ Assess degree of illness (Table 3)

Ⓑ Home
management

Office or ER visit
(Cont'd on p 571)

Treat:
    Inhale β₂-Agonist
Consider:
    Oral Steroids

Mild
(Cont'd on p 575)

Moderate
(Cont'd on p 575)

Severe
(Cont'd on p 575)

TABLE 1 Response to Therapy

Good	Incomplete	Poor
No wheezing, good air exchange	Mild to moderate wheezing, good air exchange	Severe wheezing, poor air exchange
No accessory muscle use	Moderate accessory muscle use	Severe accessory muscle use
Minimal or no dyspnea	Moderate dyspnea	Severe dyspnea
Decreased HR and RR	Unchanged HR and RR	Increased HR and RR
Pulsus paradoxus < 10 mm Hg	Pulsus paradoxus 10–15 mm Hg	Pulsus paradoxus > 15 mm Hg
PEFR > 70% baseline	PEFR 40%–70% baseline	PEFR < 40% baseline
O_2 sat > 95%	O_2 sat 90%–95%	O_2 sat < 90%

HR, heart rate; RR, respiratory rate; PEFR, peak expiratory flow rate; sat, saturation.

C. Treat acute asthma in the office or ER initially with oxygen to keep the oxygen saturation above 95%. Begin an inhaled short-acting β_2-agonist either by nebulizer or MDI with spacer. Nebulized treatments with a maskwork best for young children. Older children who know how to use an MDI should use it with a spacer, but they may require four to six puffs per treatment. If there is significant distress, nebulized treatments are more effective. Repeat doses every 20 minutes for up to an hour. Assess the peak expiratory flow-rate (PEFR) initially and after each nebulized treatment. If the PEFR is above 90% of predicted value, further treatments are not necessary. If there is no response after the first bronchodilator treatment, begin oral prednisone or parenteral methylprednisolone. Injectable β-agonists may be used if inhaled agents are not available or the child does not respond to inhaled β_2-agonists. Subcutaneous epinephrine or terbutaline may be used every 20 minutes for three doses if necessary. These drugs tend to produce more adverse effects (tachycardia, headache, tremor) than inhaled agents.

D. Assess the response to the initial treatments clinically, by PEFR, and by oxygen saturation (Table 1). If there is a good response, nebulized treatments can be changed to every 2 hours. Observe the child for at least an hour before discharge. Home medications should be resumed. Consider a short burst of steroids if they have been used in the past or if distress is significant. Make sure an adequate follow-up plan is arranged.

E. If the response is incomplete (see Table 1), begin oral prednisone or parenteral methylprednisolone. Continue nebulized β_2-agonist every 20 minutes. If the response remains good after another hour, discharge with a burst of steroids and an adequate follow-up plan. If the response is incomplete, continue for another hour; consider admission if there is no improvement at that time.

F. If the response is poor (see Table 1), hospitalize the patient. Consider the use of continuous nebulization of β_2-agonist at this point or even in patients with an incomplete response to bronchodilators prior to admission. Start parenteral methylprednisolone if not already given. Consider an injectable β-agonist (terbutaline or epinephrine) if there is poor air exchange or a poor response to inhaled agents. Also consider the use of inhaled atropine or ipratropium. Obtain an arterial blood gas (ABG) when the response is poor.

G. Before the patient is discharged after an acute attack, arrange a follow-up plan. A known asthma patient usually can resume previous asthma medications, often with a burst of steroids. If the patient has had two or more ER or office visits for acute attacks in the previous 6 months or three or more in the previous year, begin maintenance inhaled antiinflammatory therapy or step up previous therapy. Be sure to notify the primary asthma physician of the visit and any changes in therapy.

H. Early use of steroids in the ER can promote resolution of the attack and reduce the need for hospitalization or shorten the hospital stay. Start steroids upon incomplete response to the initial bronchodilator treatment. Start systemic steroids early if there has been recent use of systemic steroids or if the child is on inhaled steroids. A short course of steroids with respiratory viral infections can prevent acute attacks of asthma. Monitoring the PEFR at home allows earlier intensification of therapy and may prevent acute attacks. Courses of fewer than 7 days do not cause adrenal suppression, although repeated courses may. Other adverse effects of steroids (cataracts, osteoporosis, excessive weight gain, and so on) are unlikely with short courses. Steroid-induced myopathy with progression to severe paresis, a rare complication, can occur with the use of muscle relaxants in patients requiring mechanical ventilation.

(Continued on page 572)

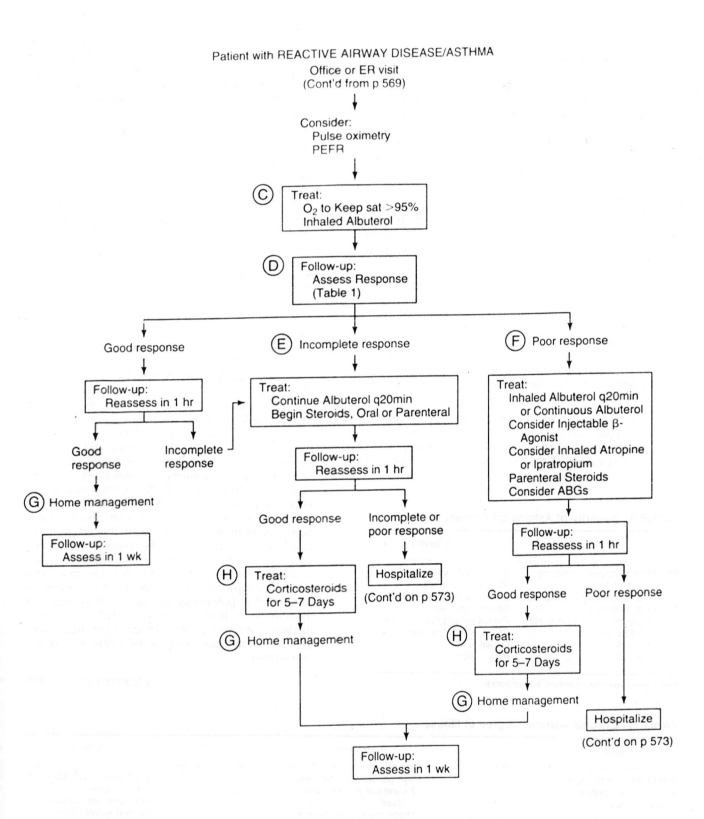

Patient with REACTIVE AIRWAY DISEASE/ASTHMA
Office or ER visit
(Cont'd from p 569)

Consider:
Pulse oximetry
PEFR

C — Treat:
O₂ to Keep sat >95%
Inhaled Albuterol

D — Follow-up:
Assess Response
(Table 1)

Good response

E — Incomplete response

F — Poor response

Follow-up:
Reassess in 1 hr

Treat:
Continue Albuterol q20min
Begin Steroids, Oral or Parenteral

Treat:
Inhaled Albuterol q20min
or Continuous Albuterol
Consider Injectable β-
Agonist
Consider Inhaled Atropine
or Ipratropium
Parenteral Steroids
Consider ABGs

Good
response

Incomplete
response

Follow-up:
Reassess in 1 hr

G — Home management

Good response

Incomplete or
poor response

Follow-up:
Reassess in 1 hr

Follow-up:
Assess in 1 wk

H — Treat:
Corticosteroids
for 5–7 Days

Hospitalize

(Cont'd on p 573)

Good response

Poor response

G — Home management

H — Treat:
Corticosteroids
for 5–7 Days

G — Home management

Hospitalize

(Cont'd on p 573)

Follow-up:
Assess in 1 wk

I. When considering hospitalization, assess the severity using clinical criteria, ABG, pulse oximetry, and PEFR (Table 2). If the P_{CO_2} is above 40 and there is poor air exchange, very severe distress, or a low O_2 saturation (sat), admit to the pediatric ICU. If the P_{CO_2} is no more than 35 and there is good air exchange, admit to the ward. Be cautious if the P_{CO_2} is 35 to 50, which may mean impending respiratory failure. Patients with P_{CO_2} above 50 are at high risk for respiratory failure and may need mechanical ventilation.

J. Give patients admitted to the ward frequent treatments with inhaled β_2-agonists. The frequency of the treatments can be decreased on improvement. Inhaled atropine or ipratropium can help. Steroids may be given PO or IV, depending on the severity. The patient should be weaned to the outpatient dose prior to discharge.

K. Since most infectious triggers of acute asthma are viruses, routine use of antibiotics is not indicated; treat only documented or suspected bacterial infections. Sinusitis may be associated with asthma. *M. pneumoniae* infections can also trigger acute attacks. If treating with erythromycin, remember to reduce the doses of theophylline and methylprednisolone. Be aware of potential allergic reactions to any medication (especially sulfa-related drugs and cefaclor).

L. If the response to inpatient treatment is poor, consider IV theophylline. If the patient is in severe distress and is likely to need ICU admission, consider IV aminophylline or theophylline in the ER. Give a loading dose and follow with a continuous infusion. Determine the theophylline level in someone already taking it as an outpatient, and adjust the loading dose accordingly. Reduce the dose when using erythromycin or other drugs that interfere with theophylline metabolism or when influenza is likely. Monitor theophylline levels at 1, 4, and 24 hours and after changing dosage.

M. In the ICU it is prudent to keep the O_2 sat above 95% by whatever means necessary. Frequent or continuous treatments with inhaled β_2-agonists may be necessary. Inhaled atropine or ipratropium, IV steroids and IV theophylline are usually necessary to prevent worsening. If the response is good, wean therapy to the level that can be administered on the ward. If the response is poor, use IV terbutaline or isoproterenol. These have some risk of myocardial necrosis, so monitor the heart rate closely to keep it under 200. Also consider monitoring cardiac enzymes with IV use of these drugs. If the patient fails to improve or the P_{CO_2} is markedly elevated, consider intubation and mechanical ventilation.

CHRONIC ASTHMA

N. Chronic asthma is classified as mild, moderate, or severe (Table 3) based on frequency of symptoms, exacerbations, and nocturnal asthma, or functional measures such as exercise tolerance and school attendance, and on objective measures of pulmonary function such as spirometry and peak flows. These are evaluated both before and after optimal treatment is established. Therapy of all degrees of chronic asthma involves child and family education about prevention, environmental controls with the emphasis on avoidance of allergens and other triggers (e.g., smoke, air pollution, chemicals), minimizing exposure to respiratory viruses, use of influenza vaccine, and allergy immunotherapy where appropriate. Some objective assessment of pulmonary function, such as peak flow measurements, is recommended to follow those with moderate or severe asthma. Treatment of triggers such as sinusitis and gastroesophageal reflux is also recommended.

(Continued on page 575)

TABLE 2 Severity of Asthma on Admission

Severe	Very Severe
Moderate to severe wheezing	Very severe wheezing
Good air exchange	Poor air exchange
Moderate accessory muscle use	Severe accessory muscle use
Moderate dyspnea	Severe dyspnea
Pulsus paradoxus ≤ 15 mm Hg	Pulsus paradoxus > 15 mm Hg
PEFR > 30% baseline	PEFR < 30% baseline
O_2 sat ≥ 90%	O_2 sat < 90%
P_{CO_2} ≤ 40 mm Hg	P_{CO_2} > 40 mm Hg

PEFR, peak expiratory flow rate; sat, saturation.

TABLE 3 Chronic Asthma: Degree of Illness

Mild	Moderate	Severe
Symptoms ≤ 2 times/wk	Symptoms > 2 times/wk	Continuous symptoms, often severe
Asymptomatic between exacerbations	Exacerbations last several days	Frequent exacerbations
Brief symptoms with activity	Moderate symptoms with activity	Limited activity level
Nocturnal symptoms < 2 times/mo	Nocturnal symptoms ≥ 2 times/mo	Frequent nocturnal symptoms
PEFR > 80% baseline varies < 20%	PEFR 60%–80% baseline varies 20%–30%	PEFR < 60% baseline varies > 30%
No emergency care	Occasional emergency care	Occasional hospitalization and emergency care

PEFR, peak expiratory flow rate.

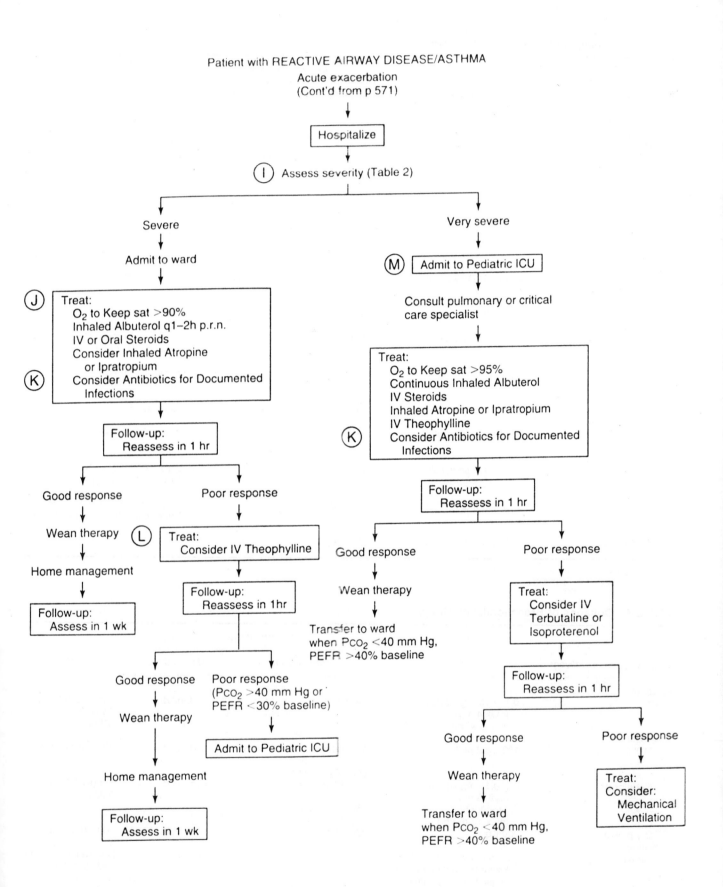

Patient with REACTIVE AIRWAY DISEASE/ASTHMA

Acute exacerbation
(Cont'd from p 571)

Hospitalize

(I) Assess severity (Table 2)

Severe

Admit to ward

(J) Treat:
O$_2$ to Keep sat >90%
Inhaled Albuterol q1–2h p.r.n.
IV or Oral Steroids
Consider Inhaled Atropine
or Ipratropium
(K) Consider Antibiotics for Documented
Infections

Follow-up:
Reassess in 1 hr

Good response

Wean therapy

Home management

Follow-up:
Assess in 1 wk

Poor response

(L) Treat:
Consider IV Theophylline

Follow-up:
Reassess in 1hr

Good response

Wean therapy

Home management

Follow-up:
Assess in 1 wk

Poor response
(Pco$_2$ >40 mm Hg or
PEFR <30% baseline)

Admit to Pediatric ICU

Very severe

(M) Admit to Pediatric ICU

Consult pulmonary or critical
care specialist

Treat:
O$_2$ to Keep sat >95%
Continuous Inhaled Albuterol
IV Steroids
Inhaled Atropine or Ipratropium
IV Theophylline
(K) Consider Antibiotics for Documented
Infections

Follow-up:
Reassess in 1 hr

Good response

Wean therapy

Transfer to ward
when Pco$_2$ <40 mm Hg,
PEFR >40% baseline

Poor response

Treat:
Consider IV
Terbutaline or
Isoproterenol

Follow-up:
Reassess in 1 hr

Good response

Wean therapy

Transfer to ward
when Pco$_2$ <40 mm Hg,
PEFR >40% baseline

Poor response

Treat:
Consider:
Mechanical
Ventilation

573

TABLE 4 Dosages of Antiinflammatory Drugs

Drug by Route of Delivery	Dosage	Dosing Intervals		Products
		Acute Episode	Maintenance	
Cromolyn sodium				
Aerosol				
MDI	1600 µg/2 puffs	—	t.i.d.-q.i.d	112, 200 puffs/canister
Dry powder†	20 mg	—	t.i.d.-q.i.d.	Caps: 20 mg
Nebulized*	20 mg/neb	—	t.i.d.-q.i.d.	20/2 ml sol
Nedocrimil				
Aerosol				
MDI	3.5 mg/2 puffs	—	t.i.d.-q.i.d.	112 puffs/canister
Beclomethasone				
Aerosol				
MDI	2–4 puffs (42 µg/puff)	—	b.i.d.-q.i.d.	200 puffs/canister
Triamcinolone				
Aerosol				
MDI	2–4 puffs (100 µg/puff)	—	b.i.d.-q.i.d.	240 puffs/canister
Flunisolide				
Aerosol				
MDI	2–4 puffs (250 µg/puff)	—	b.i.d.	100 puffs/canister
Prednisone				
Oral	0.5–1 mg/kg/dose	q6h	q.o.d.-b.i.d.	Syrup: 5, 15 mg/5 ml Tabs: 5, 10, 20 mg
Prednisolone				
Oral	0.5–1 mg/kg/dose	q6h	q.o.d.-b.i.d.	Syrup: 5, 15 mg/5 ml Tabs: 5, 10, 20 mg
Methylprednisolone				
Oral	0.5–2 mg/kg/dose	q6–12h	—	Tabs: 4, 16, 32 mg
Parenteral				
Intravenous	0.5–2 mg/kg/dose	q6–12h	—	Vials: 40, 125, 500, 1000 mg
Hydrocortisone				
Parenteral				
Intravenous	7 mg/kg/dose initially, then 3.5 mg/kg/dose	q6–12h	—	Vials: 100, 250, 500, 1000 mg Tabs: 5, 10, 20 mg
Dexamethasone				
Oral	0.15–0.3 mg/kg/dose	q12–24h	—	Liquid: 0.5 mg/5 ml, 1 mg/ml Tabs: 0.5, 0.75, 1, 1.5, 2, 4, 6 mg
Parenteral				
Intravenous	0.15–0.3 mg/kg/dose	q12–24h	—	Vials: 4, 10 mg

*Diluted in 2 ml normal saline.
†Used in a Rotahaler or Spinhaler.
MDI, metered dose inhaler.

TABLE 5 Dosages of Bronchodilating Drugs

Drug by Route of Delivery	Dosage	Dosing Intervals		Products
		Acute Episode	Maintenance	
Albuterol				
Oral	0.1–0.15 mg/kg/dose (max 4 mg)	q4–6h	t.i.d.-q.i.d.	Syrup: 2 mg/5 ml Tabs: 2, 4 mg
	> 20 kg: 4 mg	—	q12h	SR tabs: 4 mg
Aerosol				
MDI	180 µg/2 puffs	q5min p.r.n. (max 12 puffs) or q20–60min p.r.n.	t.i.d.-q.i.d.	200 puffs/canister
Nebulized*	0.1–0.15 mg/kg/neb (max 5 mg)	q20–60min p.r.n.	t.i.d.-q.i.d.	5 mg/1 ml sol 0.83 mg/ml sol
	0.5 mg/kg/hr (max 15 mg/hr)	continuous neb		
Dry powder†	200 µg	q20–60min p.r.n.	t.i.d.-q.i.d.	200 µg/capsule
Parenteral				
Intravenous	10 µg/kg over 10 min followed by continuous infusion 0.2 µg/kg/min to max 2 µg/kg/min		—	Not available in the United States
Metaproterenol				
Oral	0.4 mg/kg/dose	q4–6h	t.i.d.-q.i.d.	Syrup: 10 mg/5 ml Tabs: 10, 20 mg

*Diluted in 2 ml normal saline.
†Used in Rotahaler or Spinhaler.
MDI, metered dose inhaler.

Continued on page 576

Patient with REACTIVE AIRWAY DISEASE/CHRONIC ASTHMA

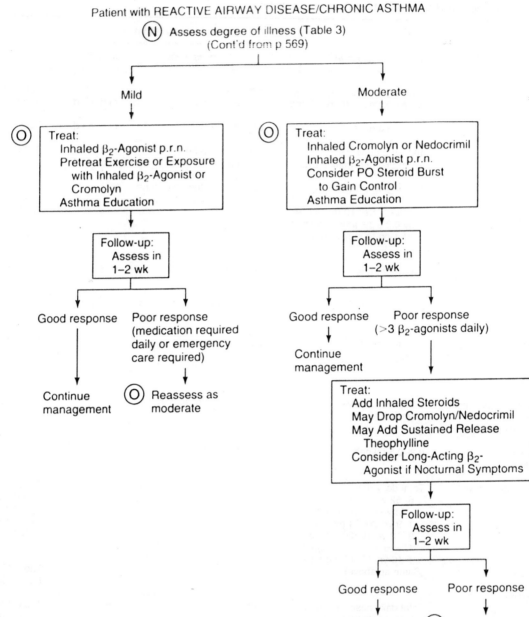

(N) Assess degree of illness (Table 3)
(Cont'd from p 569)

Mild

(O) Treat:
Inhaled β₂-Agonist p.r.n.
Pretreat Exercise or Exposure
with Inhaled β₂-Agonist or
Cromolyn
Asthma Education

Follow-up:
Assess in
1–2 wk

Good response

Poor response
(medication required
daily or emergency
care required)

Continue
management

(O) Reassess as
moderate

Moderate

(O) Treat:
Inhaled Cromolyn or Nedocrimil
Inhaled β₂-Agonist p.r.n.
Consider PO Steroid Burst
to Gain Control
Asthma Education

Follow-up:
Assess in
1–2 wk

Good response

Poor response
(>3 β₂-agonists daily)

Continue
management

Treat:
Add Inhaled Steroids
May Drop Cromolyn/Nedocrimil
May Add Sustained Release
Theophylline
Consider Long-Acting β₂-
Agonist if Nocturnal Symptoms

Follow-up:
Assess in
1–2 wk

Good response

Poor response

Continue
management

(O) Reassess as
severe

O. Pharmacologic management is done stepwise based on increasing use of antiinflammatory agents in all but the mildest asthma. Start with the appropriate antiinflammatory agent according to the level of severity and progress to the next higher step when control cannot be achieved with that agent (Table 4). If symptoms are severe or pulmonary function (PEFR or FEV₁) is reduced to 60% or less of predicted, a burst of systemic steroids is indicated along with maintenance therapy. Reduction of therapy to the next lowest level is indicated when good control is sustained for several months. Bronchodilating agents (preferably β₂-agonists) must be available for the treatment of acute episodes (Table 5), but regular use should be avoided if possible. Treat mild chronic asthma with a short-acting inhaled β₂-agonist p.r.n. up to three times a week (an oral β₂-agonist may be substituted in certain circumstances), and short-acting inhaled β₂-agonist or cromolyn before exercise or exposures to known triggers. Treat moderate chronic asthma with inhaled antiinflammatory medication daily, beginning with inhaled cromolyn or nedocrimil. Step up to inhaled corticosteroid if necessary. Increase dose of inhaled corticosteroid if necessary. Prescribe a short-acting β₂-agonist p.r.n., not to exceed three or four times a day. Add sustained-release theophylline, oral β₂-agonist, long-acting β₂-agonist, and/or inhaled anticholinergic if necessary. Treat severe chronic asthma with high-dose inhaled corticosteroid; sustained-release theophylline, oral β₂-agonist, and/or long-acting inhaled β₂-agonist as needed, especially for nocturnal symptoms; inhaled anticholinergic if necessary; short-acting β₂-agonist p.r.n., not to exceed three or four times per day; and oral corticosteroids, alternate day or daily, if necessary.

TABLE 5 Dosages of Bronchodilating Drugs *Continued*

Drug by Route of Delivery	Dosage	Dosing Intervals		Products
		Acute Episode	Maintenance	
Aerosol				
MDI	1300 µg/2 puffs	q20–60min p.r.n.	t.i.d.-q.i.d.	200 puffs/canister
Nebulized*	0.1 mg/kg/dose (max 2.5 mg)	q20–60min p.r.n.	t.i.d.-q.i.d.	5 mg/1 ml sol
Terbutaline				
Oral	0.1 mg/kg/dose	q4–6h	t.i.d.-q.i.d.	Tabs: 2.5, 5 mg
Aerosol				
MDI	400 µg/2 puffs	q20–60min p.r.n.	t.i.d.-q.i.d.	300 puffs/canister
Nebulized*	0.1 mg/kg/neb (max 2 mg)	q20–60min p.r.n.	t.i.d.-q.i.d.	1 mg/1 ml sol
Parenteral				
Subcutaneous injection	0.01 mg/kg (max 0.3 mg)	q20min × 2 then q4h p.r.n.	—	1 mg/1 ml sol
Intravenous	10 µg/kg over 10 min followed by 0.2 µg/kg/min continuous infusion to max 2 µg/kg/min		—	1 mg/1 ml sol
Bitolterol mesylate				
Aerosol				
MDI	740 µg/2 puffs	q6–8h p.r.n.	t.i.d.	300 puffs/canister
Pirbuterol acetate				
Aerosol				
MDI	400 µg/2 puffs	q4–6h p.r.n.	t.i.d.-q.i.d.	300 puffs/canister
Epinephrine				
Parenteral				
Subcutaneous injection	0.01 mg/dose (max 0.3 ml)	q20min × 2	—	1:1000 sol (1 mg/1 ml)
Aerosol				
Sus-phrine				
Parenteral				
Subcutaneous injection	0.005 ml/kg/dose (max 0.15 ml)	q6–12h × 1 dose only	—	1:200 sol (5 mg/1 ml)
Racemic epinephrine				
Aerosol				
Nebulized*	0.2–0.5 ml/neb	q20–60min p.r.n.	—	2.25% sol (20 mg/1 ml)
Theophylline				
Oral				
Sustained-release	Total daily dose: 6–52 wk: [0.3 × (age in wk) + 8] mg/kg 1–9 yr: 20–24 mg/kg 9–12 yr: 16–20 mg/kg 12–16 yr: 13–18 mg/kg >16 yr: 10–13 mg/kg		q12h	SR caps, tabs: 50, 75, 100, 125, 200, 250, 300 mg Sprinkles: 50, 75, 125, 200 mg
Non-SR	(Same as above)	—	q6h	Tabs: 100, 200 mg Liquid: 80 mg/15 ml
Aminophylline				
Oral	Total daily dose: Same as for theophylline ÷ 0.85	q6h	q6h	Tabs: 100, 200 mg Liquid: 105 mg/5 ml
Intravenous	Loading dose: 5–7 mg/kg if patient has taken no theophylline within 24 hr Bolus: 1 mg/kg to raise serum level 2 µg/ml Continuous infusion: 1–9 yr: 1 mg/kg/hr 9–12 yr: 0.9 mg/kg/hr 12–16 yr: 0.7 mg/kg/hr >16 yr: 0.5 mg/kg/hr			
Atropine				
Aerosol				
Nebulized*	0.03–0.05 mg/kg/dose (max 5 mg)	q6h	—	1 mg/1 ml sol
Ipratropium bromide				
Aerosol				
MDI	36 µg/2 puffs	q6h p.r.n.	t.i.d.-q.i.d.	200 puffs/canister
Nebulized*	0.25–0.5 mg/dose or 0.03–0.05 mg/kg/dose	q6h p.r.n.	t.i.d.-q.i.d.	0.25 mg/ml sol (0.02% sol)

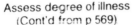

Patient with REACTIVE AIRWAY DISEASE/CHRONIC ASTHMA
Assess degree of illness
(Cont'd from p 569)

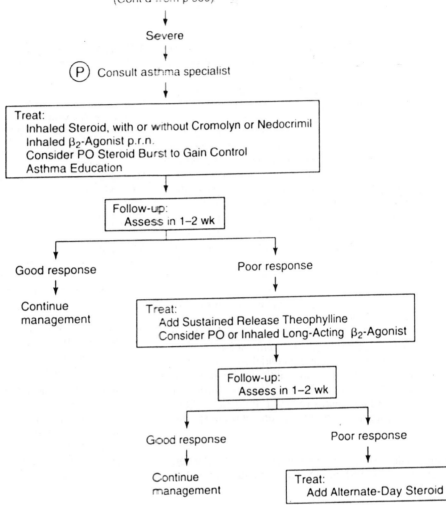

(Cont'd from p 569)

P. Consider referral to an asthma specialist (pediatric allergist or pulmonologist) for the following reasons: repeated steroid bursts, repeated ER visits, repeated hospitalizations, life-threatening episodes, mechanical ventilation for asthma, inadequate response to therapy, question of a different diagnosis (atypical signs or symptoms), to improve patient and family education, consideration of allergy immunotherapy, or a suspected complication.

References

Cockcroft DW. Therapy for airway inflammation in asthma. J Allergy Clin Immunol 1991; 87:914.

Furukawa CT. Stepping up the treatment of children with asthma. Pediatrics 1993; 92:144.

Guidelines for the diagnosis and management of asthma. National Heart, Lung and Blood Institute, National Asthma Education Program, Expert Panel Report. J Allergy Clin Immunol 1991; 88:425.

International Consensus Report of the Diagnosis and Treatment of Asthma. National Heart, Lung and Blood Institute. Eur Respir J 1992; 5:601.

Isles AF, Robertson CF. Treatment of asthma in children and adolescents: The need for a different approach. Med J Austr 1993; 158:761.

Konig P. A step-wise approach to the changing drug therapy of asthma. Am J Asthma Allergy Ped 1992; 5:69.

Larsen GL. Asthma in children. N Engl J Med 1992; 326:1540.

McWilliams B. Outpatient management of childhood asthma. Pediatr Ann 1993; 22:571.

Murphy S, Kelly HW. Evolution of Therapy for Childhood Asthma. Am Rev Respir Dis 1992; 146:544.

Patterson R. Goals in the management of asthma. Chest 1992; 101:403S.

Provisional Committee on Quality Improvement. Practice Parameter: The office management of acute exacerbations of asthma in children. Pediatrics 1994; 93:119.

Rachelefsky GS, Warner JO. International consensus of the management of pediatric asthma: A summary statement. Pediatr Pulmonol 1993; 15:125.

Van Asperen PP, Mellis CM, Sly PD. The role of corticosteroids in the management of childhood asthma. Med J Austr 1992; 156:48.

Warner JO, Gotz M, Landau LI, et al. Management of asthma: A consensus statement. Arch Dis Child 1989; 64:1065.

Warner JO, Neijens HJ, Landau LI, et al. Asthma: A follow up statement from an international paediatric asthma consensus group. Arch Dis Child 1992; 67:240.

STRIDOR

Stephen Berman, M.D.

Stridor can be acute, chronic, or recurrent. Recurrent or chronic stridor can be caused by tracheomalacia or an extrinsic lesion such as an aberrant artery. Croup is a clinical respiratory syndrome characterized by acute stridor. Inflammation of the respiratory tract above the larynx (uvula, epiglottis, and arytenoid cartilages), the larynx (false cords, aryepiglottic folds), or trachea causes narrowing of the airway and signs of upper airway obstruction. Infection of the epiglottis is usually caused by *Haemophilus influenzae* type B (HIB) , although *Streptococcus pneumoniae* and *Streptococcus pyogenes* can rarely cause acute epiglottitis. Infections of the larynx and trachea (laryngotracheitis) are usually caused by viral agents, most commonly parainfluenza viruses, followed by respiratory syncytial virus (RSV) and influenza viruses. Viral infections can be complicated by secondary bacterial tracheitis, caused by *Staphylococcus aureus, S. pneumoniae,* or *H. influenzae.*

A. In the history ask the following: When did the stridor begin? Does the child have symptoms of an upper respiratory infection or cold such as coughing? When did the cold symptoms begin? Is it difficult for the child to breathe? Is there fast breathing? Did the child recently choke on something and have difficulty breathing or turn blue? Does the child have a sore throat or hoarseness? Can the child swallow? Is there drooling or fever? Ask about access to a telephone and transportation.

B. In the physical examination listen for stridor at rest when the child is calm and during crying or coughing. Listen

TABLE 1 Degree of Respiratory Distress

Moderate	Severe	Very Severe
Intermittent stridor with crying and/or coughing and	Stridor at rest or Decreased air entry with marked retractions	Signs of impending upper airway obstruction, including cyanosis or
Good air exchange and	or Signs of toxicity	Minimal air exchange with severe retractions
Minimal or no retractions and	or Signs of dehydration	or Agitation and anxiety (air hunger)
No signs of dehydration and	or Inability to drink	
Able to drink without drooling	or Altered mental status	

for hoarseness, a barky cough, or a muffled voice. Look for retractions, cyanosis, extreme anxiety or confusion, restlessness, drooling, or a sniffing-type posture. Using a stethoscope, note air exchange, wheezing, and rales.

C. Angioedema usually presents with facial swelling, urticaria, and a history of similar allergic reactions. Foreign body aspiration can cause stridor, asymmetric breath sounds, or wheezing. The onset is sudden; and upper respiratory infection symptoms and fever are not usually present. Rarely an ingested foreign body can lodge in the esophagus and cause upper airway obstruction. A

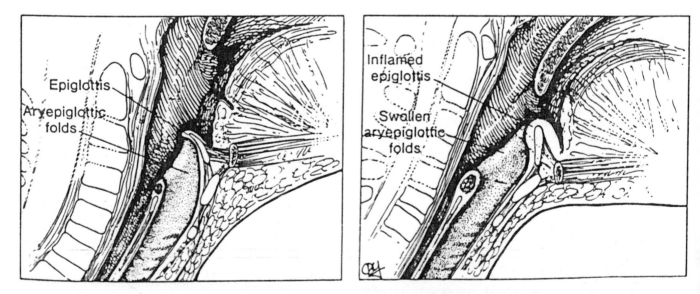

Figure 1 Diagram of the lateral neck region in a normal child **(A)** and a child with epiglottitis **(B).** (From Fleisher GR, Ludwig S, eds. Textbook of pediatric emergency medicine. 3rd ed. Baltimore: Williams & Wilkins, 1993:619; with permission.)

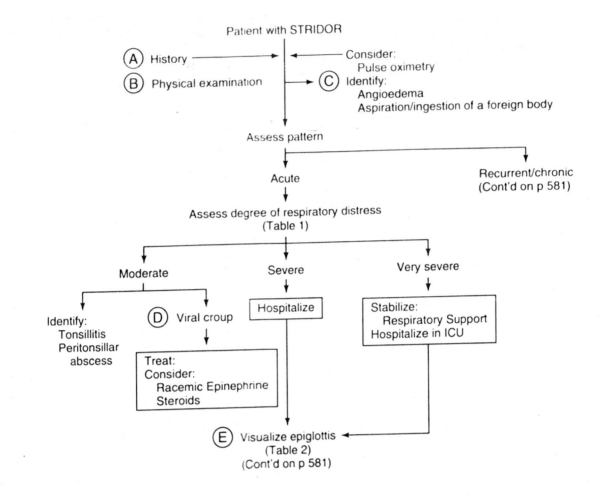

Patient with STRIDOR

(A) History ─────────────────→ ┤ ← ─── Consider:
　　　　　　　　　　　　　　　　　　　　　　　Pulse oximetry
(B) Physical examination ──→ (C) Identify:
　　　　　　　　　　　　　　　　　　　　　　Angioedema
　　　　　　　　　　　　　　　　　　　　　　Aspiration/ingestion of a foreign body

Assess pattern

Acute　　　　　　　　　　　　　　　　　　Recurrent/chronic
　　　　　　　　　　　　　　　　　　　　　(Cont'd on p 581)

Assess degree of respiratory distress
(Table 1)

Moderate　　　　　Severe　　　　Very severe

Identify:　　　(D) Viral croup　　　┌─────────┐　　┌─────────────────┐
Tonsillitis　　　　　　　　　　　　│Hospitalize│　│Stabilize:　　　　　　　　│
Peritonsillar　　　　　　　　　　└─────────┘　│　Respiratory Support │
abscess　　　　┌──────────────┐　　　│Hospitalize in ICU　　│
　　　　　　　│Treat:　　　　　　　　　│　　└─────────────────┘
　　　　　　　│Consider:　　　　　　　│
　　　　　　　│　Racemic Epinephrine│
　　　　　　　│　Steroids　　　　　　│
　　　　　　　└──────────────┘

(E) Visualize epiglottis ←
　　　(Table 2)
　　　(Cont'd on p 581)

forced expiratory chest film demonstrates air trapping and possibly a shift of the mediastinum. Endoscopy is diagnostic and therapeutic.

D. Encourage parents to give fluids to the child with viral croup. A cold mist vaporizer may be helpful. Instruct the parents to call or return if the child develops stridor at rest, chest indrawing, or becomes too ill to drink. Antibiotics should be reserved for children with associated acute otitis media. Corticosteroid treatment appears to modify the course of viral croup. The use of corticosteroids in ambulatory patients reduces the progression of the inflammation and may prevent hospitalization. Children with croup whose stridor resolves after treatment with racemic epinephrine in an ambulatory setting should be observed for at least 3 hours before returning home because stridor and respiratory distress frequently recur.

E. When acute epiglottitis is suspected, the epiglottis can be sequentially inspected by four methods until an adequate view is achieved. When visualizing the epiglottis, it is important to have available the following: oxygen, a self-inflating ambu bag, a laryngoscope, and the appropriate-size endotracheal tube (0.5 to 1 mm less than normal) in case the examination precipitates acute upper airway obstruction. Never force a distressed sitting child to lie down. This may compromise the airway and cause immediate obstruction. First, use a light alone and ask the child to open his or her mouth.

TABLE 2 Risk of Acute Airway Obstruction and Guidelines for Visualization of the Epiglottis in Children with Stridor

Risk of Acute Obstruction	Clinical Manifestations	Location and Personnel for Visualization
High (probable acute epiglottitis)	Drooling, muffled voice, severe sore throat, sniffing posture, high fever, anxiety, toxicity, no URI or cough	Operating room with airway specialist (anesthetist, otolaryngologist, pulmonologist) and surgeons
Moderate	Stridor (intermittent or constant) with minimal URI signs, high fever, age >5 yr without other signs of acute epiglottitis	Emergency room with airway specialist
Low	Stridor at rest associated with URI symptoms for 3–4 days, low-grade fever	Visualization usually not necessary; if done in emergency department or in patient ward, have present physician experienced with pediatric resuscitation
Minimal	Intermittent stridor with 2–4 days of URI, low-grade fever or no fever, no toxicity, no respiratory distress	Visualization not necessary

URI, upper respiratory infection.

TABLE 3 Drugs Used in the Treatment of Viral Croup, Bacterial Tracheitis, or Epiglottitis in Children

Drug	Dose	Product Availability
Racemic epinephrine	0.5 ml in 2 ml NS by nebulization q1–6h p.r.n.	Solution: 2.25%
Methylprednisolone (Solumedrol)	1 mg/kg/dose q12h (2–3 days)	Vials: 0.25, 0.5, 1 g
Dexamethasone (Decadron)	0.2–0.4 mg/kg/dose q12h (2–3 days)	Vials: 0.25, 0.5, 1 g
Ampicillin	50 mg/kg/dose q6h	Vials: 0.25, 0.5, 1 g
Chloramphenicol	25 mg/kg/dose q6h	Vials: 1 g
Ceftriaxone (Rocephin)	50 mg/kg/dose q12h	Vials: 0.25, 0.5, 1 g
Cefotaxime (Claforan)	50 mg/kg/dose q8h	Vials: 0.25, 0.5, 1 g
Oxacillin	25 mg/kg/dose q6h	Vials: 0.25, 0.5, 1, 2, 4 g
Nafcillin	25 mg/dose IV q6h	Vials: 0.25, 0.5, 1, 2 g

NS, normal saline.

Next, use a tongue depressor with the child sitting. If unsuccessful, perform direct pharyngoscopy with a laryngoscope while the child is sitting (Table 2). Finally, if necessary, use a laryngoscope with the child supine. Take care not to touch the epiglottis. Administer oxygen for 5 minutes prior to using a laryngoscope. Lateral neck x-ray films should not be done initially in patients at high risk for acute epiglottitis because of the danger of acute obstruction in the radiology department. The value of lateral neck films as an alternative to direct visualization in cases with a moderate risk of epiglottitis is controversial.

F. Suspect bacterial tracheitis when croup is complicated by high fever, purulent tracheal secretions, and increasing respiratory distress. Infection with *S. aureus* has been implicated in many of these cases. If endotracheal intubation is necessary, maintain adequate pulmonary toilet; abundant purulent secretions increase the risk of plugging the endotracheal tube.

G. In hospitalized children manage respiratory distress and stridor with racemic epinephrine. Corticosteroid treatment shortens the hospital stay. While mist therapy is used routinely in many centers, its efficacy has not been documented, and tents are a barrier to observation. Ribavirin therapy is not indicated for viral croup.

H. Manage acute epiglottitis with intubation in a controlled setting because of the high risk of acute airway obstruction. Initiate antibiotic therapy with an appropriate cephalosporin antibiotic or a combination of ampicillin and chloramphenicol (Table 3). Blood cultures will be positive in more than 50% of the cases caused by HIB. Identify extraepiglottic foci of infections such as pneumonia, septic arthritis, pericarditis, and meningitis. Consider bacterial pathogens other than *H. influenzae* in an HIB immunized child.

I. Causes of stridor identified by direct laryngoscopy include laryngomalacia, laryngeal web, laryngeal papilloma, redundant folds of mucous membrane in the glottic area, a floppy epiglottis, and supraglottic masses. Diagnoses associated with pharyngeal or retropharyngeal masses include enlarged adenoids, abscess or cellulitis, benign neoplasms such as cystic hygroma, hemangioma, goiter or neurofibroma, and malignancies such as neuroblastoma, lymphoma, and histiocytoma.

J. Discharge children from the hospital when stridor at rest and respiratory distress have resolved and they no longer need oxygen. They should be afebrile, eating well, and appropriately active. Schedule a follow-up visit 24 to 48 hours after discharge. Consider a visiting nurse referral. Instruct the parents to call the physician immediately if stridor or signs of respiratory distress (fast breathing or chest indrawing) return.

References

Bourchier D, Dawson KP, Fergussen DM. Humidification in viral croup: A controlled trial. Aust Paediatr J 1984; 20:289.

Cruz MN, Stewart G, Rosenberg N. Use of dexamethasone in the outpatient management of acute laryngotracheitis. Pediatrics 1995; 96:220.

Edwards KM, Dundon M, Altermeir WA. Bacterial tracheitis as a complication of viral croup. Pediatr Infect Dis J 1983; 2:390.

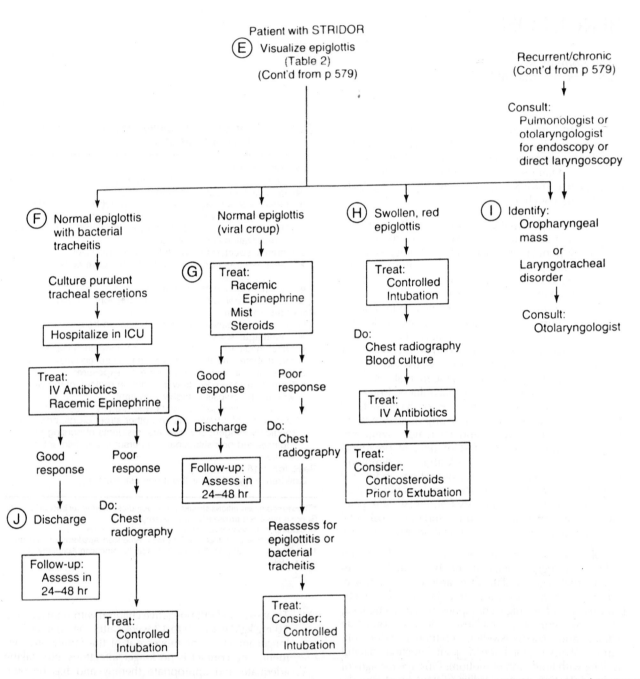

Patient with STRIDOR
(E) Visualize epiglottis
(Table 2)
(Cont'd from p 579)

Recurrent/chronic
(Cont'd from p 579)

Consult:
Pulmonologist or
otolaryngologist
for endoscopy or
direct laryngoscopy

(F) Normal epiglottis
with bacterial
tracheitis

Culture purulent
tracheal secretions

Hospitalize in ICU

Treat:
IV Antibiotics
Racemic Epinephrine

Good response / Poor response

(J) Discharge

Follow-up:
Assess in
24–48 hr

Do:
Chest
radiography

Treat:
Controlled
Intubation

Normal epiglottis
(viral croup)

(G) Treat:
Racemic
Epinephrine
Mist
Steroids

Good response / Poor response

(J) Discharge

Follow-up:
Assess in
24–48 hr

Do:
Chest
radiography

Reassess for
epiglottitis or
bacterial
tracheitis

Treat:
Consider:
Controlled
Intubation

(H) Swollen, red
epiglottis

Treat:
Controlled
Intubation

Do:
Chest radiography
Blood culture

Treat:
IV Antibiotics

Treat:
Consider:
Corticosteroids
Prior to Extubation

(I) Identify:
Oropharyngeal
mass
or
Laryngotracheal
disorder

Consult:
Otolaryngologist

Gay BB, Atkinson GO, Vanderzalin T, et al. Subglottic foreign bodies in pediatric patients. Am J Dis Child 1986; 140:165.

Hen J. Current management of upper airway obstruction. Pediatr Ann 1986; 15:274.

Husby S, Agertoft L, Mortensen S, Pederson S. Treatment of croup with nebulized steroid (budesonide): A double blind, placebo controlled study. Arch Dis Child 1993; 68:352.

Jones JL, Holland P. False-positive in lateral neck radiographs used to diagnose epiglottitis. Ann Emerg Med 1983; 12:797.

Kairys SW, Olmstead EM, O'Connor GT. Steroid treatment of laryngotracheitis: A meta-analysis of the evidence from randomized trials. Pediatrics 1989; 83:683.

Kessoon N, Mitchell I. Adverse effects of racemic epinephrine in epiglottitis. Pediatr Emerg Care 1985; 1:143.

Klassen TP, Feldman ME, Watters LK, et al. Nebulized budesonide for children with mild-to-moderate croup. N Engl J Med 1994; 331:285.

Koren G, Frand M, Barzilay Z, et al. Corticosteroid treatment of laryngotracheitis vs. spasmotic croup in children. Am J Dis Child 1983; 137:941.

Kotloff KL, Wald ER. Uvulitis in children. Pediatr Infect Dis J 1983; 2:392.

Liston SL, Gehrz RC, Siegel LG, et al. Bacterial tracheitis. Am J Dis Child 1983; 137:764.

Mauro RD, Poole SR, Lockhart CH. Differentiation of epiglottitis from laryngotracheitis in the child with stridor. Am J Dis Child 1988; 142:679.

Mills JL, Spackman TJ, Borns P, et al. The usefulness of lateral neck roentgenograms in laryngotracheobronchitis. Am J Dis Child 1979; 133:1140.

Ruddy RM. Croup: Has management changed? Contemp Pediatr 1993; 10:21.

Super DM, Cartelli NA, Brooks LJ, et al. A prospective double-blind study to evaluate the effect of dexamethasone in acute laryngotracheitis. J Pediatr 1989; 115:323.

TUBERCULOSIS

Stephen Berman, M.D.
Perla Santos Ocampo, M.D.

Tuberculosis (TB), infection with *Mycobacterium tuberculosis*, *Mycobacterium bovis,* or atypical strains, can involve the lungs, lymphatics, meninges, peritoneum, liver, kidney, bone, joints, or skin. Manifestations of tuberculosis are often nonspecific such as chronic fever, listlessness, easy fatigability, anorexia, chronic cough, or weight loss.

A. In the history ask about contact with adults, especially parents and grandparents with TB. Determine exposure to high-risk populations, including the homeless, incarcerated groups, migrant farm workers, nursing home residents, IV drug users, and HIV-positive individuals. Determine whether the patient has traveled to areas where TB is prevalent. Risk factors include immunization status, current medications, allergies, underlying conditions (such as cardiopulmonary, GI, or renal disease), sickle cell disease, and conditions and therapy that compromise immunity, especially HIV and measles infection. Ask about alterations in the mental status and normal level of activity such as playfulness, irritability, feeding and sleeping patterns, responsiveness, facial nerve paralysis, and seizures. Note any visual symptoms (vision loss, conjunctivitis) and respiratory symptoms (cough, otorrhea, earache, fast or difficult breathing, chest indrawing [retractions]). Ask about GI symptoms (vomiting, diarrhea, abdominal distention, abdominal pain, blood in stools, or jaundice), renal symptoms (pain with urination [dysuria], urinary frequency, flank pain, lower abdominal pain, hemeturia), and musculoskeletal symptoms (joint swelling, pain, limitation of movement).

B. On physical examination look, listen, and feel for findings that suggest meningitis or abscess (full fontanelle, too weak to feed, difficult to arouse, unresponsive, extremely or paradoxically irritable, nuchal rigidity, Brudzinski and Kernig signs), pneumonia (tachypnea, retractions, grunting, crackles), adenitis, soft-tissue cellulitis and abscess (swelling, erythema, induration, warmth of tissue), or bone or joint infection (painful swelling with limitation of motion). Observe for signs of cardiac infection or pericarditis (distant heart sounds, pulsus paradoxus, pericardial friction rub) and eye trouble (corneal clouding, proptosis, uveitis, retinitis, decreased extrocular movements).

C. The Mantoux method of tuberculin testing involves the subcutaneous administration of 0.1 ml of 5 tuberculin units of purified protein derivative (PPD). Skin hypersensitivity occurs 2 to 10 weeks after infection. Table 1 lists recommendations of the American Academy of Pediatrics defining a positive Mantoux skin test. A significant reaction in a child without bacille Calmette-Guérin (BCG) is induration 5 mm or larger. Induration 10 mm or larger in children who received BCG indicates infection, especially when the patient has had contact with an infectious person or lives in an area in which TB is prevalent.

TABLE 1 Definition of Positive Mantoux Skin Test (5TU-PPD) in Children*

Reaction ≥ 5 mm
Children in close contact with persons who have known or suspected infectious cases of tuberculosis:
- Households with active or previously active cases if (1) treatment cannot be verified as adequate before exposure, (2) treatment was initiated after period of child's contact, or (3) reactivation is suspected

Children suspected to have tuberculous disease:
- Chest roentgenogram consistent with active or previously active tuberculosis
- Clinical evidence of tuberculosis

Children with immunosuppressive conditionst or HIV infection

Reaction ≥ 10 mm
Children at increased risk of dissemination from:
- Young age: < 4 yr of age
- Other medical risk factors, including Hodgkin disease, lymphoma, diabetes mellitus, chronic renal failure, and malnutrition

Children with increased environmental exposure:
- Born, or whose parents were born, in regions of the world where tuberculosis is highly prevalent
- Frequently exposed to adults who are HIV infected, homeless, users of intravenous and other street drugs, poor and medically indigent city dwellers, residents of nursing homes, incarcerated or institutionalized persons, and migrant farm workers

Reaction ≥ 15 mm
Children ≥ 4 yr of age without any risk factors

---

*These recommendations should apply regardless of whether bacilli Calmette-Guérain has been previously administered.
†Including immunosuppressive doses of corticosteroids.
From Committee on Infectious Diseases, American Academy of Pediatrics: 1994 Red Book. 23rd ed. Elk Grove Village, IL: American Academy of Pediatrics, 1994.

D. Treat exposed PPD-negative children with isoniazid 5 to 10 mg/kg/day for 10 to 12 weeks after the contact is no longer infectious or moves out of the family environment. The contact is no longer infectious after taking adequate and appropriate therapy and has become smear-negative. A newborn exposed to TB should have a chest film and PPD. If findings of TB are not present, start isoniazid prophylaxis for 3 months and reapply a PPD. If the PPD is positive, continue prophylaxis; if it is negative and the contact is no longer present, isoniazid can be discontinued. (Table 2 lists recommended drugs for initial treatment of TB.)

E. Isoniazid for tuberculin-positive children without clinical disease protects against subsequent complications, especially miliary disease and meningitis. The committee on treatment, International Union Against Tuberculosis and Lung Disease, has recommended a dose of 5 mg/kg/day for 6 to 9 months.

F. Treat moderately ill patients with pulmonary infiltrate and/or mediastinal lymphadenopathy with at least two

(Continued on page 584)

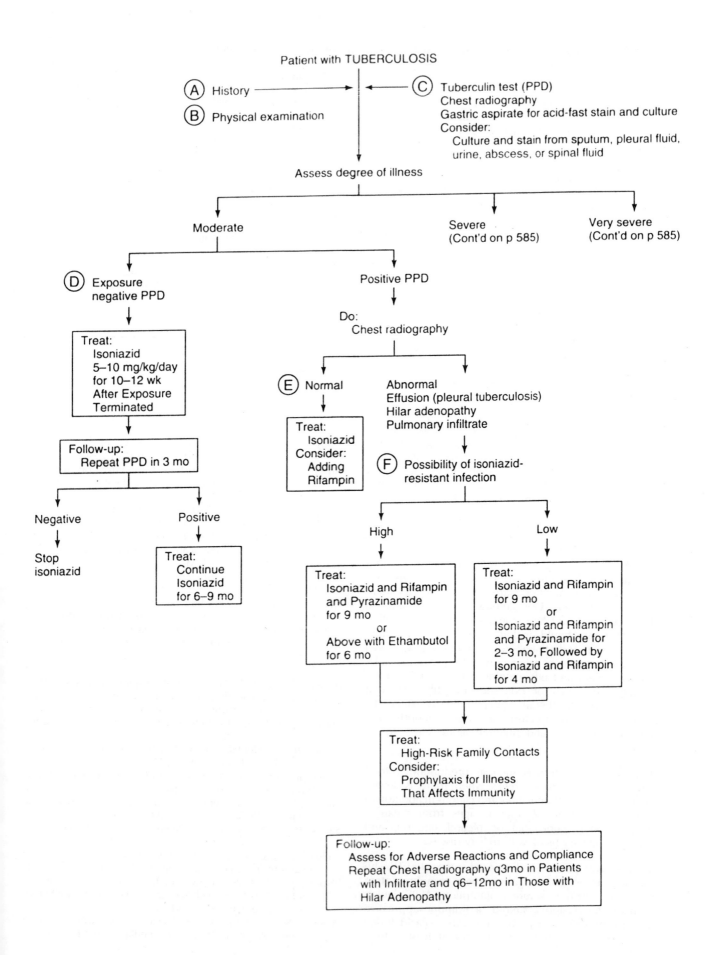

Patient with TUBERCULOSIS

(A) History

(B) Physical examination

(C) Tuberculin test (PPD)
Chest radiography
Gastric aspirate for acid-fast stain and culture
Consider:
  Culture and stain from sputum, pleural fluid,
  urine, abscess, or spinal fluid

Assess degree of illness

Moderate

Severe
(Cont'd on p 585)

Very severe
(Cont'd on p 585)

(D) Exposure
negative PPD

Positive PPD

Treat:
Isoniazid
5–10 mg/kg/day
for 10–12 wk
After Exposure
Terminated

Follow-up:
Repeat PPD in 3 mo

Negative

Stop
isoniazid

Positive

Treat:
Continue
Isoniazid
for 6–9 mo

Do:
Chest radiography

(E) Normal

Treat:
  Isoniazid
Consider:
  Adding
  Rifampin

Abnormal
Effusion (pleural tuberculosis)
Hilar adenopathy
Pulmonary infiltrate

(F) Possibility of isoniazid-
resistant infection

High

Treat:
Isoniazid and Rifampin
and Pyrazinamide
for 9 mo
    or
Above with Ethambutol
for 6 mo

Low

Treat:
  Isoniazid and Rifampin
  for 9 mo
    or
  Isoniazid and Rifampin
  and Pyrazinamide for
  2–3 mo, Followed by
  Isoniazid and Rifampin
  for 4 mo

Treat:
  High-Risk Family Contacts
Consider:
  Prophylaxis for Illness
  That Affects Immunity

Follow-up:
  Assess for Adverse Reactions and Compliance
  Repeat Chest Radiography q3mo in Patients
  with Infiltrate and q6–12mo in Those with
  Hilar Adenopathy

Drug	Forms	Daily Dose*	Maximum Daily Dose	Twice Weekly Dose	Major Adverse Reactions
Isoniazid	Tablets: 50, 100, 300 mg†‡	10–20 mg/kg PO or IM	300 mg	20–40 mg/kg max 900 mg	Hepatic enzyme elevation, peripheral neuropathy, hepatitis, hypersensitivity
Rifampin	Syrup: 50 mg/ml Vials: 1 g Capsules: 150, 300 mg†‡ Syrup: formulated from capsules 10 mg/ml	10–20 mg/kg PO or IV	600 mg	10–20 mg/kg max 600 mg	Orange discoloration of secretions and urine, nausea, vomiting, hepatitis, febrile reaction, purpura (rare)
Pyrazinamide	Tablets: 500 mg‡	15–30 mg/kg PO	2 g	50–70 mg/kg	Hepatotoxicity, hyperuricemia, arthralgias, skin rash, GI upset
Streptomycin	Vials: 1, 4 g	20–40 mg/kg IM	1 g	25–30 mg/kg IM	Ototoxicity, nephrotoxicity
Ethambutol	Tablets: 100, 400 mg	15–25 mg/kg PO	2.5 g	50 mg/kg	Optic neuritis (decreased red-green color discrimination, decreased visual acuity), skin rash

*Doses based on weight should be adjusted as weight changes.
†Isoniazid and rifampin are available as a combination capsule containing 150 mg isoniazid and 300 mg rifampin.
‡A combination of isoniazid, rifampin, and pyrazinamide in a single tablet is being introduced.
From Snider DE Jr, Rieder HL, Combs D, et al. Tuberculosis in children. Pediatr Infect Dis J 1988; 7:271.

drugs effective against the organism to prevent the development of drug resistance. When given together the isoniazid dose should not exceed 10 mg/kg/day and the rifampin dose 15 mg/kg/day because of hepatotoxicity. After several weeks of daily doses, supervised therapy is recommended twice a week if compliance may be a major problem.

G. Isolate patients with fibrocaseous TB, renal TB, and draining sinuses or abscesses.

H. Tuberculous meningitis has a high mortality rate and is associated with severe neurologic sequelae in survivors. Increased intracranial pressure must be carefully managed (see p 100). Use steroids to prevent internal hydrocephalus and basilar arachnoiditis. Initial antibiotic therapy should include three or four drugs. Streptomycin and ethambutol penetrate into CSF well only when meninges are inflamed. Isoniazid, rifampin, pyrazinamide, and ethionamide have good CSF penetration. In cases of isoniazid-susceptible TB that respond well to therapy, discontinue pyrazinamide, ethambutol, and streptomycin after 2 months and continue isoniazid and rifampin alone for 7 to 10 months.

I. Consider corticosteroids such as prednisone 1 to 2 mg/kg/day for 4 to 6 weeks when there is severe morbidity from inflammation. Indications in addition to meningitis include obstructive signs from enlarged lymph nodes, pericardial or pleural effusion, and alveolar capillary block with miliary disease.

J. Children with previously diagnosed and treated TB who develop an illness that alters their immune system (measles, pertussis, severe malnutrition, AIDS, leukemia) or start systemic steroid or immunosuppressive therapy should receive prophylaxis with isoniazid during the period of altered immunity (for at least 1 to 2 months).

References

Abughali N, Van der Kuyp F, Annable W, et al. Congenital tuberculosis. Pediatr Infect Dis J 1994; 13:748.

American Academy of Pediatrics Committee on Infectious Disease. Chemotherapy for tuberculosis in infants and children. Pediatrics 1992; 89:161.

American Academy of Pediatrics Committee on Infectious Diseases. Tuberculosis. In: Peter G, ed. 1994 Redbook: Report of the committee on infectious diseases. 23rd ed. Elk Grove Village, IL: American Academy of Pediatrics, 1994.

Girgis NI, Farid Z, Kilpatrick ME, et al. Dexamethasone adjunctive treatment for tuberculosis meningitis. Pediatr Infect Dis J 1991; 10:179.

Grossman M, Hopewell PC, Jacobs RF, et al. Consensus: Management of tuberculin-positive children without evidence of disease. Pediatr Infect Dis J 1988; 7:243.

Kendig EL Jr. Evolution of short-course antimicrobial treatment of tuberculosis in children, 1951–1984. Pediatrics 1985; 75:684.

Schaaf HS, Beyers N, Gie RP, et al. Respiratory tuberculosis in childhood: The diagnostic value of clinical features and special investigations. Pediatr Infect Dis J 1995; 14:189.

Snider DE Jr. Bacille Calmette-Guérin vaccinations and tuberculin skin tests. JAMA 1985; 253:3438.

Snider DE Jr, Rieder HL, Combs D, et al. Tuberculosis in children. Pediatr Infect Dis J 1988; 7:271.

Starke JR, Correa AG. Management of mycobacterial infection and disease in children. Pediatr Infect Dis J 1995; 14:455.

Starke JR, Jacobs RF, Jereb J. Resurgence of tuberculosis in children. J Pediatr 1992; 120:839.

Steiner P, Rao M, Mitchell M, Steiner M. Primary drug-resistant tuberculosis in children. Am J Dis Child 1985; 139:780.

Vallejo JG, Ong LT, Starke JR. Clinical features, diagnosis, and treatment of tuberculosis in infants. Pediatrics 1994; 94:1.

Visudhiphan P, Chiemchanya S. Tuberculosis meningitis in children: Treatment with isoniazid and rifampicin for twelve months. J Pediatr 1989; 114:875.

Waecker NJ, Conner JD. Central nervous system tuberculosis in children: A review of 30 cases. Pediatr Infect Dis J 1990; 9:539.

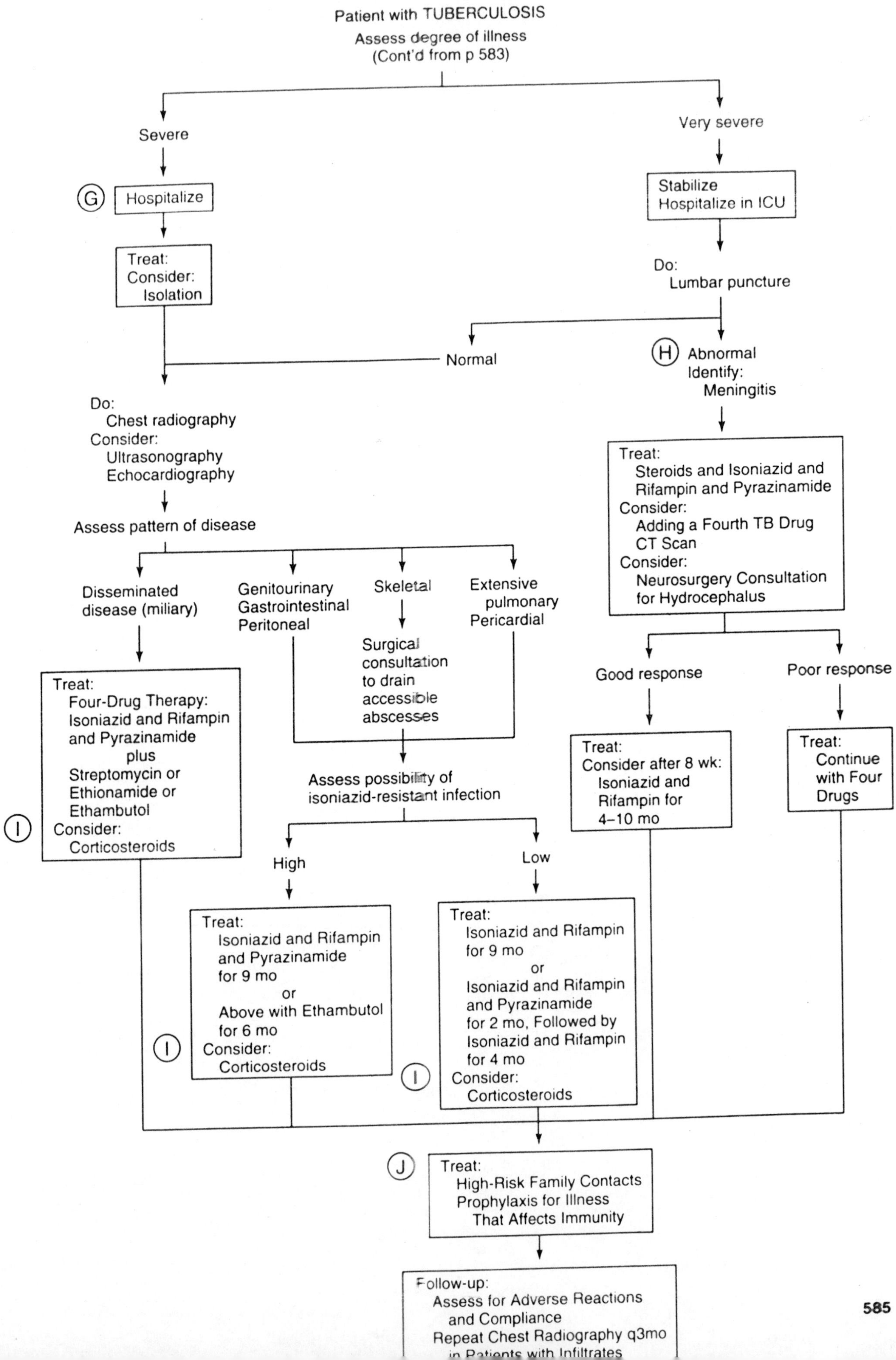

Patient with TUBERCULOSIS
Assess degree of illness
(Cont'd from p 583)

Severe

(G) Hospitalize

Treat:
Consider:
    Isolation

Very severe

Stabilize
Hospitalize in ICU

Do:
Lumbar puncture

Normal

(H) Abnormal
Identify:
    Meningitis

Do:
    Chest radiography
Consider:
    Ultrasonography
    Echocardiography

Assess pattern of disease

Treat:
    Steroids and Isoniazid and
    Rifampin and Pyrazinamide
Consider:
    Adding a Fourth TB Drug
    CT Scan
Consider:
    Neurosurgery Consultation
    for Hydrocephalus

**Disseminated
disease (miliary)**

**Genitourinary
Gastrointestinal
Peritoneal**

Skeletal

**Extensive
pulmonary
Pericardial**

Surgical
consultation
to drain
accessible
abscesses

Treat:
    Four-Drug Therapy:
    Isoniazid and Rifampin
    and Pyrazinamide
        plus
    Streptomycin or
    Ethionamide or
    Ethambutol
(I) Consider:
    Corticosteroids

Assess possibility of
isoniazid-resistant infection

Good response

Treat:
Consider after 8 wk:
    Isoniazid and
    Rifampin for
    4–10 mo

Poor response

Treat:
    Continue
    with Four
    Drugs

High

Treat:
    Isoniazid and Rifampin
    and Pyrazinamide
    for 9 mo
        or
    Above with Ethambutol
    for 6 mo
(I) Consider:
    Corticosteroids

Low

Treat:
    Isoniazid and Rifampin
    for 9 mo
        or
    Isoniazid and Rifampin
    and Pyrazinamide
    for 2 mo, Followed by
    Isoniazid and Rifampin
    for 4 mo
(I) Consider:
    Corticosteroids

(J) Treat:
    High-Risk Family Contacts
    Prophylaxis for Illness
        That Affects Immunity

Follow-up:
    Assess for Adverse Reactions
        and Compliance
    Repeat Chest Radiography q3mo
    in Patients with Infiltrates

585

RENAL AND UROLOGIC DISORDERS

Evaluation of Acute and Chronic Renal Disease
Glomerulonephritis and/or Hematuria
Nephrotic Syndrome and/or Proteinuria

Renal Failure
Scrotal Swelling/Pain
Urinary Tract Infection

EVALUATION OF ACUTE AND CHRONIC RENAL DISEASE

Gary M. Lum, M.D.
Stephen Berman, M.D.

Children with urinary tract disease may have an abnormal urinalysis (microscopic hematuria and/or proteinuria) during routine health maintenance examination, with a history of edema, hypertension or gross hematuria, and/or with abnormal renal function studies (BUN and creatinine) when evaluated for symptoms associated with a systemic illness.

A. In the history determine the onset, duration, and pattern of symptoms. Note associated factors, including streptococcal infections (poststreptococcal glomerulonephritis [PSGN]), gastroenteritis (hemolytic uremic syndrome [HUS]), trauma, toxins, medications, foods, dyes, and exercise. Identify predisposing conditions such as bleeding disorders (hemophilia), hemoglobinopathies (sickle cell disease), known familial renal disease (Alport hereditary nephritis with deafness, keratoconus), collagen vascular diseases (systemic lupus erythematosus [SLE], polyarteritis nodosa), and other vasculitides (Henoch-Schönlein purpura [HSP]). Document symptoms that suggest urinary tract infection such as dysuria, frequency, urgency, abdominal pain, and fever (see p 604).

B. In the physical examination pay special attention to any edema and hypertension. Abdominal masses raise questions of renal enlargement or tumor. Note prodromal symptoms that suggest the evolution of special conditions (bloody diarrhea—HUS) or characteristic rashes (purpura—HSP). Findings that suggest acute glomerulonephritis are coke-colored or brown-red urine and degrees of edema and/or hypertension. Signs of collagen vascular disease or malignancy include lymphadenopathy, abdominal organomegaly, skin lesions, and arthritis. Suspect a coagulation disorder when petechiae, increased bruising, or mucous membrane bleeding is present. Note signs of trauma.

C. Causes of rhabdomyolysis include trauma (crush injuries), status epilepticus, burns, electrical shock, and myositis.

D. Causes of hemoglobinuria include hemolytic anemia, paroxysmal nocturnal hemoglobinuria, septicemia, blood transfusion reactions, cardiopulmonary bypass, and ingestions (chloroform, fava beans, mushrooms, quinine, and sulfonamides). Patients with glucose-6-phosphate dehydrogenase (G6PD) are susceptible to acute hemolysis associated with ingestions.

E. Pink or reddish urine without cells can be related to foods (beets, cherries, blackberries); drugs (chloroquine, deferoxamine, ibuprofen, methyldopa, nitrofurantoin, phenazopyridine, rifampin, sulfasalazine, and pyridium); aniline dyes; urates; and metabolic disorders (alkaptonuria, homogentisic aciduria, tyrosinosis).

References

Boineau FG, Lecory JE. Evaluation of hematuria in children and adolescents. Pediatr Rev 1989; 11:101.

Jenkins RD, Fenn JP, Matsen JM. Review of urine microscopy for bacteriuria. JAMA 1986; 255:3397.

Schulman S, Kaplan BS. Hemolytic uremic syndrome: Prevention, recognition, management. Contemp Pediatr 1995; 12:61.

Patient with Suspected RENAL DISEASE AND/OR ABNORMAL URINALYSIS FINDINGS

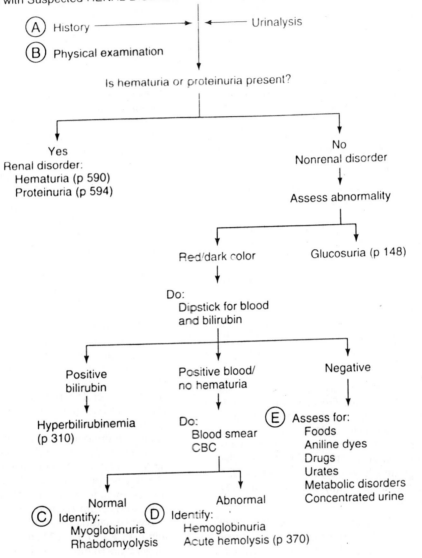

(A) History ——————→ ←—— Urinalysis

(B) Physical examination

Is hematuria or proteinuria present?

Yes
Renal disorder:
  Hematuria (p 590)
  Proteinuria (p 594)

No
Nonrenal disorder

Assess abnormality

Red/dark color   Glucosuria (p 148)

Do:
Dipstick for blood
and bilirubin

Positive bilirubin

Positive blood/ no hematuria

Negative

Hyperbilirubinemia (p 310)

Do:
Blood smear
CBC

(E) Assess for:
  Foods
  Aniline dyes
  Drugs
  Urates
  Metabolic disorders
  Concentrated urine

Normal
(C) Identify:
  Myoglobinuria
  Rhabdomyolysis

Abnormal
(D) Identify:
  Hemoglobinuria
  Acute hemolysis (p 370)

GLOMERULONEPHRITIS AND/OR HEMATURIA

Gary M. Lum, M.D.
Douglas M. Ford, M.D.

A. Findings that suggest a urinary tract or nonglomerular source of hematuria include bright red blood with or without clots, a varying degree of hematuria during stages of urination, eumorphic RBCs in the urine sediment, and no RBC casts. Typically, edema and hypertension are not present.

B. Findings that suggest a glomerular source of hematuria include brown or cola-colored urine, dysmorphic RBCs in the urine sediment, RBC casts (their absence does not rule out glomerulonephritis), significant proteinuria in the presence of microhematuria, and associated edema or hypertension.

C. Obtain radiographic studies of the urinary tract. Begin with noninvasive studies, such as ultrasound, to ascertain normal renal anatomy, then consider an intravenous pyelogram (IVP), renal scan, or CT scan. When a nonglomerular pattern of hematuria is associated with abnormal radiographic studies, obtain urologic and possibly oncologic consultation.

D. Urolithiasis, or stones in the urinary tract, usually causes abdominal and/or flank pain. Frequent or persistent urinary infections also suggest a stone. Most children with stones have hypercalciuria. Whenever possible, stone composition should be analyzed. Dietary management of children with urolithiasis depends on the cause but may include a low-sodium, low-oxalate diet with dietary calcium intake of only 400 to 600 mg/day and a high fluid intake.

E. Hypercalciuria, or high calcium urinary excretion, may be idiopathic or secondary to drugs (steroids, furosemide, vitamin D); metabolic disorders (acidosis, diabetes, hyperparathyroidism, hypothyroidism, adrenal disease); malignancy; renal tubular disorders; or rheumatoid arthritis. Idiopathic hypercalciuria appears to be related to low renal tubular reabsorption of calcium with a subsequent slight increase in parathyroid hormone. Hypercalciuria is best identified by a 24-hour urine collection. Excretion should be less than 4 mg/kg/24 hours. The ratio of calcium to creatinine measured in a spot urine should be less than 0.2. Hematuria unrelated to urolithiasis occurs in hypercalciuric patients. Urolithiasis develops within 5 years in approximately 15% of patients. Management in those patients with absorptive calciuria requires dietary restrictions to limit calcium intake to 400 to 600 mg/24 hours and increased fluid intake. Consider chlorothiazide (2 mg/kg/day) and alkali for patients with idiopathic hypercalciuria, and citrate supplement in patients with nephrocalcinosis and renal tubular acidosis.

F. Renal function tests include BUN, creatinine, electrolytes, and creatinine clearance. A functional disturbance, especially with persistently depressed serum complement, is atypical. Nephrotic syndrome or severe renal failure also makes the diagnosis of poststreptococcal glomerulonephritis (PSGN) questionable. Such atypical findings may represent membranoproliferative glomerulonephritis (MPGN), IgA glomerulonephritis, lupus glomerulonephritis, or rapidly progressive glomerulonephritis; recommend immediate pediatric nephrology consultation. The course is atypical if active glomerular disease persists beyond 2 months. Signs of active disease include decreased renal function, persistently depressed serum complement, and urinalysis with excessive hematuria (> 20 RBC hpf or RBC casts) or proteinuria (> 2 to 3 +). Microscopic hematuria persisting longer than 18 months is also unusual. Consult a pediatric nephrologist for atypical cases. Pursue percutaneous renal biopsy as part of the diagnostic work-up in all appropriate instances.

(Continued on page 592)

TABLE 1 Degree of Illness in Acute Glomerulonephritis

Moderate	Severe	Very severe
Mild to moderate elevated blood pressure and/or Decrease in renal function with creatinine < 1.5, urinine protein < 1 g/24 hr	Nephrotic syndrome or Multisystem disease or Marked elevation in blood pressure or Electrolyte abnormalities; moderate decrease in renal function with creatinine ≥ 1.5, urine problem > 1 g/24 hr	Acute renal failure or Hypertensive encephalopathy or Signs of shock/circulatory compromise

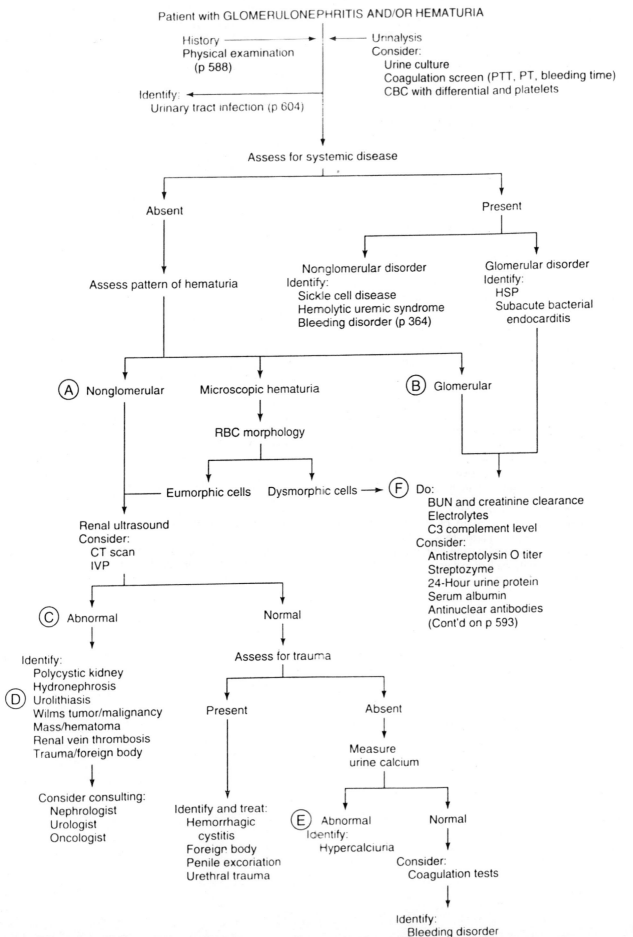

Patient with GLOMERULONEPHRITIS AND/OR HEMATURIA

History
Physical examination
(p 588)

Urinalysis
Consider:
    Urine culture
    Coagulation screen (PTT, PT, bleeding time)
    CBC with differential and platelets

Identify:
    Urinary tract infection (p 604)

Assess for systemic disease

Absent

Present

Assess pattern of hematuria

Nonglomerular disorder
Identify:
    Sickle cell disease
    Hemolytic uremic syndrome
    Bleeding disorder (p 364)

Glomerular disorder
Identify:
    HSP
    Subacute bacterial
        endocarditis

(A) Nonglomerular

Microscopic hematuria

(B) Glomerular

RBC morphology

Eumorphic cells   Dysmorphic cells → (F) Do:
                                    BUN and creatinine clearance
                                    Electrolytes
                                    C3 complement level
                                Consider:
                                    Antistreptolysin O titer
                                    Streptozyme
                                    24-Hour urine protein
                                    Serum albumin
                                    Antinuclear antibodies
                                    (Cont'd on p 593)

Renal ultrasound
Consider:
    CT scan
    IVP

(C) Abnormal

Normal

Identify:
    Polycystic kidney
    Hydronephrosis
(D) Urolithiasis
    Wilms tumor/malignancy
    Mass/hematoma
    Renal vein thrombosis
    Trauma/foreign body

Assess for trauma

Present

Absent

Consider consulting:
    Nephrologist
    Urologist
    Oncologist

Identify and treat:
    Hemorrhagic
        cystitis
    Foreign body
    Penile excoriation
    Urethral trauma

Measure
urine calcium

(E) Abnormal
Identify:
    Hypercalciuria

Normal

Consider:
    Coagulation tests

Identify:
    Bleeding disorder

591

G. Genetic conditions associated with hematuria are Alport syndrome and benign familial hematuria. Alport syndrome is a sex-linked dominant disorder involving glomerulonephritis and sensorineural deafness. Boys more often than girls develop severe progressive disease by late adolescence. Characteristic changes are present on renal biopsy. Benign familial hematuria is an autosomal dominant disorder associated with isolated hematuria without proteinuria or progressive renal disease. Renal biopsy shows a thin glomerular basement membrane with electron microscopy. Hematuria on a screening urinalysis of parents or siblings suggests this condition.

H. Acute PSGN is the most common type of acute glomerulonephritis. It usually appears in children between 3 and 7 years of age with evidence of a recent infection with *Streptococcus pyogenes* (impetigo, positive throat culture, positive streptozyme or anti-DNase B). Physical findings usually include edema and hypertension. Urinalysis reveals gross hematuria with RBCs and RBC casts. The serum complement level is transitionally decreased. Nephrotic syndrome, normal complement, acute renal failure, or a positive ANA is an atypical feature and suggests other causes.

I. IgA nephropathy associated with mesangial IgA deposition is a common cause of gross hematuria (single or recurrent episodes) and persistent asymptomatic microscopic hematuria. Gross hematuria is usually precipitated by an acute respiratory illness. Nephrotic syndrome, hypertension, or signs of acute nephritis occur in 10% to 25% of cases. Most patients have a benign course; however, progressive renal failure complicates approximately 10% of cases. There is no known effective therapy in rapidly progressive disease. Kidney transplants can be successful in patients with renal failure.

J. Henoch-Schönlein purpura (HSP) is a clinical syndrome characterized by one or more of the following: a purpuric rash, arthritis and arthralgias, abdominal pain, GI bleeding, intussusception, and glomerular involvement. Approximately half of patients with HSP have hematuria and/or proteinuria; fewer than half of these have signs of acute nephritis. HSP is also associated with mesangial IgA deposition. Asymptomatic patients (no hypertension) with normal urinalysis or minimal findings or microscopic hematuria and proteinuria less than 1 g/24 hours are at less risk for severe renal disease. Patients with acute nephritis, proteinuria more than 1 g/24 hours, or hypertensive or compromised renal function (GFR) require a kidney biopsy and follow-up for progressive renal disease.

K. If there is evidence of a decrease in renal function, treatment should include a diuretic such as furosemide. An ACE inhibitor is considered an appropriate first-line antihypertensive. Consult a pediatric nephrologist for guidance in treating the underlying renal disease with corticosteroids and/or other agents.

References

Bergstein JM. Hematuria, proteinuria, and urinary tract infections. Pediatr Clin North Am 1982; 29:55.

Boineau FG, Lewy JE. Evaluation of hematuria in children and adolescents. Pediatr Rev 1989; 11:101.

Campos A, Vernier RL. Renal Bx in children. In: Holliday MA, Barrott TM, Vernier RL, eds. Pediatric nephrology. 2nd ed. Baltimore: Williams & Wilkins, 1987:330.

Fitzwater DS, Wyatt RJ. Hematuria. Pediatr Rev 1994; 15:102.

Friedman AL. IgA nephropathy: What we've learned in 20 years. Contemp Pediatr 1987; November:53.

Havens PL, O'Rourke PP, Hahn J, et al. Laboratory and clinical variables to predict outcome in hemolytic-uremic syndrome. Am J Dis Child 1988; 142:961.

Kallen RJ. What's causing the hematuria? Contemp Pediatr 1986; June:55.

Reisman L. Renal trauma. Pediatr Rev 1983; 5:89.

Siegler RL. Management of hemolytic-uremic syndrome. J Pediatr 1988; 112:1014.

Stapleton FB. Nephrolithiasis in children. Pediatr Rev 1989; 11:21.

Welch TR, McAdams AJ, Berry A. Rapidly progressive IgA nephropathy. Am J Dis Child 1988; 142:791.

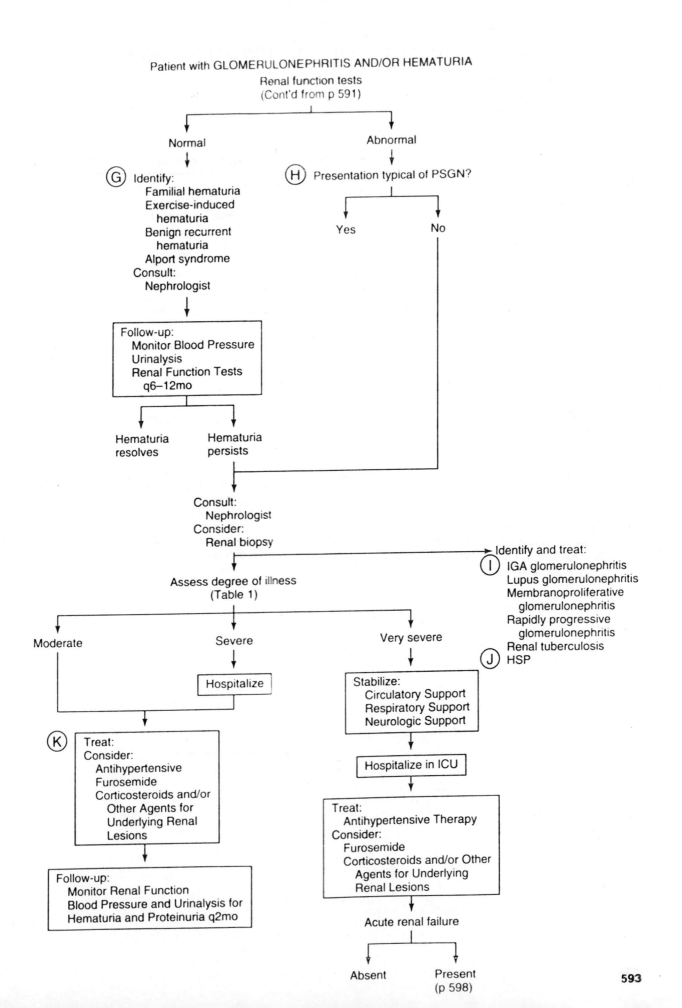

Patient with GLOMERULONEPHRITIS AND/OR HEMATURIA
Renal function tests
(Cont'd from p 591)

Normal

(G) Identify:
  Familial hematuria
  Exercise-induced
    hematuria
  Benign recurrent
    hematuria
  Alport syndrome
Consult:
  Nephrologist

Follow-up:
  Monitor Blood Pressure
  Urinalysis
  Renal Function Tests
  q6–12mo

Hematuria
resolves

Hematuria
persists

Abnormal

(H) Presentation typical of PSGN?

Yes   No

Consult:
  Nephrologist
Consider:
  Renal biopsy

Identify and treat:
(I) IGA glomerulonephritis
  Lupus glomerulonephritis
  Membranoproliferative
    glomerulonephritis
  Rapidly progressive
    glomerulonephritis
  Renal tuberculosis
(J) HSP

Assess degree of illness
(Table 1)

Moderate   Severe   Very severe

Hospitalize

Stabilize:
  Circulatory Support
  Respiratory Support
  Neurologic Support

(K) Treat:
Consider:
  Antihypertensive
  Furosemide
  Corticosteroids and/or
  Other Agents for
  Underlying Renal
  Lesions

Hospitalize in ICU

Treat:
  Antihypertensive Therapy
Consider:
  Furosemide
  Corticosteroids and/or Other
  Agents for Underlying
  Renal Lesions

Follow-up:
  Monitor Renal Function
  Blood Pressure and Urinalysis for
  Hematuria and Proteinuria q2mo

Acute renal failure

Absent   Present
                 (p 598)

593

NEPHROTIC SYNDROME AND/OR PROTEINURIA

Gary M. Lum, M.D.
Douglas M. Ford, M.D.

Proteinuria may suggest urinary tract abnormalities such as vesicoureteral reflux or obstruction, glomerular pathology such as glomerulosclerosis, or it may have a benign cause such as orthostatic proteinuria or benign persistent proteinuria (a diagnosis of exclusion). Nephrotic syndrome is severe proteinuria, hypoalbuminemia, edema, and concomitant hyperlipidemia.

Children with a persistent 4 + urinalysis for protein, 50 mg/kg/day or greater of proteinuria or 40 mg/m²/hour have nephrotic syndrome. Complications include hypertension, infection (peritonitis, sepsis, cellulitis, urinary tract infections), and coagulation disorders. Nephrotic syndrome can be associated with either hypercoagulability or hypocoagulability. Hypercoagulability is associated with increased levels of procoagulants, thrombocytosis, or increased β-thromboglobulin levels; hypocoagulation results from mild disseminated intravascular coagulation with increased fibrin split products. Idiopathic nephrotic syndrome (minimal-change nephrotic syndrome) occurs most frequently in children 1 to 7 years of age. Atypical presentations with acute renal failure, severe hypertension, hematuria, and hypocomplementemia suggest another renal parenchymal disease.

A. When nephrotic syndrome is accompanied by evidence of glomerulonephritis, take the approach described on p 590.

B. Nephrotic syndrome with features of significant renal disease or occurring in older children suggests focal glomerulosclerosis, membranous nephropathy, or mesangial nephropathy, and it requires renal biopsy documentation. Idiopathic nephrotic syndrome (minimal change disease, or nil lesion, lipoid nephrosis) occurs most frequently in children 2 to 7 years of age. Nephrotic syndrome prior to age 1 suggests congenital nephrosis with attendant renal failure and generally poor outcome. Obtain pediatric nephrology consultation for such patients.

TABLE 1   Degree of Illness in Nephrotic Syndrome

Moderate	Severe	Very Severe
Presumed minimal change disease, nephrotic syndrome without complications	Severe hypertension	Hypertensive encephalopathy
or	or	or
Decreased renal function with creatinine < 2	Cardiorespiratory complications of hypoalbuminemia related to hypovolemia, pleural effusions, and/or ascites	Acute renal failure
		or
		Shock
	or	or
	Decreased renal function with creatinine ≥ 2	Sepsis
	or	
	Infection	
	or	
	Coagulation disorder	

(Continued on page 596)

Patient with NEPHROTIC SYNDROME AND/OR PROTEINURIA

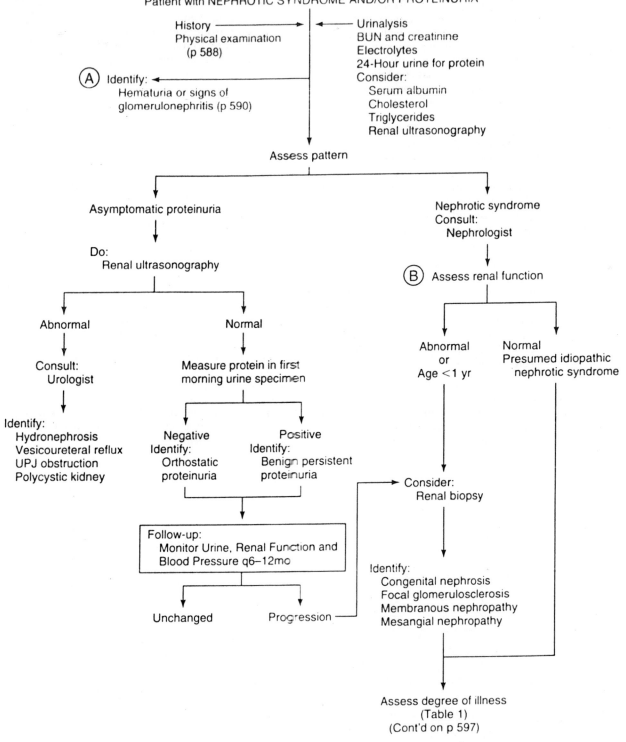

History
Physical examination
(p 588)

Urinalysis
BUN and creatinine
Electrolytes
24-Hour urine for protein
Consider:
   Serum albumin
   Cholesterol
   Triglycerides
   Renal ultrasonography

(A) Identify:
Hematuria or signs of
glomerulonephritis (p 590)

Assess pattern

Asymptomatic proteinuria

Do:
Renal ultrasonography

Abnormal

Normal

Consult:
Urologist

Measure protein in first
morning urine specimen

Identify:
  Hydronephrosis
  Vesicoureteral reflux
  UPJ obstruction
  Polycystic kidney

Negative
Identify:
  Orthostatic
  proteinuria

Positive
Identify:
  Benign persistent
  proteinuria

Follow-up:
  Monitor Urine, Renal Function and
  Blood Pressure q6–12mo

Unchanged

Progression

Nephrotic syndrome
Consult:
  Nephrologist

(B) Assess renal function

Abnormal
or
Age <1 yr

Normal
Presumed idiopathic
nephrotic syndrome

Consider:
  Renal biopsy

Identify:
  Congenital nephrosis
  Focal glomerulosclerosis
  Membranous nephropathy
  Mesangial nephropathy

Assess degree of illness
(Table 1)

(Cont'd on p 597)

C. Treat presumed minimal change disease initially with prednisone 2 mg/kg/day (maximum 60 mg) until the urine is protein free for 5 consecutive days (maximum 8 weeks). Some 73% of patients with idiopathic nephrotic syndrome respond within 2 weeks, and 85% respond within 1 month. After remission maintain the patient with 2 mg/kg on alternate days for 1 month; then decrease the dose of prednisone by 5 mg every 3 weeks. If the nephrotic syndrome recurs as the prednisone dosage is tapered, consult a pediatric nephrologist. These patients, as well as those who relapse three or more times a year, may require other drug intervention and/or long-term alternate-day prednisone. Alkylating agents, such as cyclophosphamide and chlorambucil, are the next phase of treatment in steroid-resistant or dependent cases. The side effects are dose related, hence cautiously addressed case by case. Certain patients may benefit from cyclosporine A.

D. Monitor proteinuria daily with an albumin-sensitive dipstick. Relapse is defined as 3 consecutive days with proteinuria measuring 3+ or more. Relapses are often associated with any minor acute illness, especially viral respiratory infections. Monitor patients for complications of the nephrotic syndrome such as infection (especially spontaneous peritonitis) and coagulation disorders. Hypercoagulability is associated most commonly with decreased levels of antithrombin III.

E. Hypoalbuminemia can cause severe edema, ascites, pleural effusions, and intravascular volume depletion with azotemia. The more complex cases require early pediatric nephrology consultation. Symptomatic hypoalbuminemia may be treated with 1 to 2 g/kg of 25% salt-poor albumin IV over 4 to 6 hours; if hypertension results, give furosemide 1 to 2 mg/kg IV. Although circulating volume is usually reduced, any elevated blood pressure should be treated. Oliguria is functional and relative to volume contraction. However, a cautious approach to volume expansion is important if there is any evidence of significant renal failure.

References

Feld LG, Schoeneman MJ, Kaskel FJ. Evaluation of the child with asymptomatic proteinuria. Pediatr Rev 1984; 5:248.

International Study of Kidney Disease in Children. The primary nephrotic syndrome in children. Identification of patients with minimal change nephrotic syndrome from initial response to prednisone. J Pediatr 1981; 98:561.

Kelsch RC, Sedman AB. Nephrotic syndrome. Pediatr Rev 1993; 14:30.

MacDonald NE, Wolfish N, McLaine P, et al. Role of respiratory viruses in exacerbations of primary nephrotic syndrome. J Pediatr 1986; 108:378.

McEnery PT, Strife CF. Nephrotic syndrome in children. Pediatr Clin North Am 1982; 89:875.

Oliver WJ, Kelsch RC. Nephrotic syndrome due to primary nephropathies. Pediatr Rev 1981; 2:311.

Vernier RL. Primary (idiopathic) nephrotic syndrome. In: Holiday MA, Barrott TM, Vernier RL, eds. Pediatric nephrology. 2nd ed. Baltimore: Williams & Wilkins, 1987:445.

Vernier RL, Chavers B. Glomerular permeability: New concepts. Pediatr Ann 1988; 17:590.

Yoshikawa N, Ito H, Akamatsu R, et al. Focal segmental glomerulosclerosis with and without nephrotic syndrome in children. J Pediatr 1986; 109:65.

Patient with NEPHROTIC SYNDROME AND/OR PROTEINURIA
Assess degree of illness
(Table 1)
(Cont'd from p 595)

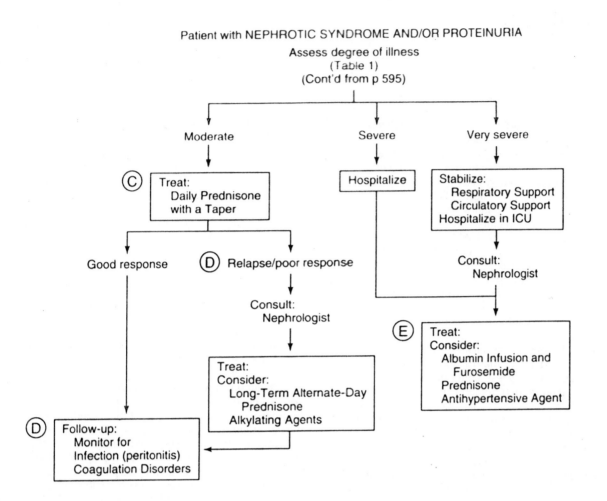

RENAL FAILURE

Gary M. Lum, M.D.
Douglas M. Ford, M.D.

Suspect acute renal failure (ARF) when there is a sudden fall in urine output and/or an acute elevation in serum BUN and creatinine (azotemia). The explanation for such changes in renal function may be grouped into three major clinical categories: (1) a condition that results in decreased renal blood flow, or a prerenal state; (2) obstruction of urine flow, or a postrenal state; and (3) renal injury or disease. All three conditions may coexist, so correctable causes of oliguria and azotemia should always be identified. ARF developing in the inpatient setting is usually caused by a prerenal or postrenal state rather than de novo primary renal disease. Nephrotoxic effects of drugs should be considered and identified.

In contrast, chronic renal failure (CRF) in children is usually a result of abnormal renal or urinary tract development. Prenatal ultrasonography may demonstrate urinary tract obstruction, abnormal renal mass, or oligohydramnios. Postnatal abnormal voiding, anomalies of the external genitalia or pinnae, abdominal masses, spontaneous pneumothorax, and azotemia suggest abnormal urinary tract development. The gradual deterioration of the glomerular filtration rate (GFR) in CRF permits adaptation to the decline in functioning nephrons, which delays the development of signs and symptoms suggesting renal failure. CRF may also arise from any of the following: (1) acute renal disease or injury; (2) hereditary disease, e.g., polycystic kidney disease, cystinosis, or hereditary glomerulonephritis; or (3) congenital renal lesions, e.g., congenital nephrotic syndrome.

A. At times it may be difficult to distinguish physiologic oliguria (prerenal) from pathophysiologic oliguria related to true renal dysfunction (with the aforementioned renal diseases ruled out). In such circumstances consider acute tubular necrosis (ATN) secondary to presumed or documented transient renal ischemic injury. Urine sodium (Na^+) and creatinine (Cr) measurements distinguish prerenal oliguria from the oliguria of ATN.

Decreased renal perfusion results in increased renal reabsorption of Na^+ (urine Na^+ < 20 mEq/L, fractional excretion [FENa] < 1%) and production of small amounts of concentrated urine (ratio of urine to plasma Cr > 40, osmolality > 450 mOsm). Thus, oliguria in the absence of concentrated urine (urine-plasma Cr ratio < 40) and inappropriate urine sodium (urine Na^+ > 20 mEq/L, FENa > 1% or [> 3% in the neonate]) support the diagnosis of ATN.

B. Renal disease producing renal insufficiency causes abnormalities of the urinary sediment. Consider (1) acute glomerulonephritis (GN), whether secondary to the immunologic renal response to streptococcal or other infections, chronic types of GN, systemic disease (systemic lupus, Henoch-Schönlein purpura), or IgA nephropathy; (2) the hemolytic uremic syndrome; and (3) acute interstitial nephritis (a renal drug allergy response). Obtain a pediatric nephrology consultation in such circumstances. Postrenal azotemia is usually the consequence of abnormal development of the genitourinary system, such as posterior urethral valves, meatal stenosis, or ureteral pelvic junction stenosis. Consider obstruction when oligoanuria is associated with an abdominal or flank mass, a palpable bladder, when a urinary catheter cannot be passed, or if there is a history of genitourinary surgery. Ultrasonographic studies are indicated. When lesions are identified, consult a urologist and/or nephrologist promptly.

C. The initial approach to ARF includes elimination of correctable causes. Dehydration with compromised circulating volume is the most common cause of prerenal azotemia in children. Other causes of decreased renal perfusion include poor cardiac function and thrombosis of renal vessels. Correct the underlying

TABLE 1 Drug Therapy for Acute Renal Failure in Children

Drug	Dosage	Product Availability
Calcium carbonate (Titralac Plus)	1 ml/kg/dose t.i.d. *or* Older children: 1 tab t.i.d.	Susp: 400 mg elemental calcium/5 ml
Calcium gluconate (10%)	100 mg/kg/dose IV slow	100 mg/ml or 0.45 mEq/ml (10 ml)
Furosemide	1–5 mg/kg/dose IV q6h	10 mg/ml (2, 4, 10 ml)
Glucose-insulin infusion	0.5–1 ml/kg $D_{50}W$ with 1 U insulin for every 4–5 g glucose (1 U for every 8–10 ml of $D_{50}W$) *or* 0.1 U insulin/kg/hr in $D_{10}W$	
Hydrochlorothiazide	1–1.5 mg/kg/dose b.i.d. (max 200 mg/day)	Sol: 50 mg/5 ml Tabs: 25, 50 mg
Kayexalate Oral: 25% sorbitol Rectal: 30%–50% in $D_{10}W$ 1% of 1% methyl cellulose or 10% sorbitol	1 g/kg/dose q16h PO or q2–6h rectally	Exchange ratio is 1 mEq K per 1 g resin
Sodium bicarbonate	1–2 mEq/kg/dose IV over 20–30 min	1 mEq/ml (8.4% sol) 10, 50 ml

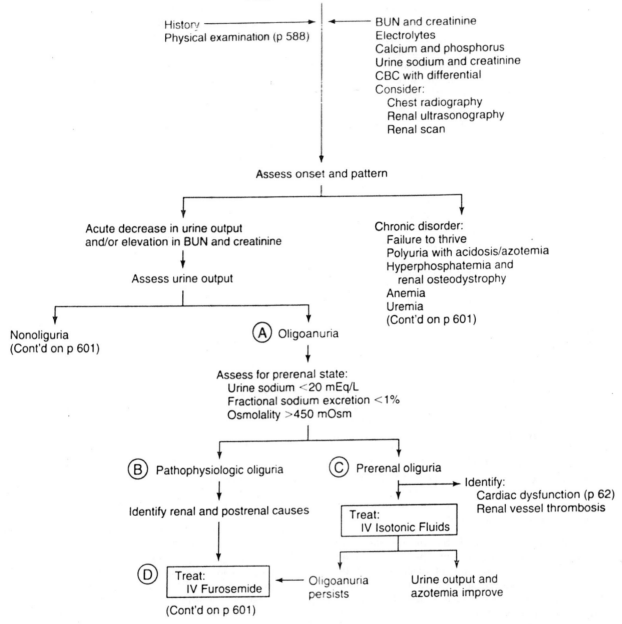

Patient with RENAL FAILURE

History ——————— BUN and creatinine
Physical examination (p 588) ←—— Electrolytes
Calcium and phosphorus
Urine sodium and creatinine
CBC with differential
Consider:
  Chest radiography
  Renal ultrasonography
  Renal scan

Assess onset and pattern

Acute decrease in urine output
and/or elevation in BUN and creatinine

Chronic disorder:
  Failure to thrive
  Polyuria with acidosis/azotemia
  Hyperphosphatemia and
    renal osteodystrophy
  Anemia
  Uremia
  (Cont'd on p 601)

Assess urine output

Nonoliguria
(Cont'd on p 601)

(A) Oligoanuria

Assess for prerenal state:
  Urine sodium <20 mEq/L
  Fractional sodium excretion <1%
  Osmolality >450 mOsm

(B) Pathophysiologic oliguria

(C) Prerenal oliguria

Identify:
  Cardiac dysfunction (p 62)
  Renal vessel thrombosis

Identify renal and postrenal causes

Treat:
IV Isotonic Fluids

(D) Treat:
IV Furosemide

Oligoanuria
persists

Urine output and
azotemia improve

(Cont'd on p 601)

condition when possible. Appropriate crystalloid is the usual choice for volume expansion unless findings suggest other deficits such as blood or albumin.

D. In some cases early intervention with diuretics may forestall oliguria. After ruling out hypovolemia, determine the renal response to a challenge dose of 2 to 5 mg/kg IV furosemide. If there is no response

to the lower dose, use a maximal dose once. Good response producing nonoliguric renal failure will ease medical management, as fluid balance can be better controlled and necessary medications, blood products, and nutrition can be safely administered, avoiding or possibly delaying dialysis. A poor response to diuretics generally heralds the need for dialysis.

E. Immediate dialysis is indicated when any of the following is present or imminent: (1) symptomatic fluid overload unresponsive to diuretics; (2) severe or unremitting acidosis where volume concerns limit the administration of sodium bicarbonate; (3) hyperkalemia in the face of limited ability to correct with infusions of sodium bicarbonate, glucose and insulin, or administration of kayexalate resin, and (4) severe azotemia (BUN >100 mg/dl—varies with age and clinical conditions); or (5) uremic symptoms (nausea, vomiting, bleeding diathesis, CNS depression).

F. Dietary restrictions depend on whether dialysis has been initiated. More stringent dietary controls are needed without dialysis; therefore, the need to provide adequate nutrition (volume of intake) must be addressed. If dialysis is part of the management, restriction of dietary protein is usually not necessary, and potassium and phosphate restriction may be lessened. Oral phosphate binders in the form of calcium carbonate or citrate aid in normalizing and controlling serum phosphorus (Table 1). Use a dose that produces a serum phosphorus of approximately 4 to 5 mg/dl. Monitor calcium with therapy. For treatment of hypertension, see p 66. Glucose and insulin as well as bicarbonate infusions are temporary measures for hyperkalemia. Kayexalate, furosemide, or dialysis removes excess potassium from the body and is more effective long-term therapy.

G. Complications of sustained ARF include fluid overload with consequent hypertension, CHF, and pulmonary edema; acidosis; hyperkalemia; and hyperphosphatemia or hypocalcemia. Anemia is a complication in prolonged ARF. Transfuse blood products under volume-controlled conditions when clinically indicated. Timely initiation of human recombinant erythropoietin 100 U/kg q.o.d. may obviate red blood cell transfusion. Treat patients with water-soluble vitamins and B complexes as well as folate and iron.

H. Complications occur in CRF but at a slower rate, permitting physiologic adjustment. The degree of renal compromise depends on time of diagnosis and any correctable cause. Radiographs can demonstrate surgically correctable problems such as ureteral reflux or obstruction, but abnormalities minimally or not immediately amenable to surgical intervention require pediatric nephrologic consultation for medical management and may prompt discussions of dialysis and renal transplantation. After the newborn period, abnormalities of the urinary system that lead to CRF may present with failure to thrive or short stature secondary to renal acidosis, azotemia, and/or renal osteodystrophy; polyuria reflecting the kidneys' inability to elaborate concentrated urine; urinary tract infection; proteinuria and/or hematuria; and if detected late, anemia and/or uremic signs and symptoms.

I. With inability to concentrate the urine, fluid overload and attendant hypertension are seldom seen. To the contrary, children with CRF are easily prone to dehydration given excessive urinary output. Abundant urine flow obviates hyperkalemia as well. Renal tubular acidosis (RTA) is one of the first biochemical abnormalities noted (RTA as an isolated renal defect is a diagnosis of exclusion). Azotemia and hyperphosphatemia ensue, with progressive deterioration in GFR. Renal osteodystrophy is primarily the result of phosphate accumulation. Although hyperphosphatemia signals increased renal excretion of phosphorus under the influence of parathyroid hormone (PTH), the sustained levels of PTH result in secondary hyperparathyroidism. Before GFR drops below 50%, effects of this mechanism can produce normal serum calcium and phosphorus, but elevated alkaline phosphatase and/or PTH measurements will reveal the secondary pathology. Early consultation and concomitant follow-up with pediatric nephrology are advisable.

References

Badr KF, Ichikawa I. Prerenal failure: A deleterious shift from renal compensation to decompensation. N Engl J Med 1988; 319:623.

Barratt TM. Acute renal failure. In: Holliday MA, Barratt TM, Vernier RL, eds. Pediatric nephrology. 2nd ed. Baltimore: Williams & Wilkins, 1987:766.

Feld LG, Springate JE, Fildes RD. Acute renal failure. I. Pathophysiology and diagnosis. J Pediatr 1986; 109:401.

Fildes RD, Springate JE, Feld LG. Acute renal failure. II. Management of suspected and established disease. J Pediatr 1986; 109:567.

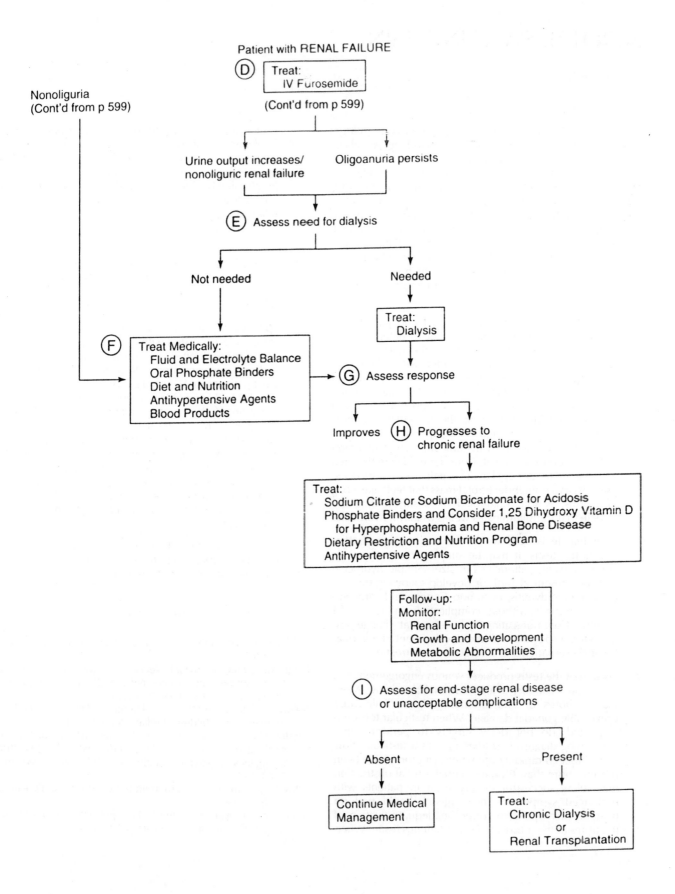

Patient with RENAL FAILURE

(D) Treat:
IV Furosemide

Nonoliguria
(Cont'd from p 599)

(Cont'd from p 599)

Urine output increases/   Oligoanuria persists
nonoliguric renal failure

(E) Assess need for dialysis

Not needed   Needed

Treat:
Dialysis

(F) Treat Medically:
   Fluid and Electrolyte Balance
   Oral Phosphate Binders
   Diet and Nutrition
   Antihypertensive Agents
   Blood Products

(G) Assess response

Improves   (H) Progresses to
chronic renal failure

Treat:
   Sodium Citrate or Sodium Bicarbonate for Acidosis
   Phosphate Binders and Consider 1,25 Dihydroxy Vitamin D
     for Hyperphosphatemia and Renal Bone Disease
   Dietary Restriction and Nutrition Program
   Antihypertensive Agents

Follow-up:
Monitor:
   Renal Function
   Growth and Development
   Metabolic Abnormalities

(I) Assess for end-stage renal disease
or unacceptable complications

Absent   Present

Continue Medical
Management

Treat:
   Chronic Dialysis
    or
   Renal Transplantation

SCROTAL SWELLING/PAIN

Stephen Berman, M.D.

A. In the history note onset, duration, pattern (intermittent or constant), and severity of scrotal swelling. Ask about associated pain radiating to the abdomen (testicular torsion), rectum (orchitis), or inguinal region (epididymitis). Sudden onset of severe pain with nausea, vomiting, and fever suggest testicular torsion. Gradual onset of pain with dysuria, urethral discharge, and fever suggests epididymitis. Note precipitating factors such as trauma, skin infection, or contact dermatitis. Patients with testicular torsion often have a history of mild trauma. Identify predisposing conditions such as Henoch-Schönlein purpura, nephrosis, liver disease, and malignancy, especially leukemia.

B. In the physical examination inspect and palpate the testis. Examine the standing patient to determine the axis of both testes. An abnormally high-lying horizontal-axis testis that is diffusely tender with discolored, edematous scrotal skin suggests testicular torsion. Elevation of the testis increases pain. Normal Doppler ultrasonography and nuclear scans do not rule out a torsion. Consider torsion of the testicular appendix when tenderness is limited to the superior lateral aspect of the testis. Occasionally the blue dot sign of infarction of the appendix is present. Consider epididymitis when an enlarged tender epididymis is palpated. A varicocele presents as a nontender scrotal mass that feels like a bag of worms. A soft, fluid-filled mass surrounding the testicle that transilluminates well is usually a hydrocele.

C. A hydrocele is fluid within the tunica vaginalis that covers the testis. It may be simple (constant size) or communicating (alterations in size). Simple hydrocele may be present at birth or develop following trauma, torsion, epididymitis, or tumor. Congenital hydroceles usually resolve without complication in 12 to 18 months. Communicating hydroceles that change size are often associated with the development of a hernia. Refer these patients to a surgeon for correction.

D. Torsion of the testis produces venous engorgement and infarction secondary to loss of arterial blood flow. More than 6 hours of total arterial occlusion will cause irreversible gonadal damage. When testicular torsion is suspected, do not delay surgery to perform time-consuming diagnostic studies such as a testicular flow scan. Proceed rapidly even when symptoms have been present more than 6 hours; partial arterial obstruction may allow successful surgery even in patients with prolonged symptoms. The surgeon should perform bilateral orchiopexy to correct inadequate fixation of the testes to the intrascrotal subcutaneous tissue. When surgery is performed within 6 hours of torsion, the gonad is always salvaged. Surgery after 7 to 12 hours is successful in 70% of cases, and after 12 hours in 20%. In emergencies consider attempting detorsion by rotating the involved testis outward towards the thigh after premedication with IV morphine (0.1 mg/kg). Dramatic relief of pain and return of the testis to its normal position indicate success. Recurrent intermittent torsion with spontaneous improvement may occur.

E. Postpubertal orchitis is associated with several viral infections (mumps, coxsackievirus, and echovirus) and with gonorrhea. In prepubertal boys obtain a urology consultation to rule out testicular torsion.

F. Epididymitis, which usually occurs after puberty, is commonly associated with *Chlamydia, Escherichia coli,* or gonorrhea. It often presents with pyuria or hematuria and may be associated with a urinary tract infection. Treat patients for *Neisseria gonorrhoeae* and *Chlamydia* (see Table 2 on p 346). Supportive measures include elevation of the scrotum, sitz baths, and analgesia. Epididymitis may have a 3 to 4 week course. When epididymitis occurs in a prepubertal boy, perform a diagnostic work-up for urinary tract abnormalities (ultrasonography, voiding cystourethrography). Bacterial pathogens are *Staphylococcus,* gram-negative enterics, *Haemophilus influenzae,* and *Salmonella.* When severe pain is present, consult a urologist and consider hospitalization.

G. Idiopathic scrotal edema may be a form of angioneurotic edema. The testes are normal, and the swelling resolves without therapy in 48 hours.

References

Hermann D. The pediatric acute scrotum. Pediatr Ann 1989; 18:198.

Likitnukul S, McCracken GH, Nelson JD, Votteler TP. Epididymitis in children and adolescents: A 20-year retrospective study. Am J Dis Child 1987; 141:41.

Nakayama DK, Rowe MI. Inguinal hernia and the acute scrotum in infants and children. Pediatr Rev 1989; 11:87.

Snyder HMcC, Caldamone AA, Duckett JW. Scrotal pain/swelling. In: Fleisher G, Ludwig S, eds. Textbook of pediatric emergency medicine. Baltimore: Williams & Wilkins, 1983:237.

Stillwell TJ, Kramer SA. Intermittent testicular torsion. Pediatrics 1986; 77:908.

Stoller MS, Kogan BA, Hricak H. Spermatic cord torsion: Diagnostic limitations. Pediatrics 1985; 76:929.

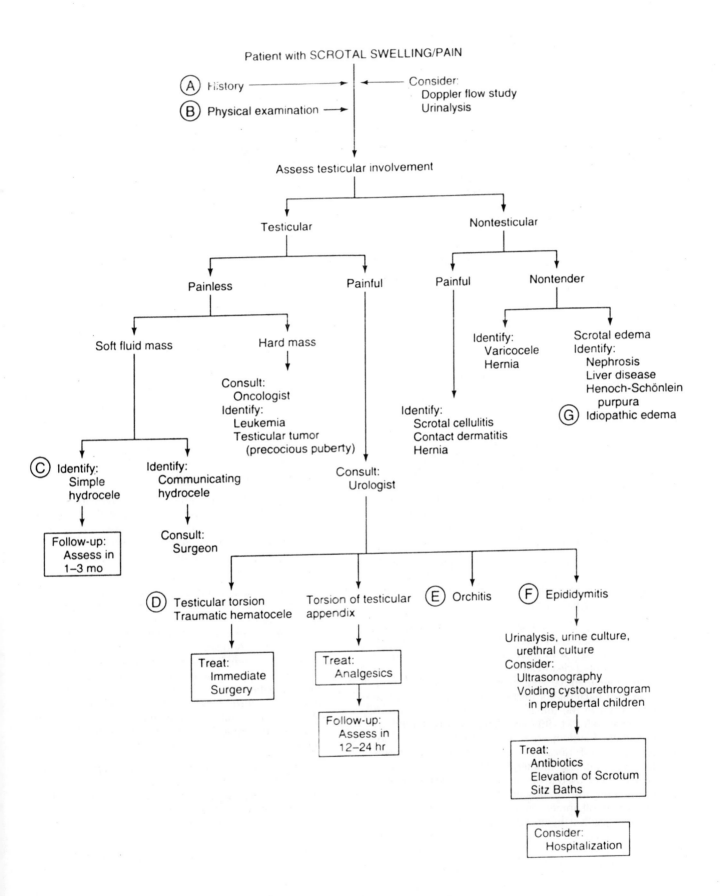

Patient with SCROTAL SWELLING/PAIN

(A) History ⟶ ← Consider:
　　　　　　　　　　　　　　Doppler flow study
(B) Physical examination ⟶ 　Urinalysis

Assess testicular involvement

Testicular　　　　　　　　　　　Nontesticular

Painless　　　　Painful　　　Painful　　　Nontender

Soft fluid mass　　Hard mass

Identify:
　Varicocele
　Hernia

Scrotal edema
Identify:
　Nephrosis
　Liver disease
　Henoch-Schönlein
　　purpura
(G) Idiopathic edema

Consult:
　Oncologist
Identify:
　Leukemia
　Testicular tumor
　　(precocious puberty)

Identify:
　Scrotal cellulitis
　Contact dermatitis
　Hernia

(C) Identify:
　　Simple
　　hydrocele

Identify:
　Communicating
　hydrocele

Consult:
　Urologist

Follow-up:
Assess in
1–3 mo

Consult:
　Surgeon

(D) Testicular torsion
　　Traumatic hematocele

Torsion of testicular
appendix

(E) Orchitis

(F) Epididymitis

Treat:
　Immediate
　Surgery

Treat:
　Analgesics

Urinalysis, urine culture,
urethral culture
Consider:
　Ultrasonography
　Voiding cystourethrogram
　　in prepubertal children

Follow-up:
Assess in
12–24 hr

Treat:
　Antibiotics
　Elevation of Scrotum
　Sitz Baths

Consider:
　Hospitalization

URINARY TRACT INFECTION

Stephen Berman, M.D.
Gary M. Lum, M.D.

Urinary tract infection (UTI) can involve the kidney (pyelonephritis or abscess), collecting system (pyonephrosis), ureter (ureteritis), bladder (cystitis), or urethra (urethritis). The most frequent organisms causing UTI are *Escherichia coli*, followed by *Klebsiella, Enterobacter, Proteus mirabilis, Pseudomonas,* and enterococci. The clinical presentation varies with age. Neonates have irritability, hypothermia or hyperthermia, poor suck, vomiting, diarrhea, and failure to thrive. Infants have fever, vomiting, diarrhea, poor feeding, and failure to thrive. Preschoolers have fever, abdominal pain, and change in urinary pattern. School-age children have fever, abdominal and/or flank pain, frequency, urgency, and dysuria. Children with a neurogenic bladder or other reason for incomplete bladder emptying have a high risk of infection.

A. In the history ask about dysuria, urgency, frequency, enuresis, abdominal pain, flank pain, or foul-smelling, cloudy urine. Ask about the frequency of recurrent episodes and document the results of prior urine cultures and radiologic studies. Note associated symptoms such as fever, chills, nausea, vomiting, vaginal or penile discharge, malaise, headaches, and visual disturbances. Identify possible predisposing factors, including poor perianal hygiene, trauma, pinworms, masturbation, chronic constipation, vaginitis or urethritis, infrequent voiding, tight clothing, exposure to chemicals (bubble bath, soaps), pregnancy, and urinary tract abnormalities. Ureteric reflux in a sibling increases the risk in the patient.

B. In the physical examination note blood pressure and do a fundoscopic examination. Determine the presence of vulvovaginitis or urethral discharge. Document suprapubic pain or flank pain.

C. Diagnosis of UTI can be based on a suprapubic aspiration that grows any organisms, a catheterized urine specimen with more than 10^3 organisms, or in older patients a clean-catch, midstream urine specimen with more than 10^5 organisms associated with more than 100 bacteria/hpf (high-power field) or a positive nitrate test in the urinalysis. A clean-catch midstream urine has an 80% to 90% correlation with a catheterized specimen. Random voids and bagged specimens are useful only if negative since contamination makes positive cultures uninterpretable; such specimens should not be used to document a UTI. The presence of bacteria on unspun, unstained urine specimens examined under oil immersion or a finding of more than five bacteria using a hemocytometer correlates well with positive cultures. Pyuria is nonspecific and occurs

TABLE 1 Degree of Illness in Urinary Tract Infection

Moderate	Severe
Signs that suggest urethritis or cystitis	Symptomatic infants <3 mo Signs of pyelonephritis: high fever, severe flank pain, toxic appearance

without UTI in appendicitis, dehydration, trauma, glomerulonephritis, renal tubular acidosis, chemical irritation, viral infection, vaginal washout, and fever.

D. A reasonable choice for initial outpatient oral antibiotic therapy is amoxicillin, TMP-SMX, nitrofurantoin, ampicillin with clavulanate, or a cephalosporin. Antibiotic therapy may require modifications based on the results of the culture and sensitivity tests. The duration of therapy is controversial; recommendations vary from 3 to 14 days, and 10 days is reasonable. Teach children proper anal hygiene. Instruct children and parents to avoid bubble baths, chemical irritants, and tight clothing. Treat any predisposing conditions such as constipation and pinworm infections.

E. Several cost-effective methods of screening for UTI are available for home use (nitrite dipstick, Microstix, glucose detection strips) or office use (Dipslide or Miniculture). Since all screening tests overdiagnose, confirm positive tests with an appropriately obtained quantitative culture.

F. Perform renal ultrasonography and voiding cystourethrography (VCUG) following a first UTI in children under 5 years of age. UTIs in children under age 5 are more likely to be associated with anomalies or reflex nephropathy. Additional risk factors include infections in boys, recurrent infections, ear anomalies, and supernumerary nipples. Unfortunately, there is no way to identify patients with serious underlying disease other than to perform renal ultrasonography and VCUG. When a renal ultrasound identifies an abnormality, radioactive renal scanning can define the anatomy (with respect to renal scarring) and function more precisely.

G. Treat hospitalized patients with suspected pyelonephritis with IV ampicillin and an aminoglycoside or third-generation cephalosporin (cefotaxime or ceftriaxone). Continue IV antibiotics until clinical signs (fever, severe pain) resolve—usually 3 to 5 days—then continue oral antibiotics for an additional 10 to 14 day course.

(Continued on page 606)

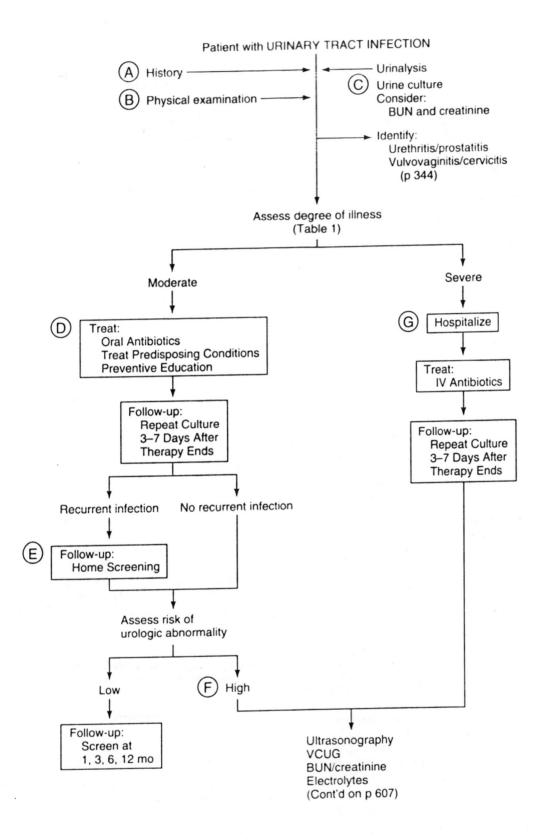

Patient with URINARY TRACT INFECTION

(A) History

(B) Physical examination

(C) Urinalysis
Urine culture
Consider:
    BUN and creatinine

Identify:
Urethritis/prostatitis
Vulvovaginitis/cervicitis
(p 344)

Assess degree of illness
(Table 1)

Moderate

(D) Treat:
Oral Antibiotics
Treat Predisposing Conditions
Preventive Education

Follow-up:
Repeat Culture
3–7 Days After
Therapy Ends

Recurrent infection   No recurrent infection

(E) Follow-up:
Home Screening

Assess risk of
urologic abnormality

Low   (F) High

Follow-up:
Screen at
1, 3, 6, 12 mo

Severe

(G) Hospitalize

Treat:
IV Antibiotics

Follow-up:
Repeat Culture
3–7 Days After
Therapy Ends

Ultrasonography
VCUG
BUN/creatinine
Electrolytes
(Cont'd on p 607)

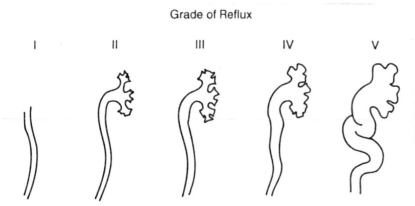

Grade of Reflux

| I | II | III | IV | V |

Figure 1 The International Classification of vesicoureteral reflux. Grade I reflux is associated with flow into a nondilated ureter. Grade II is flow into a nondilated renal pelvis. Grade III results in dilation of the collecting system. In grade IV the fornices of the collecting system are blunted. In grade V there is massive dilation and tortuosity of the collecting system. (From The International Reflux Committee. Medical versus surgical primary treatment of primary vesicoureteral reflux. Pediatrics 1987; 67:396; with permission.)

TABLE 2 Drug Therapy for Urinary Tract Infection

Drug	Dosage	Products
Outpatient Treatment		
Amoxicillin	10–15 mg/kg/dose t.i.d.	Liquid: 125 and 500/5 ml Tabs: 250, 500 mg Chewables: 125, 250 mg
TMP-SMX (Bactrim, Septra)	5 mg T/kg/dose b.i.d. or 0.5 ml/kg/dose b.i.d. Prophylaxis: 2 mg T/kg/day	Susp: 40 mg/5 ml Tabs: 80, 160 mg T:S = 1:5
Sulfisoxazole (Gantrisin)	30–40 mg/kg/dose q.i.d. Prophylaxis: 50 mg/kg/day	Susp: 500 mg/5 ml Tabs: 500 mg
Amoxicillin/Clavulanate (Augmentin)	10–15 mg/kg/dose t.i.d.	Liquid: 125, 250/5 ml Tabs: 125, 250, 500 mg
Cephalexin (Keflex)	10–15 mg/kg/dose q.i.d.	Liquid: 125, 250/5 ml Caps: 250, 500 mg
Nitrofurantoin	1.25–1.75 mg/kg/dose q.i.d. Prophylaxis: 1–2 mg/kg/day (avoid in newborns and patients with decreased renal function)	Liquid: 25 mg/5 ml Caps, tabs: 25, 50, 100 mg
IV Antibiotics for Hospitalized Patients		
Ampicillin	25–50 mg/kg/dose IV q6h	Vials: 125, 250, 50 mg; 2 g
Cefotaxime (Claforan)	50 mg/kg/dose IV q8h	Vials: 0.5, 1, 2 g
Ceftriaxone (Rocephin)	50 mg/kg/dose IV q12–24h	Vials: 0.25, 0.5, 1 g
Gentamicin	2.5 mg/kg/dose IV q8h (neonates q12h)	Vials: 20, 80 mg
Tobramycin	2.5 mg/kg/dose IV q8h (neonates q12h)	Vials: 20, 80 mg

T, trimethoprim component; S, sulfamethoxazole component.

H. Vesicoureteral reflux occurs when urine passes from the bladder to the ureter and possibly into the intrarenal collecting system (Fig. 1). Half of children studied during a UTI episode have mild or moderate reflux; 10% to 20% of these children have upper urinary tract damage. Mild or moderate reflux (grade II or less) should be allowed to resolve under protection of chemoprophylaxis. Refer patients with severe reflux (associated with any calyceal blunting or parenchymal scarring) to a pediatric urologist.

I. Antibiotics used for chemoprophylaxis include TMP-SMX, sulfisoxazole, and nitrofurantoin. They are given once daily, usually at bedtime.

J. Follow blood pressure and renal function (BUN, creatinine, and electrolytes) in any child with documented reflux due to the risk of associated renal functional disturbance, renal tubular acidosis, or hypertension. Permanent renal scarring and related proteinuria, as well as chronic renal failure and/or hypertension, may yet result from longstanding infection, so such infections require pediatric nephrologic consultation.

References

Alon U, Pery M, Davidai G, Berant M. Ultrasonography in the radiologic evaluation of children with urinary tract infection. Pediatrics 1986; 78:58.

Bailie MD, Arant BS Jr, Cho CT, et al. UTI: Long-term damage or short-term annoyance? Contemp Pediatr 1984; September:32.

Bailie MD, Arant BS Jr, Cho CT, et al. UTI: Selecting the best treatment options. Contemp Pediatr 1984; October:63.

Feld LG, Greenfield SP, Ogra PL. Urinary tract infections in infants and children. Pediatr Rev 1989; 11:71.

Landau D, Turner ME, Brennan J, Majd M. The value of urinalysis in differentiating acute pyelonephritis from lower urinary tract infection in febrile infants. Pediatr Infect Dis J 1994; 13:777.

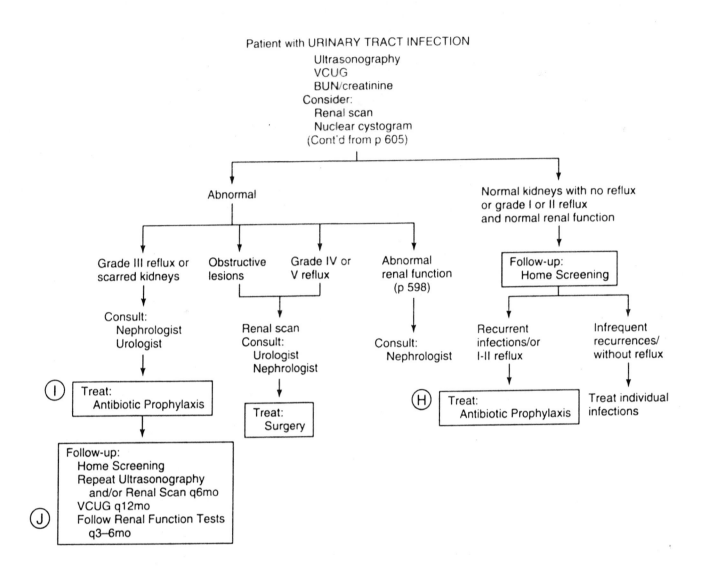

Patient with URINARY TRACT INFECTION
Ultrasonography
VCUG
BUN/creatinine
Consider:
Renal scan
Nuclear cystogram
(Cont'd from p 605)

Abnormal

Normal kidneys with no reflux
or grade I or II reflux
and normal renal function

Grade III reflux or
scarred kidneys

Obstructive
lesions

Grade IV or
V reflux

Abnormal
renal function
(p 598)

Follow-up:
Home Screening

Consult:
Nephrologist
Urologist

Renal scan
Consult:
Urologist
Nephrologist

Consult:
Nephrologist

Recurrent
infections/or
I-II reflux

Infrequent
recurrences/
without reflux

Ⓘ Treat:
Antibiotic Prophylaxis

Treat:
Surgery

Ⓗ Treat:
Antibiotic Prophylaxis

Treat individual
infections

Ⓙ Follow-up:
Home Screening
Repeat Ultrasonography
and/or Renal Scan q6mo
VCUG q12mo
Follow Renal Function Tests
q3–6mo

McCracken GH Jr. Options in antimicrobial management of urinary tract infections in infants and children. Pediatr Infect Dis J 1989; 8:552.

Moffatt M, Embree J, Grimm P, Law B. Short-course antibiotic therapy for urinary tract infections in children. Am J Dis Child 1988; 142:57.

Sheldon CA, Wacksman J. Vesicoureteral reflux. Pediatr Rev 1995; 16:22.

Sreenarasimhaiah V, Alon US. Uroradiologic evaluation of children with urinary tract infection: Are both ultrasonography and renal cortical scintigraphy necessary? J Pediatr 1995; 127:373.

Todd JK. Management of urinary tract infections: Children are different. Pediatr Rev 1995; 16:190.

TOXICOLOGIC DISORDERS

EVALUATION OF ACUTE POISONING AND OVERDOSE

Stephen Berman, M.D.

Acute poisoning may result from ingestion, eye or topical exposure, inhalation, or envenomation. The types of substances most often reported to cause poisoning are cleaning products, analgesics, cosmetics, plants, decongestants and antihistamine cold drugs, pesticides, hydrocarbons, topical medications, bites, envenomations, and foreign bodies.

A. If initial contact is by telephone, quickly obtain the patient's telephone number and address in case contact is broken. Ask about the product and amount ingested, time of ingestion, current symptoms, and medical history. Note toxins with a delayed onset of serious effects such as tricyclic antidepressants and diphenoxylate with atropine (Lomotil).

B. In the physical examination rapidly assess the airway, breathing, circulation, and the level of consciousness with the Glasgow Coma Scale (see p 104). Carefully assess the eyes for pupil size and responsiveness, nystagmus, extraocular eye movements, and fundi. Note corrosive lesions, odors, and bleeding in the mouth. Assess airway protective reflexes. Count respirations, listen for air exchange, and note retractions, grunting, and nasal flaring (signs of distress). Assess the peripheral perfusion and note heart rate and rhythm. Note skin color and any lesions such as bites, burns, or blisters.

C. Initial decontamination may include saline eye lavage, removal of contaminated clothing and washing the skin with soap and water, or GI interventions. Acute management of a toxic ingestion is activated charcoal 1 g/kg body weight with sorbitol, followed by a cathartic such as sodium or magnesium sulfate. Toxins not absorbed well to charcoal include iron, mineral acids or bases, alcohol, cyanide, solvents, hydrocarbons, and other water-insoluble compounds. The use of ipecac in awake, alert patients may not affect outcome. Gastric lavage is most effective when carried out within 1 hour of ingestion. Activated charcoal should follow gastric lavage. Use the largest nasogastric tube that can be reasonably passed and initially aspirate the gastric contents. Use half normal saline or water in older patients with volumes of 50 to 100 ml in young children and 150 to 200 in adolescents until the return is clear. This is about 2 L in adolescents and 500 ml in young children. Consider whole bowel irrigation with a polyethylene glycol-balanced electrolyte solution for iron and other heavy metal ingestions. Avoid emesis or gastric lavage when a corrosive substance or hydrocarbon petroleum distillate has been ingested.

D. When hypoglycemia is identified by dipstick, give 0.25 to 1 g/kg of glucose as 25% dextrose in water. Hypoglycemia can be associated with poisoning of ethanol, insulin, salicylates, oral hypoglycemics, and β-blocking agents. When the mental status is altered, suspect an opioid toxin and administer 1 to 2 mg of naloxone. Treat adolescent patients with a history of opioid intoxication with a 2 mg bolus every 2 minutes up to 5 times (total dose of 10 mg) if necessary for a response.

(Continued on page 612)

TABLE 1 Degree of Illness in Poisoning and Overdose

Mild	Moderate	Severe	Very Severe
Asymptomatic No risk of deterioration	Benign, self-limited toxic effects	Altered mental state (lethargy) or signs of toxicity that may worsen and become life-threatening	Unstable vital signs (shock, respiratory depression, arrhythmia) or Coma or Stupor or Seizures

Patient with ACUTE POISONING AND OVERDOSE

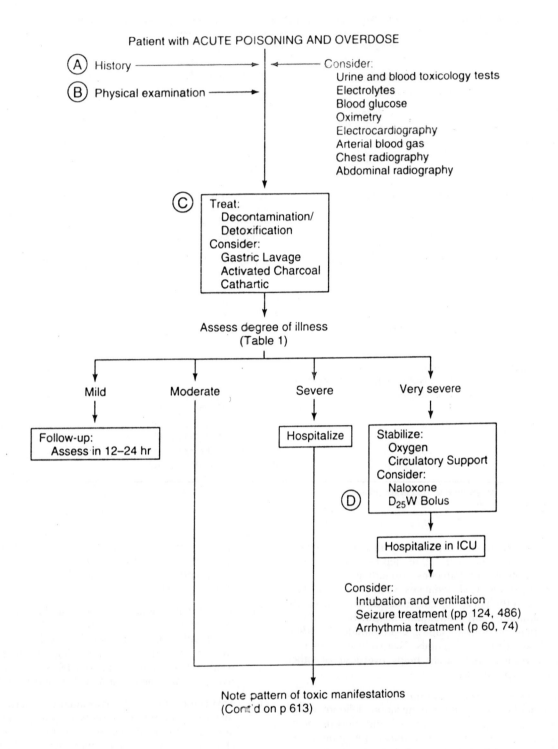

Ⓐ History ⟶ ← Consider:
                                                Urine and blood toxicology tests
Ⓑ Physical examination ⟶   Electrolytes
                                                Blood glucose
                                                Oximetry
                                                Electrocardiography
                                                Arterial blood gas
                                                Chest radiography
                                                Abdominal radiography

Ⓒ Treat:
    Decontamination/
    Detoxification
Consider:
    Gastric Lavage
    Activated Charcoal
    Cathartic

Assess degree of illness
(Table 1)

Mild   Moderate   Severe   Very severe

Follow-up:
Assess in 12–24 hr

Hospitalize

Stabilize:
    Oxygen
    Circulatory Support
Consider:
    Naloxone
Ⓓ   D$_{25}$W Bolus

Hospitalize in ICU

Consider:
    Intubation and ventilation
    Seizure treatment (pp 124, 486)
    Arrhythmia treatment (p 60, 74)

Note pattern of toxic manifestations
(Cont'd on p 613)

TABLE 2 Specific Antidotes to Acute Poisoning and Overdose in Children and Adolescents

Toxin	Antidote	Dosage	Product Availability
Opioids	Naloxone (Narcan)	1–2 mg/dose IM, IV	Solution: 0.4 mg/ml
Anticholinergics	Physostigmine	Adult: 2 mg/dose IM, IV Child: 0.5 mg/dose IM, IV May repeat q15min until improved	Solution: 1 mg/ml (2 ml)
Anticholinesterases (carbamates)	Atropine	May give q2–3h 0.05–0.1 mg/kg/dose IM or IV, repeated q15min until patient atropinized	Solution: 0.1 mg/ml or 0.3 mg/ml
Anticholinesterases (organophosphates)	Pralidoxime (Protopam)	Adult: 1–2 g IV Child: 25–50 mg/kg/dose IV Repeat in 1 hr p.r.n., then q6–8h	Solution: dilute to 10 mg/ml
Phenothiazines	Benztropine mesylate (Cogentin)	1–2 mg/dose for adults IM, IV	Inject: 1 mg/ml (2 ml) Tabs: 0.5, 1, 2 mg
	Diphenhydramine (Benadryl)	2 mg/kg/dose IM, IV, or PO q6h	Inject: 10 mg/ml Tabs: 50 mg Elixir: 12.5 mg/5 ml
Tricyclic antidepressants	Sodium bicarbonate Magnesium sulfate	1–2 mEq/kg IV 50 mg/kg IV	
Acetaminophen	N-Acetylcysteine (Mucomyst)	140 mg/kg PO initially, then 70 mg/kg q4h for 68 hr (17 doses)	10%, 20% solution
Benzodiazepines	Flumazenil (Note: Not FDA approved for pediatric use)	0.01 mg/kg IV	—
Cyanide	Sodium nitrite	Consult for recommended dose to avoid methemoglobinemia	—
Methanol and ethylene glycol	Ethanol	0.6 g/kg IV over 1 hr to achieve blood level of 100 mg/dl	—
Warfarin	Vitamin K	Child: 1–5 mg IV, IM, SC, PO Adult: 10 mg IV, IM, SC, PO	Vials: 10 mg/ml

Modified from Henretig FM, Shannon M. Toxicologic emergencies. In: Fleisher GR, Ludwig S, eds. Textbook of pediatric emergency medicine. 3rd ed. Baltimore: Williams & Wilkins, 1993:756.

E. Narcotic-sedative-hypnotic toxic syndrome is characterized by depressed mental state, depressed respirations, and hypotension. Narcotics, excluding meperidine, produce miosis. CNS sedatives, such as alcohol, barbiturates, ethchlorvynol, chlordiazepoxide, diazepam, meprobamate, and methaqualone, can be associated with small or normal pupils. Glutethimide (Doriden) overdose causes fixed pupils. Naloxone reverses narcotic overdose but rarely helps overdose of other sedative-hypnotic drugs.

F. Anticholinergic toxic syndrome is characterized by altered mental state (confusion, agitation, delirium, hallucinations, seizures, coma), dry skin and mucous membranes, mydriasis, tachycardia, urinary retention, fever, and decreased bowel sounds. Anticholinergic drugs include antihistamines, antiparkinsonism agents, belladonna alkaloids, haloperidol, tricyclic antidepressants, and toxic mushrooms and plants. Physostigmine should be given only when symptoms are life-threatening. Physostigmine is contraindicated in patients with asthma, vascular compromise, or urinary obstruction.

G. Cholinergic toxic syndrome is characterized by miosis, increased salivation, lacrimation, muscle fasciculations and weakness, sweating, vomiting, wheezing, and bradycardia. The CNS effects include irritability, headache, confusion, seizures, and coma. Chemicals and drugs that cause this syndrome include organophosphate and carbamate insecticides, physostigmine, neostigmine, and edrophonium.

H. Toxins that produce metabolic acidosis include salicylates, methanol (treat with ethanol), ethylene glycol (treat with ethanol), carbon monoxide (CO) (treat with oxygen), cyanide (treat with sodium nitrite followed by sodium thiosulfate), paraldehyde, isoniazid, formaldehyde, nalidixic acid, carbenicillin, and ticarcillin.

I. Toxins most frequently associated with cardiac arrhythmia are cyclic antidepressants, amphetamines, anticholinergics, arsenic, β-blockers, calcium channel blockers, chloral hydrate, cyanide, theophylline, digitalis, phenothiazines, quinidine, and lithium.

J. Toxins that can induce methemoglobinemia and cyanosis unresponsive to oxygen include nitrates, nitrites, aniline, phenacetin, phenols, local anesthetics, sulfonamides, phenazopyridine, antimalarials, sulfones, naphthalene, and paraaminosalicylic acid.

K. Toxins that produce extrapyramidal CNS effects (dystonic reactions or oculogyric crisis) include phenothiazines and butyrophenones. Treat with an antiparkinsonian agent (Cogentin) or an antihistamine.

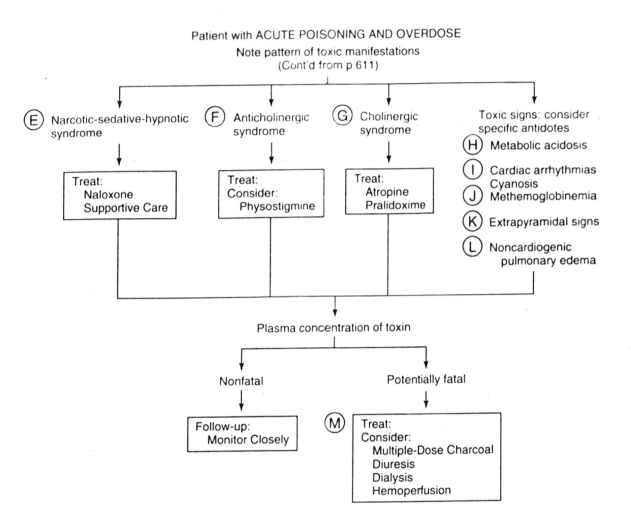

Patient with ACUTE POISONING AND OVERDOSE
Note pattern of toxic manifestations
(Cont'd from p 611)

(E) Narcotic-sedative-hypnotic syndrome

(F) Anticholinergic syndrome

(G) Cholinergic syndrome

Toxic signs: consider specific antidotes

(H) Metabolic acidosis

(I) Cardiac arrhythmias
Cyanosis
(J) Methemoglobinemia

(K) Extrapyramidal signs

(L) Noncardiogenic pulmonary edema

Treat:
Naloxone
Supportive Care

Treat:
Consider:
Physostigmine

Treat:
Atropine
Pralidoxime

Plasma concentration of toxin

Nonfatal

Potentially fatal

Follow-up:
Monitor Closely

(M) Treat:
Consider:
Multiple-Dose Charcoal
Diuresis
Dialysis
Hemoperfusion

L. Toxins that produce noncardiogenic pulmonary edema may be inhaled (CO, phosgene, hydrogen sulfide, chlorine, nitrogen oxides, and beryllium) or ingested (narcotics, salicylates, sedative hypnotics).

M. Consider additional therapies when the risk of a serious complication or a poor outcome is high. These include multiple-dose activated charcoal, diuresis with furosemide 1 mg/kg or mannitol (initial dose 0.5 g/kg), dialysis, and hemoperfusion. Indications for forced diuresis include a drug level in the potentially fatal range that is well excreted in the urine, adequate renal function, no cardiopulmonary compromise or evidence of cerebral edema, and a stable systolic blood pressure above 90 mm Hg. Multiple-dose activated charcoal is used for serious ingestions of phenobarbital, carbamazepine, phenytoin, digoxin, salicylates, and theophylline. Hemodialysis may be indicated for potentially fatal poisonings with lithium, ethylene glycol, methanol, and salicylates. Hemoperfusion may benefit poisonings with phenobarbital, theophylline, paraquat, glutethimide, methaqualone, ethchlovynol, or meprobamate.

References

Garber M. Carbamate poisoning: The other insecticide. Pediatrics 1987; 79:734.

Haddad LM. The emergency management of poisoning. Pediatr Ann 1987; 16:900.

Henretig FM, Shannon M. Toxicologic emergencies. In: Fleisher GR, Ludwig S, eds. Textbook of pediatric emergency medicine. 3rd ed. Baltimore: Williams & Wilkins, 1993:745.

Kulig K, Baro-Or D, Cantrill SV, et al. Management of acutely poisoned patients without gastric emptying. Ann Emerg Med 1985; 14:562.

Mack RB. Anticholinergic syndrome: La bella donna con il bacio di morte. Contemp Pediatr 1986; December:69.

Mack RB. Imipramine overdose: Prejudiced and proud. Contemp Pediatr 1988; August:93.

Mack RB. Methanol poisoning: When the stars threw down their spears. Contemp Pediatr 1989; April:95.

Porter GA. The treatment of ethylene glycol poisoning simplified. N Engl J Med 1988; 319:109.

Woolf AD. Poisoning in children and adolescents. Pediatr Rev 1993; 14:411.

ACETAMINOPHEN INTOXICATION

Stephen Berman, M.D.

Acetaminophen intoxication results from an ingestion of more than 140 mg/kg in a child or 7.5 g in an adult. Acetaminophen is metabolized by the liver, with a small amount excreted unchanged in the urine. The major toxic effect is on the liver. Metabolites bind to hepatocellular proteins and produce hepatic necrosis. Evidence of hepatotoxicity develops 24 to 48 hours postingestion, and damage usually peaks at 72 to 96 hours. Children are more resistant to acetaminophen hepatotoxicity because of differences in liver metabolism.

A. In the history ask about amount ingested, time of ingestion, and initial symptoms of toxicity such as nausea, vomiting, anorexia, and sweating.

B. Attempt to remove acetaminophen from the stomach with gastric lavage when large amounts have been ingested within 2 hours. Give activated charcoal and a cathartic following lavage when the ingestion occurred 2 to 4 hours earlier.

C. Assess the degree of toxicity by determining the acetaminophen level at least 4 hours after ingestion and plotting the value on the nomogram shown in Fig. 1. Patients with mild illness have ingested less than 140 mg/kg (child) or 7.5 g (adult). Those with moderate illness have ingested over 140 mg/kg (child) or 7.5 g (adult) but are under the line indicating no risk of hepatotoxicity. Severe toxicity is present in patients with possible or probable hepatic toxicity.

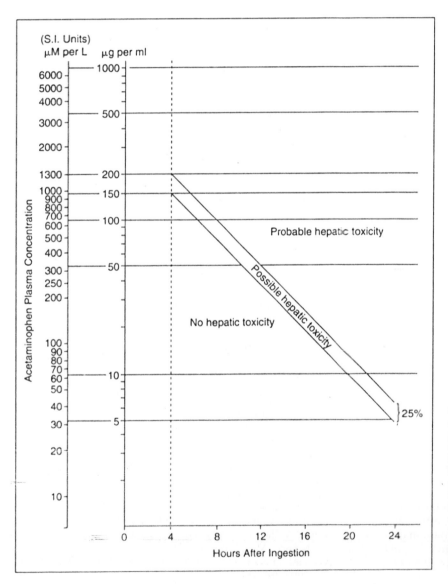

Figure 1 Rumack-Matthew nomogram for acetaminophen poisoning. Semilogarithmic plot of plasma acetaminophen levels versus time. Note: (1) Time coordinates refer to time of ingestion; (2) serum levels drawn before 4 hours may not represent peak levels; (3) the graph should be used only in relation to a single acute ingestion; and (4) the lower solid line 25% below the standard nomogram is included to allow for errors in acetaminophen plasma assays and estimated time from ingestion of an overdose. (From Riggs BS, Kulig K, Rumack BH. Current status of aspirin and acetaminophen intoxication. Pediatr Ann 1987; 16:897.)

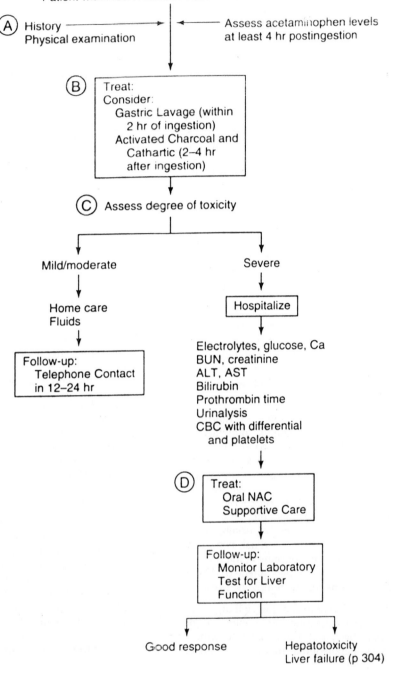

Patient with ACETAMINOPHEN INTOXICATION

Ⓐ History ──────────→ ←── Assess acetaminophen levels
Physical examination   at least 4 hr postingestion

Ⓑ Treat:
Consider:
   Gastric Lavage (within
     2 hr of ingestion)
   Activated Charcoal and
     Cathartic (2–4 hr
     after ingestion)

Ⓒ Assess degree of toxicity

Mild/moderate   Severe

Home care   Hospitalize
Fluids

Follow-up: Electrolytes, glucose, Ca
  Telephone Contact   BUN, creatinine
  in 12–24 hr   ALT, AST
                  Bilirubin
                  Prothrombin time
                  Urinalysis
                  CBC with differential
                    and platelets

Ⓓ Treat:
Oral NAC
Supportive Care

Follow-up:
  Monitor Laboratory
  Test for Liver
  Function

Good response   Hepatotoxicity
                       Liver failure (p 304)

D.   Oral *N*-acetylcysteine (NAC) should be given within 24 hours of ingestion to patients at risk for hepatotoxicity; however, results are best if treatment begins within 8 hours. If the patient cannot tolerate oral fluid because of vomiting, consider using a nasogastric or duodenal tube. Dilute the NAC solution to 5% and give an initial oral loading dose of 140 mg/kg followed by 17 maintenance doses of 70 mg/kg every 4 hours. Monitor hematologic, renal, and liver function while the patient is on NAC.

References

Mack RB. Acetaminophen overdose: Poet laureate asks a question. Contemp Pediatr 1991; June:71.

Riggs BS, Kulig K, Rumack BH. Current status of aspirin and acetaminophen intoxication. Pediatr Ann 1987; 16:886.

Smilkstein MJ, Knapp GL, Kulig KW, et al. Efficacy of oral *N*-acetylcysteine in the treatment of acetaminophen overdose. N Engl J Med 1988; 319:1557.

CARBON MONOXIDE POISONING

Jerrold M. Eichner, M.D.

Carbon monoxide (CO) is the leading cause of death by poisoning in the United States, at 3800 deaths per year. About 10,000 people each year seek medical attention for CO poisoning. The problem is grossly underdiagnosed because of its vague symptoms and unrecognized sources. Inhaled CO diffuses rapidly into the blood stream and reversibly binds to hemoglobin (Hb) with an affinity 240 times that of oxygen (O_2). The carboxyhemoglobin (COHb) decreases the amount of Hb available for O_2 transport and shifts the O_2 dissociation curve to the left, decreasing release of O_2 to the tissues. This stimulates an increase in alveolar ventilation by a reflex mechanism and increases CO uptake. The child's high metabolic rate results in rapid uptake of CO and therefore enhanced risk from exposure. Fetal Hb has a higher affinity for CO than adult Hb and the elimination half-life is longer, making the fetus and newborn more vulnerable to CO. Also, CO binds to cytochrome a3 oxidase, disrupting cellular respiration by inhibiting oxidative phosphorylation in the mitochondria, which may be its prime toxic effect. CO also binds to myoglobin, possibly causing myocardial and skeletal muscle dysfunction or necrosis. CO may cause lipid peroxidation and secondary hemorrhagic necrosis in the brain, leading to delayed neurologic sequelae.

A. In the history ask about nausea, vomiting, diarrhea, headache, weakness, fatigue, dizziness, difficulty in thinking, syncope, visual disturbance, confusion, convulsions, chest pain, and palpitations. Ask where the patient was and what the patient was doing when symptoms occurred. Describe the location: automobile (front or back seat), back of pickup truck (covered or open), home (which room), garage, etc. Ask about heaters, furnaces, stoves, fireplaces, especially those using natural gas, propane, wood, charcoal, coal, fuel oil, gasoline, kerosene; were any burning at the time or recently? Were other people or pets affected? Were methylene chloride solvents (paint removers) present?

B. In the physical examination note vomiting, lethargy, dizziness, ataxia, nystagmus, hearing loss, confusion, altered consciousness, cherry-red skin, visual disturbance, retinal hemorrhages, papilledema, motor disturbance,

TABLE 1 Symptoms of Acute CO Poisoning by Carboxyhemoglobin Level

COHb level	Symptoms
10%	Asymptomatic; may have headache, decreased exercise tolerance
20%	Fatigue, headache, nausea, vomiting, diarrhea, dizziness
30%	Visual disturbances, dyspnea, syncope, confusion, tachycardia
40%	Increased neurologic symptoms, convulsions, tachypnea
50%	Coma, Cheyne-Stokes respirations, depressed cardiovascular status
60%	Deep coma, bradycardia, hypotension, increased convulsions
70%	Respiratory failure, death

gait disturbance, convulsions, tachypnea, tachycardia, arrhythmias, depressed cardiac status (bradycardia, hypotension), and impending respiratory failure. Check any others who may have been exposed.

C. COHb levels confirm CO poisoning. The level depends on the concentration inhaled, time since removal from the source, and any treatment with O_2 in the interim. Table 1 shows the association of COHb with symptoms in acute poisoning, but a delay in drawing the sample or prior treatment with supplemental O_2 alters the correlation of symptoms with the level; patients with severe poisoning may have low or normal levels of COHb.

D. CO is a colorless, odorless, tasteless, nonirritating gas produced by incomplete combustion of organic material. The common sources are motor vehicle exhaust fumes, smoke, including cigarette smoke, and fumes from heaters, furnaces, stoves, water heaters, etc. Sterno heaters and paint removers containing methylene chloride (converted to CO by the liver) have been implicated. Poisoning can occur in automobiles, in the home, or at work, and is most frequent in northern and high-altitude states in winter.

(Continued on page 618)

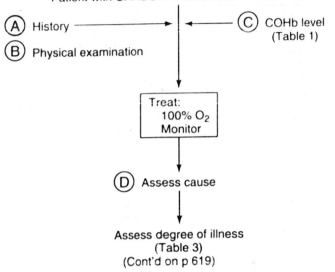

Patient with CARBON MONOXIDE POISONING

(A) History ——————→ ←—————— (C) COHb level
                                        (Table 1)

(B) Physical examination

Treat:
100% O_2
Monitor

(D) Assess cause

Assess degree of illness
(Table 3)
(Cont'd on p 619)

TABLE 2 Indications for Hyperbaric Oxygen Treatment

COHb level ≥ 25%
For pregnant patients COHb level ≥ 20% or distress on fetal monitoring
Any loss of consciousness regardless of COHb level
Any neurologic impairment regardless of COHb level
Persistence of neurologic symptoms after oxygen therapy
Arrhythmia, anginal pain, or ischemic changes on ECG
Underlying heart disease

TABLE 3 Severity According to COHb

Moderate	Severe	Very Severe (COHb >40%)
< 20% in pregnant patients	≥ 20% in pregnant patients	Shock
< 25% in other patients	≥ 25% in other patients	Cardiac arrhythmias
Symptoms that correlate with level 10%–20%	Symptoms that correlate with level ≥ 30%	Respiratory failure Coma Cerebral edema Convulsions Renal failure

E. The mainstay of treatment is supplemental O_2. High concentrations are necessary to replace CO from its tight bind to Hb, myoglobin, and cytochrome-oxidase. The half-life of COHb in room air is 4 to 5 ½ hours; with 100% O_2 it is reduced to 60 to 90 minutes; and with hyperbaric oxygen (HBO) at 3 atmospheres absolute (ATA) it is 23 minutes. Start supplemental O_2 at the first suspicion of CO poisoning; do not wait for COHb levels. Deliver O_2 with a tightly fitting nonrebreathing mask at 10 L/m, continuing until the COHb level is below 5% and symptoms resolve.

F. Careful monitoring is necessary for all patients. Cardiac arrhythmias may need treatment with antiarrhythmic agents. Hypotension may call for vascular volume expansion and/or pressor agents. Patients in a coma or with respiratory depression need tracheal intubation and mechanical ventilation. Signs of cerebral edema and increased intracranial pressure necessitate prompt management. Renal failure from myoglobinuria may demand treatment. Other respiratory injuries (smoke inhalation, chemical pneumonitis, thermal burns to the airway, aspiration, or cyanide poisoning) may be coincident and require treatment.

G. Hyperbaric oxygen (HBO) drastically increases elimination of CO from the body. Besides the reduced half-life of COHb, it speeds up the elimination of cytochrome-bound CO in tissues. In addition, 100% O_2 at 3 ATA allows for adequate tissue oxygenation by means of O_2 dissolved in plasma. There is also evidence that HBO decreases lipid peroxidation in the brain and eases cerebral edema and intracranial pressure. Table 2 lists indications for use of HBO. Starting HBO before 6 hours reduces mortality from 30% to 14%. There is enough evidence of the benefits that HBO should be attempted even if transport to an HBO facility will delay the start of treatment more than 6 hours.

H. Delayed neurologic sequelae occur in 12% to 43% of survivors of CO poisoning treated with normobaric O_2 but only up to 4% of those treated with HBO. Those sequelae include dementia, psychosis, personality alterations, memory loss, mutism, parkinsonism, cortical blindness, peripheral neuritis, perceptual deficits, and chronic headaches. Careful follow-up with neuropsychiatric examinations is important in long-term management.

I. As with all accidental poisonings and injuries, prevention is the best treatment. Comprehensive public education on the dangers of combustible material, adequate ventilation of indoor combustion, and proper maintenance of furnaces, stoves, and automobiles is necessary. Parents should be taught about the danger of having children ride in the back of pickup trucks.

References

Cobb N, Etzel RA. Unintentional carbon monoxide-related deaths in the United States, 1979 through 1988. JAMA 1991; 266:659.

Crocker PJ, Walker JS. Pediatric carbon monoxide toxicity. J Emerg Med 1985; 3:443.

Gozal D, Ziser A, Shupak A, Melamed Y. Accidental carbon monoxide poisoning. Clin Pediatr 1985; 24:132.

Hampson NB, Norkool DM. Carbon monoxide poisoning in children riding in the back of pickup trucks. JAMA 1992; 267:538.

Hardy KR, Thom SR. Pathophysiology and treatment of carbon monoxide poisoning. Clin Toxicol 1994; 32:613.

Ilano AL, Raffin TA. Management of carbon monoxide poisoning. Chest 1990; 97:165.

Mofenson HC, Caraccio TR, Brody GM. Carbon monoxide poisoning. Am J Emerg Med 1984; 2:254.

NHLBI Workshop Summary. Hyperbaric oxygenation therapy. Am Rev Resp Dis 1991; 144:1414.

Proudfoot AT. Carbon monoxide poisoning: Recent advances. Acta Clin Belg Suppl 1990; 13:61.

Raphael JC, Elkharrat D, Jars-Guincestre MC, et al. Trial of normobaric and hyperbaric oxygen for acute carbon monoxide intoxication. Lancet 1989; 2:414.

Rudge FW. Carbon monoxide poisoning in infants: Treatment with hyperbaric oxygen. South Med J 1993; 86:334.

Sanchez R, Fosarelli P, Felt B, et al: Carbon monoxide poisoning due to automobile exposure: Disparity between carboxyhemoglobin levels and symptoms of victims. Pediatrics 1988; 82:663.

Tibbles PM, Perrotta PL. Treatment of carbon monoxide poisoning: A critical review of human studies comparing normobaric oxygen with hyperbaric oxygen. Ann Emerg Med 1994; 24:269.

Tomaszewski CA, Thom SR. Use of hyperbaric oxygen in toxicology. Emerg Med Clin North Am 1994; 12:437.

Patient with CARBON MONOXIDE POISONING
Assess degree of illness
(Table 3)
(Cont'd from p 617)

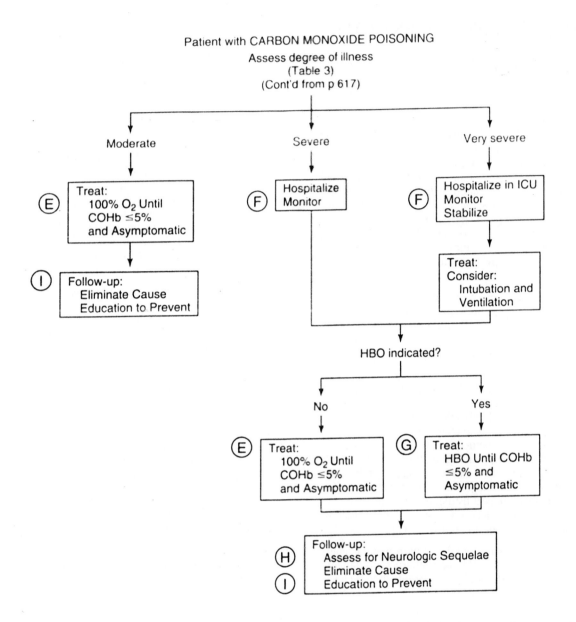

FOREIGN BODY INGESTION

Stephen Berman, M.D.

Foreign body ingestions usually are by children 6 months to 4 years of age. The child is often observed swallowing the object. The most common objects are coins, followed by safety pins (open or closed), marbles, bobbie pins, straight pins, buttons, button batteries, nails, tacks, screws, and small toys. High-risk objects associated with complications are aluminum tabs from disposable cans, objects with lead, batteries, and objects long in relation to the child's size. Over 90% of objects that pass into the stomach pass through the intestinal tract without complication. Distal sites of potential obstruction include the pylorus, duodenum, ligament of Treitz, ileocecal valve, and rectosigmoid.

A. In the history ask about symptoms associated with impaction of a foreign body in the esophagus such as dysphagia, drooling, pain, refusal to take foods, vomiting, cough, or stridor. Note congenital anomalies that may predispose to esophageal impaction (esophageal atresia).

B. Obtain anteroposterior and lateral chest radiography to locate the foreign body in the GI tract regardless of symptoms. Esophageal impaction can occur, especially with coins in asymptomatic children. The esophagus is the usual site of obstruction. The three areas of narrowing are the cricopharyngeus, the level of the arch of the aorta, and the cardioesophageal sphincter. Complications of esophageal impaction include perforation, tracheoesophageal fistula, esophageal-aortic fistula, and airway obstruction. Consider a contrast study when the ingested object is not radiopaque.

C. Mineral oil and increased intake of bran may facilitate passage by increasing stool bulk. Cathartics are dangerous, especially with sharp objects. Parents should check all stools. If the object has not been passed in 7 days, repeat the radiography.

D. Objects with lead should not be left in the stomach more than 7 days or in the small intestine more than 14 days. Batteries that do not pass within 72 hours are at a risk because of their corrosive contents. Most small batteries will pass uneventfully. Long nails and other objects may have difficulty passing the duodenal loop and ligament of Treitz. If possible, they should be endoscopically removed from the stomach and upper duodenum.

E. The method of removing a blunt esophageal foreign body is controversial. Options include the Foley catheter, bougie dilator advancement, flexible endoscopy, and rigid endoscopy. Removal of sharp objects requires endoscopy or surgery.

References

Caravati EM, Bennett DL, McElwee E. Pediatric coin ingestion: A prospective study on the utility of routine roentgenograms. Am J Dis Child 1989; 143:549.

Litovitz TL. Button battery ingestions: A review of 56 cases. JAMA 1983; 249:2495.

Neilson IR. Ingestion of coins and batteries. Pediatr Rev 1995; 16:35.

Paul RI, Christoffel KK, Binns HJ, et al. Foreign body ingestions in children: Risk of complication varies with site of initial care contact. Pediatrics 1993; 91:121.

Schunk JE, Corneli H, Bolte R. Pediatric coin ingestions: A prospective study of coin location and symptoms. Am J Dis Child 1989; 143:546.

TABLE 1   Degree of Illness in Foreign Body Ingestion

Mild	Moderate	Severe	Very Severe
Asymptomatic and Low-risk object distal to esophagus	Asymptomatic with evidence of object in esophagus or high-risk object in more distal site	Symptoms/signs of esophageal impaction or ingestion of a high-risk object	Signs of intestinal perforation, obstruction, or hemorrhage such as toxic appearance, persistent bilious vomiting, severe abdominal pain, or GI bleeding

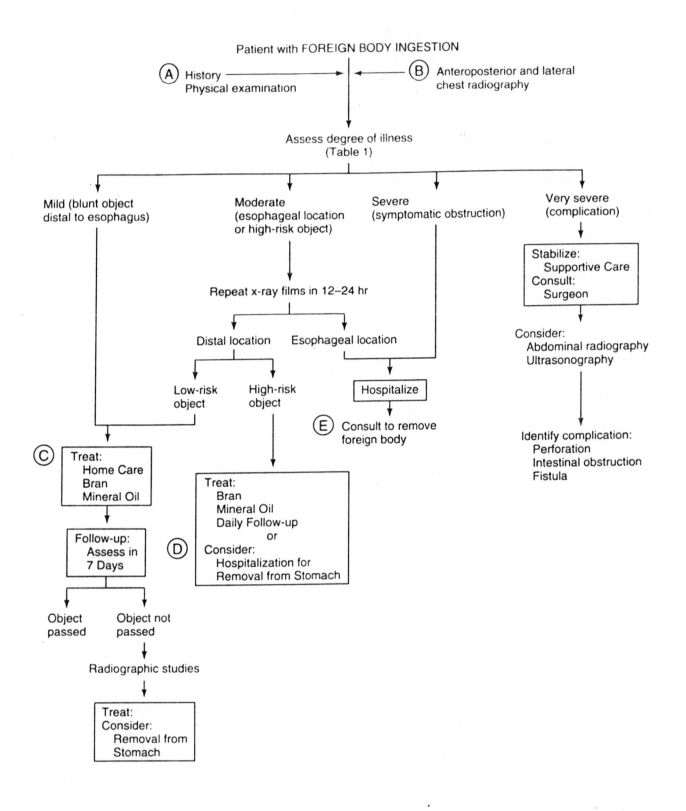

Patient with FOREIGN BODY INGESTION

(A) History —————————→ ←————— (B) Anteroposterior and lateral
Physical examination   chest radiography

Assess degree of illness
(Table 1)

| Mild (blunt object distal to esophagus) | Moderate (esophageal location or high-risk object) | Severe (symptomatic obstruction) | Very severe (complication) |

Very severe (complication)

Stabilize:
    Supportive Care
Consult:
    Surgeon

Consider:
    Abdominal radiography
    Ultrasonography

Identify complication:
    Perforation
    Intestinal obstruction
    Fistula

Moderate:
Repeat x-ray films in 12–24 hr

Distal location   Esophageal location

Low-risk   High-risk
object   object

Hospitalize

(E) Consult to remove
foreign body

(C) Treat:
Home Care
Bran
Mineral Oil

Follow-up:
Assess in
7 Days

Object   Object not
passed   passed

Radiographic studies

Treat:
Consider:
    Removal from
    Stomach

(D) Treat:
Bran
Mineral Oil
Daily Follow-up
         or
Consider:
Hospitalization for
Removal from Stomach

IBUPROFEN INTOXICATION

Stephen Berman, M.D.

Ibuprofen intoxication has become more common since the drug became available in over-the-counter preparations and in prescription form as a pediatric suspension. Ibuprofen is a nonsteroidal antiinflammatory agent that inhibits the activity of fatty acid cyclooxygenase, an enzyme involved in prostaglandin synthesis. Ibuprofen is rapidly absorbed, and in contrast to salicylates, overdosage does not appear to delay absorption. It is highly protein bound and is metabolized by the liver. The half-life is short, 0.9 to 2.5 hours. Ibuprofen and its metabolites are acids that can produce metabolic acidosis. Kidney failure in large ingestions may relate to the inhibition of renal prostaglandin synthesis. It is difficult to correlate serum ibuprofen levels with clinical toxicity.

A. Assess the degree of toxicity. Toxic symptoms develop within 4 hours of ingestion. Mildly affected patients are asymptomatic and have ingested less than 200 mg/kg. Moderately affected patients may have headache, nausea, vomiting, abdominal pain, nystagmus, diplopia, and muscle fasciculations and/or have ingested 200 to 400 mg/kg. Patients with severe symptoms have signs of CNS toxicity, liver dysfunction, renal failure or metabolic acidosis, GI bleeding, hypotension, or bradycardia and/or have ingested more than 400 mg/kg.

B. Attempt to remove ibuprofen from the stomach with ipecac in alert children 1 to 12 years of age if the ingestion occurred within 2 hours. The dose (15 ml) may be repeated if emesis has not occurred after 30 minutes. Patients who have depressed consciousness and patients with a large ingestion may need gastric lavage with a large-bore tube. Give activated charcoal and a cathartic after emesis has stopped. In severe cases consider repeating the activated charcoal dose every 4 hours until it appears in the stool. Note that the value of gastric emptying is controversial.

C. Most patients with severe toxicity respond to supportive care. Obtain liver function tests to assess dysfunction or damage. Urine alkalinization, repeated doses of activated charcoal, and hemodialysis are not necessary because of ibuprofen's short half-life, high level of protein binding, minimal enterohepatic circulation, and limited urine excretion.

References

Linden CH, Townsend PL. Metabolic acidosis after acute ibuprofen overdosage. J Pediatr 1987; 111:922.

Mack RB. Once more unto the breach: Ibuprofen toxicity. Contemp Pediatr 1988; February:127.

Patient with IBUPROFEN INTOXICATION

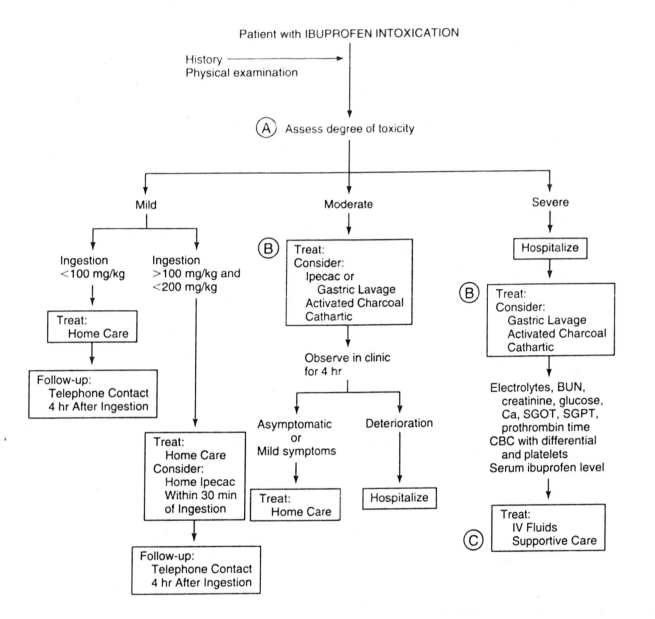

History
Physical examination

(A) Assess degree of toxicity

Mild | Moderate | Severe

Ingestion <100 mg/kg

Ingestion >100 mg/kg and <200 mg/kg

Treat:
Home Care

Follow-up:
Telephone Contact
4 hr After Ingestion

Treat:
Home Care
Consider:
Home Ipecac
Within 30 min
of Ingestion

Follow-up:
Telephone Contact
4 hr After Ingestion

(B) Treat:
Consider:
Ipecac or
Gastric Lavage
Activated Charcoal
Cathartic

Observe in clinic
for 4 hr

Asymptomatic
or
Mild symptoms

Deterioration

Treat:
Home Care

Hospitalize

Hospitalize

(B) Treat:
Consider:
Gastric Lavage
Activated Charcoal
Cathartic

Electrolytes, BUN,
creatinine, glucose,
Ca, SGOT, SGPT,
prothrombin time
CBC with differential
and platelets
Serum ibuprofen level

(C) Treat:
IV Fluids
Supportive Care

IRON POISONING

Stephen Berman, M.D.

Iron poisoning is one of the most common toxicologic emergencies in young children because of the availability of iron tablets and their candylike appearance. Ferrous sulfate tablets are routinely given to postpartum women, many of whom have toddlers in the family. Iron damages the GI mucosa and affects the lungs and liver. Excess free iron is a mitochondrial toxin leading to derangements in energy metabolism. Iron poisoning has four phases. Phase 1, the first 6 hours postingestion, is associated with vomiting, diarrhea, and GI bleeding due to mucosal injury. This phase may be complicated by shock and coma if the circulatory blood volume is sufficiently compromised. Phase 2, 6 to 24 hours postingestion, is usually associated with an improvement in symptoms, especially when supportive care is provided during phase 1. Phase 3, beginning after 24 hours, consists of marked metabolic acidosis, shock, seizures, and altered mental status caused by mitochondrial damage and hepatocellular injury. Phase 4 is characterized by late scarring of the GI tract causing pyloric obstruction.

A. Serum iron levels are useful in predicting the clinical course. Levels drawn 3 to 5 hours postingestion below 350 μg/dl are rarely associated with significant disease. Levels of 350 to 500 μg/dl are associated with symptoms in phase 1 that resolve without complication. Levels higher than 500 μg/dl are associated with phase 3 complications, including shock and severe metabolic acidosis.

B. Perform a deferoxamine challenge by administering 50 mg/kg IM to a maximum 1 g to determine whether iron-deferoxamine complexes that turn the urine pinkish orange are formed. This correlates with an elevated iron level needing treatment.

C. Decontaminate the bowel. Consider ipecac-induced emesis in an alert patient with a good gag reflex who has ingested a nonlethal amount of iron within 30 minutes. Otherwise perform gastric lavage with a 1% to 1.5% bicarbonate solution. Do not use a Fleet enema because it may cause phosphate poisoning. Obtain a postlavage abdominal film. When significant material remains, consider whole-bowel irrigation. If clumps of iron tablets remain, consider surgery, as failure to remove the iron can result in gastric perforation and severe hemorrhage.

D. Treat very severely ill patients with a continuous IV deferoxamine infusion of 15 mg/kg/hour (maximum daily dose 360 mg/kg to a total of 6 g). Monitor closely for hypotension. Maintain adequate urine output by replacing blood and other volume losses. Initiate renal dialysis if renal failure develops. Manage severely ill patients with either continuous IV infusion of deferoxamine at 5 to 10 mg/kg/hour or IM 20 mg/kg every 4 to 8 hours. Continue therapy until the patient is asymptomatic with normal-colored urine and a normal serum iron if available.

References

Henretig FM, Shannon M. Toxicologic emergencies. In: Fleisher GR, Ludwig S, eds. Textbook of pediatric emergency medicine. 3rd ed. Baltimore: Williams & Wilkins, 1993:745.

Lacouture PG, Wason S, Temple AR, et al. Emergency assessment of severity in iron overdose by clinical and laboratory methods. J Pediatr 1981; 99:89.

TABLE 1 Degree of Illness in Iron Poisoning

Mild	Moderate	Severe	Very Severe
Asymptomatic	Vomiting and diarrhea	GI blood loss	Altered mental status
and	or	or	or
No radiopaque material in stomach	Serum glucose >150 mg/dl	Metabolic acidosis	Seizures
and	or	or	or
Serum iron <350 μg/dl	WBC >15,000	Serum iron >500 μg/dl	Shock
	or	or	or
	Radiopaque material in stomach	Positive deferoxamine challenge test	Liver failure
	or		or
	Serum iron 350–500 μg/dl		Severe metabolic acidosis

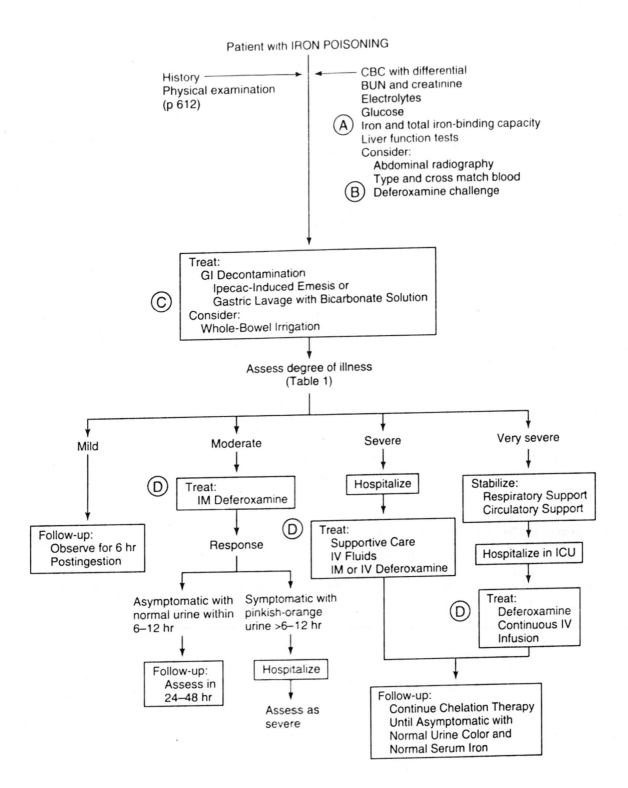

Patient with IRON POISONING

History ⟶ ⟵ CBC with differential
Physical examination　　　　BUN and creatinine
(p 612)　　　　　　　　　　Electrolytes
　　　　　　　　　　　　　　Glucose
　　　　　Ⓐ Iron and total iron-binding capacity
　　　　　　　Liver function tests
　　　　　　　Consider:
　　　　　　　　Abdominal radiography
　　　　　　　　Type and cross match blood
　　　　　Ⓑ Deferoxamine challenge

Ⓒ
Treat:
　GI Decontamination
　　Ipecac-Induced Emesis or
　　Gastric Lavage with Bicarbonate Solution
Consider:
　Whole-Bowel Irrigation

Assess degree of illness
(Table 1)

Mild　　　　　Moderate　　　　Severe　　　　Very severe

Ⓓ Treat:
　IM Deferoxamine

Hospitalize

Stabilize:
　Respiratory Support
　Circulatory Support

Follow-up:
　Observe for 6 hr
　Postingestion

Response

Ⓓ Treat:
　Supportive Care
　IV Fluids
　IM or IV Deferoxamine

Hospitalize in ICU

Asymptomatic with　　Symptomatic with
normal urine within　　pinkish-orange
6–12 hr　　　　　　　urine >6–12 hr

Ⓓ Treat:
　Deferoxamine
　Continuous IV
　Infusion

Follow-up:
　Assess in
　24–48 hr

Hospitalize

Assess as
severe

Follow-up:
　Continue Chelation Therapy
　Until Asymptomatic with
　Normal Urine Color and
　Normal Serum Iron

LEAD INTOXICATION

Stephen Berman, M.D.

Approximately 1.7 million children, or 8.9% of 1 to 5 year olds in the United States, have a blood lead level of 10 µg/dl or more. Sources of lead toxicity during childhood include ingestion of lead-based paint chips, particles, or dust; water contaminated in lead pipes; lead-glazed ceramics; contaminated dirt and dust; and polluted air from smelters and refineries. Chronic low-level lead burdens are associated with neurobehavioral dysfunction that impairs measured intelligence and academic functioning. Studies suggest that lead levels as low as 15 µg/dl have neurobehavioral effects. Elevated lead levels inhibit several enzymes, including the heme synthesis pathway, cytochrome chain in liver and adenyl cyclase in brain. Recommendations for routine lead screening are controversial where the prevalance of elevated lead levels is low.

A. In the history ask about persistent vomiting, listlessness, irritability, loss of developmental milestones, seizures, and ataxia. Note the age of the house and the last time it was painted. Does the child have a history of pica? Is there environmental pollution? Does the child have iron deficiency anemia? The value of questionnaires in selected communities to identify children at risk is unclear.

B. Confirm capillary lead determinations with a specimen obtained by venipuncture. Erythrocyte protoporphyrin is a precursor of hemeglobin, which is increased markedly (above 250 µg/dl) with high lead levels. Unfortunately, it is not sensitive enough to reliably identify children with levels between 10 and 25 µg/dl. Therefore, blood lead levels must be used to document levels in this range. The relationship between blood lead levels, which reflect recent exposure, and total body lead, soft-tissue, and bone lead, which reflect chronic exposure, is unclear. The ethylenediaminetetraacetic acid (EDTA) mobilization test can be used to assess the total body lead status. EDTA is given either IM or IV and urine is collected during the following 6 to 8 hours to measure the lead excreted. Its usefulness with elevated lead levels is unclear.

C. CDC guidelines recommend inspecting the home when a child has a confirmed lead level of 15 µg/dl or higher. It is very important to reduce lead exposure, especially when a child is receiving chelation therapy. This therapy will increase the absorption of lead in the child's environment. Recommend a diet rich in iron, zinc, and calcium for children with elevated lead levels since deficiencies in these minerals increase lead absorption. Administer iron supplementation when iron deficiency is present.

(Continued on page 628)

TABLE 1 Degree of Illness in Lead Intoxication

Mild	Moderate	Severe	Very Severe
Asymptomatic with a lead level < 25 µg/dl	Asymptomatic with lead level > 25–44 µg/dl	Symptomatic or Lead level > 45 µg/dl	Encephalopathy with erythrocyte protoporphyrin > 250

Patient with LEAD INTOXICATION

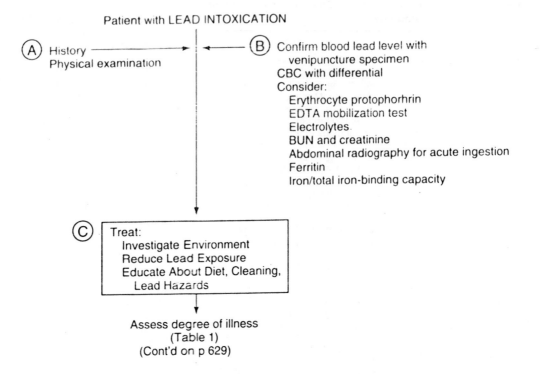

(A) History
Physical examination

(B) Confirm blood lead level with
     venipuncture specimen
CBC with differential
Consider:
     Erythrocyte protophorhrin
     EDTA mobilization test
     Electrolytes
     BUN and creatinine
     Abdominal radiography for acute ingestion
     Ferritin
     Iron/total iron-binding capacity

(C) Treat:
     Investigate Environment
     Reduce Lead Exposure
     Educate About Diet, Cleaning,
        Lead Hazards

Assess degree of illness
(Table 1)
(Cont'd on p 629)

TABLE 2 Chelation Therapy for Children with Elevated Blood Lead Levels

Lead Classification	Treatment Regimen
Symptomatic	
	BAL 75 mg/m² or 4 mg/kg/dose BAL q4h IM × 5 days
	and
	EDTA 1500 mg/m²/day continuous IV × 5 days
Asymptomatic	
Blood lead ≥ 70 μg/dl	BAL 75 mg/m² or 4 mg/kg/dose BAL q4h IM × 5 days
	and
	EDTA 1500 mg/m²/day IV × 5 days
	DMSA 10 mg/kg t.i.d. PO × 5 days
	then
	10 mg/kg b.i.d. PO × 14 days
Blood lead 45–69 μg/dl	EDTA 1000 mg/m²/day continuous IV infusion × 5 days
	DMSA 10 mg/kg t.i.d. PO × 5 days
	then
	10 mg/kg b.i.d. PO × 14 days
Blood lead 25–44 μg/dl	EDTA mobilization test followed by EDTA 1 g/m²/day by EDTA × 5 days if mobilization test is positive
	DMSA 10 mg/kg t.i.d. PO × 5 days
	then
	10 mg/kg b.i.d. PO × 14 days
	Penicillamine 10 mg/kg/day PO; increase to 30 mg/kg/day PO over 2–4 wk, treat for 6–20 wk
Blood lead 10–24 μg/dl	Chelation not recommended

BAL, dimercaprol; EDTA, ethylenediaminetetraacetic acid; DMSA, 2,3-dimercaptosuccinic acid.
Modified from Glotzer D. Management of childhood lead poisoning: Strategies for chelation. Pediatr Ann 1994; 23:610; with permission.

D. The decision to hospitalize moderately ill patients must be individualized, but it is often advisable to hospitalize the child while inspecting the home and intervening to prevent exposure while receiving chelation therapy. Treatment can be with an oral drug such as 2,3-dimercaptosuccinic acid (DMSA) or with parenteral CaEDTA.

E. Treat very severely ill children with combination chelation therapy using a continuous IV infusion of CaEDTA and IM dimercaprol (BAL) every 4 hours (Table 2). In severe cases consider treatment with CaEDTA and BAL for at least 2 days, then single-agent therapy for the remaining 3 days.

References

Berlin CM Jr, Chairperson, and the Committee on Drugs, American Academy of Pediatrics. Treatment guidelines for lead exposure in children. Pediatrics 1995; 96:155.

Besunder JB, Anderson RL, Super DM. Short-term efficacy of oral dimercaptosuccinic acid in children with low to moderate lead intoxication. Pediatrics 1995; 96:683.

Brody DJ, Pirkle JL, Kramer RA, et al. Blood lead levels in the U.S. population: Phase 1 of the third national health and nutrition examination survey (NHANES III, 1988–1991). JAMA 1994; 272:277.

Committee on Environmental Health. Lead poisoning: From screening to primary prevention. Pediatrics 1993; 92:176.

Glotzer D. Management of childhood lead poisoning: Strategies for chelation. Pediatr Ann 1994; 23:607.

Goldstein GW. Neurologic concepts of lead poisoning in children. Pediatr Ann 1992; 21:384.

Henretig FM, Shannon M. Toxicologic emergencies. In: Fleisher GR, Ludwig S, eds. Textbook of pediatric emergency medicine. 3rd ed. Baltimore: Williams & Wilkins, 1993:745.

Kimbrough RD, Levois M, Webb DR. Management of children with slightly elevated blood lead levels. Pediatrics 1994; 93:188.

Weitzman M, Glotzer D. Lead poisoning. Pediatr Rev 1992; 13:461.

Patient with LEAD INTOXICATION
Assess degree of illness
(Table 1)
(Cont'd from p 627)

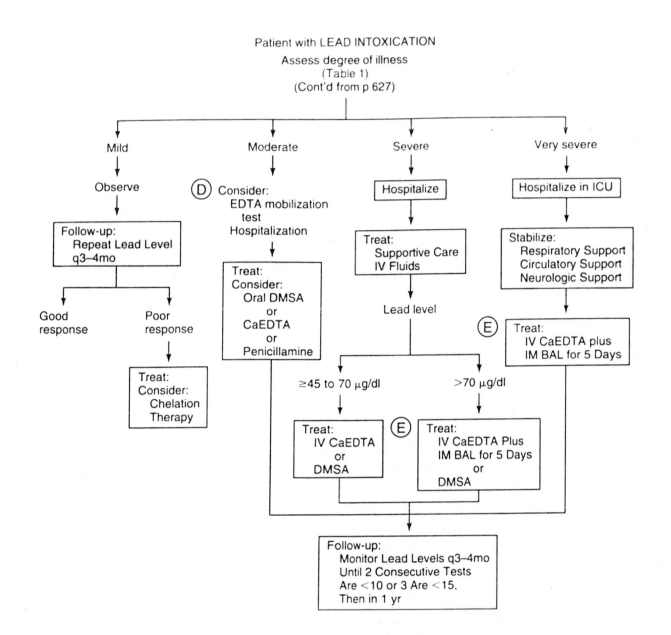

Mild	
Observe	
Follow-up: Repeat Lead Level q3–4mo	
Good response / Poor response	
Poor response → Treat: Consider: Chelation Therapy	

Moderate

Ⓓ Consider:
EDTA mobilization test
Hospitalization

Treat:
Consider:
Oral DMSA
or
CaEDTA
or
Penicillamine

Severe

Hospitalize

Treat:
Supportive Care
IV Fluids

Lead level

≥45 to 70 µg/dl

Treat:
IV CaEDTA
or
DMSA

>70 µg/dl

Ⓔ Treat:
IV CaEDTA Plus
IM BAL for 5 Days
or
DMSA

Very severe

Hospitalize in ICU

Stabilize:
Respiratory Support
Circulatory Support
Neurologic Support

Ⓔ Treat:
IV CaEDTA plus
IM BAL for 5 Days

Follow-up:
Monitor Lead Levels q3–4mo
Until 2 Consecutive Tests
Are <10 or 3 Are <15,
Then in 1 yr

METHEMOGLOBINEMIA

Jerrold M. Eichner, M.D.

Methemoglobin (MetHb) is an abnormal hemoglobin (Hb) in which the iron is oxidized from the ferrous to the ferric state. Iron in the ferric state cannot bind and transport oxygen (O_2). MetHb also shifts the oxygen dissociation curve to the left, decreasing release of O_2 to the tissues. Normally, the balance between oxidation and reduction results in about 1% of Hb being MetHb. The balance can be disrupted by excessive oxidation or deficient reduction, producing excessive MetHb. The result depends on the amount of Hb left to transport O_2, producing signs and symptoms of hypoxia, and the amount of MetHb present, giving the telltale cyanosis. Infants under 3 months of age are susceptible to methemoglobinemia because they have less than 50% of red cell reductase enzyme activity. They also have high levels of fetal Hb, which is more easily oxidized, and a higher intestinal pH than older children, which enhances the conversion of nitrates to nitrites.

A. In the history determine the onset of cyanosis. Was it from birth or later? Is the cyanosis associated with diarrhea or another illness? Is the infant formula- or breast-fed? What is the source of water used in feeding? Does anyone else in the family have cyanosis? Is there exposure to medications or chemicals that may cause methemoglobinemia (Table 1)? Ask about headache, dizziness, lethargy, fatigue, syncope, difficulty breathing, tachycardia, decreased level of consciousness, seizures, or history of pulmonary or cardiac disease.

B. In the physical examination look for visible cyanosis, especially chocolate brown color of blood. Look for signs of dehydration as well as lethargy, syncope, decreased level of consciousness, coma, seizures, respiratory distress, tachypnea, tachycardia, dyspnea, arrhythmia, cardiac failure, and respiratory failure.

C. MetHb levels are measured by cooximetry. Levels above 10% are usually associated with cyanosis. Increasing levels are associated with increasing symptoms (Table 2). Levels above 70% are frequently fatal. Measure total Hb to determine anemia; where there is less O_2 carrying capacity, any reduction by MetHb may be significant. Arterial blood gases (ABGs) usually show a normal Po_2, which responds to O_2 administration, but the cyanosis does not improve with O_2. There may be metabolic acidosis depending on the cause or effect of the hypoxia. O_2 saturation calculated with ABGs is inaccurate. Likewise, pulse oximetry gives inaccurate O_2 saturations.

D. Methemoglobinemia in childhood can be congenital or acquired (Table 3). The congenital forms, which are rare, result from an abnormal Hb or a deficiency

TABLE 1   Selected Inducers of Methemoglobinemia

Nitrates/nitrites	Local anesthetics
Sodium nitrite	Lidocaine
Amyl nitrite	Cetacaine
Bismuth subnitrite	Benzocaine
Butyl nitrite	Prilocaine
Nitroglycerine	**Antibacterials**
Silver nitrate	Sulfonamides
Nitrate salts	Dapsone
Sodium nitroprusside	Paraaminosalicylic acid
Analgesics	Chloroquine
Acetanilid	Primaquine
Phenacetin	Phenazopyridine
Other medications	**Miscellaneous**
Metoclopramide	Aniline dyes, inks
Phenytoin	Naphthalene
Resorcinol	Copper sulfate
	Chlorate salts
	Nitrobenzene
	Nitrogen dioxide
	Trinitrotoluene
	Spinach

TABLE 2   Signs and Symptoms of Methemoglobinemia

Methemoglobin Concentration (%)	Signs and Symptoms
<10	None
10–20	Visible cyanosis, chocolate brown color of blood
20–45	Headache, dizziness, lethargy, fatigue, syncope, dyspnea, tachycardia
45–55	Decreased consciousness, coma, convulsions, arrhythmia, shock
55–70	Coma, acidosis, cardiac failure, respiratory failure
>70	High risk of death

in NADH- or NADPH-dependent MetHb-reducing enzymes. NADH-dependent reductase is responsible for 95% of MetHb reduction activity, and its deficiency produces cyanosis at birth. Acquired forms, which are more common, occur when the oxidation of heme to the ferric form occurs faster than the enzymes can reduce it. Numerous chemicals and medications are oxidants known to cause methemoglobinemia (see Table 1). These are primarily nitrite and aniline compounds such as local anesthetics, sulfonamides, and

(Continued on page 632)

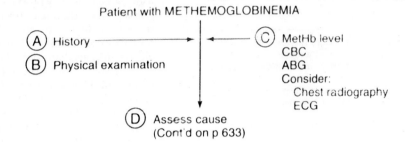

Patient with METHEMOGLOBINEMIA

(A) History ⟶

(B) Physical examination

(C) MetHb level
CBC
ABG
Consider:
  Chest radiography
  ECG

(D) Assess cause
(Cont'd on p 633)

TABLE 3 Causes of Methemoglobinemia

Congenital	Acquired
NADH-dependent methomoglobin reductase deficiency	Exposure to chemical inducers of methemoglobin
Hemoglobin M	Diarrhea and acidosis in young infants
Unstable hemoglobins	Infectious causes
	Cow or soy milk protein intolerance
	UTI with nitrite-forming bacteria
	Renal tubular acidosis

UTI, urinary tract infection.

TABLE 4 Classification by Severity

Mild/moderate	MetHb level <20% and asymptomatic
Severe	MetHb level 20%–45%
	MetHb level <20% with symptoms
Very severe	MetHb level >45%
	MetHb level <45% with acidosis, coma, convulsions, cardiac failure, or respiratory failure

nitrates. Well water, especially from less than 30 feet deep, may contain high levels of nitrates from fertilizers. This water mixed with infant formulas has caused methemoglobinemia in over 2000 reported cases, with a 10% mortality. A more common but underdiagnosed cause of methemoglobinemia in infancy is diarrhea with acidosis. The rate of MetHb reduction is reduced as the blood pH falls. The cause of the diarrhea may be infection or dietary cow milk or soy milk protein intolerance associated with increased nitrite production in the intestinal tract. There may also be an association with nitrite-producing bacteria in the intestinal or urinary tract. One infant reported with diarrhea and renal tubular acidosis developed methemoglobinemia. Infants with diarrhea and acidosis have a more severe illness than those with equivalent blood MetHb levels secondary to chemical exposure.

E. Consider chest radiography and an ECG to identify pulmonary or cardiac disease.

F. Supplemental 100% O_2 is the initial treatment for all degrees of severity. Continue O_2 until the real Sao_2 is adequate in room air and symptoms resolve. When exposure to chemicals is the cause, removal of the offending agent is essential. For skin contact, remove all clothing and wash the skin with soap and water. For oral contact consider gastric emptying and activated charcoal, as with other poisonings.

G. Treat patients with severe and very severe illness with 1% solution of methylene blue 1 to 2 mg/kg IV over 5 to 10 minutes. Repeat in 1 hour if cyanosis and symptoms persist. The total dose should not exceed 7 mg/kg. Methylene blue is reduced to leukomethylene blue by NADPH and MetHb reductase. The leukometh-

ylene blue reduces MetHb to Hb without enzymes. Methylene blue may produce side effects including precordial pain, dyspnea, restlessness, or tremor. High doses may directly oxidize Hb to MetHb. It may cause MetHb production and hemolysis in patients with glucose-6-phosphate dehydrogenase (G6PD) deficiency, and should not be used in those patients. When methylene blue fails to resolve the cyanosis, consider G6PD deficiency or NADPH reductase deficiency and test for these. If either is found, treat with ascorbic acid. Large doses of ascorbic acid will reduce MetHb nonenzymatically, although too slowly for emergency use.

H. With severe methemoglobinemia from either an enzyme deficiency or failure of methylene blue to work, consider exchange transfusion or hyperbaric oxygen. In the presence of anemia consider simple transfusion.

I. Follow-up includes elimination of the cause. Remove MetHb-producing chemicals from the child's environment. For unknown causes test the water for nitrates and nitrites and avoid ingestion of any contaminated water until the source of the nitrates or nitrites can be removed. For formula-fed infants with diarrhea as the cause, change to a noncow and nonsoy protein—containing formula. Look for urinary tract infections caused by nitrite forming bacteria such as *E. coli*.

References

Askew GL, Finelli L, Genese CA, et al. Boilerbaisse: An outbreak of methemoglobinemia in New Jersey in 1992. Pediatrics 1994; 94:381.

Avner JR, Henretig FM, McAneney CM. Acquired methemoglobinemia: The relationship of cause to course of illness. Am J Dis Child 1990; 144:1229.

Curry S. Methemoglobinemia. Ann Emerg Med 1982; 11:214.

Dagan R, Zaltzstein E, Gorodischer R. Methaemoglobinaemia in young infants with diarrhoea. Eur J Pediatr 1988; 147:87.

Dean BS, Lopez G, Krenzelok EP. Environmentally-induced methemoglobinemia in an infant. Clin Toxicol 1992; 30:127.

Gebara BM, Goetting MG. Life-threatening methemoglobinemia in infants with diarrhea and acidosis. Clin Pediatr 1994; 33:370.

Kross BC, Ayebo AD, Fuortes LJ. Methemoglobinemia: Nitrate toxicity in rural America. Am Fam Physician 1992; 46:183.

Luk G, Riggs D, Luque M. Severe methemoglobinemia in a 3-week-old infant with a urinary tract infection. Crit Care Med 1991; 19:1325.

Mansouri A, Lurie AA. Concise review: Methemoglobinemia. Am J Hematol 1993; 42:7.

Murray KF, Christie DL. Dietary protein intolerance in infants with transient methemoglobinemia and diarrhea. J Pediatr 1993; 122:90.

Pollack ES, Pollack CV. Incidence of subclinical methemoglobinemia in infants with diarrhea. Ann Emerg Med 1994; 24:652.

Sager S, Grayson GH, Feig SA. Methemoglobinemia associated with acidosis of probable renal origin. J Pediatr 1995; 126:59.

Yano SS, Danish EH, Hsia YE. Transient methemoglobinemia with acidosis in infants. J Pediatr 1982; 100:415.

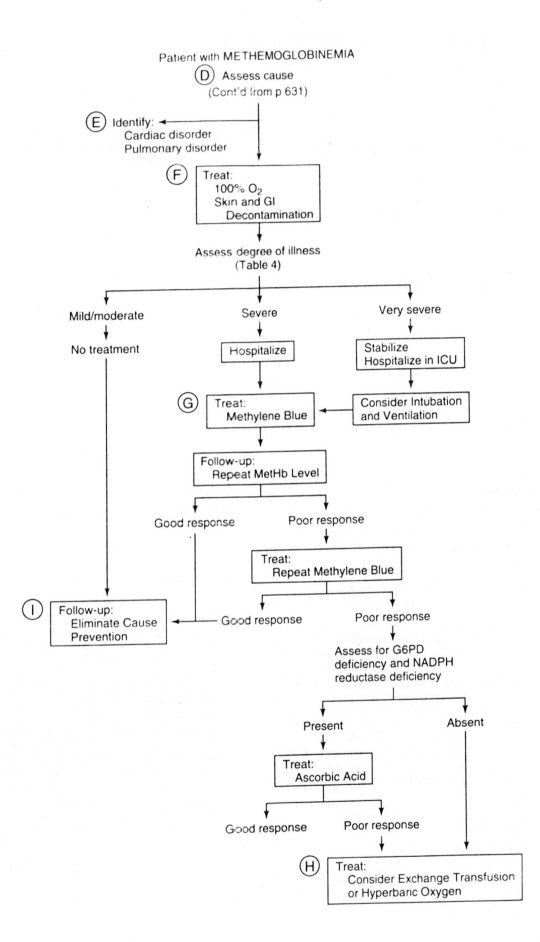

Patient with METHEMOGLOBINEMIA

(D) Assess cause
(Cont'd from p 631)

(E) Identify:
Cardiac disorder
Pulmonary disorder

(F) Treat:
100% O$_2$
Skin and GI
Decontamination

Assess degree of illness
(Table 4)

Mild/moderate | Severe | Very severe

No treatment

Hospitalize

Stabilize
Hospitalize in ICU

Consider Intubation
and Ventilation

(G) Treat:
Methylene Blue

Follow-up:
Repeat MetHb Level

Good response | Poor response

Treat:
Repeat Methylene Blue

(I) Follow-up:
Eliminate Cause
Prevention

Good response | Poor response

Assess for G6PD
deficiency and NADPH
reductase deficiency

Present | Absent

Treat:
Ascorbic Acid

Good response | Poor response

(H) Treat:
Consider Exchange Transfusion
or Hyperbaric Oxygen

PENICILLIN-ALLERGIC REACTIONS

Stephen Berman, M.D.

Allergic penicillin reactions are classified as immediate, accelerated, or late. Immediate allergic reactions occur within 30 minutes of administering penicillin. Anaphylaxis, the most severe immediate reaction, is associated with hypotension, stridor (laryngeal edema), or wheezing (bronchospasm). Most fatal cases of anaphylaxis develop within 15 minutes of parenteral administration. Fatal reactions are very rare; one to two deaths occur in every 100,000 patients who receive penicillin. Severe reactions are less likely with oral therapy. It is not clear whether the form of injectable penicillin—aqueous benzylpenicillin, procaine penicillin, and benzathine penicillin—affects the frequency of fatal anaphylaxis. Mild allergic reactions occur in 5% to 10% of patients treated with penicillin. Swelling (angioedema) and hives (urticaria) are common immediate reactions. Accelerated reactions occur 30 minutes to 3 days after receiving penicillin. Clinical signs include wheezing, stridor, swelling, hives, and swollen joints. Late reactions occur more than 3 days after starting penicillin. Any of the clinical signs described in accelerated reactions can develop, but a rash is the most frequent sign. It is often difficult to know if the development of a rash in children treated with penicillin is caused by a viral infection or a late allergic reaction.

A. A penicillin-allergic reaction occurs in approximately 6% of individuals with a history of any type of prior reaction, as compared with 2% without an allergic history. Individuals who have had an immediate-type reaction are at highest risk. Some 10% to 30% of patients with a history of anaphylaxis or hives will have an allergic reaction on a subsequent exposure to penicillin. Anaphylactic reactions appear to be the least frequent in children under 12 years of age. The risk of a repeat reaction is higher within 1 year of a previous one.

B. Acute confusion, dizziness, hallucinations, or seizures can immediately follow IM injection of procaine penicillin G. These signs are usually associated with tachycardia and elevated blood pressure. This acute nonallergic reaction called Hoigne syndrome is said to be caused by a sudden elevation of free procaine in the CNS. The incidence is estimated at 3 to 18 cases/1000 injections. The condition is self-limited and resolves without specific treatment. The inadvertent intraarterial injection of long-acting benzathine penicillin can produce persistent arterial vasospasm and arterial thrombus that can cause vascular insufficiency, limb gangrene, or myelitis.

C. Treat mild reactions with an antihistamine. A reasonable initial choice is oral diphenhydramine or hydroxyzine (Table 1).

TABLE 1 Drugs Used in the Treatment of Penicillin-Allergic Reaction in Infants and Children

Drug	Dosage	Product Availability
Epinephrine	Infants < 1 yr: 0.1 ml/dose Children 1–2 yr: 0.2 ml/dose Children >2 yr: 0.3 ml/dose or 0.01 ml/kg/dose (max 0.3 ml/dose) All doses should be taken q15–30min p.r.n.	Vials: 1 : 1000
Diphenhydramine	IV: 25–50 mg/dose PO: 1.25 mg/kg/dose q6h	Elixir: 12.5 mg/5 ml Caps: 25, 50 mg Injection: 10, 50 mg/ml
Hydroxyzine	0.6 mg/kg/dose q6h PO	Caps: 25, 50, 100 mg Susp: 25 mg/5 ml Syrup: 10 mg/5 ml
Methylprednisolone	1–2 mg/kg/dose (max 40 mg/dose)	Injection: 40, 62.5, 125 mg/ml
Hydrocortisone (Cortef, Solu-cortef, Cortisol)	4–8 mg/kg/dose (max 200 mg/dose)	Injection: 50, 125 mg/ml
Prednisone	1 mg/kg/dose b.i.d. for 3–5 days (max 30 mg/dose)	Tabs: 5, 10, 20, 50 mg Syrup: 5 mg/5 ml

D. A positive skin test identifies patients at high risk for an allergic reaction; 50% to 75% of patients with positive-skin tests will have an allergic reaction compared with 3% to 4% of patients with negative skin tests. Properly done and interpreted negative skin tests to major determinant penicilloyl polylysine (PPL) and penicillin G show the chances of an allergic reaction in a patient with a prior allergic reaction to be very rare. Skin testing with only penicillin G will fail to identify over half of patients who would be positive if both penicilloyl polylysine and penicillin G were used. Unfortunately, skin testing with only penicillin G will also miss approximately 25% of the patients who will have immediate reactions, including anaphylaxis. Therefore, a negative skin test with penicillin G does not mean that a patient with a prior allergic reaction will not have another reaction. Given the low rate of anaphylaxis (4 to 15 cases/100,000 patients), it

(Continued on page 636)

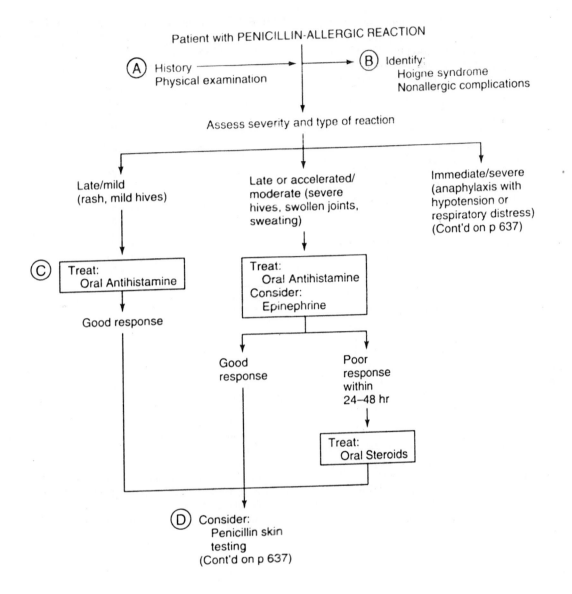

Patient with PENICILLIN-ALLERGIC REACTION

(A) History
Physical examination

(B) Identify:
Hoigne syndrome
Nonallergic complications

Assess severity and type of reaction

Late/mild
(rash, mild hives)

Late or accelerated/
moderate (severe
hives, swollen joints,
sweating)

Immediate/severe
(anaphylaxis with
hypotension or
respiratory distress)
(Cont'd on p 637)

(C) Treat:
Oral Antihistamine

Good response

Treat:
Oral Antihistamine
Consider:
Epinephrine

Good
response

Poor
response
within
24–48 hr

Treat:
Oral Steroids

(D) Consider:
Penicillin skin
testing
(Cont'd on p 637)

is not necessary or feasible to routinely skin test all patients with PPL and penicillin G prior to giving penicillin. Skin testing with PPL and penicillin G is most useful when it is important to administer penicillin to a patient with a history compatible with a prior allergic reaction.

E. Administer epinephrine SC or IM. The dose may be repeated every 15 to 30 minutes as needed. If anaphylaxis follows an IM penicillin injection, do not administer epinephrine in the same limb. When shock is present, stabilize the circulation with 20 ml/kg of an isotonic solution administered as rapidly as needed. Consider IV or IM diphenhydramine and methylprednisolone or hydrocortisone.

F. Patients allergic to penicillin may have a cross-reaction to other β-lactam antibiotics such as cephalosporins, carbapenems, and monobactams.

G. Effective alternative antibiotics that can be used to treat serious infections (bacteremia, meningitis) in penicillin-allergic patients are vancomycin for staphylococcal and other gram-positive infections, chloramphenicol for *Haemophilus influenzae,* gram-positive and gram-negative enterics, and clindamycin for gram-positive organisms and anaerobes. Erythromycin, TMP-SMX, and erythromycin-sulfisoxazole are oral antibiotics useful in treating less severe infections such as acute otitis media.

H. Several methods of penicillin desensitization are available. In an emergency begin with 1 U of penicillin IV and double the dose at 15 minute intervals. A safe oral desensitization protocol is shown in Table 2. Remember to have epinephrine available to treat an immediate reaction.

TABLE 2 Oral Penicillin Desensitization Protocol*

Dose	Units	Route
1	100	PO
2	200	PO
3	400	PO
4	800	PO
5	1,600	PO
6	3,200	PO
7	6,400	PO
8	12,800	PO
9	25,000	PO
10	50,000	PO
11	100,000	PO
12	200,000	PO
13	400,000	PO
14	200,000	SC
15	400,000	SC
16	800,000	SC
17	1,000,000	IM

*Interval between doses, 15 minutes. The total regimen requires 4 hours. IV therapy if indicated may be started 15 minutes after completing this schedule.

References

Idsoe O, Guthe T, Willcox RR, DeWeck AL. Nature and extent of penicillin side reactions, with particular reference to fatalities from anaphylactic shock. Bull WHO 1968; 38:159.

Sieber TY, D'Angelo M. Psychosis and seizures following the injection of penicillin G procaine. Am J Dis Child 1985; 139:335.

Sullivan TJ, Wedner HJ, Shatz GS, et al. Skin testing to detect penicillin allergy. J Allergy Clin Immunol 1981; 68:171.

Sullivan TJ, Yecies LD, Shatz GS, et al. Desensitization of patients allergic to penicillin using orally administered β-lactam antibodies. J Allergy Clin Immunol 1982; 69:275.

Patient with PENICILLIN-ALLERGIC REACTION

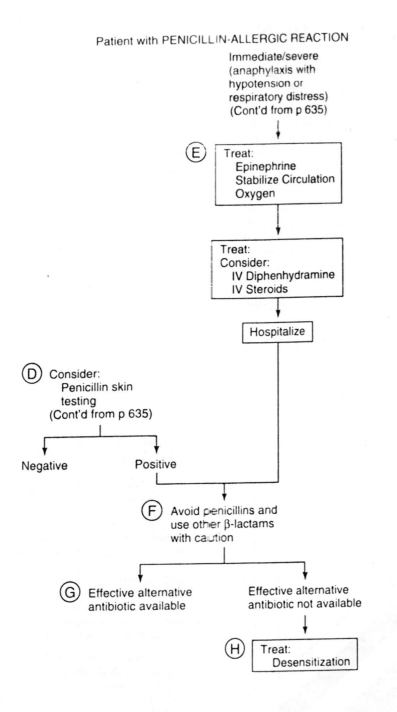

Immediate/severe
(anaphylaxis with
hypotension or
respiratory distress)
(Cont'd from p 635)

E Treat:
Epinephrine
Stabilize Circulation
Oxygen

Treat:
Consider:
IV Diphenhydramine
IV Steroids

Hospitalize

D Consider:
Penicillin skin
testing
(Cont'd from p 635)

Negative   Positive

F Avoid penicillins and
use other β-lactams
with caution

G Effective alternative
antibiotic available

Effective alternative
antibiotic not available

H Treat:
Desensitization

SALICYLATE INTOXICATION

Stephen Berman, M.D.

Salicylate intoxication can result from ingestion of aspirin, bismuth subsalicylate (Pepto Bismol), oil of wintergreen, or skin absorption of salicylic acid ointments. While regular doses of aspirin are rapidly absorbed, large overdoses and enteric coated preparations are absorbed more slowly. Toxic effects of salicylates are related to the following: (1) direct stimulation of the CNS respiratory center, producing respiratory alkalosis; (2) uncoupling of oxidative phosphorylation producing metabolic acidosis; (3) interference with glucose metabolism that can cause hypoglycemia or hyperglycemia; (4) local irritation of gastric mucosa, producing nausea and vomiting; and (5) decreased hemostasis related to increased capillary fragility, thrombocytopenia, hypoprothrombinemia, and decreased platelet aggregation. Salicylate toxicity is characterized by three phases. In phase 1 patients have respiratory alkalosis with an alkaline urine and renal loss of Na^+, K^+, and bicarbonate; in phase 2 patients have respiratory alkalosis with an acid urine because of potassium depletion; in phase 3 patients have metabolic acidosis and acid urine.

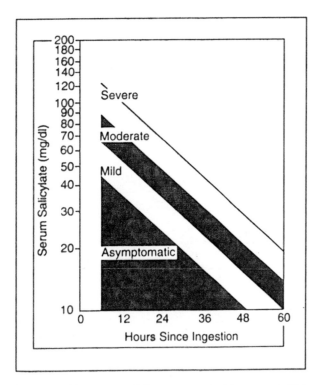

Figure 1 Nomogram relating serum salicylate concentration and expected severity of intoxication at varying intervals following the ingestion of a single dose of salicylate. (From Riggs BS, Kulig K, Rumack BH. Current status of aspirin and acetaminophen intoxication. Pediatr Ann 1987; 16:886.)

A. The assessment of the degree of toxicity depends on whether the intoxication is acute or chronic. When the amount of salicylate ingested acutely can be determined, the degree of toxicity reflects the dose. Mild toxicity is associated with ingestions less than 150 mg/kg, moderate toxicity with ingestions of 150 to 300 mg/kg, and severe toxicity with ingestion of more than 300 mg/kg. When the amount of the acute ingestion is uncertain or confirmation is desired, a serum salicylate should be drawn initially and at least 6 hours after an ingestion. A nomogram (Fig. 1) is used to determine the degree of toxicity for acute ingestions. Ingestions of more than 100 mg/kg/day for several days can cause chronic salicylate toxicity, and salicylate levels do not correlate with clinical severity. Severe toxicity is present in patients with acidosis, dehydration, CNS manifestations, or marked hyperventilation. Patients with very severe toxicity related to acute or chronic ingestion develop noncardiogenic pulmonary edema, intractable seizures, coma, or renal failure.

B. Urine alkalinization is effective because the amount of ionized salicylate increases with an alkaline urine pH. Less ionized salicylate is reabsorbed across the distal tubule than the nonionized form. Administer an isotonic IV solution (0.45% NaCl with 88 mEq of sodium bicarbonate/L) at 10 to 20 ml/kg/hour to maintain a urine output of 1 to 2 m/kg/hour. Add 20 to 40 mEq/L of potassium to the solution because potassium depletion will prevent urine alkalinization. Alkalinization rather than forced diuresis is recommended. Monitor electrolytes, calcium, and glucose closely. Consider multiple-dose charcoal. A cathartic should be given only with the first dose of charcoal. The charcoal appears to bind and remove salicylate that diffuses from the circulation into the intestine. Continue urine alkalinization and multiple-dose charcoal until the salicylate concentration is below 40 mg/dl.

C. Indications for hemodialysis include (1) an acute ingestion with serum salicylate level greater than 100 mg/dl or chronic ingestion with a salicylate level of 60 to 70 mg/dl or higher, (2) renal failure, (3) severe acidosis and electrolyte abnormalities, (4) neurologic deteriorations, and (5) clinical deterioration despite other therapy.

References

Hennetig FM, Shannon M. Toxicologic emergencies. In: Fleisher G, Ludwig S, eds. Pediatric emergency medicine. 3rd ed. Baltimore: Williams & Wilkins, 1993:745.
Riggs BS, Kulig K, Rumack BH. Current status of aspirin and acetaminophen intoxication. Pediatr Ann 1987; 16:886.

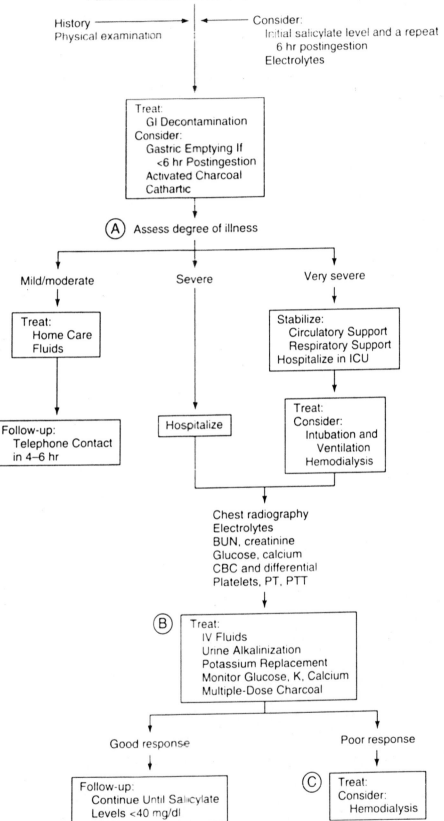

Patient with SALICYLATE INTOXICATION

History ⟶ ⟵ Consider:
Physical examination Initial salicylate level and a repeat
6 hr postingestion
Electrolytes

Treat:
GI Decontamination
Consider:
Gastric Emptying If
<6 hr Postingestion
Activated Charcoal
Cathartic

(A) Assess degree of illness

Mild/moderate | Severe | Very severe

Treat:
Home Care
Fluids

Stabilize:
Circulatory Support
Respiratory Support
Hospitalize in ICU

Follow-up:
Telephone Contact
in 4–6 hr

Hospitalize

Treat:
Consider:
Intubation and
Ventilation
Hemodialysis

Chest radiography
Electrolytes
BUN, creatinine
Glucose, calcium
CBC and differential
Platelets, PT, PTT

(B) Treat:
IV Fluids
Urine Alkalinization
Potassium Replacement
Monitor Glucose, K, Calcium
Multiple-Dose Charcoal

Good response | Poor response

Follow-up:
Continue Until Salicylate
Levels <40 mg/dl

(C) Treat:
Consider:
Hemodialysis

TRAUMA

BITES

Rachelle Nuss, M.D.

Bites are most frequently caused by dogs, cats, and humans, less frequently by rodents, bats, and wild carnivores. Infections of dog and cat bites are usually due to *Staphylococcus aureus*, *Streptococcus viridans*, and *Pasteurella multocida*, although at least 25% of such wounds involve anaerobes. Infections caused by human bites are associated with *S. aureus*, α-hemolytic *Streptococcus*, *Eikenella corrodens*, and in 50% of infections, anaerobes.

A. If a dog or cat bit the victim, inquire about the animal. Is its owner known to the victim? Does it appear well? Are its immunizations current? Was the attack provoked? Is it safely restrained where it can be observed for the next 10 to 14 days? If it is a human bite, was it administered by another child or was the victim abused by an adult? Inquire about the health status of the perpetrator. How old is the wound? What measures have been taken to care for it? When was the last tetanus immunization?

B. Assess the extent of the bite wound and whether bleeding is under control. Note scratches, abrasions, contusions, punctures, and lacerations and determine the wound's depth. Examine the wound for lacerated tendons, ligaments, and nerves. Note signs of infection.

C. Obtain a culture for aerobic and anaerobic bacteria if the bite is on the hand or face or appears infected.

D. Radiography is indicated for suspected periosteal penetration or fracture or if there is a possibility that foreign material, such as teeth, may be embedded in tissue.

E. Wild carnivores and bats may be rabid, but rodents and rabbits are generally not. Rabies prophylaxis is not indicated for bites by healthy dogs with known owners who can observe the animal over the next 10 to 14 days. Bites by strays and other mammals should be discussed with the local health department. If indicated, postexposure prophylaxis for rabies includes administration of human rabies immunoglobulin at 20 IU/kg, half locally around the wound and the rest IM, and human diploid cell rabies vaccine. Initially 1 ml IM is given followed by similar doses on days 3, 7, 14, and 28.
    The human assailant should be tested for hepatitis and HIV. If the assailant is strongly suspected of having hepatitis A, the victim should immediately be given immune serum globulin pending results of testing. If the assailant is suspected of having hepatitis B, hepatitis B immunoglobulin and hepatitis B vaccine should be given. If the assailant is subsequently documented to have hepatitis B, immunoglobulin and vaccine are repeated at 1 month. A third hepatitis B vaccine is given 6 months after the initial dose. The exact risk of

transmission of HIV through a bite has not been determined; however, there is at least one case report suggesting that it is a possibility.

F. Irrigation with 150 to 200 ml of normal saline using a 25 ml syringe and 19 gauge needle is indicated in nonpuncture wounds. This decreases the incidence of dog bite wound infection. Since cat bites are usually puncture wounds, irrigation is not indicated. Careful trimming of the wound edge in nonpuncture wounds may decrease the infection rate. Individuals who have had fewer than two tetanus immunizations and those with two immunizations but a wound 24 or more hours old require tetanus immunoglobulin and tetanus toxoid. Individuals who have received three or more immunizations but the last booster was more than 5 years prior to the bite require a booster.

G. Severe wounds include those that have extensive damage, sometimes involving lacerated arteries, tendons, ligaments, or nerves; occur in an immunocompromised host; cause signs of systemic toxicity; and occur at sites at high risk for functional or significant cosmetic morbidity.

H. The use of prophylactic antibiotics is controversial. Consider antibiotic prophylaxis for all human, dog, and cat bites that are more than 8 hours old; deep puncture wounds for which adequate cleaning is difficult; hand and face wounds; wounds that will have a delayed primary closure; and wounds occurring in an immunoincompetent host. Augmentin is recommended because of its broad coverage. Patients allergic to penicillin can be treated with cephalexin (Keflex), erythromycin, or tetracycline, but their coverage is not so wide.

I. For cosmetic reasons, suturing of facial bites may be warranted; this may be done the same day as the bite, or a delayed primary closure may be performed. The risk of infection is relatively low in the face because of the rich vascular supply, but these wounds still require diligent observation. Do not suture puncture wounds, bites seen after 12 hours, or bites in immunocompromised hosts.

J. Obtain a wound and blood culture prior to beginning treatment with antibiotics. The initial choice of IV antibiotics prior to culture results for dog, cat, and human bites should be penicillin and a penicillinase-resistant penicillin or clindamycin. For those with a dog or cat bite who are allergic to penicillin, vancomycin and cepholathin are good alternatives. For the penicillin-allergic victim of a human bite, vancomycin and cefoxitin are acceptable.

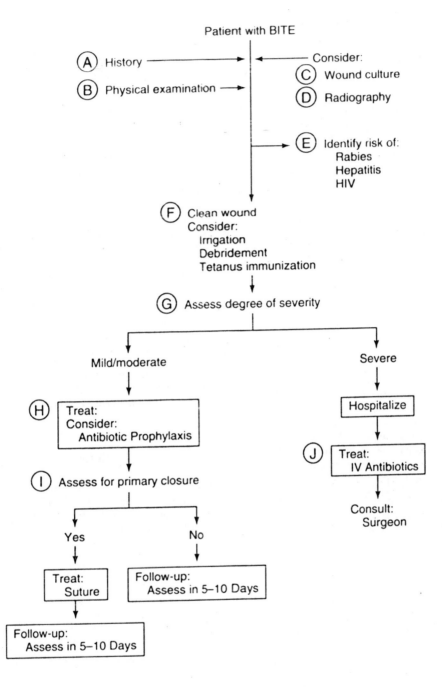

Patient with BITE

(A) History

(B) Physical examination

Consider:
(C) Wound culture
(D) Radiography

(E) Identify risk of:
Rabies
Hepatitis
HIV

(F) Clean wound
Consider:
Irrigation
Debridement
Tetanus immunization

(G) Assess degree of severity

Mild/moderate

Severe

(H) Treat:
Consider:
Antibiotic Prophylaxis

Hospitalize

(J) Treat:
IV Antibiotics

(I) Assess for primary closure

Consult:
Surgeon

Yes

No

Treat:
Suture

Follow-up:
Assess in 5–10 Days

Follow-up:
Assess in 5–10 Days

References

Andersen C. Animal bites. Guidelines to current management. Postgrad Med 1992; 92:134.

Avner J, Baker D. Dog bites in urban children. Pediatrics 1991; 88:55.

Brook I. Microbiology of human and animal bite wounds in children. Pediatr Infect Dis J 1987; 6:29.

Edwards M. Infections due to human and animal bites. In: Feigin RD, Cherry JD, eds. Textbook of pediatric infectious diseases. Philadelphia: Saunders, 1992:2334.

Shirley L, Ross S. Risk of transmission of human immunodeficiency virus by bite of an infected toddler. J Pediatr 1989; 114:425.

BURNS

Michael R. Clemmens, M.D.

A. The first step in the evaluation of a burned child is careful attention to the adequacy of the airway, breathing, and circulation (ABC). The child should be assessed for associated injuries. A history that is inconsistent with the examination or an unusual burn pattern should raise suspicions of child abuse.

B. Burns are considered severe to very severe (major burn) if any of the following criteria are met: (1) Body surface area (BSA) burned is more than 15% partial thickness. (2) BSA burned is 10% full thickness. (3) The face, eyes, ears, hands, feet, or perineum is involved. (4) There is associated major trauma. (5) There are inhalation burns. (6) There are electrical burns. The palm of the child's hand is approximately 1% of BSA and can be used as a rough guide to estimating burned area. In general, the younger the child, the smaller the degree of injury required to classify a burn as major. A surgeon familiar with pediatric burns should be consulted in all but the most minor cases.

C. Mild or moderate (minor) burns are usually treated on an outpatient basis. Cleanse the wound with a dilute mild soap and rinse it with saline. Debride ruptured vesicles. Intact blisters are generally left alone. Apply a thin layer of 1% sulfadiazine cream and a sterile dressing. Give a tetanus booster if needed. Some children require codeine for pain control. Most burns should be reexamined and redressed in 24 hours.

D. In children with major burns the first priority is to maintain a patent airway. Respiratory distress, cyanosis, facial burns, cough, or voice changes suggest the need for aggressive airway management. Administer oxygen in all such cases or if the history suggests smoke inhalation. Provide ventilatory support as needed.

E. Vigorous fluid administration is indicated for patients with major burns. Initial therapy is normal saline or lactated Ringer's solution 20 ml/kg IV, repeated until perfusion is adequate. Subsequent fluid is given at 4 ml/kg/percentage BSA burned, with half of that amount given over the first 8 hours. Calculate maintenance fluid as usual and add it to this replacement. A Foley catheter will help follow urine output. IV morphine may be needed for pain control.

F. Baseline laboratory tests include CBC, arterial blood gas, carboxyhemoglobin level, type and cross-match blood, electrolytes, BUN, creatinine, and a urinalysis. Obtain a baseline chest radiograph.

G. All major pediatric burns should be treated in consultation with a surgeon familiar with their care. Most major burns should be treated at a pediatric burn center.

References

Fleisher G, Ludwig S, eds. Textbook of pediatric emergency medicine. Baltimore: Williams & Wilkins, 1988.

O'Neill JA. Evaluation and treatment of the burned child. Pediatr Clin North Am 1975; 22:407.

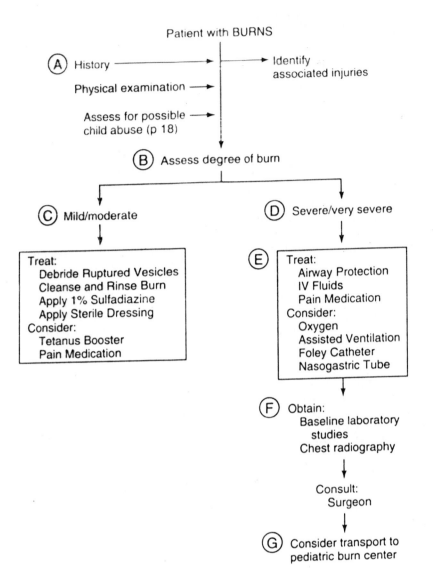

Patient with BURNS

(A) History ──────────────→ ┤──→ Identify
                                   associated injuries

Physical examination ──→

Assess for possible ──→
child abuse (p 18)

(B) Assess degree of burn

(C) Mild/moderate   (D) Severe/very severe

(E) Treat:
      Debride Ruptured Vesicles
      Cleanse and Rinse Burn
      Apply 1% Sulfadiazine
      Apply Sterile Dressing
    Consider:
      Tetanus Booster
      Pain Medication

(E) Treat:
      Airway Protection
      IV Fluids
      Pain Medication
    Consider:
      Oxygen
      Assisted Ventilation
      Foley Catheter
      Nasogastric Tube

(F) Obtain:
      Baseline laboratory
        studies
      Chest radiography

    Consult:
      Surgeon

(G) Consider transport to
    pediatric burn center

DENTAL AND ORAL TRAUMA

Michael R. Clemmens, M.D.

A. Determine the mechanism of injury, symptoms since the injury, and any associated injuries. Determine whether the teeth involved are primary or secondary. Account for all teeth.

B. Injuries to the teeth are considered complicated if the pulp is involved, uncomplicated if only the enamel and dentin are involved. Bleeding from the center of the tooth suggests pulp involvement. All tooth injuries should be referred to a dentist; however, complicated tooth fractures require immediate consultation.

C. Teeth are held in place by a fine periodontal filament. Injury to this structure will cause teeth to loosen or even to avulse. Account for all teeth. If teeth are missing, consider an intrusion injury (which can be identified with intraoral radiographs), aspiration, or ingestion (identified with routine radiographs). If permanent teeth have been avulsed, they should be gently cleaned and soaked in milk, saline, or saliva (under the tongue) and replaced within 30 minutes. Obtain an immediate dental consultation. Increased tooth mobility likewise requires consultation, but the type of injury determines the degree of urgency. Teeth with significantly increased mobility should be seen within 24 hours, whereas those with minimal to no movement may be seen within days.

D. Carefully examine the lips, gums, tongue, and the floor of the mouth. Lip lacerations through the vermilion border require careful approximation to avoid disfigurement; consider consultation with a plastic surgeon. Tears of the frenulum rarely require suturing, but when noted in an infant should alert the examiner to the possibility of child abuse. Tongue lacerations are often left unrepaired unless they are gaping or unless bleeding cannot be controlled with ice and pressure. Large tongue lacerations may require surgical consultation. Hematomas on the floor of the mouth should raise the suspicion of fracture.

E. The mandible is most often broken at the condyles. Look for swelling, deformity, or malocclusion. Mandibular radiographs, including Panarex views, are critical. Obtain oral surgery consultation when a fracture is present.

References

Berkowitz R, Ludwig S, Johnson R. Dental trauma in children and adolescents. Clin Pediatr 1980; 19:3.

McCarthy F. Emergencies in dental practice. Prevention and treatment. Philadelphia: Saunders, 1979.

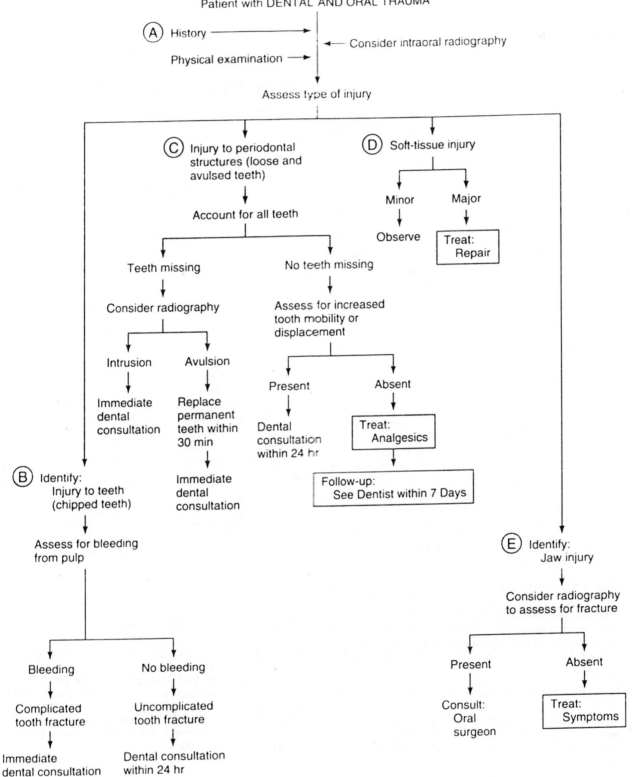

Patient with DENTAL AND ORAL TRAUMA

(A) History ⟶

⟵ Consider intraoral radiography

Physical examination ⟶

Assess type of injury

(C) Injury to periodontal structures (loose and avulsed teeth)

Account for all teeth

Teeth missing

Consider radiography

Intrusion

Immediate dental consultation

Avulsion

Replace permanent teeth within 30 min

Immediate dental consultation

No teeth missing

Assess for increased tooth mobility or displacement

Present

Dental consultation within 24 hr

Absent

Treat: Analgesics

Follow-up: See Dentist within 7 Days

(D) Soft-tissue injury

Minor

Observe

Major

Treat: Repair

(B) Identify: Injury to teeth (chipped teeth)

Assess for bleeding from pulp

Bleeding

Complicated tooth fracture

Immediate dental consultation

No bleeding

Uncomplicated tooth fracture

Dental consultation within 24 hr

(E) Identify: Jaw injury

Consider radiography to assess for fracture

Present

Consult: Oral surgeon

Absent

Treat: Symptoms

FROSTBITE

Stephen Berman, M.D.

DEFINITION

Frostbite is a lesion caused by exposure to freezing temperatures. The most frequent areas affected are the feet (especially the big toes), hands, and face (ears, nose, and cheeks).

PATHOPHYSIOLOGY

Exposure to cold freezes the tissue, leading to the formation of ice crystals and cellular disruption. The cold also causes local vasoconstriction leading to stasis and hypercoagulability. This results in formation of microthrombi, which produce anoxia, local metabolic acidosis, inflammation, and edema. The tissue edema further reduces blood flow and contributes to a spiraling effect. If the process is not interrupted in time, necrosis and tissue loss occur.

A. In the history determine the circumstances of the injury. Factors that increase the risk of injury include constrictive clothing, previous cold injury, diabetes mellitus, hypothermia, and immobilization.

B. In the initial physical examination it is usually difficult to determine the severity of the injury. The extent of the freezing and tissue loss may not be apparent for 4 to 5 days. The skin may appear waxy yellow or pale mottled blue. It will appear hyperemic when rewarmed regardless of the severity of the damage. In severely affected lesions vesicles or bullae form within 6 to 24 hours and a black dry eschar can develop within 9 to 15 days. Note the appearance of the skin, sensation to pinprick, and whether the vesicles are clear or hemorrhagic. In severe cases the extent of the necrosis may not be apparent for 45 days. Identify signs of dehydration, hypothermia, altitude effects (pulmonary edema), and exhaustion.

C. During transportation replace wet clothing with dry clothing and do not allow the affected area to thaw and refreeze. Institute rapid rewarming as soon as possible after removal from the cold when there is no chance of refreezing. If appropriate, immerse the injury in a water bath at 36° to 40° C (96.8° to 104° F) for about 20 to 30 minutes.

D. Debride clear bullae but leave hemorrhagic blisters intact and apply aloe vera cream every 6 hours. If feasible, splint and elevate affected areas to reduce edema. Administer tetanus prophylaxis if indicated. Adequate pain medication is important. Consider IV or IM morphine or meperidine to keep the patient comfortable. Give ibuprofen or another nonsteroidal antiinflammatory agent to reduce the inflammation and edema and promote blood flow. Consider low-dose heparin to prevent microthrombosis when the damage is severe. Additional therapies for extensive injuries—in consultation with critical care and other specialists—include plasma volume expanders (dextran), vasodilating agents (tolazoline), hypotensive agents (guanethidine, reserpine), sympatholytic agents (phenoxybenzamine), and thrombolytic enzymes (streptokinase, tissue plasminogen activator).

E. Consider daily hydrotherapy in warm water for patients with tissue loss. A fasciotomy may be needed to treat a compartment syndrome and ischemia. Amputation should not be considered until 3 to 4 weeks after the injury. The value of prophylactic antibiotics is unclear. However, monitor the injury closely for signs of infection.

TABLE 1 Degree of Illness in Frostbite

Moderate	Severe	Very Severe
Sensation to pinprick intact and Healthy-appearing skin color and Absent or clear vesicles/bullae	Absent sensation to pinprick or Frozen appearance of tissue/skin or Hemorrhagic vesicles/bullae or Cyanosis of skin	Severe frostbite with systemic signs of dehydration, hypothermia, altitude effects (sickness or pulmonary edema), or exhaustion

References

Bracker MD. Environmental and thermal injury. Clin Sports Med 1992; 11:419.

Britt LD, Dascombe WH, Rodriguez A. New horizons in the management of hypothermia and frostbite injury. Surg Clin North Am 1991; 71:345.

Foray J. Mountain frostbite: Current trends in prognosis and treatment (from results concerning 1261 cases). Int J Sports Med 1992; 13:S193.

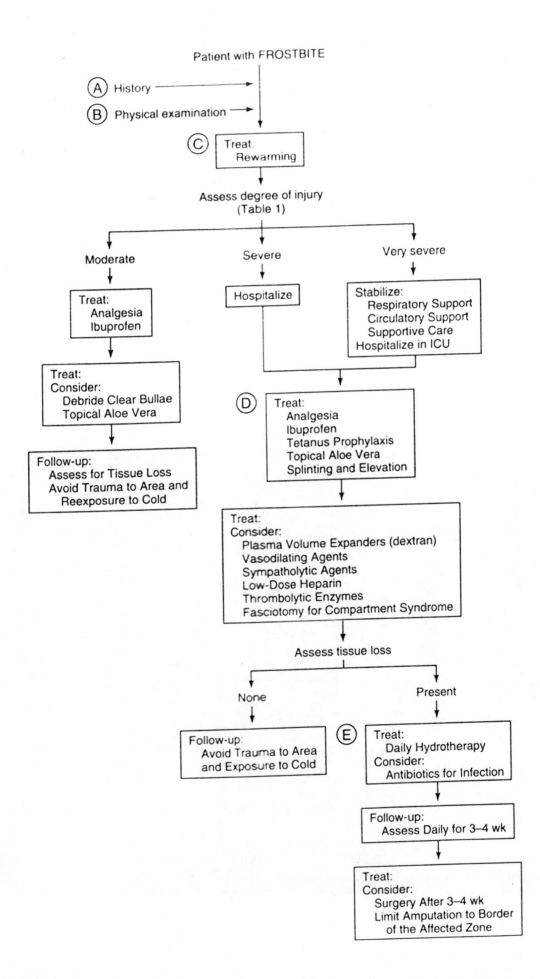

Patient with FROSTBITE

(A) History

(B) Physical examination

(C) Treat:
Rewarming

Assess degree of injury
(Table 1)

Moderate

Treat:
Analgesia
Ibuprofen

Treat:
Consider:
Debride Clear Bullae
Topical Aloe Vera

Follow-up:
Assess for Tissue Loss
Avoid Trauma to Area and
Reexposure to Cold

Severe

Hospitalize

Very severe

Stabilize:
Respiratory Support
Circulatory Support
Supportive Care
Hospitalize in ICU

(D) Treat:
Analgesia
Ibuprofen
Tetanus Prophylaxis
Topical Aloe Vera
Splinting and Elevation

Treat:
Consider:
Plasma Volume Expanders (dextran)
Vasodilating Agents
Sympatholytic Agents
Low-Dose Heparin
Thrombolytic Enzymes
Fasciotomy for Compartment Syndrome

Assess tissue loss

None

Follow-up:
Avoid Trauma to Area
and Exposure to Cold

Present

(E) Treat:
Daily Hydrotherapy
Consider:
Antibiotics for Infection

Follow-up:
Assess Daily for 3–4 wk

Treat:
Consider:
Surgery After 3–4 wk
Limit Amputation to Border
of the Affected Zone

HAND INJURIES

Richard C. Fisher, M.D.

A. In the history determine the mechanism of injury. Because of their intrinsically inquisitive nature, children injure their hands by the most unlikely means. The injuries involve soft-tissue, bone, and epiphyseal plates. Lacerations may involve skin, nerve, or tendons. Crush injuries often injure soft-tissues and bone. Fractures and dislocations are the result of falls or abduction of the digits.

B. In the physical examination observe for swelling, contusions, lacerations, and bony deformity. In young children the examination of the intricate functions of the hand is difficult. Often it is best to watch the child use the hand to play or grasp objects. A sensory examination should be performed if possible.

C. If a fracture, dislocation, or foreign body is suspected, radiographs are indicated.

D. Superficial lacerations are most common and can usually be safely sutured after cleansing the wound. It is important to determine the status of tendon and nerve function at the time of initial treatment, as injuries to these structures may require surgical treatment.

E. Most crush injuries occur when fingers are caught in a closing door. There are three typical injuries. Subungual hematoma may be treated with ice packs if mild or open drainage with a sterile #11 scapel blade, a needle, or a heated paper clip. Nail bed lacerations should be repaired using a fine suture technique. Fractures of the distal phalanx, tuft fractures, are usually minimally displaced and can be treated by splinting for several weeks until healed.

F. Carpal bone fractures are uncommon in younger children, but with adolescence scaphoid fractures occur

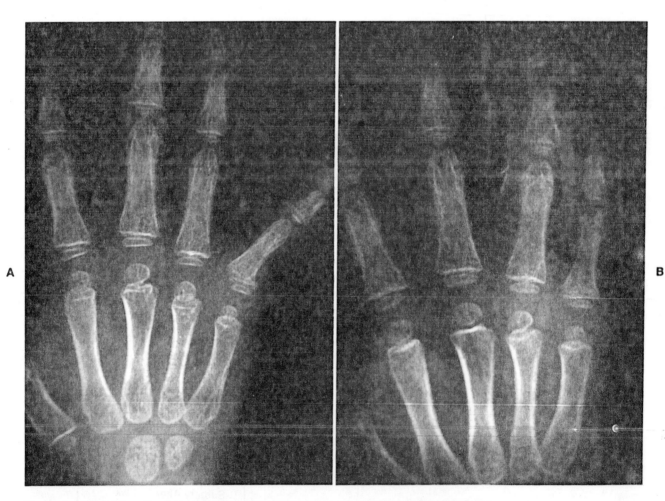

Figure 1 **A,** Salter type II epiphyseal fracture of the base of the proximal phalanx of the little finger.
B, Postreduction showing the bone in satisfactory position.

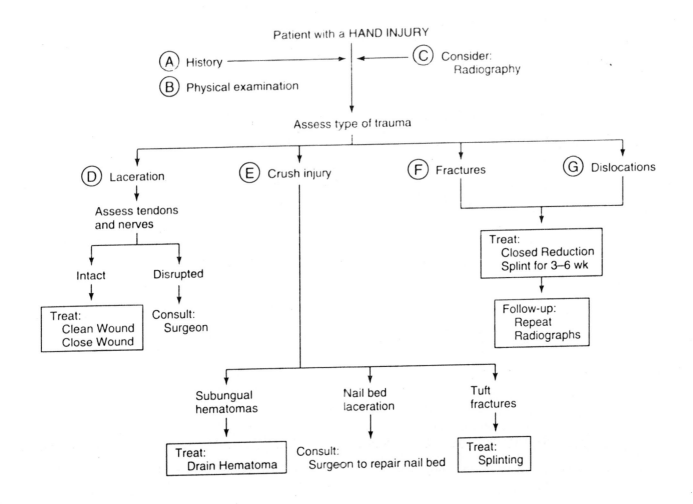

Patient with a HAND INJURY

(A) History ——————————→ ←—————— (C) Consider: Radiography

(B) Physical examination

Assess type of trauma

(D) Laceration — (E) Crush injury — (F) Fractures — (G) Dislocations

Laceration (D)
Assess tendons and nerves

Intact → Treat: Clean Wound / Close Wound

Disrupted → Consult: Surgeon

Fractures (F) / Dislocations (G)
Treat: Closed Reduction / Splint for 3–6 wk

Follow-up: Repeat Radiographs

Crush injury (E)
Subungual hematomas → Treat: Drain Hematoma

Nail bed laceration → Consult: Surgeon to repair nail bed

Tuft fractures → Treat: Splinting

---

with increasing frequency. Metacarpal fractures are common in older children from falls or punching injuries. An acceptable deformity of metacarpal neck fractures is 10 degrees at the index metacarpal and up to 40 degrees at the little finger. Rotational deformity is unacceptable and should be carefully evaluated. Fractures of the digits occur in falls or by catching the finger on an object, causing abduction. Fractures through the growth plate are often the result of the latter mechanism (Fig. 1). They can be reduced by placing a round object, such as a pencil, between the digits and correcting the deformity. These injuries should be treated by closed reduction and splinting for 3 to 6 weeks.

G. Dislocations at the proximal and distal interphalangeal joints are often associated with athletics. It is important to rule out adjacent fractures, which can result in joint instability or tendon avulsion injuries.

References

American Society for Surgery of the Hand, Burgess L, ed. The hand: Examination and diagnosis. New York: Churchill Livingstone, 1990.

Bhende MS, Dandrea LA, Davis HW. Hand injuries in children presenting to a pediatric emergency department. Ann Emerg Med 1993; 22:1519.

Tolo VT, Wood B. Pediatric orthopaedics in primary care. Baltimore: Williams & Wilkins, 1993.

HEAD INJURIES

Stephen Berman, M.D.

Acute head trauma results in approximately 100,000 pediatric hospital admissions a year. Most brain injuries involve concussion, contusion, hemorrhage, or laceration (with or without an associated skull fracture).

A. Determine the time, circumstances, and severity of the trauma. Note duration of any loss of consciousness, altered mental status, retrograde amnesia, seizure activity, vomiting, ataxia, or headache. Identify predisposing conditions, especially bleeding disorders and underlying CNS pathology (hydrocephalus, arteriovenous malformations). Consider the possibility of nonaccidental trauma.

B. Assess the patient for multiple trauma. A slow respiratory rate, elevated blood pressure, and slow pulse rate suggest increased intracranial pressure. Hypotension and fast pulse and respiratory rate suggest shock. Orbital ecchymosis (raccoon sign), mastoid erythema and swelling (battle sign), or hemotympaneum suggests a basilar skull fracture. Carefully palpate the skull for evidence of a depressed skull fracture. Note any CSF discharge from the nose or ears. Examine the optic fundi to identify papilledema, hemorrhages, and absence of venous pulsations. Retinal hemorrhages suggest inflicted head injury when the history does not suggest a serious accidental trauma. Perform a thorough neurologic evaluation to identify neurologic signs (paralysis, paresis, ataxia, pathologic reflexes, meningeal signs). In patients with altered consciousness determine the level of brain dysfunction and the Glasgow Coma Score (Table 1). Patients with scores of 8 or less have a poor prognosis and if they survive are likely to suffer severe sequelae. Findings that suggest a subdural hematoma include increased head size, bulging fontanelle, retinal hemorrhages, extraocular palsy, hemiparesis, and anemia. Suspect an acute epidural hematoma when rapid deterioration in level of consciousness follows a 12 to 48 hour lucid period.

C. Indications for skull radiography include open head injury, possible depressed compound or basilar fracture, possible foreign body, suspicion of child abuse, and moderate to severe injury in which a CT scan cannot be performed.

D. Sideline evaluation and guidelines for return to competition are summarized in the form developed by the Colorado Trauma Institute (box).

E. Home follow-up includes instructing the parents to waken the child during the night, to check the pupils for size and response to light, and to note any alteration in mental status, difficulty in speaking, blurring of vision,

(Continued on page 654)

TABLE 1   The Glasgow Coma Scale

The scale provides an easy to use, standardized scoring system for evaluating neurologic function in severely injured patients. To calculate the patient's total score, add up the best scores for each subscale. If you are unable to test a subscale, mark it U and assign it no score. A score of 7 or below indicates severe compromise of brain function.

Subscale	Response	Score
Best eye opening	Spontaneous	4
	To voice	3
	To pain	2
	None	1
Best verbal response	Oriented	5
	Confused conversation	4
	Inappropriate words	3
	Incomprehensible sounds	2
	None	1
Best motor response, upper limb	Obeys commands	6
	Localizes pain	5
	Flexor withdrawal (decorticate posturing)	4
	Abnormal flexion (decerebrate posturing)	3
	Extension	2
	Flaccid	1

From Rosman NP. Pediatric emergencies: Managing acute head trauma. Contemp Pediatr 1986; 3:30; reprinted with permission.

TABLE 2   Degree of Illness in the Patient with Head Injury

Mild	Moderate	Severe
Asymptomatic or No loss of consciousness and rapid clearing of mental status	>10 min posttraumatic unconsciousness or Posttraumatic seizures or Focal neurologic deficits or Retrograde amnesia lasting >30 min or Evidence of depressed skull fracture, basilar skull fracture, or CSF leak or Signs of severe headache or Persistent vomiting or Irritability	Respiratory distress or Circulatory instability or Altered mental status (unresponsiveness, coma) or Marked irritability or Signs of increased intracranial pressure (severe headache, protracted vomiting, altered mental status)

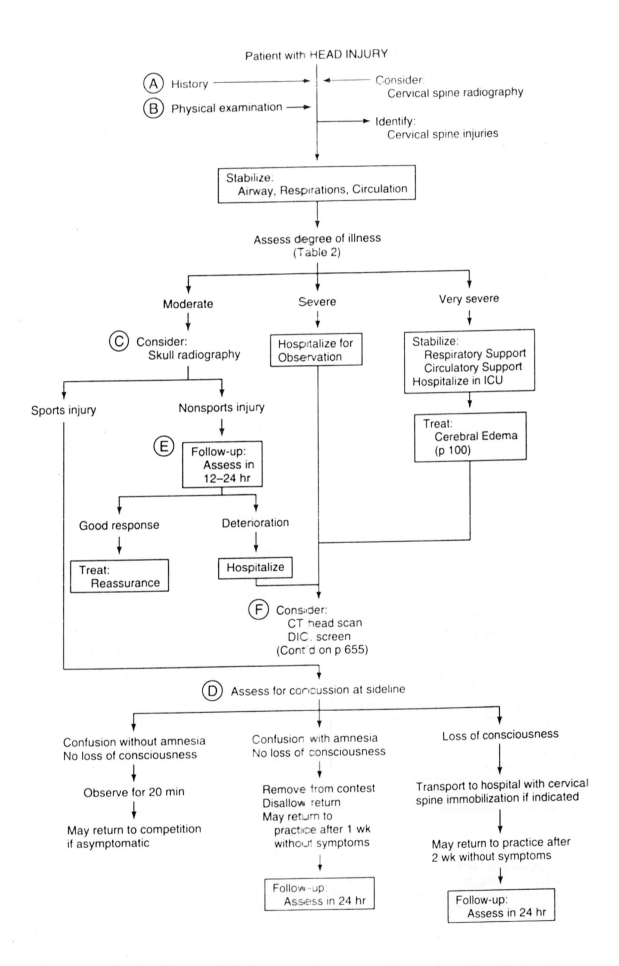

Patient with HEAD INJURY

(A) History ⟶ ← Consider:
    Cervical spine radiography

(B) Physical examination ⟶

⟶ Identify:
    Cervical spine injuries

Stabilize:
Airway, Respirations, Circulation

Assess degree of illness
(Table 2)

Moderate   Severe   Very severe

(C) Consider: Hospitalize for   Stabilize:
    Skull radiography   Observation   Respiratory Support
                                                    Circulatory Support
                                                    Hospitalize in ICU

Sports injury   Nonsports injury

(E) Follow-up: Treat:
    Assess in   Cerebral Edema
    12–24 hr   (p 100)

Good response   Deterioration

Treat: Hospitalize
Reassurance

(F) Consider:
    CT head scan
    DIC screen
    (Cont'd on p 655)

(D) Assess for concussion at sideline

Confusion without amnesia   Confusion with amnesia   Loss of consciousness
No loss of consciousness   No loss of consciousness

Observe for 20 min   Remove from contest   Transport to hospital with cervical
                                   Disallow return   spine immobilization if indicated
                                   May return to
May return to competition   practice after 1 wk
if asymptomatic   without symptoms   May return to practice after
                                                                    2 wk without symptoms

                                   Follow-up:
                                   Assess in 24 hr   Follow-up:
                                                                    Assess in 24 hr

F. A Glasgow Coma score of 12 or less, altered mental status, and focal neurologic signs increase the likelihood of an abnormal CT scan. However, clinical findings cannot identify a low-risk group within the moderate (symptomatic) category. CT scans should be done initially without contrast and preferably without sedation. Skull fractures are associated with a higher risk of brain contusion or laceration. In addition, skull fractures that involve the area of the middle meningeal artery or the venous sinus predispose to an intracranial bleed.

G. Disseminated intravascular coagulation (DIC) is common in severe brain injury and increases the case fatality rate and risk of a neurologic disability. CSF leaks usually heal spontaneously within 2 weeks of trauma. Prophylactic antibiotics do not prevent secondary infection. When signs of meningeal irritation or fever develop, perform a spinal tap to diagnose meningitis. Consider surgical repair when a CSF leak has failed to resolve within 2 weeks. Skull fractures may be complicated by a leptomeningeal cyst when CSF accumulates under the scalp because of a tear in the dura and arachnoid membranes. Refer these patients to a neurosurgeon. Severe head trauma may be associated with a postconcussion syndrome characterized by behavior disturbances (aggressiveness), poor impulse control, emotional lability, phobias, headaches, vertigo, dizziness, and deteriorating school performance.

H. The case fatality rate of children with brain tissue contusion, hemorrhage, or laceration is 48%. Moderate or severe disability occurs in almost all patients with a Glasgow Coma score of 3 or 4 on admission, in 65% with a score of 5 to 8, in 5% with a score of 9 to 12, and in 4% with a score of 13 to 14. Disability is rare (1 in 500) in cases with concussion alone.

I. Posttraumatic seizures may be immediate, early, or late. Impact seizures that occur immediately with head trauma are benign and not associated with subsequent epilepsy. Early posttraumatic seizures occur during the first week after head trauma; of these, 35% occur within the first hour, 40% within 24 hours, and 25% within 1 week. Treat early posttraumatic seizures with anticonvulsants for 6 months. Late posttraumatic seizures, which occur after 1 week, have a high rate of recurrence and may require treatment for 3 to 4 seizure-free years.

References

Casey R, Ludwig S, McCormick M. Minor head trauma in children: An intervention to decrease functional morbidity. Pediatrics 1987; 80:159.

Duhaime AC, Alario AJ, Lewander WJ, et al. Head injury in very young children: Mechanisms, injury types, and ophthalmologic findings in 100 hospitalized patients younger than 2 years of age. Pediatrics 1992; 90:179.

Gerring JP. Psychiatric sequelae of severe closed head injury. Pediatr Rev 1986; 8:115.

Greenspan AI, MacKenzie EJ. Functional outcome after pediatric head injury. Pediatrics 1994; 94:425.

Hennes H, Lee M, Smith D, et al. Clinical predictors of severe head trauma in children. Am J Dis Child 1988; 142: 1045.

unsteadiness in walking, difficulty in using the arms, fever, persistent vomiting, or seizures. Recommend a clear liquid diet until the child has gone 6 hours without vomiting. Reassurance and instructions for return to usual routine are important.

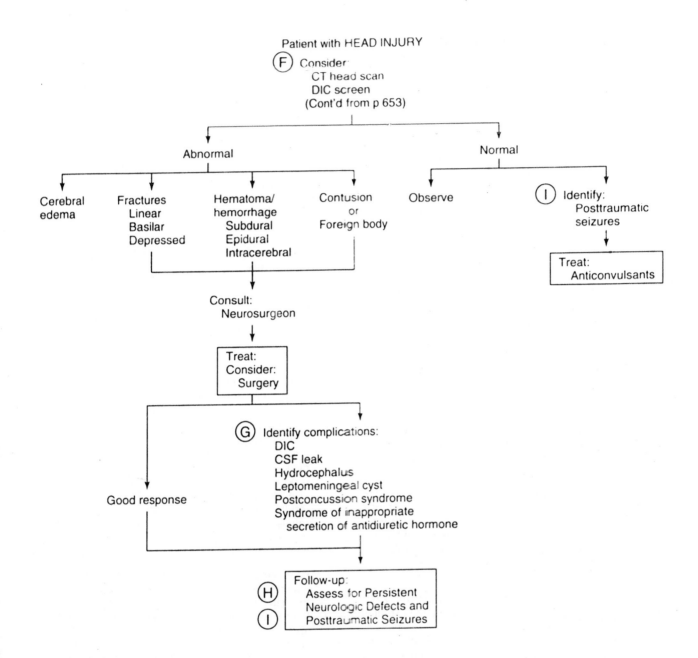

Patient with HEAD INJURY

(F) Consider:
CT head scan
DIC screen
(Cont'd from p 653)

Abnormal

- Cerebral edema
- Fractures
  Linear
  Basilar
  Depressed
- Hematoma/ hemorrhage
  Subdural
  Epidural
  Intracerebral
- Contusion
  or
  Foreign body

Consult:
Neurosurgeon

Treat:
Consider:
Surgery

Good response

(G) Identify complications:
DIC
CSF leak
Hydrocephalus
Leptomeningeal cyst
Postconcussion syndrome
Syndrome of inappropriate
secretion of antidiuretic hormone

(H)
(I) Follow-up:
Assess for Persistent
Neurologic Defects and
Posttraumatic Seizures

Normal

- Observe
- (I) Identify:
  Posttraumatic
  seizures

  Treat:
  Anticonvulsants

Kaufman BA, Dacey RG Jr. Acute care management of closed head injury in childhood. Pediatr Ann 1994; 23:18.

Kraus JF, Fife D, Conroy C. Pediatric brain injuries: The nature, clinical course, and early outcomes in a defined United States population. Pediatrics 1987; 79:501.

Masters SJ, McClean PM, Arcarese JS, et al: Skull x-ray examinations after head trauma: Recommendations by a multidisciplinary panel and validation study. N Engl J Med 1987; 316:84.

Miner ME, Kaufman HH, Graham SH, et al: Disseminated intravascular coagulation fibrinolytic syndrome following head injury in children: Frequency and prognostic implications. J Pediatr 1982; 100:687.

Rachesky I, Boyce WT, Duncan B, et al: Clinical prediction of cervical spine injuries in children: Radiographic abnormalities. Am J Dis Child 1987; 141:199.

Rivara F, Tanaguchi D, Parish RA, et al: Poor prediction of positive computed tomographic scans by clinical criteria in symptomatic pediatric head trauma. Pediatrics 1987; 80:579.

Rosenthal BW, Bergman I. Intracranial injury after moderate head trauma in children. J Pediatr 1989; 115:346.

Rosman NP. Pediatric emergencies: Managing acute head trauma. Contemp Pediatr 1986; 3:24.

Tyler JS, Mira MP, Hollowell JG. Head injury training for pediatric residents. Am J Dis Child 1989; 143:930.

LOWER EXTREMITY TRAUMA

Richard C. Fisher, M.D.
Stephen Berman, M.D.

A. A careful history will help determine the nature and severity of the injury. Simple falls often result in mild or moderate injuries. High-energy trauma, such as traffic accidents and falls from heights, cause severe injuries. Be alert for the signs of nonaccidental trauma. These include multiple fractures of different ages in an infant, a questionable or inconsistent history of injury, children presenting late for care, and rotational fractures of the long bones.

B. Assess the degree of injury by clinical examination and appropriate radiography. Severe injuries are characterized by deformity, a rapid onset of hemarthrosis or effusion, joint instability, or mechanical blockage. Moderate injuries generally have small, slowly developing effusions, minimal ecchymosis, no gross deformity, and pain or tenderness specific to the site of injury. Mild injuries have diffuse, poorly localized pain and tenderness without an effusion or hemarthrosis. Gross deformity, point tenderness, and painful motion indicate fracture. Associated findings indicating severe injury include vascular impairment from a major vessel injury, fractures through a preexisting bone lesion (pathologic fractures), and skin wounds in the vicinity of a fracture. The latter indicates a possible open fracture, an emergency.

C. Torus fractures and nondisplaced distal tibial fractures may appear as mild injuries with minimal radiographic changes on initial films. The young child may present only with unwillingness to use the extremity. If fracture is suspected, the extremity should be immobilized. Follow-up films in about 2 weeks will show new bone formation.

D. Treat acute injuries as outlined for upper extremity injuries (see p 660). Be sure to determine the extent of injury about the knee and ankle before allowing unrestricted weight-bearing activities. Hemarthrosis immediately after injury suggests a severe ligament injury or intraarticular fracture. The latter should be evident on radiograph. Assess the integrity of the medial and lateral collateral ligaments by noting a definite end point when medial and lateral stress is applied to the knee both extended and flexed (20 to 25 degrees). Document the integrity of the anterior cruciate ligament by assessing forward movement of the tibia when stressed with the knee flexed 90 degrees (anterior drawer) and 30 degrees (Lachman test). Document the integrity of the posterior cruciate by observing whether the tibia sags backward with the knee flexed to 90 degrees and the heel resting on the examination table (posterior drawer sign). Assess the ankle by stabilizing the lower leg and holding the heel firmly in the opposite hand. Test the integrity of the anterior talofibular ligament by pulling forward on the heel, causing anterior subluxation of the calcaneus and talus if it is ruptured, and by eliciting pain while stressing the ankle in the equinovarus position. Evaluate the integrity of the fibulocalcaneal ligament by inverting the heel and palpating for tenderness and laxity over the ligament. Increased inversion with this maneuver indicates a possible grade 3 sprain. Tenderness specifically between the tibia and fibula and widening of this distance on the radiograph suggests a third-degree tear of the syndesmosis. Epiphyseal fractures about the knee and ankle are more common than ligament ruptures in young children. If joint laxity is suspected from the clinical examination, radiographs taken while stressing the joint will help differentiate ligament from epiphyseal plate injuries.

E. Consider other more serious causes of a painful extremity, especially tumor and infection. Radiography, bone scan, and the erythrocyte sedimentation rate are helpful.

F. Shin splints is a generic term for anterior calf pain associated with activity. The causes include periostitis at the insertion of the posterior tibial tendon along the tibia. Stress fractures are characterized by pain with activity and point tenderness. A recent increase in activity level is frequent. Common areas of stress fracture are the metatarsals, distal fibula, proximal tibia, and femoral neck. Initial radiographs may be normal; the bone scan is positive earlier. Pain over the Achilles tendon and its insertion into the os calcis apophysis (Sever syndrome) results from a combination of a tight gastrocnemius-soleus mechanism and overuse. Pain at the insertion of the posterior tibial tendon accompanies an accessory navicular, usually after minimal trauma or overuse.

G. Patellofemoral pain is extremely common in the adolescent knee. Symptoms, which include pain beneath the patella with walking stairs, kneeling, or sitting for a long time, may be accompanied by mild effusions, abnormal tracking, and crepitus. Osteochondritis dissecans presents as vague knee pain, at times with effusions. If the fragment becomes dislodged, knee motion is blocked. The lesion is apparent on the radiograph, usually on the lateral aspect of the medial femoral condyle. Excessive stress on the patella tendon mechanism results in pain at either the patella insertion (jumper's knee) or the tibial insertion (Osgood-Schlatter disease). Both manifest as local tenderness, swelling, and pain with use or resisted stress. Radiographic examination is usually not diagnostic. Serious nontraumatic hip abnormalities, such as Legg-Perthes syndrome and slipped capital femoral epiphysis, often have knee pain as the initial symptom.

H. Rehabilitation should include active range-of-motion, muscle strengthening, and stretching exercises. Knee rehabilitation should stress hamstring stretching and short arc quadriceps strengthening exercises, limiting the arc to the last 20 to 30 degrees before full extension. Resumption of activities should be gradual, staying below the pain threshold.

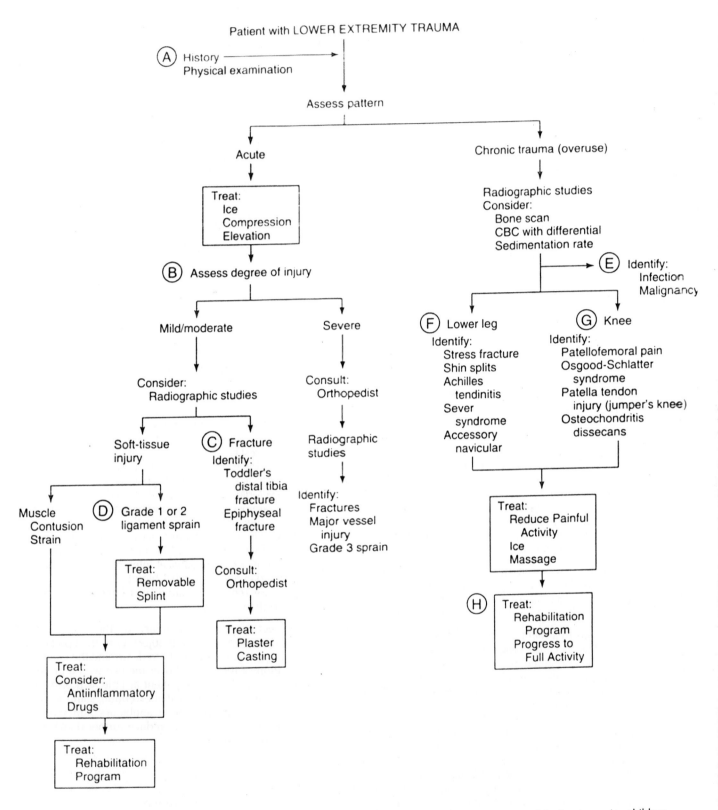

Patient with LOWER EXTREMITY TRAUMA

(A) History — Physical examination

Assess pattern

Acute

Treat:
Ice
Compression
Elevation

(B) Assess degree of injury

Mild/moderate

Consider:
Radiographic studies

Soft-tissue injury

Muscle
Contusion
Strain

(D) Grade 1 or 2
ligament sprain

Treat:
Removable
Splint

Treat:
Consider:
Antiinflammatory
Drugs

Treat:
Rehabilitation
Program

(C) Fracture
Identify:
Toddler's
distal tibia
fracture
Epiphyseal
fracture

Consult:
Orthopedist

Treat:
Plaster
Casting

Severe

Consult:
Orthopedist

Radiographic
studies

Identify:
Fractures
Major vessel
injury
Grade 3 sprain

Chronic trauma (overuse)

Radiographic studies
Consider:
Bone scan
CBC with differential
Sedimentation rate

(E) Identify:
Infection
Malignancy

(F) Lower leg
Identify:
Stress fracture
Shin splits
Achilles
tendinitis
Sever
syndrome
Accessory
navicular

(G) Knee
Identify:
Patellofemoral pain
Osgood-Schlatter
syndrome
Patella tendon
injury (jumper's knee)
Osteochondritis
dissecans

Treat:
Reduce Painful
Activity
Ice
Massage

(H) Treat:
Rehabilitation
Program
Progress to
Full Activity

References

Cooper RR. Fractures in children. In: Clark CR, Bonfiglio M, eds. Orthopaedics: Essentials of diagnosis and treatment. New York: Churchill Livingstone, 1994:215.

Rivara FP, Pansh RA, Meuller BA. Extremity injuries in children: Predictive value of clinical findings. Pediatrics 1986; 78:803.

Rockwood CA, Wilkins KE, King RE. Fractures in children. Philadelphia: Lippincott, 1991.

Staheli LT. Fundamentals of pediatric orthopedics. New York: Raven Press, 1992.

Tanner SM. Putting children with knee injuries back in the game. Contemp Pediatr 1995; 12:114.

OCULAR INJURY

Robert D. Gross, M.D.
Joel N. Leffler, M.D.

A. In a traumatized child even a seemingly trivial injury may be serious. Assess the physical findings and presume that the injury is more involved than the presenting signs suggest. For example, an eyelid laceration may be associated with a penetrating injury to the globe. Instillation of a sterile topical anesthetic facilitates examination of the injured eye. Assess visual acuity using a pinhole lens to overcome any refractive error. After checking the eyelids for signs of laceration, examine the eye using a penlight. Check the cornea for laceration and the anterior chamber for bleeding (hyphema). Shallowness of the anterior chamber (as compared with the normal eye) suggests a leaking wound (corneal laceration). A peaked pupil indicates iris prolapse into the wound. An irregular pupil may be seen after a contusion injury in association with blood in the anterior chamber. Examine the sclera carefully. A scleral perforation may be obscured by an overlying subconjunctival hemorrhage. Examine the eye with the ophthalmoscope, checking for media opacities (disturbance of the red reflex) suggestive of a corneal perforation, cataract, or vitreous hemorrhage. If there is media opacity, examine the retina for hemorrhage or edema. Test ocular mobility in all fields of gaze and ask the patient about any double vision. Double vision after blunt trauma to the eye may be a sign of an orbital floor fracture. An afferent pupillary defect is a sign of optic nerve damage. Traumatic mydriasis may accompany blunt trauma and hyphema. Pupillary involvement in addition to ptosis and restricted eye movements suggests a third nerve palsy.

B. X-rays or CT scan can identify and localize intraocular foreign bodies and rule out orbital fracture or head injury. MRI may also be useful if suspected retained material is nonmetallic or if CT resolution is inadequate.

C. Immediate treatment of chemical burns to the eye is mandatory because progressive damage may accompany the continued presence of a chemical agent, especially an alkali. Alkali burns are more severe than acid burns because of their rapid penetration through the cornea and anterior chamber. Acids precipitate tissue proteins that form barriers to further tissue penetration. Treat chemical burns immediately with copious irrigation of the eyes with readily available fluid, followed by normal saline solution lavage in the emergency room for at least 1 hour. Continue irrigation until pH paper indicates a physiologic pH. Check pH again in 30 minutes and repeat lavage if pH is elevated. If eversion of the lids reveals retained particles, swab the fornices with cotton-tipped applicators under topical anesthesia. Recheck pH. When pH is stable, administer cycloplegics and antibiotics. Use analgesics during the immediate treatment period. Follow-up includes monitoring and treatment of intraocular pressure elevation and secondary iridocyclitis.

D. Corneal abrasions are extremely painful, and examination can be aided by the use of tetracaine, a topical anesthetic. Fluorescein dye will confirm the presence of an epithelial defect. Most abrasions heal within 24 to 48 hours with a pressure patch, cycloplegic drops, and antibiotic ointment.

E. Embedded corneal foreign bodies require prompt referral to an ophthalmologist for removal using a fine needle or burr drill. Metallic foreign bodies may leave a rust ring, which requires removal to prevent inflammation and prolonged healing time.

F. Hyphema is bleeding into the anterior chamber following blunt or lacerating trauma. A history should exclude bleeding disorders; sickle cell, kidney, and liver disease; and aspirin or other anticoagulant therapy. Hyphema is a sight-threatening condition that requires close monitoring and ophthalmic consultation. Treatment is geared to prevent rebleeds during the first 5 days after injury. Clinical outcomes and rebleeding rates do not vary significantly in patients who are hospitalized versus those who are homebound. In addition to limiting the patient's activity, elevating the head to 30 degrees during rest can hasten settling of the hyphema, thereby facilitating examination of the posterior segment of the eye. Medical treatment of hyphema may include the use of cycloplegics and topical steroids. Antifibrinolytics (e.g., aminocaproic acid) and systemic steroids have also been suggested for medical therapy and may be of benefit in certain circumstances. Patients should receive close follow-up during the first 5 days of treatment. Some may require surgical intervention to avoid optic nerve damage or corneal blood staining if intraocular pressure remains elevated or if large clots persist for more than 10 days.

G. Suspect a penetrating injury to the eye when an accident involves a sharp object. Perform a preliminary examination with penlight to determine the extent and location of the injury. Cover the eye with a protective shield and disturb the patient as little as possible prior to repair. Prior to surgical intervention, start the patient on appropriate parenteral antibiotics and give analgesics and antiemetics to reduce further damage from agitation or emesis.

References

Eagling EM, Roper-Hall MJ. Eye injuries: An illustrated guide. Philadelphia: Lippincott, 1986.
Fraunfelder FT, Hampton RF. Current ocular therapy. Philadelphia: Saunders, 1995.
Shingleton BJ, Hersh PS, Kenyon KR. Eye trauma. St. Louis: Mosby, 1991.

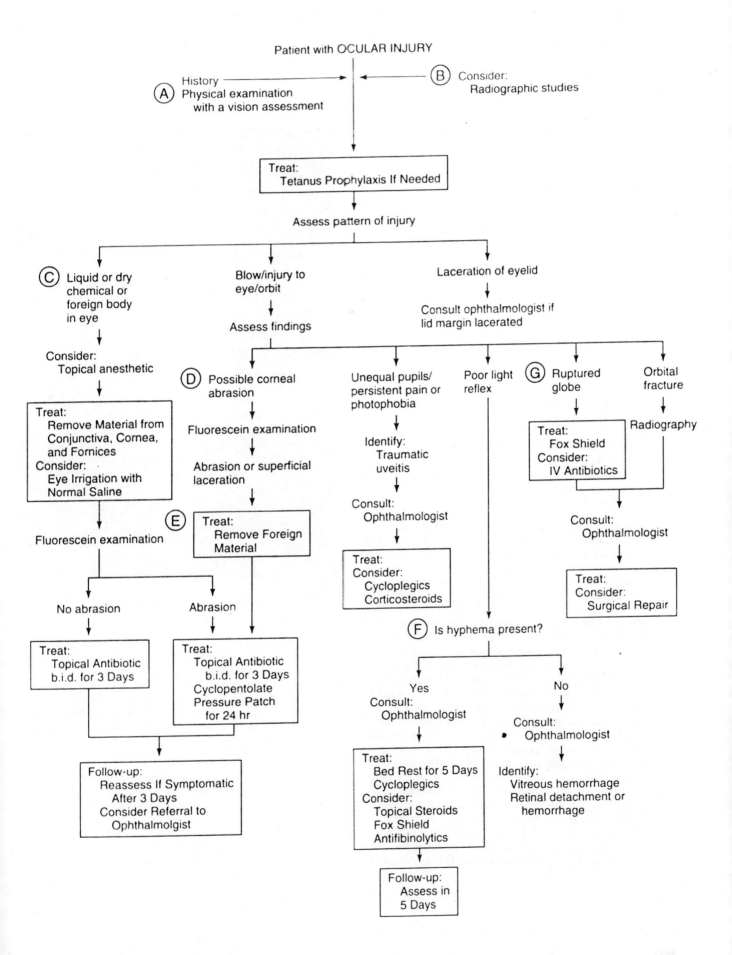

Patient with OCULAR INJURY

(A) History
Physical examination
with a vision assessment

(B) Consider:
Radiographic studies

Treat:
Tetanus Prophylaxis If Needed

Assess pattern of injury

(C) Liquid or dry
chemical or
foreign body
in eye

Blow/injury to
eye/orbit

Laceration of eyelid

Consult ophthalmologist if
lid margin lacerated

Consider:
Topical anesthetic

Assess findings

Treat:
Remove Material from
Conjunctiva, Cornea,
and Fornices
Consider:
Eye Irrigation with
Normal Saline

(D) Possible corneal
abrasion

Fluorescein examination

Abrasion or superficial
laceration

Unequal pupils/
persistent pain or
photophobia

Poor light
reflex

(G) Ruptured
globe

Orbital
fracture

Identify:
Traumatic
uveitis

Treat:
Fox Shield
Consider:
IV Antibiotics

Radiography

Fluorescein examination

(E) Treat:
Remove Foreign
Material

Consult:
Ophthalmologist

Consult:
Ophthalmologist

No abrasion

Abrasion

Treat:
Consider:
Cycloplegics
Corticosteroids

Treat:
Consider:
Surgical Repair

Treat:
Topical Antibiotic
b.i.d. for 3 Days

Treat:
Topical Antibiotic
b.i.d. for 3 Days
Cyclopentolate
Pressure Patch
for 24 hr

(F) Is hyphema present?

Follow-up:
Reassess If Symptomatic
After 3 Days
Consider Referral to
Ophthalmolgist

Yes
Consult:
Ophthalmologist

No

Consult:
• Ophthalmologist

Treat:
Bed Rest for 5 Days
Cycloplegics
Consider:
Topical Steroids
Fox Shield
Antifibinolytics

Identify:
Vitreous hemorrhage
Retinal detachment or
hemorrhage

Follow-up:
Assess in
5 Days

UPPER EXTREMITY FRACTURES

Richard C. Fisher, M.D.

A. Although fractures of the upper extremity vary in complexity, several types may be treated in the primary care setting. Evaluation should include history, physical examination, and routine radiographs (see p 382). Most injuries of the upper extremity result from a fall onto the arm or the outstretched hand. Common fractures include the clavicle, elbow region, forearm, and distal radius. The signs of injuries in these areas are swelling, possibly deformity, point tenderness, and reluctance to use or move the extremity. Radiographs are important for accurate diagnosis. Special imaging is usually not indicated.

B. Fractures of the clavicle usually occur in the middle and outer third and cause mild, diffuse swelling over the clavicle with point tenderness. On occasion mild deformity may be seen. Perform careful neurovascular examination of the upper extremity to be certain that underlying vessels and the brachial plexus are not injured, although such injuries are rare. Most clavicle fractures in children need no reduction, as healing and remodeling will take place with even moderate deformities. The shoulder girdle is best immobilized in a sling to relieve the weight of the arm. A figure 8 dressing may help reduce motion across the fracture site. These fractures generally heal sufficiently to remove the support in 3 to 4 weeks, and full function returns by 4 to 8 weeks.

C. Elbow injuries may be complex and fraught with complications. X-ray films are often difficult to interpret. Displaced fractures and dislocations are probably best referred for orthopedic care. Some can be treated in the primary care setting. The three most common are nondisplaced supracondylar fractures, torus type fractures of the radial neck, and nursemaid's elbow. Most elbow injuries cause swelling, and the patient is reluctant to use the arm. No deformity is visible with the three injuries mentioned. Supracondylar fractures without displacement are graded type I (Fig. 1). Treat these with posterior splint, ice, elevation, and frequent checks of the neurovascular system. Repeat films in a week to 10 days to be certain that no displacement of the fracture has occurred; the splint can be changed at that time to a long arm cast for an additional 3 to 5 weeks. Healing shows as periosteal new bone formation. Injuries to the radial neck and head are often difficult to interpret by x-ray. A small buckle fracture at the radial neck indicates a torus fracture. The mechanism of injury is a fall on the outstretched hand; up to 20 degrees of angulation is acceptable without reduction. Treat these similarly to supracondylar fractures. Nursemaid's elbow is a traction injury usually resulting from lifting the child by one arm. Radiographs are normal. The injury consists

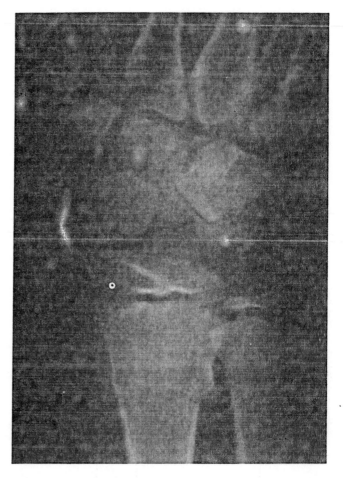

Figure 1 Anteroposterior radiograph of a torus fracture of the distal radius.

of displacement of the annular ligament about the radial head. Reduction, accomplished by supination of the forearm, usually is accompanied by a click felt over the radial head area. This is usually all that is necessary; the child gradually resumes function. If function does not return in a short time, apply a splint for a day or two with the arm in supination. The parents should be aware of the mechanism and that it may be a recurrent injury.

D. Fractures of the mid and distal portions of the radius and ulna are one of the most common childhood fractures. They occur generally from a fall on the outstretched arm and are accompanied by pain, swelling, and at times deformity. Displaced fractures should be reduced under appropriate anesthesia. Acceptable angulation is 25 to 30 degrees dorsal in the distal radius and 10 degrees as

(Continued on page 662)

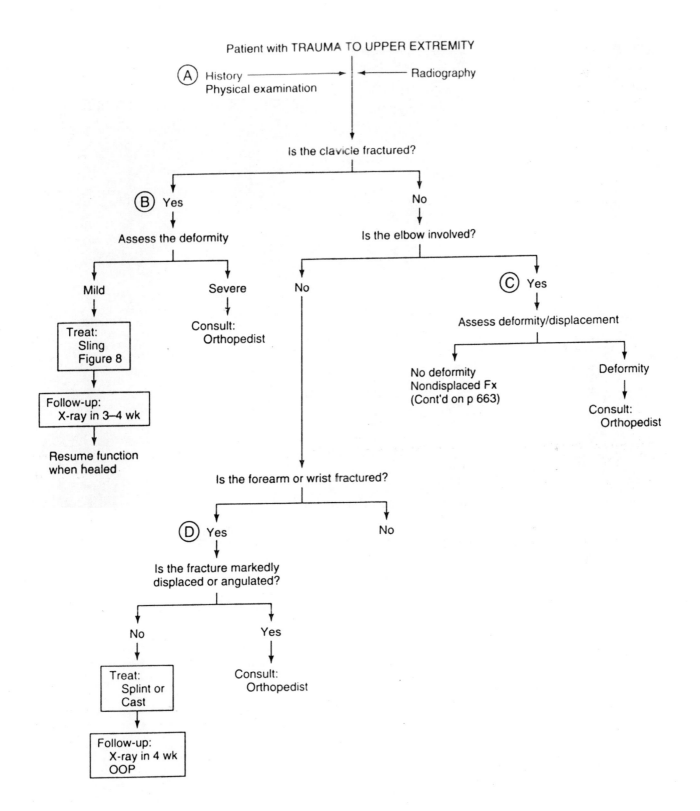

Patient with TRAUMA TO UPPER EXTREMITY

Ⓐ History ——————→ ←—————— Radiography
Physical examination

Is the clavicle fractured?

Ⓑ Yes

No

Assess the deformity

Is the elbow involved?

Mild

Severe

No

Ⓒ Yes

Treat:
Sling
Figure 8

Consult:
Orthopedist

Assess deformity/displacement

Follow-up:
X-ray in 3–4 wk

No deformity
Nondisplaced Fx
(Cont'd on p 663)

Deformity

Resume function
when healed

Consult:
Orthopedist

Is the forearm or wrist fractured?

Ⓓ Yes

No

Is the fracture markedly
displaced or angulated?

No

Yes

Treat:
Splint or
Cast

Consult:
Orthopedist

Follow-up:
X-ray in 4 wk
OOP

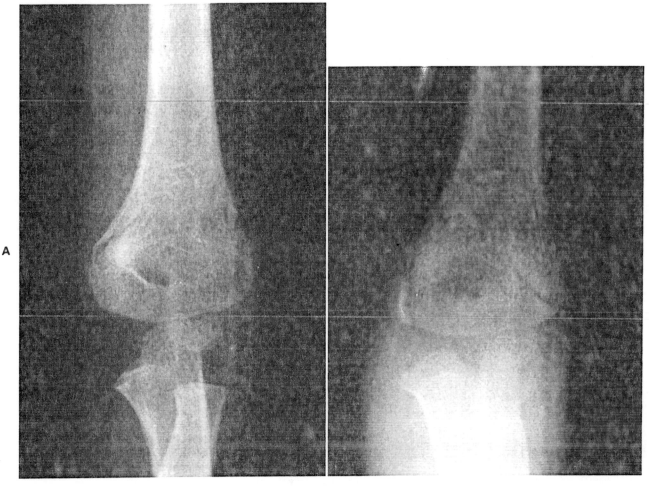

Figure 2 A, Anteroposterior radiograph of the elbow of a child with a minimally displaced supracondylar fracture of the distal humerus. **B,** An x-ray taken 3 weeks later shows periosteal new bone.

as one nears the mid shaft. Torus fractures are stable injuries without a break in the periosteum (Fig. 2). Treat with plaster splint or, if swelling and deformity are minimal, a short arm cast. Healing takes about 4 weeks; x-ray film taken at the time of plaster removal shows evidence of periosteal new bone. If the fracture is significantly displaced or significantly angulated, reduction under appropriate anesthetic is necessary.

E. Common injuries to the distal humerus include supracondylar and lateral condyle fractures (Fig. 3). These may be nondisplaced and difficult to see on initial x-rays. If the clinical examination includes swelling and tenderness with a nondisplaced fracture or no apparent fracture by radiography, the elbow should be placed in a long arm splint and reexamined in a week to 10 days. Repeat x-ray films are usually indicated at that time.

Patient with TRAUMA TO UPPER EXTREMITY

No deformity
Nondisplaced Fx
(Cont'd from p 661)

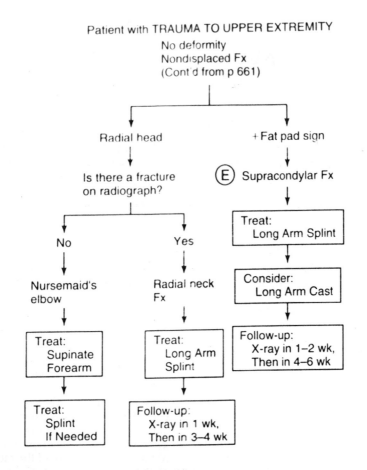

Radial head

Is there a fracture
on radiograph?

No → Nursemaid's elbow

Treat:
Supinate
Forearm

Treat:
Splint
If Needed

Yes → Radial neck Fx

Treat:
Long Arm
Splint

Follow-up:
X-ray in 1 wk,
Then in 3–4 wk

+ Fat pad sign

(E) Supracondylar Fx

Treat:
Long Arm Splint

Consider:
Long Arm Cast

Follow-up:
X-ray in 1–2 wk,
Then in 4–6 wk

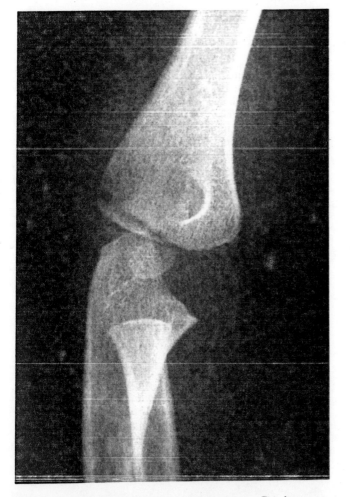

Figure 3 Lateral condyle fracture of distal humerus. This fracture is commonly missed.

References

Cooper RR. Fractures in children. In: Clark CR, Bonfiglio M, eds. Orthopaedics: Essentials of diagnosis and treatment. New York: Churchill Livingstone, 1994:215.

Dicke TE, Nunley JA. Distal forearm fractures in children. Orthop Clin North Am 1993; 24:333.

Green NE, Swiontkowski MF. Skeletal trauma in children. Philadelphia: Saunders, 1994.

Rockwood CA, Wilkins KE, King RE. Fractures in children. Philadelphia: Lippincott, 1991.

UPPER EXTREMITY TRAUMA

Richard C. Fisher, M.D.

A. A careful history will help to determine the nature of the injury. Simple falls often result in mild or moderate injuries; high-energy trauma such as traffic accidents and falls from heights cause severe injuries. Be alert for the signs of nonaccidental trauma. These include multiple fractures of different ages, a questionable or inconsistent history of injury, children presenting late for care, and rotational fractures of the long bones.

B. Treat acute injuries with ice, elevation, and mild compression during the first 24 to 36 hours. This provides mild analgesia, helps to control swelling and bleeding, and reduces the inflammatory response to the injury. Elevate the extremity and wrap with an Ace bandage or Ace-foam composite. Apply an ice bag with this dressing for 30 minutes each hour for 2 to 3 hours.

C. Assess the degree of injury. Mild injuries have diffuse, poorly localized pain without effusion or hemarthrosis. Moderate injuries generally have small, slowly developing effusions, minimal ecchymosis or swelling, no gross deformity, and pain and tenderness specific to the site of injury. Severe injuries are characterized by deformity, a rapid onset of hemarthrosis or effusion, ligamentous instability, or mechanical blockage of the joint. Gross deformity, point tenderness, and painful motion indicate fracture. Associated findings indicating severe injury include vascular impairment from a major vessel injury, fractures through a preexisting bone lesion (pathologic fractures), and skin wounds in the vicinity of a fracture. The latter indicates a possible open fracture, which requires emergency treatment.

D. Implement a rehabilitation program to include active range-of-motion exercises, muscle strengthening to provide for muscle balance, and stretching exercises. There should be gradual resumption of activities.

E. Torus fracture, nondisplaced supracondylar fractures at the elbow, and nursemaid's elbow may all appear clinically as mild injuries and show minimal or no abnormality on radiography. Often the child presents only with unwillingness to use the arm. Torus and supracondylar fractures need rigid immobilization. Nursemaid's elbow (pulled elbow) is caused by longitudinal traction on the outstretched arm, resulting in subluxation of the annular ligament about the radial head. It will reduce with forearm supination. (See p 660.)

F. More serious causes of a painful extremity, especially tumor and infection, should be considered. Radiography and the erythrocyte sedimentation rate, WBC, and any fever are often helpful.

G. Little League shoulder and pitcher's elbow both are the result of repetitive throwing. Shoulder injuries may result from either a stress fracture at the epiphyseal plate or an impingement of the rotator cuff beneath the acromion. Pitcher's elbow has any of several causes, including osteochondritis of the capitellum, early fusion and overgrowth of the proximal radius, and avulsion injury to the medial epicondyle. Young gymnasts may develop painful stress changes at the distal epiphyseal plate of the radius and stress fractures of the ulnar shaft.

References

Cooper RR. Fractures in children. In: Clark CR, Bonfiglio M, eds. Orthopaedics: Essentials of diagnosis and treatment. New York: Churchill Livingstone, 1994:215.

Rockwood CA, Wilkins KE, King RE. Fractures in children. Philadelphia: Lippincott, 1991.

Staheli LT. Fundamentals of pediatric orthopedics. New York: Raven Press, 1992.

Younger ASE, Tredwell MD, Mackenzie WG, et al. Accurate prediction of outcome after pediatric forearm fracture. J Pediatr Orthop 1994; 14:200.

Patient with UPPER EXTREMITY TRAUMA

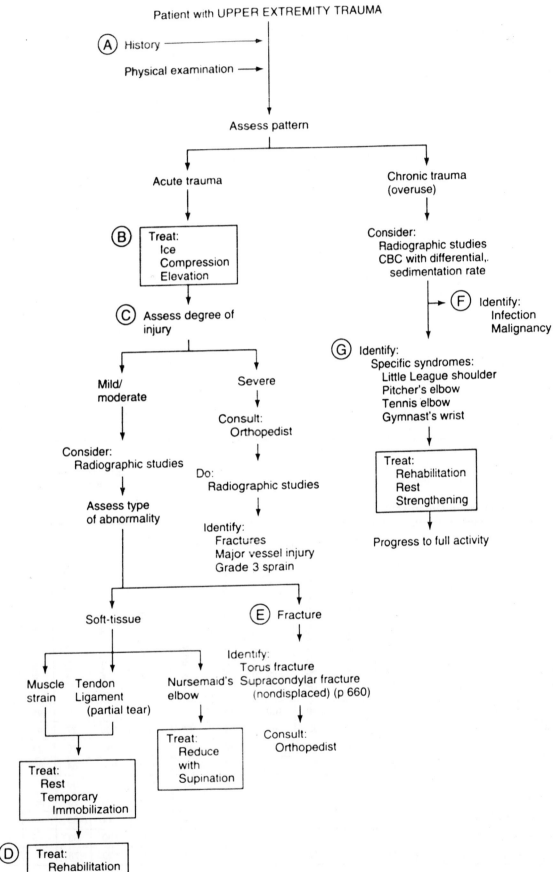

(A) History

Physical examination

Assess pattern

Acute trauma

Chronic trauma (overuse)

(B) Treat:
Ice
Compression
Elevation

Consider:
Radiographic studies
CBC with differential,
sedimentation rate

(F) Identify:
Infection
Malignancy

(C) Assess degree of injury

(G) Identify:
Specific syndromes:
Little League shoulder
Pitcher's elbow
Tennis elbow
Gymnast's wrist

Mild/ moderate

Severe

Consult:
Orthopedist

Treat:
Rehabilitation
Rest
Strengthening

Consider:
Radiographic studies

Do:
Radiographic studies

Progress to full activity

Assess type
of abnormality

Identify:
Fractures
Major vessel injury
Grade 3 sprain

Soft-tissue

(E) Fracture

Identify:
Torus fracture
Supracondylar fracture
(nondisplaced) (p 660)

Muscle
strain

Tendon
Ligament
(partial tear)

Nursemaid's
elbow

Treat:
Reduce
with
Supination

Consult:
Orthopedist

Treat:
Rest
Temporary
Immobilization

(D) Treat:
Rehabilitation

APPENDIX

ANTIMICROBIAL SUSCEPTIBILITIES AT THE CHILDREN'S HOSPITAL

Chris Paap, Pharm.D.
Marti Roe, S.M. (ASCP)

TABLE 1 Gram-positive Organisms (% Susceptible)

Organisms and (# of Isolates)	Penicillin (IV/PO)	Ampicillin/amoxicillin (IV/PO)	Amp/sulb and Amox/clav (IV/PO)	Oxa-/Naf-/Dicloxacillin (IV/PO)	Cefazolin/cephalexin (IV/PO)	Cefuroxime (IV/PO)	Cefotaxime/ceftriaxone (IV)	Trimethoprim/sulfa (IV/PO)	Erythromycin (IV/PO)	Clindamycin (IV/PO)	Gentamicin (IV)	Vancomycin (IV)
Staph aureus (131)	10	14	99	95	98	99	90	100	85	96		100
Coag Negative Staph (107)		10		51	50	50		68	35	66		100
Strept viridans (44)	36	65		21	76			61		92		100
Strept pneumoniae (124)	61						67	56		78		100
Enterococcus (59)	85	89	90		R	R	R	80		45	99*	93

*99% of isolates were sensitive for gentamicin synergy (1994 data).
R, resistant.
Small italic values represent literature/populational estimates of sensitivity and may not reflect The Children's Hospital sensitivities.
From Contagious Comments, The Children's Hospital Department of Epidemiology and Quality Performance, March 1996:3.

TABLE 2 Gram-negative Organisms (% Susceptible)

Organisms and (# of Isolates)	Ampicillin/amoxicillin (IV/PO)	Amp/sulb and Amox/clav (IV/PO)	Cefazolin/cephalexin (IV/PO)	Cefuroxime/cefaclor (IV/PO)	Cefotaxime/ceftriaxone (IV)	Gentamicin (IV)	Tobramyicin (IV)	Amikacin (IV)	Trimethoprim/sulfa (IV/PO)	Chloramphenicol (IV/PO)	Nitrofurantoin (PO)	Ciprofloxacin (IV/PO)
Haemophilus species (46)	42	100	50	100	96				95	95		99
E. coli (447)	50	75	92	95	99	97	98	100	77	90	99	100
Klebsiella pneum/oxyt (93)	1	71	77	94	97	95	92	98	70	80	68	98
Proteus mirabilis (11)	55	95	82	95	100	91	100	100	64	80	R	100
Enterobacter cloacae (40)	8	57	3	38	68	95	95	100	90	70	32	100
Citrobacter freundii (23)	23	71	9	43	65	95	91	100	73	95	93	100
Xanthomonas maltophilia (9)	14	20			13	44	56	44	89			100
Salmonella species (15)	73	73	100	100	100	93	93	100	93			100
Shigella species (18)	22	39	72	78	100	100	100	100	78			100

R, resistant.
Small italic values represent literature/populational estimates of sensitivity and may not reflect The Children's Hospital sensitivities.
From Contagious Comments, The Children's Hospital Department of Epidemiology and Quality Performance, March 1996:3.

TABLE 3 *Pseudomonas aeruginosa* (% Susceptible)

Organisms and (# of Isolates)	ANTIMICROBIALS	Ticarcillin (IV)	Ticarcillin/clav [Timentin] (IV)	Piperacillin (IV)	Ceftazidime (IV)	Aztreonam (IV)	Imipenem/cilastatin (IV)	Trimethoprim/sulfa (IV/PO)	Ciprofloxacin (IV/PO)	AMINOGLYCOSIDES	Gentamicin (IV)	Tobramycin (IV)	Amikacin (IV)
NONMUCOID strains (232)		*80*	*80*	93	87	74	71	23	88		86	94	92
MUCOID strains (126)		*80*	*80*	91	90	64	95	18	67		65	90	59

Small italic values represent literature/populational estimates of sensitivity and may not reflect The Children's Hospital sensitivities.
From Contagious Comments, The Children's Hospital Department of Epidemiology and Quality Performance, March 1996:3.

TABLE 4 Anaerobic Organisms (% Susceptible)

(Not tested at The Children's Hospital)	ANTIMICROBIALS	Penicillin (IV/PO)	Ampicillin/amoxicillin (IV/PO)	Amp/sulb and Amox/clav (IV/PO)	Ticar/clav [Timentin] (IV)	Ticarcillin (IV)	Piperacillin (IV)	Cefoxitin/cefotetan (IV)	Imipenem/cilastatin (IV)	Clindamycin (IV/PO)	Metronidazole (IV/PO)	Chloramphenicol (IV/PO)	Erythromycin (IV/PO)
Oral anaerobes		+ + +	+ + +	+ + +	+ + +	+ + +	+ + +	+ + +	+ + +	+ + +	+ +	+ + +	+ +
Abdominal anaerobes				+ + +	+ + +			+ +	+ + +	+ +	+ + +	+ + +	

+, 50%–75% susceptible; + +, 76%–90% susceptible; + + +, >90% susceptible.
Values represent literature/populational estimates of sensitivity and may not reflect The Children's Hospital sensitivities.
From Contagious Comments, The Children's Hospital Department of Epidemiology and Quality Performance, March 1996:3.

TABLE 5 Intravenous Antimicrobials: Relative Cost Comparison

Drug	Dose Regimen	10 Day Course Relative Cost*	Adult Dose (>40 kg Child)
Penicillin and Ampicillin			
Ampicillin	200 mg/kg/day div q6h	3.80	1–2 g q6h
Ampicillin/sulbactam (Unasyn)	200 mg/kg/day div q6h	6.14	1–2 g q6h
Penicillin G	200,000 U/kg/day div q6h	3.74	2–5 MU q4–6h
Antistaphylococcal agents			
Cefazolin	100 mg/kg/day div q8h	2.69	1 g q8h
Cephaparin	80 mg/kg/day div q6h	3.48	0.5–1 g q6h
Cephalothin	125 mg/kg/day div q6h	3.63	1–2 g q6h
Nafcillin	150 mg/kg/day div q6h	3.51	1–2 g q6h
Vancomycin†	40 mg/kg/day div q6h	4.06	1 g q8–12h
Broad spectrum β-lactams			
Cefuroxime	150 mg/kg/day div q8h	4.31	0.75–1.5 g q8h
Cefotaxime	150 mg/kg/day div q8h	5.47	1–2 g q6–8h
Ceftriaxone	100 mg/kg/day div q12h	8.10	1–2 g q12h
Ceftriaxone	75 mg/kg/day div q24h	5.68	1–2 g q24h
Antianaerobic agents			
Cefoxitin	160 mg/kg/day div q6h	5.92	1–2 g q6–8h
Cefotetan	80 mg/kg/day div q12h	3.67	1–2 g q12h
Clindamycin	40 mg/kg/day div q8h	2.66	600–900 mg q8h
Metronidazole	30 mg/kg/day div q6h	3.43	0.5 to 1 g q6h
Antipseudomonal agents			
Ceftazidime	150 mg/kg/day div q8h	5.86	1–2 g q8–12h
Ticarcillin	300 mg/kg/day div q6h	5.21	3 g q4–6h
Ticarcillin/clavulanate (Timentin)	300 mg/kg/day div q6h	6.23	3.1 g q4–6h
Piperacillin	300 mg/kg/day div q6h	5.63	3 g q4–6h
Piperacillin/tazobactam (Zosyn)	300 mg/kg/day div q6h	6.51	2.25 g q4–6h
Aztreonam	120 mg/kg/day div q8h	6.05	1–2 g q6–12h
Imipenem/cilastatin (Primaxin)	60 mg/kg/day div q6h	9.85	0.5–1 g q6–8h
Ciprofloxacin	10 mg/kg/day div q12h	3.38	200–400 mg q12h
Aminoglycosides			
Gentamicin†	7.5 mg/kg/day div q8h	2.49	5 mg/kg/day div q8h
Tobramycin†	7.5 mg/kg/day div q8h	3.33	5 mg/kg/day div q8h
Amikacin†	22.5 mg/kg/day div q8h	5.41	15 mg/kg/day div q8h
Miscellaneous agents			
Doxycycline	4 mg/kg/day div q24h	1.00	50–100 mg q12–24h
Erythromycin	40 mg/kg/day div q6h	3.36	0.5–1 g q6h
Trimethoprim/sulfa (Bactrim)	10 mg/kg/day div q12h	3.47	80–160 mg q12h
Chloramphenicol†	75 mg/kg/day div q6h	4.64	500 mg q6h

*Relative cost includes drug cost plus IV supplies and personnel time for the preparation and administration of the drug ($8.00/dose); based on a 30 kg child.
†Additional costs of serum concentration and toxicity monitoring included.
All costs are based on *actual costs* to The Children's Hospital, not patient charge.
From Contagious Comments, The Children's Hospital Department of Epidemiology and Quality Performance, March 1996:3.

INDEX

---

* Page numbers in *italics* indicate figures; *t* indicates tables.

Nipple discharge in adolescent girls, 342-343
Nocturnal enuresis, 38
Nodule, 80
Nonallergic rhinitis, 530
Nonblistering, nonerythematous skin lesions, 90-91
Nonfebrile seizures, 486-491
   drugs in treating, 488t
   side effects of drugs used to treat, 490t
Nonketotic hyperosmolar coma, 138
Nonspecific colitis, 272
Noonan syndrome, 132
Normocytic anemia, 376-377
Nummular eczema, 84
Nursemaid's elbow, 664
Nutritional therapy; see also Diet
   for eating disorders, 32
   for encopresis, 36
   for growth deficiency, 218, 220
Nystagmus, 501

O

Obesity, 166-169
Obstructive apnea, 538, 550
Obstructive lesions, 58t
Ocular injury, 658-659
Ophthalmic gonorrhea, 504
Ophthalmologic disorders
   conjunctivitis/red, painful eyes, 502-506, 504t
   evaluation of poor vision, 500-501, 500t
   orbital cellulitis or abscess, 508-509
   periorbital (preseptal) cellulitis, 510-511
   strabismus, 512, 513
Ophthalmoplegia, 502
Ophthalmoscopy, 501
Oral trauma, 646
Orbital cellulitis or abscess, 508-509
   intravenous antibiotics for, 508t
Orchitis, postpubertal, 602
Orthostatic syncope, 250
Osgood-Schlatter disease, 656
Osteochondritis, 664
Osteochondritis dissecans, 388, 656
Osteomyelitis, 398-401, 400t
Otitis media, 522-523, 525, 527, 554
   with complications, 522
   definitions, 522
   with effusion, 522
   etiology, 522, 524, 526
   and language disorder, 42
   therapy for, 524t
Otolaryngologic disorders
   mastoiditis, 516-517
   neck mass/cervical adenitis, 518-521
   otitis media, 522-527
   parotid swelling/parotitis, 528-529
   rhinitis-chronic, 530-533
   sinusitis, 534-537
   snoring/adenoidal hypertrophy, 538-539
   sore throat/pharyngitis/tonsillitis, 540-545
Ovarian torsion, acute, 264
Ovaries
   malignancies of, 260
   polycystic, 356

P

Pacemakers, in treating bradyarrhythmias, 60
Pain
   abdominal
      acute, 262-265
         degree of illness in, 262t
      persistent or recurrent, 266-269
         definitions, 266
         etiology, 266, 268
   foot, 388-389
   musculoskeletal, 200
   patellofemoral, 656
   pelvic, degree of illness in, 348t
   pelvic pain, 348, 350
   school phobia as cause of, 8
Palmar grasp, 456
Pancreatitis, 264, 314-315
   severity of illness in, 314t
Panhypopituitarism, 148
Papilloma intraductal, 342
Papillomatosis, juvenile, in breast, 336
Papule, 80
Papulosquamous disorders, 92-93
Parainfluenza viruses as cause of pneumonia, 564
Paramyotonia congenita, 464
Paranasal sinuses; see Sinusitis
Parapsoriasis, 92
Paronychia, 388
Parotid swelling, 528-529
   drugs in treating, 528t
Parotitis; see Parotid swelling
Paroxysmal coughing, 250
Partial thromboplastin time (PTT)
   in detecting bleeding in newborn, 410
   in detecting hemolytic anemia, 370
   in detecting thrombocytopenia in newborn, 444
Pasteurella multocida and infection of bites, 642
Pastia's sign, 86
Patellofemoral pain, 656
Patent ductus arteriosus (PDA), 426
Pelvic inflammatory disease (PID), 344-347
   degree of illness in, 344t
   drugs in treating, 346t
Pelvic pain, 348-351
   degree of illness in, 348t
Pemoline for attention deficit hyperactivity disorder,
     13t, 14
Penicillin-allergic reactions, 634-637
   drugs in treating, 634t
   oral desensitization protocol, 636t
Peptic ulcer disease, 316-319
   antacid preparations for, 318t
   degree of illness in, 316t
   drug therapy for, 300t, 316t
Perinatal asphyxia, 432, 434
Periodic breathing, 550
Periorbital (preseptal) cellulitis
   antibiotic therapy for, 510t
   degree of illness in, 510t
Peripheral cyanosis, 56
Peripheral (GnRH-independent) precocity in boys, 170
Pertussis, 558, 560
Peutz-Jeghers syndrome, 274

Pharyngitis; *see* Sore throat
Pharyngococonjunctival fever, 502
Pharyngoconjunctivial fever, 502
Phlyctenular keratoconjunctivitis, 502
Phobia, school, 8, 44
Pierre Robin syndrome, 118, 550, 562
Pitcher's elbow, 664
Pityriasis alba, 90
Pityriasis rosea, 92
Plantar grasp, 456
Plantar warts, 388
Plaque, 80
PLEVA (pityriasis lichenoides et varioliformis acuta), 92
Pneumonia, 564-567
    antibiotic treatment of, 564t, 566t
    bacterial, 110
    and congestive heart failure, 62
    degree of illness in, 564t
        Pneumocystitis carinii, 224
Pneumoperitoneum, 422
Poisoning; *see also* Intoxication
    acute drug, 612-615
        degree of illness in, 612t
        specific antidotes to, 614t
    carbon monoxide, 616-619
        symptoms of acute, 616t
    food
        Clostridium perfringens, 282
        staphylococcal, 282
    iron, 624-625
        degree of illness in, 624t
    lead, 372
        and foreign body ingestion, 620
Polycystic ovaries, 356
Polycystic ovary syndrome and obesity, 168
Polyps, 274
Port wine stains, 94
Positive-pressure ventilation (PPV), 428, 430
Postpubertal orchitis, 602
Postresuscitation management, 430
Posttraumatic seizures, 654
Prader-Willi syndrome, 132
Precocity
    peripheral (GnRH-independent), 170
    true or central, 170
Precordial catch syndrome, 200
Pregnancy, prevention of, in sexual abuse, 24
Prehospital basic life support, 116-117, *116*
Premature adrenarche, 170, 172
Premature thelarche, 172
Prematurity, apnea of, 552
Preschool children
    developmental delay in, 28-31
    vision scoring guidelines for, 500t
Proteinuria, 594-597
Prothrombin time (PT)
    in detecting bleeding in newborn, 410
    in detecting thrombocytopenia in newborn, 444
Pseudohypoparathyroidism, 146
Pseudomembranous colitis, 274
Pseudomonas aeruginosa, 667t
Pseudopseudohypoparathyroidism, 146
Pseudotumor cerebri, 472
Psoriasis, 92

Psychogenic symptoms, evaluation of, 8-9
Psychotherapy for attention deficit hyperactivity disorder, 14
Puberty
    delayed, 132-133, *132*
    precocious
        in boys, 170-171
            drug therapy for, 170t
        in girls, 172-173
            treatment of, 172t
Pulmonary disease/respiratory distress
    in chest pain, 198, 200
    cyanosis related to, 562-563
Pulmonary disorders, 548-549
    apnea and sudden infant death syndrome, 550-553
    bronchiolitis, 554-557
    chronic cough, 558-561
    cyanosis related to pulmonary disease/respiratory
        distress, 562-563
    and evaluation of cough, 548-549
    pneumonia, 564-567
    reactive airway disease, 568-577, 570t, 572t
    stridor, 578-581, *578*
    tuberculosis, 582-585
Pulmonary edema, 118, 562
Pulmonary infarctions, 110
Pulmonary masses, 560
Pulse oximetry, 554, 565
Pyelonephritis, 604

R

Radiographs
    in assessing arthritis, 384
    in assessing bronchiolitis, 554
    in assessing chronic cough, 560
    in assessing dental and oral trauma, 646
    in assessing foot pain, 388
    in assessing methemoglobinemia, 632
    in assessing musculoskeletal disorders, 382
    in assessing ocular injury, 658
    in assessing peptic ulcer disease, 316-318
    in assessing pneumonia, 565
    in assessing sepsis, 436, 438
    in assessing septic arthritis, 402
    in assessing upper extremity fractures, 660, 662
Radius, fractures of, 660, 662
Rash
    diaper, 84
    in erythematous maculopapular lesions, 86
    in evaluating skin lesions, 80
    in measles, 212, 244
    in rubella, 212
Raynaud phenomenon, 386
Reactive airway disease (RAD), 558, 568-577
    dosages of antiinflammatory drugs for, 574t
    dosages of bronchodilating drugs for, 574t, 576t
    response to therapy, 570t
Reactive arthritis, 386
Receptive disorder, 40
Recurrent acute otitis media, 522
Red cell fragmentation, 370
Reflux
    gastric, 550
    gastroesophageal, 550

Trauma — cont'd
  ocular injury, 658-659
  upper extremity, 664-665
    fractures, 660-663, *660, 662, 663*
Treacher Collins syndrome, 40
Tremors, 492-495
  drug therapy for, 492*t*
Tretinoin, 82
Trigonocephaly (metopic suture), 452, *454*
Tropics, acute fever in, 188-191
True precocity, 170
Tuberculin skin test, 246
Tuberculosis, 582-585
Tuberculous masses, 260
Tuberculous meningitis, 584
Tumors; *see also* Cancer; Carcinoma; Masses
  brain, 472
  breast, 200, 336-337
  choroid plexus, 472
  hepatocellular, 308
  Wilms, 260
Turner syndrome, 132, 178, 274
Tympanocentesis, 522
Typhoid fever, 252-253, 255
  degree of illness in, 252*t*
  drugs in treating, 254*t*
Typhus
  murine, 190, 248
  scrub, 190, 248
Tyrosinemia, 312

U

Ulcer, peptic, 316-319
  antacid preparations for, 318*t*
  degree of illness in, 316*t*
  drug therapy for, 300*t*, 316*t*
Ulcerative colitis, 322-325
  degree of illness in, 322*t*
Ultrasonography
  in assessing osteomyelitis, 398
  breast, 336
  in confirming ascites, 270
  in diagnosing abdominal pain, 262, 264
Uncal herniation syndrome, 104
Unresponsive acute otitis media, 522
Upper airway obstruction, diagnoses of, 550
Upper extremity fractures, 660-663, *660, 662, 663*
Upper extremity trauma, 664-665
Urinary tract infection, 604-607
  degree of illness in, 604*t*
  drug therapy for, 606*t*
  and urinalysis, 588
Urine alkalinization, 638
Urolithiasis, 590
Urticaria lesions, 86
Urticaria pigmentosa, 96
Uterine bleeding, dysfunctional, 340-341, 340*t*

V

Vaginoplasty, 128
Vaginosis, bacterial, 359
Valgus angulation, 390

Valsalva maneuver, 258
Varicella, 96
Vascular birthmarks, 94-95
Vascular malformation, 274
Vascular rings, 550, 562
Vasogenic edema, 102
Vasoocclusive crises, 110
Vasovagal syncope, 250
Vertical talus, 388
Vertigo, 496-497
  chronic or progressive, 496
  recurrent, 496
Vesicle, 80
Vesicoureteral reflux, 606, *606*
Vesiculobullous disorders, 96-97
Vision screening guidelines, 500-501, 500*t*
  for children ages 3 to 5 years, 500*t*
  for children ages 6 years and older, 500*t*
Vitamin B_{12} deficiency, 160
Vitamin K deficiency, 364
Vocal cord paralysis, 118, 562
Voiding cystourethrography, 604
Vomiting
  after infancy, 326-329
    degree of illness in, 326*t*
  during infancy, 33, 330-333
    degree of illness in, 330*t*
von Willebrand disease, 364
Vulvovaginitis, 358-361
  drugs in treating, 358*t*

W

Waardenburg syndrome, 40
Warts, 90
  plantar, 388
Werdnig-Hoffman syndrome, 449
Western blot test, 225
West Nile fever, 206
West Nile virus, 190
Wheal, 80
Wide Range Achievement Test (WRAT)
  in assessing attention deficit hyperactivity disorder, 10
  in assessing learning problems, 46
Wildervanck syndrome, 40
Williams syndrome, 136
Wilms tumor, 260
  staging classification for, 258*t*
Wiskott-Aldrich syndrome, 378
Wolff-Parkinson-White (WPW) syndrome, 74

X

Xanthogranuloma, juvenile, 90
Xerophthalmis, 244
Xyphoid process syndrome, 200

Y

Yellow fever, 190

Z

Zidovudine, 226